DEVELOPMENT OF
SENSORY SYSTEMS
IN MAMMALS

WILEY SERIES IN NEUROBIOLOGY
R. Glenn Northcutt, Editor

DEVELOPMENT OF SENSORY SYSTEMS IN MAMMALS

Edited by

James R. Coleman

University of South Carolina
Columbia, South Carolina

A Wiley-Interscience Publication
JOHN WILEY & SONS
New York · Chichester · Brisbane · Toronto · Singapore

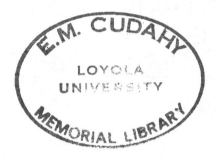
Copyright © 1990 by John Wiley & Sons, Inc.

All rights reserved. Published simultaneously in Canada.

Reproduction or translation of any part of this work
beyond that permitted by Section 107 or 108 of the
1976 United States Copyright Act without the permission
of the copyright owner is unlawful. Requests for
permission or further information should be addressed to
the Permissions Department, John Wiley & Sons, Inc.

Library of Congress Cataloging in Publication Data:

Development of sensory systems in mammals / edited by James R.
   Coleman.
       p.   cm. — (Wiley series in neurobiology)
   Includes bibliographical references.
   ISBN 0-471-85271-6
   1. Senses and sensation.   2. Developmental neurobiology.
3. Mammals—Physiology.   I. Coleman, James R. (James Roland)
II. Series.
   [DNLM: 1. Mammals—growth & development.   2. Neural Pathways—
growth & development.   3. Neurobiology.   4. Sense Organs—growth &
development.   WL 700 D4892]
QP431.D38   1990
599'.0182—dc20
DNLM/DLC
for Library of Congress   89-24787
                                                                 CIP

Printed in the United States of America

10 9 8 7 6 5 4 3 2 1

CONTRIBUTORS

Matti Anniko, Department of Oto-Rhino-Laryngology & Head and Neck Surgery, Otologic Research Laboratories, University of Umeå, University Hospital, Umeå, Sweden

Leo M. Chalupa, Department of Psychology, University of California, Davis, California 95616

Nicolas L. Chiaia, Department of Anatomy, Medical College of Ohio, Toledo, Ohio 43699

Benjamin M. Clopton, Kresge Hearing Research Institute, University of Michigan, Ann Arbor, Michigan 48109

James R. Coleman, Departments of Psychology and Physiology, University of South Carolina, Columbia, South Carolina 29208

Günter Ehret,* Zoologisches Institut, Universitat Bonn, Bonn, Federal Republic of Germany

* *Present address:* Abteilung Biologie IV, Universität Ulm, D-79 Ulm

Michael J. Friedlander, Neurobiology Center and Department of Physiology and Biophysics, University of Alabama at Birmingham, Birmingham, Alabama 35294

Pasquale P. Graziadei, Department of Biological Science, Florida State University, Tallahassee, Florida 32306

Mark F. Jacquin, Department of Anatomy, St. Louis University, St. Louis, Missouri 63104

Herbert P. Killackey, Department of Psychobiology, University of California, Irvine, California 92717

Lynne Kiorpes, Department of Psychology and Center for Neural Science, New York University, New York, New York 10003

Leonard M. Kitzes, Department of Anatomy and Neurobiology, University of California, Irvine, California 92717

Charlotte M. Mistretta,
Department of Biologic and
Materials Sciences, School of
Dentistry, University of
Michigan, Ann Arbor, Michigan
48109

J. Anthony Movshon, Department
of Psychology and Center for
Neural Science, New York
University, New York, New
York 10003

Robert W. Rhoades, Department
of Anatomy, Medical College of
Ohio, Toledo, Ohio 43699

Colleen R. Snead, Kresge Hearing
Research Institute, University of
Michigan, Ann Arbor, Michigan
48109

John S. Tootle, Neurobiology
Center and Department of
Physiology and Biophysics,
University of Alabama at
Birmingham, Birmingham,
Alabama 35294

Cheryl A. White, Department of
Psychology, University of
California, Davis, California
95616

Thomas A. Woolsey, James L.
O'Leary Division of
Experimental Neurology and
Neurosurgery, Department of
Neurology and Neurosurgery,
and McDonnell Center for
Studies of Higher Brain
Function, Washington
University School of Medicine,
St. Louis, Missouri 63110

*All knowledge of things obtained from pure intellect
or pure reason is nothing but mere illusion;
only experience yields truth.*

IMMANUEL KANT
Prolegomena, 1783

SERIES PREFACE

Neuroscience is a rapidly expanding interdisciplinary field that is yielding significant insights into the organization and function of nervous systems. An outgrowth of several more traditional disciplines—Animal Behavior, Comparative Biology, Cybernetics, Neuroanatomy, Neurochemistry, Neurophysiology, and Physiological Psychology—Neuroscience arose because of many reasons, but central to the focus of Neuroscience is the growing realization that no single approach or discipline can fully explain how nervous systems are organized; how they come into being ontogenetically, as well as phylogenetically; how a specific nervous system works and what operational principles are applicable to most, if not all, nervous systems.

From subcellular organelles and processes to entire networks mediating behavior, the complexity and diversity exhibited by nervous systems is staggering. The goal of Neuroscience is to understand how these complex and diverse systems work as devices for information processing, control, and communication. Unlike artificial devices that are man-made and thus specifically designed to solve limited, well-defined sets of problems, nervous systems are the result of a historical process called evolution. Thus their analysis is further confounded by the fact that they have arisen opportunistically and without optimal design. Understanding how they have arisen, how they have adapted to solve problems that are virtually unlimited, is a challenge that can not be met by a single discipline. Although individual neuroscientists will continue to focus on specific questions related to a particular facet of neural organization or a single species, achievement of the goals of Neuroscience demands an eclectic approach that is rapidly becoming its hallmark.

The Wiley Series in Neurobiology reflects this eclecticism, and the Series will present work ranging from subcellular to behavioral topics, from specialized monographs to contributions spanning several disciplines. As a forum in which nervous systems are viewed and analyzed from widely different perspectives, it is hoped that these offerings will not only provide information to researchers in all disciplines of Neuroscience, but will also provide further stimulation for an eclectic approach to the evolution, organization, and function of nervous systems.

R. GLENN NORTHCUTT

Ann Arbor, Michigan
March 1983

PREFACE

Within the past two decades there has been an extraordinary burst of new information on the organization of sensory systems in vertebrate animals. This volume of the Wiley-Interscience Series in Neurobiology is specifically intended to summarize the growing body of literature on the mechanisms by which the sensory systems of mammalian species develop. Early scientists, including von Helmholtz, recognized that sensory receptors and associated neural pathways provide the interface between the physical world of stimuli and perceptual responses in mammals and other organisms. Study of sensory system development is now providing answers to how and why sensory processing that leads to these perceptual responses is acquired. Not only do these findings illustrate both genetically controlled and environmentally contingent patterns of sensory system development, but they also reveal major principles generalizable to other regions of the developing nervous system. This volume also offers insights into comparative development of structure and function among mammals, including humans.

The present volume provides a valuable synopsis of major findings in sensory systems of mammals presented by leading workers in the field. Organizational features imposed on each chapter create elements of a textbook format. However, the authors have also retained some individual flavor and have typically placed emphasis on the most important and exciting research recently conducted in that specialty. As a result of these efforts, this book is expected to be useful to advanced undergraduates, graduate students, and more senior investigators in the fields of neuroscience, psychobiology, sensation and perception, and related disciplines.

The first chapter in the section on the visual system, by Leo Chalupa and Cheryl White, describes the development of visual structures from the eye to cortex. Included is recent work on the overproduction of cells and axons, and redistribution of axon projections and synaptic formations during prenatal and early postnatal life. In the second chapter, Michael Friedlander and John Tootle summarize the physiological development of visual system structures including the relationship between onset of photoreceptor activity and that of retinal or central neurons. Characterizations of early response properties to light are compared with adult properties, including changes in receptive field size and acuity. In Chapter 3, Lynne Kiorpes and Anthony Movshon discuss development of behavioral responses to patterned light with emphasis on findings in cat, monkey, and human. Their survey accents the roles of receptor–neural changes relative to those of accessory eye structures on behavioral maturation of visual response behavior. Anthony Movshon and Lynne Kiorpes next describe in Chapter 4 how experiential variables influence the maturation of structure, physiological response properties, and behavioral responses in the visual system.

In the section on the auditory system the volume editor describes the development of ear structures and central auditory pathways in Chapter 5. There is discussion of the independence of generation and initial development of auditory system neurons from other levels of the neuraxis, as well as aspects of later parallel and centripetal patterns of structural growth that are influenced by cochlear and accessory ear maturation. In Chapter 6, Leonard Kitzes summarizes age-related changes of absolute thresholds, frequency shifts, and localization mechanisms of neurons of the auditory pathway. He discusses the role of the various ear structures in maturation of neuronal sensitivity to acoustic stimuli. In the following chapter, Günther Ehret surveys major findings of behavioral responses to sound in various developing mammals and compares maturation of behavioral sensitivity to underlying anatomical and physiological changes in the auditory system. In Chapter 8, the influences of experiential factors on development of auditory response mechanisms are explored by Benjamin Clopton and Colleen Snead. Discussion accentuates the impact of acoustic deprivation on structure and binaural response properties of neurons of the central auditory system.

In the next section, Matti Anniko, in Chapter 9, describes developmental events in the vestibular system. Anniko discusses preprogrammed features of the inner ear, as well as the competition of fibers on sensory hairs and the formation of temporary synapses. Details of structural descriptions are provided in the context of contemporary methods, which include the use of tissue cultures.

The section on the somatosensory system begins with Chapter 10 by Herbert Killackey, Mark Jacquin, and Robert Rhoades. This chapter describes structural connections of somatosensory pathways with emphasis on formation of vibrissal representation. A peripheral-to-central sequence of maturational events is depicted after early cell generation and growth along this axis, and the timing of cortical connectional patterns is traced. In Chapter 11, Robert Rhoades, Herbert Killackey, Nicolas Chiaia, and Mark Jacquin summarize the physiology of development in the somatosensory system. They discuss maturational differences in receptive field size in peripheral and central neurons. These authors also provide insight into central alterations in somatotopy after peripheral damage. In Chapter 12,

Thomas Woolsey further explicates the effects of early postnatal nerve damage on survival and organization of central vibrissal organization. Woolsey describes "barrel" compensation patterns after vibrissal damage and underscores the importance of nerve growth factor in maintenance of trigeminal ganglia.

The last major section, which embraces the chemical senses, includes a discourse on development of the olfactory system in Chapter 13 by Pasquale Graziadei. This chapter describes neurogenesis and plasticity in a system possessing special features of neural regeneration into adulthood, although like other sensory systems these pathways are sensitive to stimulus deprivation procedures during postnatal life. A note of particular interest in this chapter is the inclusion of a previously unpublished photograph from the work of Antonio Scarpa (1782) showing the human olfactory nerves and bulb and a reproduced original illustration drawn by Camillo Golgi of the structure of the olfactory bulb using the then (1875) newly discovered silver dichromate impregnation method. In Chapter 14, Charlotte Mistretta discusses the many interesting features of taste development. This system exhibits ongoing receptor turnover and constant reformation of synapses. Gustatory pathways of mammals display distinct qualitative and quantitative physiological and behavioral modifications in sensitivity to taste stimuli during development.

The final chapter provides a brief synopsis of some of the major issues and findings detailed in the first 14 chapters of this volume. Each sensory system possesses unique stimulus-processing features by receptors, but many principles of neural development are exhibited in parallel across these systems, and various maturational gradients can also be compared. This volume emphasizes that beyond the genetic programming of early development, all systems show a sensitive period in which exposure to the sensory environment influences final progression to mature central organization and perceptual capability.

In short, these chapters serve as a valuable source of information on development of the major sensory systems. Discussion of important issues, findings, and contemporary methods are all brought out within a single volume. The excitement generated by research on sensory system ontogeny are concisely presented by principal authors in the field who provide a framework for understanding mechanisms of development. Research on development of sensory systems described in this volume includes major contributions to the broader scope of developmental neurobiology and psychobiology, and should be of interest to readers in these areas.

JAMES R. COLEMAN

Columbia, South Carolina
May 1990

CONTENTS

DEVELOPMENT OF
SENSORY SYSTEMS
IN MAMMALS

Part One

THE VISUAL SYSTEM

Chapter One

PRENATAL DEVELOPMENT OF VISUAL SYSTEM STRUCTURES

LEO M. CHALUPA AND CHERYL A. WHITE

Department of Psychology
University of California
Davis, California

I INTRODUCTION

The visual system has long been a favorite model for developmental studies, but until recently little was known about prenatal development of the mammalian retina and visual pathways. To a large degree this was due to the formidable technical challenges that needed to be overcome before undertaking such studies. These included the perfection of *in utero* surgical methods as well as the modification of various anatomical protocols to deal with problems inherent to fetal material. Additionally, during the late 1960s and into the mid-1970s, the major emphasis was placed on the role of experience in the development of sensory systems. In the case of the visual system, it appeared plausible to assume that experience commences with eye opening, that is, at birth or shortly thereafter. As our knowledge of early postnatal events accumulated, however, it became obvious that at least some of the key events responsible for the development and plasticityof the newborn visual system are initiated before parturition.

Much of the initial research on prenatal development of the mammalian visual system was devoted to tracing connections between visual centers of the fetal brain. This work led to the consideration of such phenomena as cell death, retraction of exuberant axon collaterals, and restructuring of axon terminals. More recently, investigators have begun to consider some of the mechanisms that may be responsible for such remarkable developmental events. Of particular relevance are competition among ingrowing axons, interactions among dendrites within a given class of cells, and the role of neuronal activity before the onset of visual experience (i.e., spontaneous discharge of fetal cells).

In this chapter we will review what is currently known about the prenatal development of the mammalian visual system. For the most part, we will be concerned with recent studies dealing with the cat and monkey, although information on other species will also be included. Our ultimate goal is to understand the normal as well as the abnormal development of the human brain. It is our firm belief that such animal research provides an appropriate vehicle for achieving this long-term objective. Discussion of anatomical and physiological events occurring during postnatal development of the visual system of mammals is presented in Chapter 2 of this volume.

For readers not familiar with the mammalian visual system, we will first provide a brief overview of the structural organization of the retina and the main components of the central visual pathways. In particular, we will emphasize those fundamental features of the mature visual system that have figured prominently in recent studies of prenatal development.

II ANATOMICAL OVERVIEW OF THE MATURE VISUAL SYSTEM

A The Mammalian Retina

The mature retina is a thin transparent sheet composed of three layers of cell bodies separated by two plexiform layers containing synaptic connections (see Figure 1). In mammals, the layer of cells farthest from the center of the eye consists of photoreceptors (the rods and cones), which absorb light and

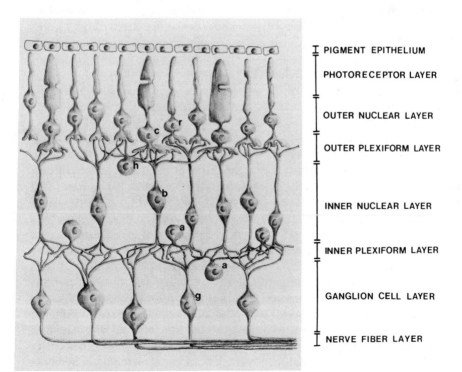

PIGMENT EPITHELIUM

PHOTORECEPTOR LAYER

OUTER NUCLEAR LAYER

OUTER PLEXIFORM LAYER

INNER NUCLEAR LAYER

INNER PLEXIFORM LAYER

GANGLION CELL LAYER

NERVE FIBER LAYER

FIGURE 1. Schematic illustration of the nuclear and plexiform layers of the retina. r, rod; c, cone; h, horizontal cell; b, bipolar cell; a, amacrine cell; g, retinal ganglion cell.

transduce it into electrical responses. The cell bodies of the receptors form the outer nuclear layer. The next cell layer, the inner nuclear layer, contains the somata of three distinct cell types: horizontal, bipolar, and amacrine. Horizontal and amacrine cells provide a mechanism for lateral interconnections within the retina, while bipolar cells convey information from the receptors to the ganglion cells. Photoreceptors make synaptic contact with bipolar and horizontal cells in the outer plexiform layer, whereas synaptic contacts between bipolar cells and ganglion cells as well as those of amacrine cells are made in the inner plexiform layer. Ganglion cell bodies are situated in the ganglion cell layer, a layer that also contains numerous "displaced" amacrine cells. The axons of ganglion cells traverse the retinal surface toward the optic disk to form the optic nerve. The number of optic nerve fibers varies markedly across species: in the cat there are about 150,000 fibers (e.g., Williams et al., 1983), while in the rhesus monkey and in the human there are about 1.5 million (Potts et al., 1972; Rakic and Riley, 1983a). At maturity, each ganglion cell body contributes only a single axon to the optic nerve population, but some of these fibers branch beyond the nerve, in the optic tract, to innervate more than one retinorecipient region.

To the foregoing simplified overview of retinal anatomy two important points must be added. First, the five major retinal cell types noted above can be further distinguished on the basis of morphological and functional criteria into different classes of cells. For instance, in the cat retina three broad classes of ganglion cells have historically been delineated (Boycott and Wässle, 1974). Although this tripartite classification of the cat's ganglion cells is still quite useful, recent evidence points to many more classes of ganglion cells in this species (Kolb et al., 1981). This is of clear relevance for developmental studies since different classes of retinal ganglion cells project in a differential manner to the visual centers of the brain (e.g., Wässle, 1982). Furthermore, it is quite likely that each class of cell also possesses specialized presynaptic circuitry that provides the class with distinct functional properties.

The second point to be noted is that the distribution of cells is not uniform across the retinal surface. To a certain degree this appears to be true of all mammals, but such nonuniformity is particularly striking in species with well-developed focal vision, such as cat and primate. To use ganglion cells as an example, in the adult cat the density of ganglion cells is about 80 times greater in the region of the retina specialized for detailed vision, the area centralis, than it is in the retinal periphery (see Figure 2). This difference is even more pronounced when ganglion cell densities in equivalent regions of the primate retina are compared. Numerous studies have systematically plotted the density of a given cell type across the retinal surface and related the resulting gradients to basic features of visual function (e.g., Fukuda and Stone, 1974; Rowe and Stone, 1976). For instance, ganglion cell density gradients dominate the visual map representations at virtually all levels of the visual system. Typically, the high-density region (area centralis of the

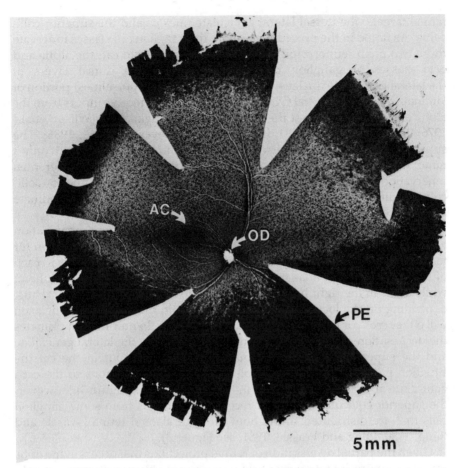

FIGURE 2. Retinal wholemount from an adult cat in which the lateral geniculate nucleus and the superior colliculus received bilateral injections of horseradish peroxidase. The density of retrogradely labeled ganglion cells is greatest at the area centralis (AC) and declines markedly toward the periphery. OD, optic disk; PE, pigment epithelium. (From Chalupa et al., 1984.)

cat and the foveal region of the primate) is substantially overrepresented (i.e., magnified) in retinorecipient structures as well as in the multiple areas of the visual cortex. As will be discussed in a later section, recent studies from our laboratory have provided a surprisingly simple (and we think a correct) explanation of how such regional gradients in the mammalian retina are established during ontogeny.

B Central Visual Pathways

The mammalian retina projects directly to a large number of nuclei, but studies of prenatal development have focused primarily on the two major retinal targets: the dorsal lateral geniculate nucleus and the superior colliculus. As noted in the preceding section, the ganglion cell classes innervate these two main retinorecipient centers differentially. In cat, the alpha and beta classes of ganglion cells project to the two dorsal layers of the lateral geniculate nucleus, the A laminae, and the dorsalmost portion of laminaC, while the ventral C layers of the geniculate receive inputs from the alpha and gamma, but not the beta, classes of ganglion cell (Wilson et al., 1976; Illing and Wässle, 1981; Itoh et al., 1981; Leventhal et al., 1985). The superior colliculus is also innervated by alpha and gamma cells, with only a minor beta cell input (Wässle and Illing, 1980; Itoh et al., 1981). Differential innervation of the dorsal lateral geniculate nucleus and the superior colliculus by different classes of retinal ganglion cells also occurs in the primate brain (Leventhal et al., 1981).

Another fundamental feature of mammalian visual system organization is the decussation pattern of the retinal projections. It has been known for more than a century (cf. Polyak, 1957) that in humans ganglion cells in each of the two left hemiretinas project to visual centers in the left hemisphere, while those in the right hemiretinas project to the right hemisphere. Thus, depending on the location of its cell body within the retina, an optic axon will either cross or remain uncrossed at the chiasm. In non-human primates the decussation pattern of ganglion cells innervating the lateral geniculate and the superior colliculus is thought to be similar, but in the cat the situation is somewhat more complex. The retinal projections to the cat's geniculate appear to be like those in the primate brain (Figure 3); however, the superior colliculus of the cat receives projections from some ganglion cells that are distributed throughout the contralateral retina (Wässle and Illing, 1980; Illing and Wässle, 1981; see Figure 3).

Given the partial decussation of retinal projections that occurs at the optic chiasm, retinorecipient nuclei could be innervated by projections from both eyes. This is in fact the case. Both the lateral geniculate nucleus and the superior colliculus receive binocular inputs, but in the mature animal the projections from each eye are largely segregated. In the geniculate, this segregation into ocular domains is reflected in terms of the laminar organization of the nucleus. In the cat, the most dorsal layer of the geniculate, the A layer, receives projections exclusively from the contralateral eye, while the underlying A1 layer is innervated by axons stemming from the ipsilateral retina (Figure 3). Such laminar separation of ocular inputs is also evident in the C laminae of the geniculate. Although the superior colliculus is also a laminated structure, ocular segregation in the colliculus is not defined on the basis of laminar boundaries. Rather, within the visual layers there are small gaps in the projection from the contralateral eye, and these gaps are filled by ipsilateral retinotectal input (Graybiel, 1975, 1976; Harting and Guillery, 1976).

Axons of lateral geniculate neurons innervate the visual cortex (area 17 of the primate and areas 17 and 18 of the cat), with the bulk of the these

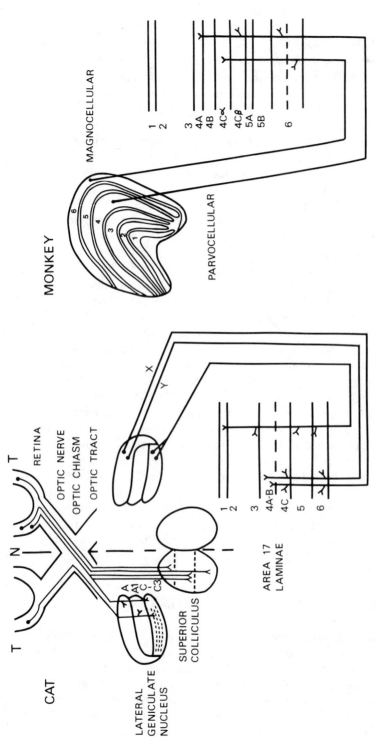

FIGURE 3. A schematic drawing of retinal projections to the lateral geniculate nucleus and the superior colliculus in the cat and projection patterns of geniculate fibers to cortical area 17 in cat and monkey. Both target nuclei of optic tract fibers receive input from the contralateral nasal retina and the ipsilateral temporal retina. In addition, the superior colliculus receives input from the contralateral temporal retina. Geniculocortical input is primarily to sublaminae of layer 4 in cat and monkey. Major cortical projection from the A and Al laminae of cat geniculate are from X- and Y-cells, while output from C laminae are from Y- and W-cells. (See also Chapter 2, Figure 8.) The geniculocortical projections from magnocellular and parvocellular laminae of monkey are shown at right.

afferents terminating in layer IV (Figure 3). Here, again, there is a substantial degree of binocular segregation in the mature organism. In the large binocular portion of the visual cortex, geniculate projections terminate in distinct patches within layer IV, with alternate patches representing input from a given eye. This adult organization has been elegantly described by its discoverers, Hubel and Wiesel (1972).

The last attribute of central visual system organization we will discuss is topographic organization. This refers to the fact that at maturity there is an orderly representation of the receptor surface (i.e., the retina) in the various visual centers of the brain. A map of the retinal surface is found at virtually all levels of the visual system, but the complexity of such maps and the set of rules that a given retinotopic map appears to follow vary considerably. Topographic order is, of course, not unique to the visual system. Such organization is fundamental to all the major sensory modalities, and it is also prevalent in numerous nonsensory pathways in the brain.

A complete explanation of mammalian visual system development would account for each of the fundamental attributes of the mature visual system noted above. To review these key points, imagine a newborn ganglion cell in the mammalian retina. As the growth cone of this cell navigates along the optic pathway, several critical events must occur to ensure the long-term survival of the neuron and its utility in the subsequent processing of visual information. Once the axon of the ganglion cell reaches the optic chiasm, the proper decussation choice must be made. Subsequently, the appropriate retinorecipient target must be invaded, a topographically correct region in the target innervated, and particular types of cells within the region selected for formation of stabilized synaptic contacts. As the central connections of the retinal ganglion cell are being established, its dendrites must grow to establish contact with appropriate presynaptic neurons (i.e., amacrine and bipolar cells).

At present, we do not have a complete description of these developmental events. Nor do we possess adequate theoretical explanations of the factors underlying the ontogeny of the mammalian visual system. However, in the last decade or so, considerable progress has been achieved.

III   PRENATAL DEVELOPMENT OF THE RETINA

The retina is unique among sensory organs: it is a part of the brain, formed by the evagination of the forebrain. This evagination can first be recognized as depressions in the rostral portion of the neural plate (see Figure 4). As these depressions deepen, they form the optic vesicles. With the closing of the neural tube the optic vesicles become rounded protuberances on the lateral walls of the forebrain. At this stage the lumen of the optic vesicle is continuous with that of the forebrain. As embryonic development proceeds, each optic vesicle begins to flatten and gradually becomes invagi-

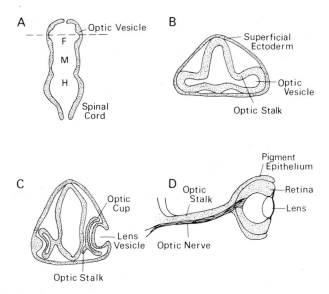

FIGURE 4. Embryogenesis of the retina. (*A*) Dorsal view of the neural tube, the precursor of the brain, showing the plane of section for (*B*), (*C*), and (*D*). F, forebrain; M, midbrain; H, hindbrain. (*B*) The optic vesicles are formed by evagination of the lateral walls of the forebrain. (*C*) Invagination of the optic vesicles creates a two-layered optic cup while the lens vesicle forms from invagination of the overlying ectoderm. (*D*) The optic cup differentiates into the pigment epithelium and neural layer of the retina. (Adapted from Lund, 1978.)

nated to transform the single-walled vesicle into a double-layered optic cup (Figure 4C). The inner wall of the cup will form the neural layer of the retina, while the outer wall will differentiate into the pigment layer (Figure 4D). As invagination of the optic cup continues, the opening to the forebrain (the lumen) becomes progressively constricted, forming the optic stalk through which pioneer optic axons will subsequently grow toward their central targets.

A   Cell Proliferation

Two methods have been used to study retinal cell proliferation: thymidine autoradiography and nuclear staining. With thymidine autoradiography a pulse of tritiated thymidine is injected directly into the vitreous chamber of the fetal eye. The radioactive thymidine is cleared rapidly from the animal (in about 1 h), but before clearance some of it is taken in by mitotic cells and incorporated into their nuclear material. If the cells continue dividing, the thymidine becomes diluted. However, if the cells are in their final cycle of division at the time of the injection, they remain heavily labeled. The other procedure for studying cell proliferation, the nuclear staining method, involves staining chromosomal material so that mitotic figures can be detected (e.g., Rapaport and Stone, 1983b).

In the developing retina, as in other regions of the central nervous system, neuroblasts undergoing mitosis are largely confined to the ventricular zone (Angevine et al., 1970), the most external layer of the neural retina. As cells leave the mitotic cycle, they migrate from the ventricular layer to their final positions, where they differentiate and grow to maturity. There is a rough inverse sequence of cell formation (inverse to the direction in which visual information will be processed): ganglion cells attain their adult complement first and photoreceptors last (e.g., Sidman, 1961). In the cat, the available evidence indicates that ganglion cells, A-type horizontal cells, amacrine cells, and cones are among the first born, whereas rods, B-type horizontal cells, and bipolar cells are born later (Polley et al., 1981, 1985; Zimmerman et al., 1985). In the monkey, retinal ganglion and horizontal cells appear to be the first to form, followed by cones and then rods, amacrine cells, and bipolar cells (LaVail et al., 1983).

Studies from Stone's laboratory (Rapaport et al., 1985; Robinson et al., 1985) have demonstrated that cytogenesis of neurons in the developing cat retina actually occurs in two distinct zones: ventricular and "subventricular." Cell division occurs concurrently in these two zones, but it persists for a longer period in the subventricular zone. The subventricular zone corresponds to the inner nuclear layer, which can be recognized after the formation of the outer plexiform layer. It is not certain which cell types are formed in this inner zone of cell division. These may be bipolar cells or Müller cells as well as some photoreceptors that migrate across the outer plexiform layer.

The rough inside-to-outside pattern of retinal cell birth would be expected if cell identify were specified by mitotic lineage. A recent study by Turner and Cepko (1987), however, indicates that a single progenitor cell can give rise to more than one retinal cell type, possibly as late as the final mitosis. These findings suggested to Turner and Cepko that determination of retinal cell type is guided by extrinsic factors rather than strict lineage. The investigators carried out their work on postnatal rat retinas, in which only rods, bipolar, amacrine, and nonneuronal cells are still mitotic. It will be of interest to apply the lineage marker method to fetal tissue in which ganglion cell and other retinal cell types are being born.

A gradient across the retinal surface in the cytogenesis of retinal neurons has been observed in primates (LaVail et al., 1983) as well as cat, the species for which the greatest detail is known. Gestation in the cat is about 65 days. Tritiated thymidine studies have demonstrated that the first retinal ganglion cells in this species are born at about day 21 after conception (E21) in the central retina (Kliot and Shatz, 1982; Walsh et al., 1983) and that the last ganglion cells are generated some 15 days later (E36) in the peripheral regions of the retina. It should be noted that these studies provide information only about those neurons that have survived to the time that the animals were sacrificed. Given the massive degree of ganglion cell loss that occurs during the normal development of the mammalian retina (see below), it is likely that the thymidine method, as it has been used to date, has not provided an accurate starting date of cell proliferation. This reservation is supported by the recent observation of Williams et al. (1986) that growing axons are seen in the optic stalk of the fetal cat as early as E19.

Examination of mitotic cells at the ventricular layer has demonstrated that there is also a central-to-peripheral pattern in the termination of mitotic activity (Rapaport and Stone, 1983b). These investigators found that by E50 mitosis has ceased at the area centralis but is continuing in peripheral retina. By birth it has ceased over the central 50% of the retina, and 10 days after birth no mitotic profiles are observed at the ventricular surface. Recently, a similar regional sequence in the termination of mitotic activity has been reported in the human fetal retina (Provis et al., 1985a).

Curiously, the studies that have stained for mitotic figures have not found a regional gradient across the retina in the initiation of cytogenesis, as observed in the tritiated thymidine experiments summarized above. This may reflect the fact that the two methods of studying cytogenesis are evaluating different aspects of the cell division process. Staining for mitotic figures permits examination of cells at several stages of mitosis, and with this method the fate of the daughter cells is unknown. Thus, some of the cells containing mitotic profiles may undergo several additional cycles of cell division. In contrast, tritiated thymidine is incorporated only by cells in the S phase (the DNA synthetic phase) of the cell cycle and labels most heavily those cells undergoing their final division.

Within the ganglion cell layer, there is also a difference in the timing and pattern of cell birth of small, medium, and large neurons that survive to adulthood (Kliot and Shatz, 1982; Walsh et al., 1983). Medium-sized cells are produced before the largest ganglion cells, and small ganglion cells are produced throughout the period of ganglion cell generation. Medium cell production becomes restricted to peripheral retina by E29 (Walsh et al., 1983) and appears to be completed by E32, an age when large cell cytogenesis has ceased in central retina but is continuing in the periphery. No large cells are labeled in tritiated thymidine studies after E34 in the cat's retina (Walsh et al., 1983), but small cells, thought to be displaced amacrine cells, continue to be labeled as late as E56 (Kliot and Shatz, 1982).

These results are of considerable interest because they imply a differential schedule of production, and presumably maturation, of the three main classes of ganglion cells found in the mature cat's retina. Such timing differences could have important implications for the organization of retinofugal pathways as well as for retinal innervation patterns of central targets.

B   Formation of Retinal Layers

The first indication of nuclear layers during the development of the mammalian retina occurs when newborn cells migrate from the ventricular margin of the neuroblast layer to an inner zone that will form the ganglion cell layer. The beginning of a laminated retina can be seen in the cat as early as E30 (Rapaport and Stone, 1982). Initially, the neuroblast and ganglion cell layers are separated by a presumptive inner plexiform layer containing numerous migrating cells (Rapaport and Stone, 1982). The immature inner plexiform layer has a unistratified appearance at E35 and contains ganglion cell and amacrine cell processes (Zimmerman et al., 1985). The degree of separation between the two nuclear layers increases with age but does not appear to vary with retinal position (Rapaport and Stone, 1982). At about the time the separation of the neuroblast layer and ganglion cell layer appears clear, at E50, the outer plexiform layer begins to emerge (Rapaport and Stone, 1982). The outer plexiform layer divides the neuroblast layer into inner and outer nuclear layers. The outer plexiform layer first forms in the central retina and spreads to the entire retina some 5 to 10 days after birth (Donovan, 1966; Rapaport and Stone, 1982).

A similar sequence of events occurs in the formation of layers in the primate retina. As in the cat, the ganglion cell layer in the fetal monkey becomes distinguished before the emergence of other nuclear layers (Nishimura and Rakic, 1985). Gestation in the rhesus monkey is about 165 days. The inner plexiform layer can be recognized around E65 (Smelser et al., 1974; Nishimura and Rakic, 1985), and by E74 all three nuclear layers are present in the retinal region that will correspond to the fovea centralis (Hendrickson and Kupfer, 1976). By E156, about 9 days before birth, the inner and outer nuclear layers have emerged in the periphery of the monkey retina. Thus, retinal layers are formed in the monkey before birth, whereas in the cat this process is not completed until about 1 week after birth, near the time of eye opening.

C Synaptogenesis

In both the cat (Greiner and Weidman, 1980; Maslim and Stone, 1986) and monkey (Nishimura and Rakic, 1983) synaptic contacts are first seen in the inner plexiform layer. At maturity this retinal layer contains two general types of synapses: ribbon synapses that are characteristic of bipolar input to amacrine and ganglion cells and conventional synapses characteristic of amacrine cell input to ganglion, bipolar, and other amacrine cells (Dowling and Boycott, 1966; Dowling, 1970). In the cat, conventional synapses are observed as early as E45 whereas ribbon synapses are noted near birth (Maslim and Stone, 1986). In the monkey, the first conventional synapses appear at E78, while ribbon synapses emerge at E99 (Nishimura and Rakic, 1985). These observations suggest that synapses conveying information laterally in the inner plexiform layer are established substantially earlier than those contacts that carry information centripetally. Later in fetal development, this sequence also occurs in the outer plexiform layer, where the first synaptic contacts are between receptors and horizontal cells (Maslim and Stone, 1986). Rods form synaptic contacts with horizontal cells a few days earlier than cones. Maslim and Stone (1986) noted that all synapses in the outer plexiform layer show a pronounced central-to-peripheral gradient of development. Such a gradient is also seen in the formation of bipolar cell synapses in the inner plexiform layer but not in the establishment of the initial synapses, presumably between amacrine cells, in this layer.

The foregoing studies indicate that visual experience cannot be a factor in the establishment of synaptic circuitry in the retina of the cat and monkey. This is certainly the case in the primate, where the density of synapses in the inner plexiform layer is comparable to that of the adult some 2 months before birth. While in the cat the photoreceptor and bipolar contacts are largely established after birth, synaptogenesis is virtually completed by the time the optical quality of the eye has attained adultlike quality, about 4–5 weeks after birth (Bonds and Freeman, 1978).

D   Ganglion Cell Differentiation and Growth

As noted previously, in the adult cat's retina three main classes of retinal ganglion cells—alpha, beta, and gamma—have been differentiated on the basis of soma size, dendritic field size, and dendritic branching pattern (Boycott and Wässle, 1974). These morphological classes of ganglion cells have been shown to correspond to the physiological cell types Y, X, and W, respectively (e.g., Saito, 1983). Each cell type projects selectively to the major retinorecipient nuclei (e.g., Wässle, 1982). From a developmental perspective, it would be of great interest to determine when the different classes of retinal ganglion cells attain their specialized morphological and functional properties as well as their selective patterns of central projections. It is obviously not possible to determine the visual responses of these cells in the fetal retina, although it should be feasible to examine the prenatal developmental of any specialized membrane properties.

Until recently, little was known about the differentiation and growth of retinal ganglion cells in the fetal retina. Work from Stone and colleagues indicated that soma size groupings emerge quite late in fetal development, at E57 (Rapaport and Stone, 1983a), but that cell classes based on dendritic morphologies can be distinguished somewhat earlier, around E50 (Maslim et al., 1986). A recent study by Ramoa et al. (1987) has added much to our descriptive understanding of prenatal ganglion cell development. Using Lucifer yellow filling of identified ganglion cells, these investigators found that ganglion cells undergo significant remodeling during fetal and early postnatal stages. Among the changes that take place during the last 2 weeks of gestation and the first postnatal weeks are growth of somata and dendritic fields, elimination of dendritic and occasional somatic spines, simplification of dendritic branching patterns, and loss of intraretinal axon collaterals and side branches. Despite the expression of transient features such as spines and exuberant dendritic branching, some of the ganglion cells could be grouped into one of three morphological classes as early as E52 based on relative soma size, dendritic branching, and dendritic spread.

E   Ganglion Cell Dendrites

In the adult cat, cell bodies of on- and off-alpha ganglion cells are distributed across the retinal surface in two independent mosaic patterns (Wässle et al., 1981b,c). Furthermore, the dendrites of these two subpopulations of alpha cells provide complete coverage of the retina with only a small amount of overlap between dendrites of the same functional subclass. A similar mosaic pattern has been described for the beta cell class (Wassle et al., 1981a). These elegant observations led Wassle and colleagues (Wässle and Rieman, 1978; Wässle et al., 1981b) to hypothesize that during early development interactions among neighboring ganglion cells of the same functional sub-class regulate dendritic growth. There are two somewhat different ways in which this important hypothesis has been viewed in the literature on dendritic development. Studies on the rat retina (Linden and Perry, 1982; Perry and Linden, 1982) have been interpreted as showing that developing ganglion cell dendrites compete for afferent input, presumably from bipolar and amacrine cells. The other possibility is that growing dendrites may recognize the membrane of "conspecific" cells and that such recognition could cause the slowing or termination of dendritic growth.

Several recent studies have demonstrated that experimental manipulations that modify the normal density of retinal ganglion cells are accompanied by morphological alterations in dendritic fields of these cells (Ault et al., 1985; Eysel et al., 1985; Kirby and Chalupa, 1985, 1986). For instance, Kirby and Chalupa (1985, 1986) found that when retinal ganglion cell density is increased by prenatal unilateral enucleation, alpha ganglion cells in the remaining retina develop smaller than normal dendritic fields. Correspondingly, manipulations that reduce the density of ganglion cells (Ault et al., 1985) have been noted to result in an increase in the size of dendritic fields. These findings support the idea that interactions among developing ganglion cells dendrites are a factor in regulating the dendritic field size of individual retinal ganglion cells as originally postulated by Wassle and colleagues (Wässle and Rieman, 1978; Wässle et al., 1981b). However, it is unknown whether a change in the density of ganglion cells is accompanied by corresponding changes in the density of retinal neurons presynaptic to ganglion cells. Thus, the degree to which dendritic growth is dependent upon afferent input and/or some type of membrane recognition mechanism is still unresolved.

It is known that afferent input cannot be a factor in the initial growth of ganglion cell dendrites since in the fetal cat some of these neurons have extensive dendritic arbors as early as E36 (Lia et al., 1983; Maslim et al., 1986; Shatz and Sretavan, 1986; Ramoa et al., 1987), much before the formation of synaptic contacts in the inner plexiform layer. A role for synaptic factors in the elaboration of ganglion cell dendrites is suggested, however, by the observation that the dendritic arbors of cells become segregated into sublaminae of the inner plexiform layer around birth, coincident with the formation of bipolar–ganglion cell synapses (Maslim and Stone, 1986).

F Loss of Retinal Ganglion Cells

During normal development of the mammalian retina there is a massive overproduction of retinal ganglion cells followed by a period of ganglion cell loss. This is also the case in the avian retina (Rager and Rager, 1976; Hughes and McLoon, 1979). Three types of evidence have documented this intriguing phenomenon. First, pyknotic profiles have been recognized in the ganglion cell layer of the developing retina, and this has been interpreted as evidence for the death of retinal ganglion cells (e.g., Cunningham et al., 1982; Sengelaub and Finlay, 1982). However, it is not easy to ascertain from such material whether the degenerating profiles are indeed ganglion cells or the other cell type within the ganglion cell layer, displaced amacrine cells. Second, counts have been made of presumed ganglion cells in Nissl-stained tissue at different stages of development and have been found to be much higher during ontogeny than at maturity (Stone et al., 1982). In Nissl-stained material it is not possible to differentiate unequivocally ganglion cells from other cell types, and thus studies (e.g., Stone et al., 1982) relying on this approach are subject to the same criticism indicated in the preceding sentences. Several laboratories have sought to overcome this potential pitfall by retrograde labeling of ganglion cells following injections of tracers into the developing brain (e.g., Potts et al., 1982; Dreher et al., 1983; Lia et al., 1983, 1987b; Perry et al., 1983). There is no guarantee, however, that such injections label the entire population of ganglion cells in the developing retina, and most likely this approach underestimates the degree of normal cell loss. Still another approach, to be considered below, is to count the number of axons in the developing optic nerve. The assumption here is that each fiber in the optic nerve stems from a single retinal ganglion cell.

An alternative hypothesis for ganglion cell loss has been proposed by Hinds and Hinds (1978, 1983). On the basis of electron microscopic serial reconstruction of sections through the developing mouse retina, these investigators suggested that displaced amacrine cells develop from immature ganglion cells that lose their axon without degeneration of the soma. However, the transformation hypothesis has not been supported by two studies of developing rat retina (Dreher et al., 1983; Perry et al., 1983). At present it is generally assumed that loss of ganglion cells in the developing retina is due to neuronal death rather than to transformation of immature cells. The possible causes of retinal ganglion cell death will be considered in subsequent sections.

G Formation of Retinal Topography

Retinal topography refers to the distribution of cells across the retinal surface. In all mammals, and particularly in those with good focal vision such as the cat, the monkey, and humans, the density of ganglion cells is nonuniform. The highest density of these cells is found at or near the center of gaze (i.e., region of highest visual acuity) and declines toward the retinal periphery. Topography of the prenatal retina differs markedly from that of the mature retina in that early in fetal development the distribution of ganglion cells is relatively uniform across the retina (Stone et al., 1982).

What underlies the change in distribution of ganglion cells during ontogeny? In their study of the fetal cat retina, Stone et al. (1982) first suggested that ganglion cell death may be an important factor in this process. This would be the case if during early development more ganglion cells died in peripheral regions than in the central region of the retina. (Note that the designation "central" retina does not refer to the geometric center but rather to the retinal region functionally specialized for central vision.) Subsequently, Stone et al. (1984) plotted the loci of dying cells in the ganglion cell layer of the fetal cat retina and found their distribution to be "diffuse." This was interpreted as showing that cell death could not be a major factor in establishing retinal topography. By a process of elimination, these investigators reasoned that the decrease of ganglion cells from the peripheral retina might result from the transformation mechanism discussed above.

The retina grows enormously during fetal development, and this suggests an alternative explanation for the formation of retinal topography. If the peripheral regions of the retina were to expand substantially more than the central region, this would effectively dilute the peripheral population of ganglion cells to a greater degree than the central population. Such a nonuniform pattern of growth has been documented in the retina of the postnatal cat (Mastronarde et al., 1984).

A recent study from our laboratory (Lia et al., 1987b) has shown unequivocally that the fetal cat's retina also expands in a nonuniform manner. More importantly, this differential expansion of the growing fetal retina was shown to be the dominant factor in regulating overall retinal topography. A recent histological study of the developing cat retina has also suggested the importance of retinal growth in ontogeny of the area centralis (Robinson, 1987). Observations from other laboratories indicate that this may be a common feature of mammalian retinal development (Sengelaub et al., 1986; Robinson et al., 1986; Dreher et al., 1984).

IV   DEVELOPMENT OF THE FETAL OPTIC NERVE AND TRACT

Since the retina is a part of the brain, the optic nerve is actually a fiber tract within the central nervous system. It is largely a matter of convenience and historical precedence, then, that the collection of ganglion cell axons rostral to the optic chiasm is referred to as "nerve" and caudal to the chiasm as "tract." From a technical perspective it is simpler to perform an ultrastructural analysis of the optic nerve than the tract because the nerve can be readily separated from the brain, while much of the optic tract is embedded in neural tissue. There is also reason to believe that the overall organization of the adult optic nerve differs from that of the optic tract. Other than the fact that the nerve contains optic fibers from one eye and the tract from both eyes, there is evidence that the retinotopic organization is different in the nerve than in the tract (Horton et al., 1979; Aebersold et al., 1981) as is the grouping of axons by caliber (Guillery et al., 1982; Williams and Chalupa, 1983a; Walsh, 1986).

A   Overproduction of Optic Nerve Fibers

It is generally assumed that each axon in the optic nerve corresponds to a single ganglion cell. As a consequence, several laboratories have recently quantified the rise and fall in the number of fibers within the nerve for the purpose of assessing changes in the retinal ganglion cell population during early development. There is good evidence that this assumption is valid in mature animals (e.g., Chalupa et al., 1984) and a high probability that it is also largely correct in the developing nerve. While there is evidence for the presence of a transient retinoretinal projection during early development (Bunt and Lund, 1981), the number of cells involved is exceedingly small (Kirby et al., 1988). Furthermore, Lia et al. (1986) have demonstrated that ganglion cell axons do not branch in the developing optic nerve. There are some ganglion cells that possess branched axons within the retina (Dacey, 1985; Ramoa et al., 1987), but in these cases it appears that only one axonal branch enters the optic nerve.

Quantitative analysis of the fiber population in the developing optic nerve has been performed for various species, including rat (Lam et al., 1982; Perry et al., 1983; Sefton and Lam, 1984; Crespo et al., 1985), opossum (Kirby and Wilson, 1984), cat (Ng and Stone, 1982; Williams et al., 1983, 1986), rhesus monkey (Rakic and Riley, 1983a), and human (Provis et al., 1985b). These studies permit two generalizations. First, the overproduction and subsequent elimination of optic nerve axons appear to be basic developmental features of the mammalian visual system. Second, the overall temporal pattern of axon elimination appears similar across mammalian species. There is an initial period of rapid fiber loss followed by a longer period during which axon number decreases at a slow rate (see Figure 5). Parenthetically, it should be noted that these phenomena are not unique to mammals as they have also been documented in the optic nerve of the chick (Rager and Rager, 1976; Rager, 1980). There are substantial differences among species in the degree of ganglion cell overproduction, but the reasons for this are unclear. For example, Williams et al. (1986) have estimated that in cat there is a five- to sixfold overproduction of ganglion cell axons, while in primates this overproduction is about half as great, that is, two- to threefold (Rakic and Riley, 1983a).

B   Growth Cones and Necrotic Optic Nerve Fibers

A detailed description of the ultrastructure in the mammalian optic nerve has been provided by Williams et al. (1986) in work from our laboratory on

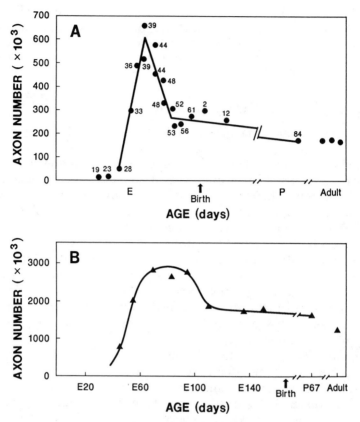

FIGURE 5. Axon number in the optic nerve as a function of gestational age in the cat (*A*) and monkey (*B*). Numbers associated with dots in (*A*) indicate prenatal or postnatal age in days. In both species there is an overproduction and subsequent elimination of optic fibers during fetal development. [(*A*) Adapted from Williams et al., 1986; (*B*) adapted from Rakic and Riley, 1983a.]

the fetal cat. The information in this section will largely rely on these findings.

Axons enter the optic stalk, the precursor of the optic nerve, shortly after the first ganglion cells are generated. At this stage, the optic stalk consists largely of neuroepithelial cells as well as a substantial number of intercellular spaces or ducts, some of which contain the "pioneer" ganglion cell axons (Figure 6). In the fetal cat, the early fibers are preferentially distributed around the perimeter of the stalk and, as in other species (e.g., Silver and Sapiro, 1981), are mostly within the ventral portion.

During this time that axons are being added to the optic nerve, growth cones can be recognized as large processes that possess a specialized organellar composition (see Figure 7). Recently, Williams and Rakic (1984) have

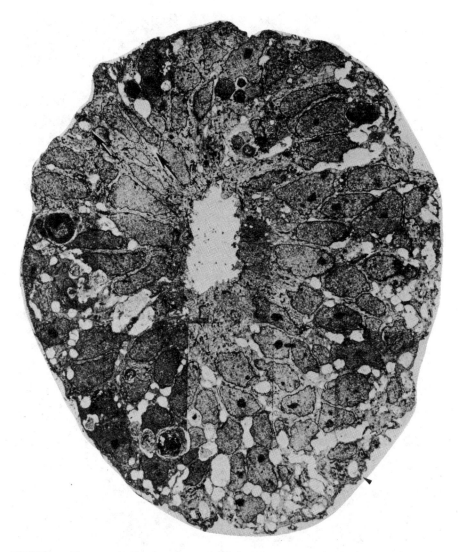

FIGURE 6. The optic stalk, the precursor of the optic nerve, of a fetal cat 19 days after conception. At this stage the stalk consists principally of neuroepithelial cells and large inter-cellular spaces or ducts, some of which contain optic nerve fibers (arrows) and growth cones (arrowhead). Dark-appearing necrotic cells can be seen at the 7-, 9-, and 11-o'clock positions. ×2200. (From Williams et al., 1986.)

provided three-dimensional reconstruction of ganglion cell growth cones in the optic nerve of the fetal rhesus monkey. Growth cones in the mammalian optic nerve, in common with growth cones in a variety of other species and systems (e.g., Yamada et al., 1971; Bunge, 1973), are characterized by a distal fringe made up largely of sheetlike extensions termed lamellipodia

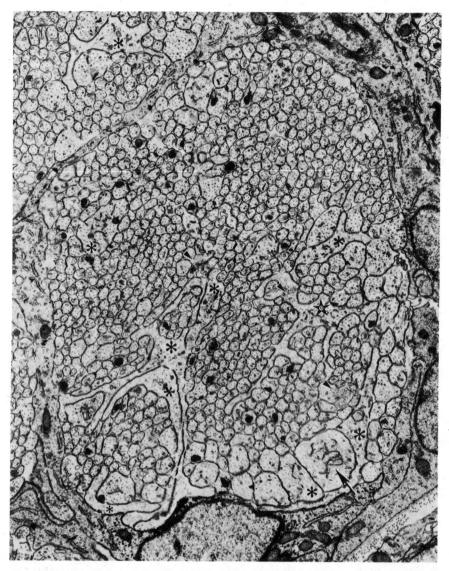

FIGURE 7. A fascicle containing 752 fibers from the optic nerve of an E33 cat. Growth cones are marked by asterisks. One (star) has elaborate lamellipodia and borders 58 fibers. In another growth cone a labyrinthine smooth endoplasmic reticulum can be seen (arrow). Vesicular aggregates (arrowheads) are found in both growth cones and axons. ×13,600. (From Williams et al., 1986.)

and a central core region containing a variety of organelles, some of which are undoubtedly required for the extension and retraction of the growing axon.

At all stages of development, but particularly during the late phase of axon addition, growth cones are preferentially distributed in the periphery of the developing nerve (Silver and Sapiro, 1981; Rager, 1983; Silver and Rutishauser, 1984; Williams and Rakic, 1983a,b; Williams et al., 1986). This distribution of growth cones may reflect the corresponding central-to-peripheral gradient in the generation of retinal ganglion cells discussed above. Alternatively, it may simply reflect the tendency for growth cones normally to grow near the outer margins of the optic nerve (Silver and Rutishauser, 1984), where they would presumably encounter less mechanical resistance.

In the fetal cat, growth cones are present in the optic nerve only during the period when fibers are being added to the nerve, from E19 to E39. Their number is always quite small, ranging from 2.0% of the population at E28 to about 0.3% at E39. In contrast, necrotic fibers are observed over a broader period, ranging in cat from as early as E28 until several weeks after birth, and are distributed throughout the developing optic nerve. The dying fibers can be distinguished by their dark and mottled axoplasm and, in presumably more advanced stages of necrosis, by their disintegrating membrane (Figure 8). Thus, some axons are undergoing necrosis while other fibers are still being added to the optic nerve. This indicates that the peak number of axons observed during the development of the optic nerve actually underestimates the total production of these fibers. The observations of Williams et al. (1986) also suggest that some of the very large dying fibers may be degenerating growth cones (see Figure 9). This would indicate that some of the fiber population in the optic nerve is eliminated without ever reaching the vicinity of target cells in the various retinorecipient nuclei.

C   Organization of the Optic Tract

A detailed ultrastructural analysis of the developing optic tract in mammals has yet to be carried out. However, a series of elegant papers by Guillery and colleagues (Torrealba et al., 1982; Walsh and Guillery, 1985; Walsh, 1986; Reese and Guillery, 1987) demonstrates that fibers are arranged within the tract on the basis of age-related groupings. This is indicated by developmental evidence from work on the ferret (Walsh and Guillery, 1985; Walsh, 1986) as well as by the organization of axon calibers evident in the optic tract of adult cats (Torrealba et al., 1982) and monkeys (Reese and Guillery, 1987). For instance, in cat and ferret, the oldest fibers in the tract (those whose ganglion cells were presumably generated first) lie farthest from the pial surface of the brain (i.e., deepest in the tract), while the newer fibers are near the pia (i.e., most superficial in the tract). The ordering in the optic tract by fiber caliber (Figure 10A) presumably results from the fact that different

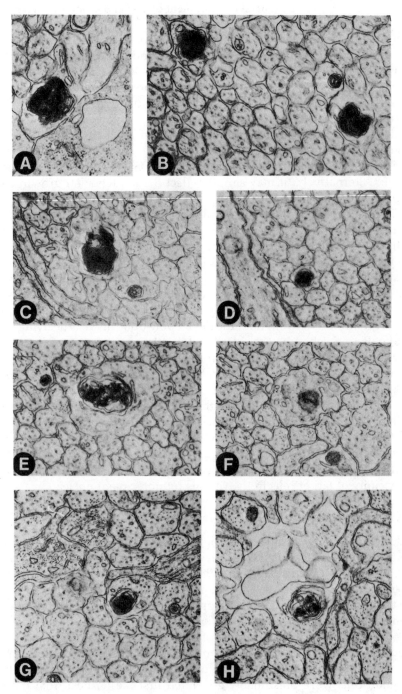

FIGURE 8. Necrotic axons from fetal cats at E33 (*A, B*); E39 (*C, D*); E53 (*E, F*); and E61 (*G, H*). Necrotic fibers were identified as those with dark, mottled axoplasm. Some (*B, C, H*) are partly disintegrated, while others (*A, B, D*) have accumulated dense material. ×30,000. (From Williams et al., 1986.)

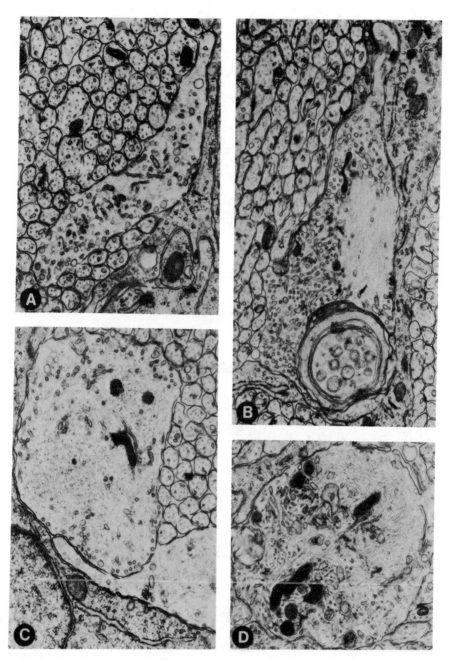

FIGURE 9. Unusual growth cones possibly undergoing necrosis in the optic nerve of an E33 cat. (*A*) Growth cone with an abnormally high vesicular count. ×25,000. (*B*) A large inclusion and accumulation of intermediate filaments are indications of necrosis. ×25,000. (*C*) A dilated growth cone with large, dark-rimmed vesicles and hyperplasia of neurofilaments. ×26,000. (*D*) A large fiber that has accumulated neurofilaments. ×26,000. (From Williams et al., 1986.)

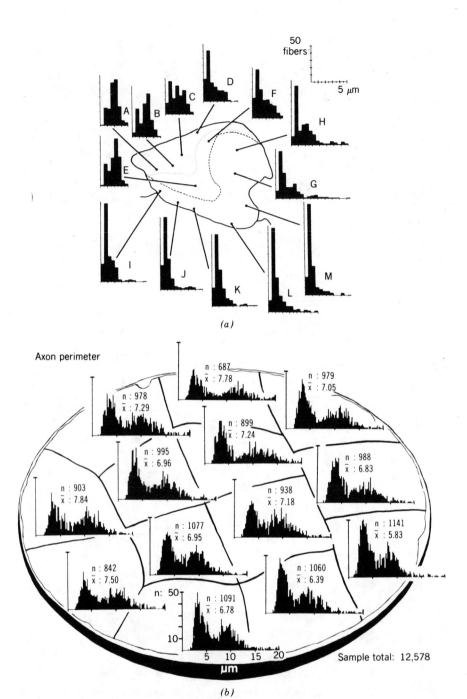

FIGURE 10. Distribution of axon size in the optic tract and nerve of the adult cat. (A) Histograms of fiber diameter are superimposed on a schematic drawing of a cross section through the optic tract. Dorsomedial is to the upper left, rostrolateral to the lower left. (B) Regional distribution of inner axon perimeters is shown in a schematic drawing of the optic nerve. The number of axons and their mean perimeter are given above the histograms. Lateral is to the right, dorsal is up. [(A) From Guillery et al., 1982; (B) from Williams and Chalupa, 1983a.]

size classes of retinal ganglion cells are produced during distinct developmental periods (see above). Since all axon diameter classes are intermingled within the optic nerve (Williams and Chalupa, 1983a), this indicates that during development a pronounced change occurs in the arrangement of these fibers as they grow through the chiasm (Figure 10B). What causes such a pronounced developmental rearrangement is unknown, but it has been suggested that this may reflect changes in the glial structure along the retinal pathway (Walsh, 1986).

V CYTOGENESIS AND MATURATION OF RETINORECIPIENT NUCLEI

Tritiated thymidine has been used to examine the patterns of cell birth in the two main retinorecipient targets: the dorsal lateral geniculate nucleus and the superior colliculus. In this section we will summarize these observations and also deal with related issues of cell growth and differentiation.

A Lateral Geniculate Nucleus

Cells destined to form the lateral geniculate nucleus are generated at a germinal zone lining the third ventricle of the developing brain. Detailed information regarding the generation of geniculate cells in the cat has been provided by Hickey and colleagues (Hickey and Cox, 1979; Hickey and Hitchcock, 1984; Weber et al., 1986). Geniculate neurons in this species are born from E22 to E32. There appears to be little if any relation between the birth dates of geniculate cells and the somal size, structural class, lamina, or retinotopic location attained at maturity (Hickey and Hitchcock, 1984; Hitchcock et al., 1984). Recently, this laboratory also found (Weber et al., 1986) that interneurons in the lateral geniculate are born over the same period as relay cells (i.e., those that project to the cortex). A gradient was observed, however, in the termination of cell birth within the cat's geniculate: the genesis of larger neurons ends significantly earlier than the genesis of smaller cells (Hickey and Hitchcock, 1984).

A different account of the pattern of neurogenesis in the cat's lateral geniculate nucleus has been provided by Shatz (1981). She reported (in abstract form) that geniculate neurons in the cat are born in an inside-to-outside spatiotemporal gradient such that the earliest neurons migrate the least distance from the ventricular zone and form the A layers, while the last-born cells migrate through the older cells to form the C layers. The reasons for the apparent discrepancy with the findings of Hickey et al. are unclear. A notable difference between the approach of these two laboratories, however, is the survival period of the embryos following the thymidine injections. Hickey and colleagues charted labeled cells in neonatal cats some 2 months after birth while Shatz did so in prenatal animals. Substantial cell

death does occur during early development of the mammalian lateral geniculate nucleus (e.g., Sengelaub et al., 1985), but it is unlikely that this factor
could have obscured the spatial pattern of cell birth evident in the fetal
animals.

In Nissl material, the morphology and size of geniculate neurons appear
quite uniform in fetal cats 20 days before birth (Kalil, 1978). By 10 days
before birth, cells have assumed a variety of shapes, but clear variations in
somal size do not become apparent until about 1 week after birth (Kalil,
1978). In the first postnatal week, geniculate cells of the cat lack dendrites
and are marked instead by multiple somatic processes or a few short thick
extensions (Mason, 1983). An active period of dendritic growth does not
begin in this species until the second postnatal week.

Lamination also develops quite late. An interlaminar zone between the A
and A1 layers is first seen around E60 (Shatz, 1983) and is clearly present by
birth (Kalil, 1978). The interlaminar zone between the A1 and C layers
emerges even later, at about postnatal day 3. By 2 weeks after birth, the
interlaminar regions of the cat's geniculate have widened and assumed
their cell-sparse character (Kalil, 1978).

The cat's lateral geniculate rotates 90° in the horizontal plane between
E40 and E60 (Shatz, 1983) followed by a shift in the sagittal plane that
continues for a few months after birth (Kalil, 1978).

A detailed study of the genesis of the dorsal lateral geniculate nucleus of
the rhesus monkey has been provided by Rakic (1977a). In monkey geniculate cells are born between E36 and E43, near the end of the first quarter of
the 165-day gestational period. A clear spatiotemporal gradient of cell proliferation was observed. The cells born earliest migrate to the outermost
surface of the diencephalon, while cells born later achieve progressively
more inner positions so that there is an outside-in gradient of cell birth in the
nucleus. This means that neurons in the magnocellular layers of the mature
monkey's lateral geniculate are generated before cells that ultimately form
the parvocellular layers of the nucleus. An outside-in pattern of cell proliferation has also been noted in the lateral geniculate nucleus of the mouse
(Angevine, 1970) and the albino rat (Lund and Mustari, 1977) but apparently not in the pigmented rat (Bruckner et al., 1976). In rodents, the
generation of these cells is relatively late in fetal development in comparison
to the primate or cat, occurring at about the beginning of the final quarter of
gestation.

As in cat, in the rhesus monkey the laminar organization of the lateral
geniculate nucleus emerges relatively late, about 2 months after the completion of the genesis of geniculate neurons. What underlies the formation
of layers in the dorsal lateral geniculate is unknown, although a combination of intrinsic and extrinsic factors has been implicated (cf. Casagrande
and Brunso-Bechtold, 1985).

Unlike cat, in monkey substantial dendritic growth of lateral geniculate
neurons occurs before birth (Garey and Saini, 1981), so that most of the

neuronal types evident in the adult geniculate can be recognized in the late fetal monkey. The relatively advanced maturation in the morphology of these cells probably relates to the recent finding that the receptive field properties of monkey lateral geniculate neurons are already well developed on the day of birth (Blakemore and Vital-Durand, 1986). In contrast, the functional properties of the cat's lateral geniculate neurons mature over a period several weeks after birth (e.g., Daniels et al., 1978; see also Chapter 2, this volume, by Friedlander and Tootle).

B Superior Colliculus

In comparison to lateral geniculate neurons, cells in the superior colliculus are generated over a somewhat broader period. In cat, collicular cells are born between E22 and at least E37 (Ragland and Hickey, 1982), while in rhesus monkey this occurs from E30 to E56 (Cooper and Rakic, 1981). In both species cells destined for all laminae and for all positions within the laminae are produced at about the same time, except that neurogenesis of the superficial layers continues for a longer period than neurogenesis in the intermediate and deep layers. Since cells in the superficial layers of the mammalian superior colliculus respond exclusively to visual stimuli (Chalupa, 1984), then some visual neurons of the superior colliculus are likely generated later than the extravisual and polysensory cells that are confined to the intermediate and deep layers.

Interestingly, Cooper and Rakic (1983) have demonstrated a clear gradient in cellular differentiation and synaptogenesis in the superior colliculus of the rhesus monkey. In terms of both cell size and synaptic density, the middle region of the superficial gray layer matures significantly earlier than other regions in the superficial layer. These results indicate that the pattern of neurogenesis is not necessarily related to the subsequent pattern of maturation in the developing brain.

VI DEVELOPMENT OF RETINAL PROJECTIONS

Until the mid-1970s virtually all of our knowledge of projection patterns within the central nervous system was derived from studies that relied on degeneration methods. This classic approach was employed to study the early development of connections in the mammalian visual system (e.g., Anker, 1977; Lund and Bunt, 1976). The degeneration method, however, was not well suited to provide detailed information regarding the characteristics of developing pathways. The substantial normal degeneration of cells and terminals in the developing brain made it problematic to clearly distinguish "noise" from the lesion-induced degeneration. This technical difficulty was resolved with the introduction of neuroanatomical tracing methods based on the axoplasmic transport of tritiated amino acids and horseradish peroxidase. As a consequence, within the last decade or so a great deal of information has accumulated regarding the organization of retinofugal and other projections in the mammalian brain. Before summarizing the results of these studies, it should be noted that the axoplasmic tracing methods as applied to developing systems are not without potential pitfalls.

Two concerns are of particular relevance. First, in the mature brain, it is possible to demonstrate (under certain conditions) "spillage" of anterograde tracers from axonal terminals and the subsequent incorporation and transport of the tracer by second-order neurons. For instance, this property has been used effectively by numerous investigators in transneuronal autoradiographic tracing studies to study the organization of ocular dominance columns in the visual cortex (e.g., Rakic, 1976; Shatz and Stryker, 1978; Stryker and Harris, 1986). What distinguishes "standard" autoradiographic tracing from transneuronal tracing is that in the latter a greater amount of the tracer is injected and longer survival periods are employed after the injection. Ascertaining these parameters in the fetal brain, however, is not a trivial matter as the rate of tracer incorporation and transport as well as the leakiness of axonal terminals all undoubtedly vary during the course of development. For the most part, these considerations have been ignored in the developmental literature. A second methodological concern is that cytoarchitectural boundaries are often difficult to discern in fetal tissue so that the localization of anterograde label to specific regions of the developing brain cannot be made with the same degree of confidence as at maturity. For instance, the laminar organization of the lateral geniculate and the superior colliculus is poorly differentiated even during late fetal development so that it is difficult to specify precisely the retinorecipient layers of these structures. These reservations notwithstanding, the use of the anterograde tracing methods has clearly provided a plethora of valuable information on the development of connections in the mammalian visual system.

A   Description of Early Retinal Projections

In 1976 Rakic reported that projections from each eye are completely intermingled in the lateral geniculate nucleus and the superior colliculus of the fetal rhesus monkey before gradually segregating during the second half of gestation into the eye-specific domains characteristic of the mature animal. This was done by injecting tritiated amino acids into the vitreous body of one eye, allowing the fetus to survive for a number of days after the injection and then removing the animal by cesarean section. Sections were processed by the standard autoradiography method. Although these results were initially viewed with some skepticism, analogous observations have subsequently been made in a number of other species, including the opossum (Cavalcante and Rocha-Miranda, 1978), hamster (So et al., 1978;

Frost et al., 1979), rat (Land and Lund, 1979; Bunt et al., 1983), ferret (Linden et al., 1981), grey squirrel (Cusick and Kaas, 1982) and cat (Williams and Chalupa, 1982, 1983b; Shatz, 1983; Chalupa and Williams, 1984b). Thus, it is now well established that a fundamental property of mammalian retinal projections is that they are more widespread during early development than at maturity. Three qualifiers should be added to this generalization. First, there appear to be species differences in the extent to which crossed and uncrossed retinal projections overlap during ontogeny. In general, species with substantial binocular vision appear to show a greater degree of early overlap than those with limited binocular vision. Second, the time course of this overlap and segregation process differs across species. For instance, in the rhesus monkey segregation is largely complete in both the lateral geniculate and the superior colliculus about 3 weeks before birth. In cat this is achieved a few days before birth (see Figure 11), while in rodents segregation of retinal projections occurs after birth. Third, even during the period of maximum overlap, the inputs from the two eyes are not equivalent in density. Early projections from the retina, which is innervating appropriate territory (appropriate in terms of the mature pattern), appear substantially denser than the projections stemming from the other retina.

B   Factors Underlying Early Widespread Retinal Projections

Two factors have been implicated in this developmental process: overproduction of retinal ganglion cells and reorganization of retinal ganglion cell terminals.

As discussed in a previous section, during early development there is a massive overproduction of ganglion cells in the mammalian retina. Assuming that the axons of a substantial subpopulation of these neurons innervate the retinorecipient nuclei, overproduction could account for the more widespread projections evident during early development. It would follow, then, that to a certain degree ocular segregation is achieved by the normal loss of retinal ganglion cells. A substantial degree of ganglion cell loss does occur during the period when retinal projections become segregated. For instance, in the cat (Chalupa and Williams, 1985; Williams et al., 1986) some 200,000 ganglion cells, as judged by axon counts in the optic nerve, are eliminated from E46 until birth, the period during which ocular domains are established in the dorsal lateral geniculate, superior colliculus, and pretectal complex. It is important to stress, however, that this does not mean that all ganglion cell loss is related to this developmental process. In fact, as will be discussed in a later section, there is good reason to believe that multiple factors account for the loss of retinal ganglion cells.

A more direct approach has also implicated ganglion cell death in the segregation process. Removal of one eye during early development, when the projections from the two eyes are intermingled, results in a widespread projection pattern from the remaining eye in mature enucleated animals

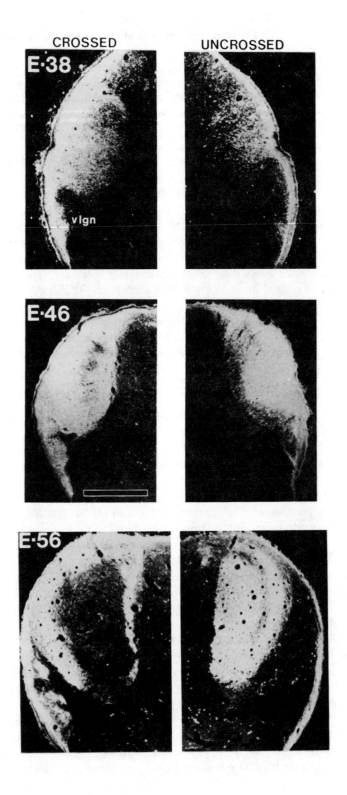

CROSSED UNCROSSED

E·38

vlgn

E·46

E·56

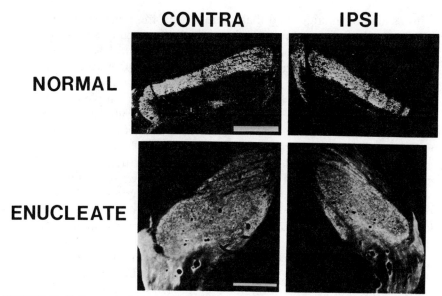

FIGURE 12. Retinogeniculate projection patterns in a normal and a prenatally enucleated adult cat. Above, the normal projection from the retina to the lateral geniculate nucleus is segregated by eye of origin. Below, unilateral enucleation during the fetal period in which projections from the two eyes overlap results in a widespread projection from the remaining eye. (Bottom micrographs reproduced from Chalupa and Williams, 1984a.)

(Land and Lund, 1979; Rakic, 1981; Chalupa and Williams, 1984a). An example of the phenomenon is shown in Figure 12. It is generally assumed that the widespread input is due to the maintenance of the exuberant retinal projections that were present at the time of the monocular enucleation. If retraction of early retinal projections is due to cell loss, then procedures that apparently stem retraction, such as monocular enucleation, should be expected also to attenuate cell death in the retina. This prediction has been confirmed in both monkey (Rakic and Riley, 1983b) and cat (Williams et al., 1983; Chalupa et al., 1984). It should be noted that the increase in the population of ganglion cells in the remaining eye of unilaterally enucleated animals, while significant, is considerably less than double that of the normal complement of cells. It is about 20% greater than normal in the cat and about 30% greater in the monkey.

FIGURE 11. Development of the retinogeniculate projection in the fetal cat as seen in cross sections of the lateral geniculate nucleus. At E38 HRP-labeled retinogeniculate afferents from the injected eye project throughout both the contralateral and ipsilateral lateral geniculate nucleus; vlgn, ventral lateral geniculate nucleus, ×100. At E46 the density of label has increased but initiation of segregation is seen in the less dense areas in the center of the crossed projection and medial border of the uncrossed projection. ×67. By E56 segregation of retinal fibers by eye of origin is well advanced, ×55. (From Chalupa and Williams, 1985.)

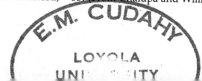

It has also been suggested that alterations in the morphology of retinal ganglion cell terminals underlie the early intermingling and subsequent segregation of retinal projections. Sretavan and Shatz (1986b) have filled retinogeniculate axon terminals by deposits of horseradish peroxidase (HRP) into the optic tract of fetal cats using an *in vitro* preparation. The earliest terminals studied in detail, at E38, possess a simple morphology. Most end in growth cones, although a few display a limited number of short side branches along their main trunk within the geniculate. By E43, the period of maximum overlap of retinal projection to the geniculate, the number of such side branches has increased markedly. Between E55 and birth, when segregation of retinal projections is achieved, retinogeniculate axons lose their side branches, so that by birth they tend to have smooth trunks but quite elaborate terminal arbors. On the basis of these observations Sretavan and Shatz (1986b) proposed that the transient side branches provide the substrate for the intermingling of inputs from the two eyes.

Collectively, the results of the foregoing studies indicate that both overproduction of retinal ganglion cells as well as restructuring of retinogeniculate axon terminals could underlie the changes seen in retinal projections during the early development of the mammalian visual system.

C Formation of Retinofugal Synapses

Electron microscopic studies have revealed that the first synapses in the lateral geniculate nucleus and the superior colliculus are formed several days after retinal afferents invade these targets (Lund and Lund, 1972; Cragg, 1975; Hendrickson and Rakic, 1977; Cooper and Rakic, 1983) Interestingly, in both cat and monkey, retinogeniculate synaptogenesis precedes the formation of retinal synapses. For instance, in the cat retina (as reviewed in a preceding section) the earliest retinal synapses reported to date are found in the inner plexiform layer at E45 (Maslim and Stone, 1986). By comparison, Shatz and Kirkwood (1984) have demonstrated functional retinogeniculate connections using an *in vitro* assay as early as E39. Similarly, in the rhesus monkey, the first retinal synapses (Nishimura and Rakic, 1985) are established at least 2 weeks later than those in the dorsal lateral geniculate nucleus (Hendrickson and Rakic, 1977) and the superior colliculus (Cooper and Rakic, 1983). Thus, synaptic development commences in the major subcortical visual centers well before the formation of functional circuits within the retina.

The density of central synapses increases progressively during ontogeny to attain levels that are even higher than at maturity, so that there is a period of synapse elimination that largely takes place after birth (Cragg, 1975; Holstein et al., 1985). However, even during the postnatal period of synaptic reorganization, the majority of synaptic contacts are immature and the profiles typical of retinal synapses are not fully established until several weeks after birth.

One question of considerable interest is whether or not the retinal projections demonstrated by anterograde transport of HRP following intravitreal injections of the tracer form synaptic contacts in inappropriate regions of the target nuclei. The term "inappropriate" designates that region from which the retinal afferents will subsequently withdraw during normal development. A brief report dealing with the exuberant ipsilateral retinocollicular projection in the neonatal rat (Jeffery et al., 1984) concluded that such transient retinal projections form no or few synaptic contacts. However, a comprehensive treatment of this problem from the same laboratory (Campbell et al., 1984) revealed that during the development of the hamster's retinal projections, transient inappropriate synapses are in fact established with lateral geniculate neurons. The data of Shatz and Kirkwood (1984) further suggest that such transient retinogeniculate synapses in the fetal cat form functional contacts. Thus some degree of synapse elimination must be taking place in central targets during the time that other synaptic contacts are being formed.

D Precision of Early Retinal Projections

The results of studies summarized in the preceding sections clearly demonstrate that retinal connections are more widespread during ontogeny than at maturity, but the studies do not deal with the question of the degree of order exhibited by such developing pathways. In other words, how does the detailed organization of developing projections compare with the exquisite pattern evident in the mature brain? In particular, information regarding two fundamental attributes of the mammalian visual system is of prime importance: retinal decussation patterns and topography of retinofugal pathways. We will deal with these two issues in this section.

1 Establishment of Retinal Decussation Patterns

As described in an earlier section, in each mammalian species there is a partial decussation of optic nerve fibers at the optic chiasm, the particular pattern of decussation and the degree of decussation showing species-typical variations. How then does the pattern evident in the adult of a given species compare with that found during early development. Several studies have addressed this issue by making unilateral injections of retrograde tracers into the optic tract or retinorecipient centers and subsequently examining the resulting distribution of labeled ganglion cells in the ipsilateral and contralateral retinas. In general, it has been demonstrated that early retinal decussation patterns are less precise than at maturity, but the degree of imprecision appears to vary across species. For instance, in adult rodents the ipsilateral retinal projection is normally quite limited, arising from a relatively small population of cells located predominantly in the lower temporal retina (the temporal crescent). In contrast, in the developing rodent visual system, there is a greater number of such ipsilaterally projecting cells (Figure 13), and further, they are distributed throughout the retina (Insausti et al., 1984; Jeffery, 1984). The decline in the number of such ipsilaterally projecting cells and their restriction to the temporal crescent could be due to either cell death or the retraction of transient axonal collaterals. The available evidence from dye labeling experiments suggests that the former mechanism is the key factor (Jeffery and Perry, 1982; Insausti et al., 1984).

In the developing cat visual system the available evidence indicates that the decussation pattern is established with a lesser degree of error than is the case in rodents. Recent experiments from our laboratory (Lia et al., 1987a) have shown that during fetal development some retinal ganglion cells do project to the inappropriate hemisphere. However, the number of such neurons appears to be relatively small in comparison to that described from the developing rodent. Thus, as early as E35, unilateral injections of various retrograde tracers have revealed that the vast majority of retinal ganglion cells in the fetal cats are confined to the appropriate hemiretina. The proportion of cells decussating in an "inappropriate" manner is no more than about 2–4% of the overall ganglion cell population. A few of the cells forming the uncrossed retinal projection are still found in the nasal retina in the postnatal cat as late as 10 days after birth (Jacobs et al., 1984), so that some imprecision in the decussation pattern is evident even after the establishment of ocular domains within the dorsal lateral geniculate nucleus and the superior colliculus. Finally, prenatal monocular enucleation in the cat, which results in the "maintenance" of the early widespread retinal projections, does not result in the maintenance of ganglion cells in the inappropriate hemiretina (Chalupa and Williams, 1984a).

Research in progress in this laboratory (Lia et al., 1988) indicates that the precision of the retinal decussation is even greater in the fetal rhesus monkey. A clear and remarkably mature decussation pattern is evident even before the onset of retinal ganglion cell loss, at about midgestation (see Figure 14).

The foregoing observations suggest that decussation patterns are established with considerable precision during early development in species that possess a high degree of binocular vision. It may be that in species characterized by a large binocular field, such as cat and even more so primate, the mechanisms underlying the formation of decussation patterns have become highly evolved to provide guidance for the appropriate ingrowth of retinal axons. At present, little is known about such mechanisms. However, it is probably the case that factors at the optic chiasm as well as fiber–fiber interactions both contribute to the formation of appropriate decussation patterns.

2   Topography of Developing Retinofugal Projections

Several recent studies have dealt with the question of retinotopic order in developing retinal pathways. Jeffery (1985) showed that in the ferret the

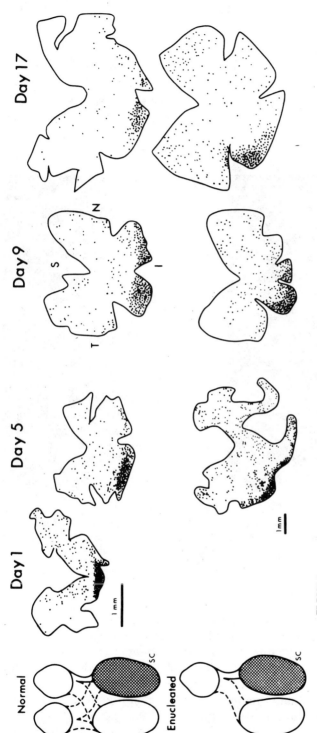

FIGURE 13. Distribution of retinal ganglion cells projecting to the ipsilateral superior colliculus in the normal and enucleated golden hamster. Left, cross hatching indicates the injected colliculus; upper, normal retinas; lower, retinas from animals that had the other eye removed on the day of birth. In the normal animal, the ipsilateral projection gradually becomes restricted to a site of origin in the temporal crescent of the retina. Unilateral enucleation appears to save ipsilaterally projecting cells outside the temporal crescent. T, temporal; N, nasal; S, superior, I, inferior; SC, superior colliculus. (From Insausti et al., 1984.)

IPSI   CONTRA

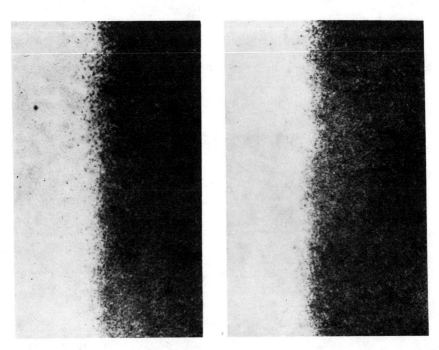

FIGURE 14. Sharp demarcation between ipsilaterally and contralaterally projecting retinal regions in the fetal monkey at E83/85. Retinal ganglion cells retrogradely labeled by unilateral injections of horseradish peroxidase into the optic tract are found almost entirely within the appropriate hemiretinas both ipsilateral and contralateral to the injection sites.

contralateral retinal projections to the dorsal lateral geniculate and the superior colliculus are organized in an orderly manner prior to the segregation of retinal afferents. The method he employed involved making a small retinal lesion prior to injection of HRP into the damaged eye. This permitted the localization of a limited region in the two main retinorecipient nuclei that showed an interruption in the pattern of label (corresponding to the damaged area of the retina). While this approach was suitable for demonstrating that the topography of the contralateral retinal projection is similar in early development to that of the adult ferret, it precluded the study of more subtle targeting errors. A substantial degree of topographic order in the early retinogeniculate projection is also suggested by the recent observations of Sretavan and Shatz (1987). Following labeling of optic tract axons in the fetal cat using an *in vitro* preparation, these investigators observed clear gradients in axon arbor maturation and stereotypic trajectories about 2 weeks before birth, which was interpreted as demonstrating "a fair degree of topographic order."

Perhaps the most direct approach for tackling the problem of topographic organization in developing retinal pathways is to make focal deposits of retrograde tracers into a target structure for the purpose of subsequently mapping the distribution of labeled ganglion cells within the retina. This method has been used to study the retinocollicular projection of the developing rat (O'Leary et al., 1986) and the fetal cat (Ostrach et al., 1986). O'Leary et al. (1986) made focal deposits of the fluorescent tracer fast blue into the caudal portion of the superior colliculus, which revealed a substantial degree of topographic error during the early development of the rat's contralateral retinocollicular pathway. These investigators also showed that topographic errors are normally eliminated by ganglion cell death. In contrast, experiments in our laboratory (Ostrach et al., 1986) have shown that in the fetal cat there is a remarkable degree of precision in the topographic organization of the contralateral and ipsilateral retinocollicular pathways (Figure 15). At all fetal ages focal injections of a variety of retrograde tracers resulted in a well-defined and localized region in both the ipsilateral and contralateral retina that contained a high density of labeled cells. Outside of this retinal area, some retinal cells were also found to be labeled with the tracer. Presumably these represent topographic errors in the developing retinocollicular projection of the fetal cat, but the number of such "ectopic" neurons was quite small (even as early as E38), representing about 1% of the total population of ganglion cells in the fetal retina.

It is conceivable, but we think unlikely, that the difference in the precision of the retinocollicular pathway between the developing rodent and cat could be due to methodological factors. Rather, as seems to be the case with the decussation pattern, the degree of order exhibited in early retinofugal projections of rodents is less precise than that found in mammals with a more highly developed visual system. This viewpoint is also supported by other observations. In particular, it has been reported by Frost (1984) that early retinal projections in the hamster transiently innervate thalamic regions beyond the lateral geniculate (the ventrobasal complex and the medial geniculate) and beyond the superior colliculus (the inferior colliculus and the midbrain tegmentum). In contrast, such aberrant retinal inputs are not observed in the fetal cat (Williams and Chalupa, 1982; Shatz, 1983), nor in the fetal monkey (Rakic, 1977b). Additionally, early monocular enucleation, which "maintains" the widespread retinal projection of the remaining eye, results in gross topographic disorders in the retinal projections of the re-

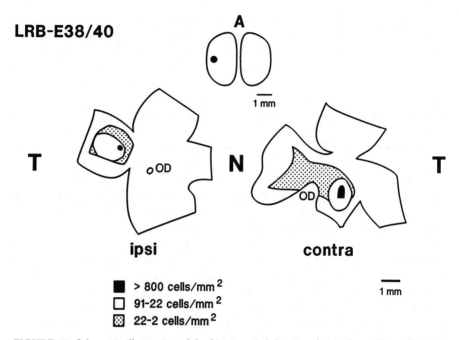

FIGURE 15. Schematic illustration of the location and density of retinal ganglion cells retrogradely labeled by unilateral injection of latex rhodamine beads (LRB) into a small region of fetal cat superior colliculus. Both ipsilateral and contralateral to the injection, labeled cells are restricted to topographically appropriate regions, indicating a high degree of precision in retinal projections as early as E38/40. A, anterior; T, temporal; N, nasal.

maining eye in rodents (e.g., Finlay et al., 1979; Thompson, 1979; Rhoades and Chalupa, 1980), while a normal retinotopic organization is evident in central targets innervated by the remaining eye of prenatally enucleated cats (Chalupa and Williams, 1984a; White et al., 1989).

The apparent species differences indicated in the foregoing should not detract from the main overall conclusions regarding the precision of early retinal projections. In all mammalian species studied to date, the overall pattern of early retinal inputs resembles that found at maturity. Additionally, some degree of error is normally present in the early projection patterns, both in terms of retinal decussations as well as topography. These incorrect connections are eliminated during the course of normal development. Most probably this is largely due to the death of retinal ganglion cells.

E   Interruption of Early Binocular Interactions

It has been known for over a decade that early monocular enucleation results at maturity in a more widespread than normal projection from the remaining eye (Chow et al., 1973; Lund and Lund, 1976). Initially, it was commonly assumed that this reflected an expansion of retinal projections due to the sprouting of retinal ganglion cell afferents. However, following the introduction of anterograde tracing methods for the study of the normal organization of developing retinofugal projections (Rakic, 1977b, 1981; Land and Lund, 1979), it became apparent that the effects of monocular enucleation are largely due to the maintenance of the widespread retinal projection present at the time of the enucleation. In animals such as cat and monkey whose visual cortex is normally organized in ocular dominance columns, this manipulation also prevents the formation of cortical ocular domains (Rakic, 1981; Shook and Chalupa, 1986). As a consequence, these monocular enucleation experiments suggest that prenatal binocular competition is involved in the restriction of the initially intermingled retinal projections. The evidence for this viewpoint has been recently summarized by Rakic (1986).

In recent years, considerable information has accumulated regarding the anatomical and functional consequence of interrupting *in utero* binocular interactions. In the studies to be discussed next, monocular enucleations were performed early in development when projections from the two eyes are largely intermingled. At maturity the remaining retina of these pre-natally enucleated animals projects to the entire ipsilateral and contralateral lateral geniculate nucleus and then via the geniculate in a continuous fashion to layer IV of the visual cortex (area 17 of the monkey and areas 17 and 18 of the cat). In the cat, prenatal enucleation also results in a sparse aberrant projection from the A laminae of the dorsal lateral geniculate nucleus to area 19 of the visual cortex (Shook and Chalupa, 1986).

Additionally, interruption of early binocular interactions results in a greater than normal population of ganglion cells in the remaining retina (Rakic and Riley, 1983b; Williams et al., 1983; Chalupa et al., 1984). This is due to a decrease in the severity of ganglion cell death. However, the size of the remaining retina does not change appreciably so that the density of ganglion cells is increased compared to normal. As a consequence of the greater density of ganglion cells, the dendritic fields of at least one class of retinal cells, the alpha type, is reduced in size (see Figure 16). This is thought to reflect a greater degree of competitive dendritic interactions in the remaining "crowded" retina (Kirby and Chalupa, 1986).

In view of these pronounced anatomical differences between the normal visual system and that of animals in which binocular interactions are interrupted prenatally, it is of obvious interest to determine the functional consequences of this manipulation. In prenatally enucleated cats, it has been found that the retinotopic organization of the dorsal lateral geniculate (Chalupa and Williams, 1984a) and of cortical area 17 (Shook et al., 1985) appear normal (Figure 17). Furthermore, tangential penetrations through the cortex show that orientation columns develop in the absence of ocular dominance columns. In the cortex of the prenatal enucleates, small recep-

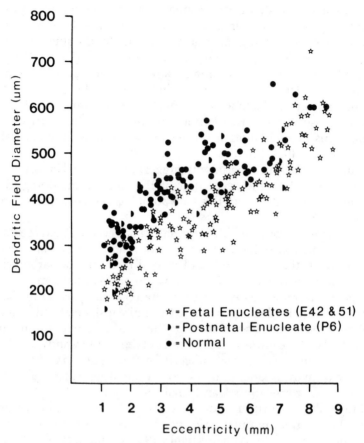

FIGURE 16. Retinal ganglion cell dendritic spread as a function of distance from the area centralis. In normal and both prenatally and postnatally enucleated adult cats dendritic field size of alpha cells increases with eccentricity. However, in prenatally enucleated, but not postnatally enucleated, animals, dendritic field diameter is lower than normal except at far peripheral locations. (From Kirby and Chalupa, 1986.)

tive fields are significantly more numerous than in the normal animal (Shook et al., 1985). It has been hypothesized that this could result from the smaller dimensions of dendritic fields in the remaining retina. However, recent studies in our laboratory (White et al., 1987) suggest a different interpretation. In a quantitative analysis of receptive fields within the dorsal lateral geniculate of adult cats monocularly enucleated *in utero*, White et al. (1987, 1989) have found that there is a change in the proportion of Y and X geniculate neurons: the number of Y-cells is significantly lower than normal and the number of X-cells is higher. Assuming that the relative density of Y and X projections to the cortex changes in a corresponding manner, this would provide the visual cortex with a greater than normal X-type

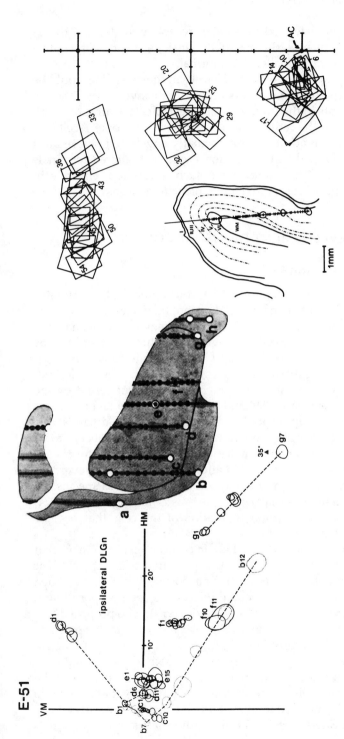

FIGURE 17. Normal topographic organization of receptive fields in the visual centers of adult cats that were monocularly enucleated during gestation. Above left, electrode penetrations through the geniculate of an adult cat enucleated on E51. The loci of recorded cells are indicated in dark circles. White circles represent electrolytic lesions. The geniculate was ipsilateral to the remaining eye. At far left are the locations of receptive fields of cells recorded in the dorsal lateral geniculate nucleus, from the most medial penetration (b) to the most lateral penetration (g). Penetration (a) was in the medial interlaminar nucleus; penetration (h) in the ventral lateral geniculate nucleus. VM, vertical meridian; HM, horizontal meridian. At right, a reconstruction of an electrode penetration through area 17 of an adult cat that was enucleated on E49. Recorded cells are indicated by lines and electrolytic lesions by circles. WM, white matter. At far right, orderly topography of receptive fields. The numbers indicate the order in which cells were recorded. Ordinate divisions are 1°. (Top reproduced from Chalupa and Williams, 1984a; bottom from Shook et al., 1985.)

43

projection, an input characterized by smaller receptive fields than the Y-type input. Reflecting this bias, the overall dimensions of cortical receptive fields would be significantly smaller than normal.

The change in the proportion of X- and Y-cells in the geniculate could be due to alterations in the terminal arbors and/or the convergence ratios of retinogeniculate afferents in the prenatally enucleated cats. Garraghty et al. (1988) have reported that the retinogeniculate terminals of some Y-cells are much more widespread in adult cats monocularly enucleated before birth than in normal animals. If the synaptic density of such altered terminals were lower than normal, this could make such inputs less effective in activating a given subpopulation of lateral geniculate neurons.

VII   PRENATAL DEVELOPMENT OF VISUAL CORTEX

A   Cytogenesis of Cortical Cells

Cortical cells undergo mitosis in a proliferative zone lining the lateral ventricles. When these cells complete their final division, they migrate away from the germinal zone to form the cortical plate, the region that at maturity becomes the neocortex. Of the cells surviving to maturity, the first to be born are destined for the deepest cortical layers, while those born last become situated in the most superficial layers of the cortex. This inside-first, outside-last sequence of cortical development was first suggested by the irradiation study of Hicks et al. (1959) and was subsequently demonstrated clearly with the autoradiographic method by Angevine and Sidman (1961). These findings on the developing rodent neocortex have since been documented in a number of other mammalian species, including the rhesus monkey (Rakic, 1974) and the cat (Luskin and Shatz, 1985a). However, the steepness of this neurogenetic gradient appears to vary across species. Of the species studied to date, it is sharpest in the rhesus monkey (Rakic, 1974) where there is substantial temporal separation of the cells that become distributed in different layers of the cortex.

The presence of the "inside-out" gradient in cortical cell birth means that later born cells must migrate through earlier generated cells to reach their final destination within the layers of the neocortex. What guides such neuronal migration is unknown. Several models have been proposed, and perhaps the most interesting idea is that of Rakic (1974), who proposed that radial glia, a transient class of neuroglial cells, play a key role in this process.

In animals with relatively prolonged gestation periods, such as the cat and monkey, the use of the tritiated thymidine method has permitted a reasonably precise analysis of the temporal sequence of neurogenesis in the visual cortex. In the cat, cells in the primary visual cortex that survive to maturity are almost all generated in the latter half of gestation, between E31 and E57 (Luskin and Shatz, 1985a). While in the rhesus monkey, with a

165-day gestation period, these neurons are born between E45 and E102 (Rakic, 1974). Although the overall period of cortical neurogenesis is longer in monkey than in cat, in both species it takes about 1 week to produce the cells of each cortical layer.

B Ingrowth of Afferents and Synaptogenesis

An issue of considerable importance is how the ingrowth of afferents to the visual cortex relates to the period of cell generation and migration. The available evidence indicates that projections from the lateral geniculate nucleus reach the vicinity of the cortical plate while many neurons are still being born and others are in the process of migrating to their final destination (Rakic, 1974, 1975, 1976). However, these afferents do not invade the cortical plate immediately; rather they wait for several weeks in the underlying cortical subplate and the overlying marginal zone (Rakic, 1977b). (In this regard, geniculocortical afferents differ from retinal afferents since there is no indication of such a delay by ganglion cell axons in their innervation of retinorecipient nuclei.) It has been suggested that during this waiting period, the ascending projections to the developing cortex make synaptic contacts with cells distributed within the marginal and subplate zones (Marin-Padilla, 1978; Kostovic and Rakic, 1980; Bourgeois and Rakic, 1983).

Recently, Shatz and her colleagues (Luskin and Shatz, 1985b; Chun et al., 1987) have documented two key observations concerning the properties of these cells in the fetal cat. First, almost all are generated in a 6-day period (E24–E30) before the birth of neocortical neurons (Luskin and Shatz, 1985b). Second, Chun et al. (1987) identified these cells as neurons by examining their ultrastructural appearance and showed further that these neurons comprise several subpopulations on the basis of their immunoreactivity for different neuropeptides. These findings confirm and extend the observations of Kostovic and Rakic (1980) on the origin of interstitial neurons in the fetal cortex of the primate.

As gestation proceeds, virtually all the neurons in the marginal and subplate zones disappear. Their disappearance coincides with the invasion of the cortical plate by the visual afferents. In cat the geniculocortical afferents innervate layer 4 shortly before birth (Luskin and Shatz, 1984), and synaptogenesis in the cat visual cortex takes place largely after birth (Cragg, 1975). In the rhesus monkey geniculocortical afferents invade the visual cortex by E124, more than a month before birth (Rakic, 1976), and by birth synaptic density is similar to that of the adult animal (Rakic et al., 1986). Interestingly, Rakic et al. (1986) have recently shown that synapses develop at virtually identical rates in all the layers of the visual cortex. As noted by these investigators, this observation was unexpected given the pronounced inside-out pattern of cortical neurogenesis evident in this species.

Cortical synaptogenesis continues postnatally, and as is the case in the lateral geniculate nucleus and the superior colliculus, there is a substantially higher density of synapses in the neonatal than in the mature visual cortex (Cragg, 1975; Rakic et al., 1986). The decrease in synaptic density that follows is due to the elimination of synapses rather than to dilution stemming from an increase in cortical volume. In addition to synapse elimination, cell loss due to neuronal death also takes place within the developing visual cortex as well as in other areas of the cortex (Finlay and Slattery, 1983). However, it is still a matter largely of conjecture as to what factors control the viability of cortical synapses as well as cell survival.

VIII   CONCLUSIONS

On the basis of the information that has accumulated over the past decade or so, several broad generalizations can be made regarding our current understanding of the events that occur during prenatal development of the mammalian visual system. We will conclude this chapter by delineating what we consider to be some of the more salient points. Our intent here is not simply to summarize the information already presented in this chapter. Rather, we wish to provide our impressions and interpretations, which, while admittedly biased by experience of our research program, should still provide a fair account of this subarea within developmental neurobiology.

First, while the initial studies in this field typically emphasized the degree to which early connections of the mammalian visual system are more widespread than those found at maturity, it is now clear that several fundamental features of prenatal visual pathways are in fact remarkably precise in their organization. When the pioneer retinal ganglion cell axons first innervate their target nuclei, with few exceptions these fibers terminate in the appropriate regions of the fetal brain, that is, in the retinorecipient nuclei. Furthermore, the overall decussation pattern and the topography of these early projections are, at least at a gross level, fundamentally similar to what is present at maturity. Unquestionably, elimination of inappropriate projections does occur during early development of the mammalian visual system. We wish to stress, however, that in all mammals studied to date, and particularly in species such as cat and monkey, which are highly dependent on vision, such projection errors in toto represent only a small fraction of the entire population of projection neurons in any given pathway. From this perspective, we believe that many of the papers dealing with the formation of early connections in the mammalian birth (including some from this laboratory) have been overly profuse in emphasizing the exuberant nature of early connections in the developing visual system.

Related to the foregoing is the second point that deserves emphasis: the regressive events that have been documented during the formation of the visual system may not be entirely relevant to the establishment of mature projection patterns. A notable example is the seemingly ubiquitous phenomenon of cell death. It is astounding that five of six ganglion cells generated during the fetal development of the cat's retina fail to survive to maturity. Yet such massive loss of cells may have little to do with refinement of early retinofugal projection patterns. Undoubtedly, some ganglion cell loss results from early binocular interactions or competition at the retinorecipient nuclei, while some reflects correction of inappropriate decussation patterns and topographic errors as well as the elimination of transient retinoretinal projections. But again, in our judgment, the available evidence clearly indicates that the vast majority of ganglion cell loss does not represent developmental refinements of early projections. Retinal events such as the establishment of regional gradients in ganglion cell density across the retina also appear to account for only a minimal degree of ganglion cell death. To explain the massive loss of ganglion cells that normally occurs during the development of the mammalian retina, it has been proposed that both interactions among ganglion cells as well as events occurring at the target nuclei must be taken into account (Kirby and Chalupa, 1986). A model of this proposal has been recently formulated (Chalupa, 1988).

The third point we wish to emphasize also deals with our current knowledge regarding the regressive events that take place during early development. In general, three types of phenomena have been shown to occur during the formation of the mammalian visual system. As depicted diagrammatically in Figure 18, these are restructuring of terminal arbors, the elimination of supernumerary axonal branches, and cell death. In the recent past it has not been uncommon to assume that one of these factors was principally, if not solely, responsible for restructuring the developmental pattern of projections at a given level of the visual system. For instance, cell death and the concomitant elimination of optic axons was initially implicated in the segregation of early retinal projections (Rakic and Riley, 1983b; Williams et al., 1983; Chalupa et al., 1984). As we noted in this chapter, the available evidence now indicates that restructuring of immature axon terminals (Sretavan and Shatz, 1986b) as well as the elimination of ganglion cells both play a role in the formation of ocular domains within the cat's dorsal lateral geniculate nucleus. We believe that this is also likely to be the case at other levels of the mammalian visual system. For instance, while retraction of supernumerary axon collaterals has been shown to be involved in the establishment of connections among heterotopic and homotopic cortical visual areas (Clarke and Innocenti, 1986), none of the available evidence eliminates the involvement of other factors (i.e., cell death and restructuring of terminal arbors) in this developmental process. Indeed, the recent observations of Price and Blakemore (1985) indicate that in the neonatal cat both axonal retraction and cell death are involved in the elimination of a transient projection between area 17 and area 18. We are not suggesting that all connections within the developing visual system arise as a consequence of the equal involvement of multiple factors. Rather, we think that some revision is warranted of the seemingly prevalent attitude that restructuring of projections at a particular level of the visual system is due, for the most part, to a sole developmental factor.

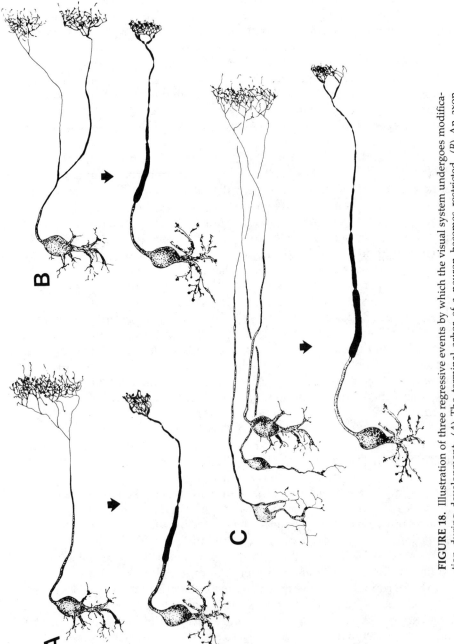

FIGURE 18. Illustration of three regressive events by which the visual system undergoes modification during development. (*A*) The terminal arbor of a neuron becomes restricted. (*B*) An axon collateral is lost. (*C*) Neurons die and their axons atrophy. (From Chalupa and Williams, 1985.)

As yet little is known about the mechanisms underlying the developmental events we have considered. Trophic factors, competitive interactions, and activity-dependent stabilization of synapses are among the "mechanisms" currently in vogue that could soon yield greater insight into the causes of the dramatic changes that have been described during the early development of the visual system. Studies such as those of Meyer on the retinotectal system of the goldfish (1982) as well as those from the laboratories of Dubin (e.g., Dubin et al., 1986) and Stryker (e.g., Stryker and Harris, 1986) on the visual system of the neonatal cat clearly attest to the wealth of information that can be garnered when an appropriate tool (in this case tetrodotoxin) is utilized to examine specific developmental problems from a mechanistic perspective. A promising start on this problem has been achieved in the prenatal cat (Shatz and Stryker, 1988), and there is every reason to believe that future studies will provide further documentation of the functional status of fetal neurons in the mammalian visual system (cf. Fitzgerald, 1987).

We hope we have succeeded in conveying some of the exciting and dramatic progress that has been attained in our understanding of the prenatal development of the mammalian visual system. Such progress has been achieved in a reasonably short period, a little over a decade, and by the efforts of relatively few laboratories. Barring a catastrophic change in research resources, we believe that the next decade will surpass the achievements of the past. We base this optimism on the vast expansion in the arsenal of tools that has become available to cellular neurobiologists. Even more important is the increase in the number of highly competent young investigators, from a variety of disciplines, who have become interested in the prenatal development of the mammalian visual system.

ACKNOWLEDGMENTS

The research from our laboratory has been supported by grants EY03991 from the National Eye Institute of the National Institutes of Health and INT-83220440 from the National Science Foundation. C. A. White is a predoctoral trainee in cellular neurobiology supported by grant NINCDS T32 NS07300 from NIH.

We wish to thank the following colleagues in our laboratory for work contributing to this chapter: Michael A. Kirby, Barry Lia, Louis H. Ostrach, Brenda L. Shook, and Robert W. Williams. We would also like to thank Cara Snider for preparing the illustrations.

REFERENCES

Aebersold, H., O. D. Creutzfeldt, U. Kuhnt, and D. Sanides (1981) Representation of the visual field in the optic tract and optic chiasma of the cat. Exp. Brain Res. 42:127–145.

Angevine, J. B., Jr. (1970) Time of neuron origin in the diencephalon of the mouse. An autoradiographic study. J. Comp. Neurol. 139:129–188.

Angevine, J. B., Jr., and R. L. Sidman (1961) Autoradiographic study of cell migration during histogenesis of cerebral cortex in the mouse. Nature 192:766–768.

Angevine, J. B., Jr., D. Bodian, A. J. Coulombre, M. V. Edds, Jr., V. Hamburger, M. Jacobson, K. M. Lyser, M. C. Prestige, R. L. Sidman, S. Varon, and P. A. Weiss (1970) Embryonic vertebrate central nervous system: Revised terminology. Anat. Rec. 166:257–262.

Anker, R. L. (1977) The prenatal development of some of the visual pathways in the cat. J. Comp. Neurol. 173:185–204.

Ault, S. J., J. D. Schall, and A. G. Leventhal (1985) Experimental alteration of cat retinal ganglion cell dendritic field structure. Soc. Neurosci. Abstr. 11:15.

Blakemore, C., and F. Vital-Durand (1986) Organization and post-natal development of the monkey's lateral geniculate nucleus. J. Physiol. 380:453–491.

Bonds, A. B., and R. D. Freeman (1978) Development of optical quality in the kitten eye. Vision Res. 18:391–398.

Bourgeois, J. P. and P. Rakic (1983) Synaptogenesis in the primary visual cortex: Quantitative analysis in pre- and postnatal rhesus monkeys. Soc. Neurosci. Abstr. 9:692.

Boycott, B. B., and H. Wässle (1974) The morphological types of ganglion cells of the domestic cat's retina. J. Physiol. 240:397–419.

Bruckner, G., V. Mareš, and D. Biesold (1976) Neurogenesis in the visual system of the rat. An autoradiographic investigation. J. Comp. Neurol. 166:245–256.

Bunge, M. B. (1973) Fine structure of nerve fibers and growth cones of isolated sympathetic neurons in culture. J. Cell Biol. 56:713–735.

Bunt, S. M., and R. D. Lund (1981) Development of a transient retino-retinal pathway in hooded and albino rats. Brain Res. 211:399–404.

Bunt, S. M., R. D. Lund, and P. W. Land (1983) Prenatal development of the optic projection in albino and hooded rats. Dev. Brain Res. 6:149–168.

Campbell, G., K.-F. So, and A. R. Lieberman (1984) Normal postnatal development of retinogeniculate axons and terminals and identification of inappropriately located transient synapses: Electron microscope studies of horseradish peroxidase-labelled retinal axons in the hamster. Neuroscience 13:743–759.

Casagrande, V. A., and J. K. Brunso-Bechtold (1985) Development of lamination in the lateral geniculate nucleus: Critical factors. In R. N. Aslin (ed.): Advances in Neural and Behavioral Development, Vol. 1. Norwood, NJ: Ablex Publishing, pp. 33–78.

Cavalcante, L. A., and C. E. Rocha-Miranda (1978) Postnatal development of retinogeniculate, retinopretectal and retinotectal projections in the opossum. Brain Res. 146:231–248.

Chalupa, L. M. (1984) Visual physiology of the mammalian superior colliculus. In H. Vanegas (ed.): Comparative Neurology of the Optic Tectum New York: Plenum Publishing, pp. 775–818.

Chalupa, L. M. (1988) Factors underlying the loss of ganglion cells in the developing mammalian retina. In S. R. Hilfer and J. B. Sheffield (eds.): Cell and Developmental Biology of the Eye. New York: Springer-Verlag.

Chalupa, L. M., and R. W. Williams (1984a) Organization of the cat's lateral geniculate nucleus following interruption of prenatal binocular competition. Human Neurobiol. 3:103–107.

Chalupa, L. M., and R. W. Williams (1984b) Prenatal development and reorganization in the visual system of the cat. In J. Stone, B. Dreher, and D. H. Rapaport (eds.): Development of the Visual Pathways in Mammals. New York: Alan R. Liss, pp. 89–102.

Chalupa, L. M., and R. W. Williams (1985) Formation of retinal projections in the cat. In R. W. Aslin (ed.): Advances in Neuronal and Behavioral Development, Vol. 1. Norwood, NJ: Ablex Publishing Corp., pp. 1–32.

Chalupa, L. M., R. W. Williams, and Z. Henderson (1984) Binocular interaction in the fetal cat regulates the size of the ganglion cell population. Neuroscience 12:1139–1146.

Chow, K. L., L. H. Mathers, and P. D. Spear (1973) Spreading of uncrossed retinal projection in superior colliculus of neonatally enucleated rabbits. J. Comp. Neurol. 151:307–321.

Chun, J. J. M., M. J. Nakamura, and C. J. Shatz (1987) Transient cells of the developing mammalian telencephalon are peptide-immunoreactive neurons. Nature 325:617–620.

Clarke, S., and G. M. Innocenti (1986) Organization of immature intrahemispheric connections. J. Comp. Neurol. 251:1–22.

Cooper, M. L., and P. Rakic (1981) Neurogenetic gradients in the superior and inferior colliculi of the rhesus monkey. J. Comp. Neurol. 202:309–334.

Cooper, M. L., and P. Rakic (1983) Gradients of cellular maturation and synaptogenesis in the superior colliculus of the fetal rhesus monkey. J. Comp. Neurol. 215:165–186.

Cragg, B. G. (1975) The development of synapses in the visual system of the cat. J. Comp. Neurol. 160:147–166.

Crespo, D., D. D. M. O'Leary, and W. M. Cowan (1985) Changes in the numbers of optic nerve fibers during late prenatal and postnatal development in the albino rat. Dev. Brain Res. 19:129–134.

Cunningham, T. J., I. M. Mohler, and D. L. Giordano (1982) Naturally occurring neuron death in the ganglion cell layer of the neonatal rat: Morphology and evidence for regional correspondence with neuron death in superior colliculus. Dev. Brain Res. 2:203–215.

Cusick, C. G., and J. H. Kaas (1982) Retinal projections in adult and newborn grey squirrels. Dev. Brain Res. 4:275–284.

Dacey, D. M. (1985) Wide-spreading terminal axons in the inner plexiform layer of the cat's retina: Evidence for intrinsic axon collaterals of ganglion cells. J. Comp. Neurol. 242:247–262.

Daniels, J. D., J. D. Pettigrew, and J. L. Norman (1978) Development of single-neuron responses in kitten's lateral geniculate nucleus. J. Neurophysiol. 41:1373–1393.

Donovan, A. (1966) The postnatal development of the cat retina. Exp. Eye Res. 5:249–254.

Dowling, J. E. (1970) Organization of vertebrate retinas. Invest. Ophthalmol. 9:655–680.

Dowling, J. E., and B. B. Boycott (1966) Organization of the primate retina: Electron microscopy. Proc. Roy. Soc. Lond. B. 166:80–111.

Dreher, B., R. A. Potts, and M. R. Bennett (1983) Evidence that the early postnatal reduction in the number of rat retinal ganglion cells is due to a wave of ganglion cell death. Neurosci. Lett. 36:255–260.

Dreher, B., R. A. Potts, S. Y. K. Ni, and M. R. Bennett (1984) The development of heterogeneities in distribution and soma sizes of rat retinal ganglion cells. In J. Stone, B. Dreher, and D. H. Rapaport (eds.): Development of Visual Pathways in Mammals. New York: Alan R. Liss, pp. 39–57.

Dubin, M. W., L. A. Stark, and S. M. Archer (1986) A role for action-potential activity in the development of neuronal connections in the kitten retinogeniculate pathway. J. Neurosci. 6:1021–1036.

Eysel, U. T., L. Piechl, and H. Wässle (1985) Dendritic plasticity in the early postnatal feline retina: Quantitative characteristics and sensitive period. J. Comp. Neurol. 242:134–145.

Finlay, B. L., and M. Slattery (1983) Local differences in the amount of early cell death in neocortex predict adult local specializations. Science 219:1349–1351.

Finlay, B. L., K. G. Wilson, and G. E. Schneider (1979) Anomalous ipsilateral retinotectal projections in Syrian hamsters with early lesions: Topography and functional capacity. J. Comp. Neurol. 183:721–740.

Fitzgerald, M. (1987) Spontaneous and evoked activity of fetal primary afferents in vivo. Nature 326:603–605.

Frost, D. O. (1984) Axonal growth and target selection during development: Retinal projections to the ventrobasal complex and other "nonvisual" structures in neonatal Syrian hamsters. J. Comp. Neurol. 230:576–592.

Frost, D. O., K.-F. So, and G. E. Schneider (1979) Postnatal development of retinal projections in Syrian hamsters: A study using autoradiographic and anterograde degeneration techniques. Neuroscience 4:1649–1677.

Fukuda, Y., and J. Stone (1974) Reginal distribution and central projections of Y-, X- and W-cells of the cat's retina. J. Neurophysiol. 37:749–772.

Garey, L. J., and K. D. Saini (1981) Golgi studies of the normal development of neurons in the lateral geniculate nucleus of the monkey. Exp. Brain Res. 44:117–128.

Garraghty, P. E., C. J. Shatz, D. W. Sretavan, and M. Sur (1988) Axon arbors of X and Y retinal ganglion cells are differentially affected by prenatal disruption of binocular inputs. Proc. Natl. Acad. Sci. USA 85:7361–7365.

Graybiel, A. M. (1975) Anatomical organization of retinotectal afferents in the cat: An autoradiographic study. Brain Res. 96:1–23.

Graybiel, A. M. (1976) Evidence for banding of the cat's ipsilateral retinotectal connection. Brain Res. 114:318–327.

Greiner, J. V., and T. A. Weidman (1980) Histogenesis of the cat retina. Exp. Eye Res. 30:439–453.

Guillery, R. W., E. H. Polley, and F. Torrealba (1982) The arrangement of axons according to fiber diameter in the optic tract of the cat. J. Neurosci. 2:714–721.

Harting, J. K., and R. W. Guillery (1976) Organization of retinocollicular pathways in the cat. J. Comp. Neurol. *166*:133–144.

Hendrickson, A., and C. Kupfer (1976) The histogenesis of the fovea in the macaque monkey. Invest. Ophthalmol. *15*:746–756.

Hendrickson, A., and P. Rakic (1977) Histogenesis and synaptogenesis in the dorsal lateral geniculate nucleus (LGd) of the fetal monkey brain. Anat. Rec. *187*:602.

Hickey, T. L., and N. R. Cox (1979) Cell birth in the dorsal lateral geniculate nucleus of the cat: A H^3-thymidine study. Soc. Neurosci. Abstr. *5*:788.

Hickey, T. L., and P. F. Hitchcock (1984) Genesis of neurons in the dorsal lateral geniculate nucleus of the cat. J. Comp. Neurol. *228*:186–199.

Hicks, S. P., C. J. D'Amato, and M. J. Lowe (1959) The development of the mammalian nervous system. I. Malformation of the brain, especially the cerbral cortex, induced in rats by radiation. II. Some mechanisms of the malformations of the cortex. J. Comp. Neurol. *113*:435–469.

Hinds, J. W., and P. L. Hinds (1978) Early development of amacrine cells in the mouse retina: An electron microscope, serial section analysis. J. Comp. Neurol. *179*:277–300.

Hinds, J. W., and P. L. Hinds (1983) Development of retinal amacrine cells in the mouse embryo: Evidence for two modes of formation. J. Comp. Neurol. *213*: 1–23.

Hitchcock, P. F., T. L. Hickey, and C. G. Dunkel (1984) Genesis of morphologically identified neurons in the dorsal lateral geniculate nucleus of the cat. J. Comp. Neurol. *228*:200–209.

Holstein, G. R., T. Pasik, P. Pasik, and J. Hámori (1985) Early postnatal development of the monkey visual system. II. Elimination of retinogeniculate synapses. Dev. Brain Res. *20*:15–31.

Horton, J. C., M. M. Greenwood, and D. H. Hubel (1979) Nonretinotopic arrangement of fibres in cat optic nerve. Nature *282*:720–722.

Hubel, D. H., and T. N. Wiesel (1972) Laminar and columnar distribution of geniculo-cortical fibers in the macaque monkey. J. Comp. Neurol. *146*:421–450.

Hughes, W. F., and S. C. McLoon (1979) Ganglion cell death during normal retinal development in the chick: Comparisons with cell death induced by early target field destruction. Exp. Neurol. *66*:587–601.

Illing, R.-B., and H. Wässle (1981) The retinal projection to the thalamus in the cat: A quantitative investigation and a comparison with the retinotectal pathway. J. Comp. Neurol. *202*:265–285.

Insausti, R., C. Blakemore, and W. M. Cowan (1984) Ganglion cell death during development of ipsilateral retinocollicular projection in golden hamster. Nature *308*:362–365.

Itoh, K., M. Conley, and I. T. Diamond (1981) Different distributions of large and small retinal ganglion cells in the cat after HRP injections of single layers of the lateral geniculate body and the superior colliculus. Brain Res. *207*:147–152.

Jacobs, D. S., V. H. Perry, and M. J. Hawken (1984) The postnatal reduction of the uncrossed projection from the nasal retina in the cat. J. Neurosci. *4*:2425–2433.

Jeffery, G. (1984) Retinal ganglion cell death and terminal field retraction in the developing rodent visual system. Dev. Brain Res. *13*:81–96.

Jeffery, G. (1985) Retinotopic order appears before ocular separation in developing visual pathways. Nature 313:575–576.

Jeffery, G., and V. H. Perry (1982) Evidence for ganglion cell death during development of the ipsilateral retinal projection in the rat. Dev. Brain Res. 2:176–180.

Jeffery, G., B. J. Arzymanow, and A. R. Lieberman (1984) Does the early exuberant retinal projection to the superior colliculus in the neonatal rat develop synaptic connections? Dev. Brain Res. 14:135–138.

Kalil, R. (1978) Development of the dorsal lateral geniculate nucleus in the cat. J. Comp. Neurol. 182:265–292.

Kirby, M. A., and L. M. Chalupa (1985) Retinal crowding reduces the size of dendritic fields of alpha ganglion cells. Soc. Neurosci. Abstr. 11:222.

Kirby, M. A., and L. M. Chalupa (1986) Retinal crowding alters the morphology of alpha ganglion cells. J. Comp. Neurol. 251:532–541.

Kirby, M. A., and P. D. Wilson (1984) Axon count in the developing optic nerve of the North American opossum: Overproduction and elimination. Soc. Neurosci. Abstr. 10:467.

Kirby, M. A., B. Lia, and L. M. Chalupa (1988) Retino-retinal projections in the fetal cat. Invest. Ophthalmol. Vis. Sci. Supp. 29:206.

Kliot, M., and C. J. Shatz (1982) Genesis of different retinal ganglion cell types in the cat. Soc. Neurosci. Abstr. 8:815.

Kolb, H., R. Nelson, and A. Mariani (1981) Amacrine cells, bipolar cells and ganglion cells of the cat retina: A Golgi study. Vision Res. 21:1081–1114.

Kostovic, I., and P. Rakic (1980) Cytology and time of origin of interstitial neurons in the white matter in infant and adult human and monkey telencephalon. J. Neurocytol. 9:219–242.

Lam, K., A. J. Sefton, and M. R. Bennett (1982) Loss of axons from the optic nerve of the rat during early postnatal development. Dev. Brain Res. 3:487–491.

Land, P. W., and R. D. Lund (1979) Development of the rat's uncrossed retinotectal pathway and its relation to plasticity studies. Science 205:698–700.

LaVail, M. M., D. Yasumura, and P. Rakic (1983) Cell genesis in the rhesus monkey retina. Invest. Ophthalmol. Vis. Sci. Supp. 24:7.

Leventhal, A. G., R. W. Rodieck, and B. Dreher (1981) Retinal ganglion cell classes in the Old World monkey: Morphology and central projections. Science 213:1139–1142.

Leventhal, A. G., R. W. Rodieck, and B. Dreher (1985) Central projections of cat retinal ganglion cells. J. Comp. Neurol. 237:216–226.

Lia, B., R. W. Williams, and L. M. Chalupa (1983) Early development of retinal specialization: The distribution and decussation patterns of ganglion cells in the prenatal cat demonstrated by retrograde peroxidase labeling. Soc. Neurosci. Abstr. 9:702.

Lia, B., R. W. Williams, and L. M. Chalupa (1986) Does axonal branching contribute to the overproduction of optic nerve fibers during early development of the cat's visual system? Dev. Brain Res. 25:296–301.

Lia, B., M. A. Kirby, and L. M. Chalupa (1987a) Decussation of retinal ganglion cell projections during prenatal development of the cat. Soc. Neurosci. Abstr. 13:1690.

Lia, B., R. W. Williams, and L. M. Chalupa (1987b) Formation of retinal ganglion cell topography during prenatal development. Science 236:848–851.

Lia, B., C. J. Snider, and L. M. Chalupa (1988) The nasotemporal division of the retinal ganglion cell decussation pattern in the fetal rhesus monkey. Soc. Neurosci. Abstr. 14:458.

Linden, R., and V. H. Perry (1982) Ganglion cell death within the developing retina: A regulatory role for retinal dendrites? Neuroscience 7:2813–2827.

Linden, D. C., R. W. Guillery, and J. Cucchiaro (1981) The dorsal lateral geniculate nucleus of the normal ferret and its postnatal development. J. Comp. Neurol. 203:189–211.

Lund, R. D. (1978) Development and Plasticity of the Brain. New York: Oxford University Press.

Lund, R. D., and A. H. Bunt (1976) Prenatal development of central optic pathways in albino rats. J. Comp. Neurol. 165:247–264.

Lund, R. D., and J. S. Lund (1972) Development of synaptic patterns in the superior colliculus of the rat. Brain Res. 42:1–20.

Lund, R. D., and J. S. Lund (1976) Plasticity in the developing visual system: The effects of retinal lesions made in young rats. J. Comp. Neurol. 169:133–154.

Lund, R. D., and M. J. Mustari (1977) Development of the geniculocortical pathway in rats. J. Comp. Neurol. 173:289–306.

Luskin, M. B., and C. J. Shatz (1984) Spatio-temporal relations between the cells of layers 4 & 6 and their geniculocortical afferent input during development. Soc. Neurosci. Abstr. 10:1079.

Luskin, M. B., and C. J. Shatz (1985a) Neurogenesis of the cat's primary visual cortex. J. Comp. Neurol. 242:611–631.

Luskin, M. B., and C. J. Shatz (1985b) Studies of the earliest generated cells of the cat's visual cortex: Cogeneration of subplate and marginal zones. J. Neurosci. 5:1062–1075.

Marin-Padilla, M. (1978) Dual origin of the mammalian neocortex and evolution of the cortical plate. Anat. Embryol. 152:109–126.

Maslim, J., and J. Stone (1986) Synaptogenesis in the retina of the cat. Brain Res. 373:35–48.

Maslim, J., M. Webster, and J. Stone (1986) Stages in the structural differentiation of retinal ganglion cells. J. Comp. Neurol. 254:382–402.

Mason, C. A. (1983) Postnatal maturation of neurons in the cat's lateral geniculate nucleus. J. Comp. Neurol. 217:458–469.

Mastronarde, D. N., M. A. Thibeault, and M. W. Dubin (1984) Non-uniform postnatal growth of the cat retina. J. Comp. Neurol. 228:598–608.

Meyer, R. L. (1982) Tetrodotoxin blocks the formation of ocular dominance columns in goldfish. Science 218:589–591.

Ng, A. Y. K., and J. Stone (1982) The optic nerve of the cat: Appearance and loss of axons during normal development. Dev. Brain Res. 5:263–271.

Nishimura, Y., and P. Rakic (1983) Sequence of synaptic formation in the perifoveal region of the rhesus monkey retina: Quantitative and serial section electron microscopic analyses. Soc. Neurosci. Abstr. 9:700.

Nishimura, Y., and P. Rakic (1985) Development of the rhesus monkey retina. I. Emergence of the inner plexiform layer and its synapses. J. Comp. Neurol. *241*:420–434.

O'Leary, D. D. M., J. W. Fawcett, and W. M. Cowan (1986) Topographic targeting errors in the retinocollicular projection and their elimination by selective ganglion cell death. J. Neurosci. *6*:3692–3705.

Ostrach, L. H., M. A. Kirby, and L. M. Chalupa (1986) Topographic organization of retinocollicular projections in the fetal cat. Soc. Neurosci. Abstr. *12*:119.

Perry, V. H., and R. Linden (1982) Evidence for dendritic competition in the developing retina. Nature *297*:683–685.

Perry, V. H., Z. Henderson, and R. Linden (1983) Postnatal changes in retinal ganglion cell and optic axon populations in the pigmented rat. J. Comp. Neurol. *219*:356–368.

Polley, E. H., C. Walsh, and T. L. Hickey (1981) Neurogenesis in cat retina. A study using ^{3}H-thymidine autoradiography. Soc. Neurosci. Abstr. *7*:672.

Polley, E. H., R. P. Zimmerman, and R. L. Fortney (1985) Development of the outer plexiform layer (OPL) of the cat retina. Soc. Neurosci. Abstr. *11*:14.

Polyak, S. (1957) The Vertebrate Visual System. Chicago: University of Chicago Press.

Potts, A. M., D. Hodges, C. B. Shelman, K. J. Fritz, N. S. Levy, and Y. Mangnall (1972) Morphology of the primate optic nerve. I. Method and total fiber count. Invest. Ophthalmol. *11*:980–988.

Potts, R. A., B. Dreher, and M. R. Bennett (1982) The loss of ganglion cells in the developing retina of the rat. Dev. Brain Res. *3*:481–486.

Price, D. J., and C. Blakemore (1985) Regressive events in the postnatal development of association projections in the visual cortex. Nature *316*:721–724.

Provis, J. M., D. Van Driel, F. A. Billson, and P. Russell (1985a) Development of the human retina: Patterns of cell distribution and redistribution in the ganglion cell layer. J. Comp. Neurol. *233*:429–451.

Provis, J. M., D. Van Driel, F. A. Billson, and P. Russell (1985b) Human fetal optic nerve: Overproduction and elimination of retinal axons during development. J. Comp. Neurol. *238*:92–100.

Rager, G. H. (1980) Development of the retinotectal projection in the chicken. Adv. Anat. Embryol. Cell Biol. *63*:1–92.

Rager, G. (1983) Structural analysis of fiber organization during development. In J.-P. Changeux, J. Glowinski, M. Imbert and F. E. Bloom (eds.): Molecular and Cellular Interactions underlying Higher Brain Functions. Prog. Brain Res. *58*:313–319.

Rager, G., and U. Rager (1976) Generation and degeneration of retinal ganglion cells in the chicken. Exp. Brain Res. *25*:551–553.

Ragland, I. M., and T. L. Hickey (1982) Neurogenesis of the cat's superior colliculus: A ^{3}H-thymidine study. ARVO Abstr. *22*:245.

Rakic, P. (1974) Neurons in rhesus monkey visual cortex: Systematic relation between time of origin and eventual disposition. Science *183*:425–427.

Rakic, P. (1975) Timing of major ontogenetic events in the visual cortex of the rhesus monkey. In N. A. Buchwald and M. A. B. Brazier (eds.): Brain Mechanisms in Mental Retardation. New York: Academic Press, pp. 3–40.

Rakic, P. (1976) Prenatal genesis of connections subserving ocular dominance in the rhesus monkey. Nature 261:467–471.

Rakic, P. (1977a) Genesis of the dorsal lateral geniculate nucleus in the rhesus monkey: Site and time of origin, kinetics of proliferation, routes of migration and pattern of distribution of neurons. J. Comp. Neurol. 176:23–52.

Rakic, P. (1977b) Prenatal development of the visual system in the rhesus monkey. Phil. Trans. Roy. Soc. Lond. B. 278:245–260.

Rakic, P. (1981) Development of visual centers in the primate brain depends on binocular competition before birth. Science 214:928–931.

Rakic, P. (1986) Mechanism of ocular dominance segregation in the lateral geniculate nucleus: Competitive elimination hypothesis. TINS 9:11–15.

Rakic, P., and K. P. Riley (1983a) Overproduction and elimination of retinal axons in the fetal rhesus monkey. Science 219:1441–1444.

Rakic, P., and K. P. Riley (1983b) Regulation of axon number in primate optic nerve by prenatal binocular competition. Nature 305:135–137.

Rakic, P., J.-P. Bourgeois, M. F. Eckenhoff, N. Zecevic, and P. S. Goldman-Rakic (1986) Concurrent overproduction of synapses in diverse regions of the primate cerebral cortex. Science 232:232–235.

Ramoa, A. S., G. Campbell, and C. J. Shatz (1987) Transient morphological features of identified ganglion cells in living fetal and neonatal retina. Science 237:522–525.

Rapaport, D. H., and J. Stone (1982) The site of commencement of maturation in mammalian retina: Observations in the cat. Dev. Brain Res. 5:273–279.

Rapaport, D. H., and J. Stone (1983a) Time course of morphological differentiation of cat retinal ganglion cells: Influences on soma size. J. Comp. Neurol. 221:42–52.

Rapaport, D. H., and J. Stone (1983b) The topography of cytogenesis in the developing retina of the cat. J. Neurosci. 3:1824–1834.

Rapaport, D. H., S. R. Robinson, and J. Stone (1985) Cytogenesis in the developing retina of the cat. Austral. New Zeal. J. Ophthalmol. 13:113–124.

Reese, B. E., and R. W. Guillery (1987) Distribution of axons according to diameter in the monkey's optic tract. J. Comp. Neurol. 260:453–460.

Rhoades, R. W., and L. M. Chalupa (1980) Effects of neonatal enucleation on receptive-field properties of visual neurons in superior colliculus of the golden hamster. J. Neurophysiol. 43:595–611.

Robinson, S. R. (1987) Ontogeny of the area centralis in the cat. J. Comp. Neurol. 255:50–67.

Robinson, S. R., D. H. Rapaport, and J. Stone (1985) Cell division in the developing cat retina occurs in two zones. Dev. Brain Res. 19:101–109.

Robinson, S. R., B. Dreher, G. M. Horsburgh, and M. J. McCall (1986) Development of the ganglion cell density gradient in the rabbit retina. Soc. Neurosci. Abstr. 12:985.

Rowe, M. H., and J. Stone (1976) Properties of ganglion cells in the visual streak of the cat's retina. J. Comp. Neurol. 169:99–126.

Saito, H.-A. (1983) Morphology of physiologically identified X-, Y-, and W-type retinal ganglion cells of the cat. J. Comp. Neurol. 221:279–288.

Sefton, A. J., and K. Lam (1984) Quantitative and morphological studies on developing optic axons in normal and enucleated albino rats. Exp. Brain Res. 57:107–117.

Sengelaub, D. R., and B. L. Finlay (1982) Cell death in the mammalian visual system during normal development: I. Retinal ganglion cells. J. Comp. Neurol. 204:311–317.

Sengelaub, D. R., L. F. Jacobs, and B. L. Finlay (1985) Regional differences in normally occurring cell death in the developing hamster lateral geniculate nuclei. Neurosci. Lett. 55:103–108.

Sengelaub, D. R., R. P. Dolan, and B. L. Finlay (1986). Cell generation, death, and retinal growth in the development of the hamster retinal ganglion cell layer. J. Comp. Neurol. 246:527–543.

Shatz, C. J. (1981) Inside-out pattern of neurogenesis of the cat's lateral geniculate nucleus. Soc. Neurosci. Abstr. 7:140.

Shatz, C. J. (1983) The prenatal development of the cat's retinogeniculate pathway. J. Neurosci. 3:482–499.

Shatz, C. J., and P. A. Kirkwood (1984) Prenatal development of functional connections in the cat's retinogeniculate pathway. J. Neurosci. 4:1378–1397.

Shatz, C. J., and D. W. Sretavan (1986) Interactions between retinal ganglion cells during the development of the mammalian visual system. Ann. Rev. Neurosci. 9:171–207.

Shatz, C. J., and M. P. Stryker (1978) Ocular dominance in layer IV of the cat's visual cortex and the effects of monocular deprivation. J. Physiol. 281:267–283.

Shatz, C. J., and M. P. Stryker (1988) Prenatal tetrodotoxin infusion blocks segregation of retinogeniculate afferents. Science 242:87–89.

Shook, B. L., and L. M. Chalupa (1986) Organization of geniculocortical connections following prenatal interruption of binocular interactions. Dev. Brain Res. 28:47–62.

Shook, B. L., L. Maffei, and L. M. Chalupa (1985) Functional organization of the cat's visual cortex after prenatal interruption of binocular interactions. Proc. Natl. Acad. Sci. USA 82:3901–3905.

Sidman, R. L. (1961) Histogenesis of mouse retina studied with thymidine-H³. In G. K. Smelser (ed.): Structure of the Eye. New York. Academic Press, pp. 487–586.

Silver, J., and U. Rutishauser (1984) Guidance of optic axons in vivo by a preformed adhesive pathway on neuroepithelial endfeet. Dev. Biol. 106:485–499.

Silver, J., and J. Sapiro (1981) Axonal guidance during development of the optic nerve: The role of pigmented epithelia and other extrinsic factors. J. Comp. Neurol. 202:521–538.

Smelser, G. K., V. Ozanics, M. Rayborn, and D. Sagun (1974) Retinal synaptogenesis in the primate. Invest. Ophthalmol. 13:340–361.

So, K.-F., G. E. Schneider, and D. O. Frost (1978) Postnatal development of retinal projections to the lateral geniculate body in Syrian hamsters. Brain Res. 142:343–352.

Sretavan, D. W., and C. J. Shatz (1986a) Prenatal development of cat retinogeniculate axon arbors in the absence of binocular interactions. J. Neurosci. 6:990–1003.

Sretavan, D. W., and C. J. Shatz (1986b) Prenatal development of retinal ganglion cell axons: Segregation into eye-specific layers within the cat's lateral geniculate nucleus. J. Neurosci. 6:234–.251

Sretavan, D. W., and C. J. Shatz (1987) Axon trajectories and pattern of terminal arborization during the prenatal development of the cat's retinogeniculate pathway. J. Comp. Neurol. 255:386–400.

Stone, J., D. H. Rapaport, R. W. Williams, and L. M. Chalupa (1982) Uniformity of cell distribution in the ganglion cell layer of prenatal cat retina: Implications for mechanisms of retinal development. Dev. Brain Res. 2:231–242.

Stone, J., J. Maslim, and D. Rapaport (1984) The development of the topographical organization of the cat's retina. In J. Stone, B. Dreher, and D. H. Rapaport (eds.): Development of Visual Pathways in Mammals. New York: Alan R. Liss, pp. 3–21.

Stryker, M. P., and W. A. Harris (1986) Binocular impulse blockade prevents the formation of ocular dominance columns in cat visual cortex. J. Neurosci. 6:2117–2133.

Thompson, I. D. (1979) Changes in the uncrossed retinotectal projection after removal of the other eye at birth. Nature 279:63–66.

Torrealba, F., R. W. Guillery, U. Eysel, E. H. Polley, and C. A. Mason (1982) Studies of retinal representations within the cat's optic tract. J. Comp. Neurol. 211:377–396.

Turner, D. L., and C. L. Cepko (1987) A common progenitor for neurons and glia persists in rat retina late in development. Nature 328:131–136.

Walsh, C. (1986) Age-related fiber order in the ferret's optic nerve and optic chiasm. J. Neurosci. 6:1635–1642.

Walsh, C., and R. W. Guillery (1985) Age-related fiber order in the optic tract of the ferret. J. Neurosci. 5:3061–3069.

Walsh, C., E. H. Polley, T. L. Hickey, and R. W. Guillery (1983) Generation of cat retinal ganglion cells in relation to central pathways. Nature 302:611–614.

Wässle, H. (1982) Morphological types and central projections of ganglion cells in the cat retina. In N. Osborne and G. Chader (eds.): Progress in Retinal Research. New York: Pergamon Press, pp. 125–152.

Wässle, H., and R.-B. Illing (1980) The retinal projection to the superior colliculus in the cat: A quantitative study with HRP. J. Comp. Neurol. 190:333–356.

Wässle, H., and H. J. Riemann (1978) The mosaic of nerve cells in the mammalian retina. Proc. Roy. Soc. Lond. B. 200:441–461.

Wässle, H., B. B. Boycott, and R.-B. Illing (1981a) Morphology and mosaic of on- and off-beta cells in the cat retina and some functional considerations. Proc. Roy. Soc. Lond. B. 212:177–195.

Wässle, H., L. Peichl, and B. B. Boycott (1981b) Dendritic territories of cat retinal ganglion cells. Nature 292:344–345.

Wässle, H., L. Peichl, and B. B. Boycott (1981c) Morphology and topography of on- and off-alpha cells in the cat retina. Proc. Roy. Soc. Lond. B. 212:157–175.

Weber, A. J., R. E. Kalil, and T. L. Hickey (1986) Genesis of interneurons in the dorsal lateral geniculate nucleus of the cat. J. Comp. Neurol. 252:385–391.

White, C., L. M. Chalupa, M. A. Kirby, B. Lia, and L. Maffei (1987) Functional consequences of interrupting prenatal binocular interactions in the dorsal lateral geniculate nucleus of the cat. Soc. Neurosci. Abstr. *13*:1536.

White, C. A., L. M. Chalupa, L. Maffei, M. A. Kirby, and B. Lia (1989) Response properties in the dorsal lateral geniculate nucleus of the adult cat after interruption of prenatal binocular interactions. J. Neurophysiol. *62*:1039–1051.

Williams, R. W., and L. M. Chalupa (1982) Prenatal development of retinocollicular projections in the cat: An anterograde tracer transport study. J. Neurosci. *2*:604–622.

Williams, R. W., and L. M. Chalupa (1983a) An analysis of axon caliber within the optic nerve of the cat: Evidence of size groupings and regional organization. J. Neurosci. *3*:1554–1564.

Williams, R. W., and L. M. Chalupa (1983b) Development of the retinal pathway to the pretectum of the cat. Neuroscience *10*:1249–1267.

Williams, R. W., and P. Rakic (1984) Form, ultrastructure, and selectivity of growth cones in the developing primate optic nerve: 3-dimensional reconstructions from serial electron micrographs. Soc. Neurosci. Abstr. *10*:373.

Williams, R. W., and P. Rakic (1985a) Deployment of ganglion cell growth cones in retina, optic nerve, and optic tract of rhesus monkeys. Invest. Ophthalmol. Vis. Sci. Suppl. *26*:286.

Williams, R. W., and P. Rakic (1985b) Dispersion of growing axons within the optic nerve of the embryonic monkey. Proc. Natl. Acad. Sci. USA *82*:3906–3910.

Williams, R. W., M. J. Bastiani, and L. M. Chalupa (1983) Loss of axons in the cat optic nerve following fetal unilateral enucleation: An electron microscopic analysis. J. Neurosci. *3*:133–144.

Williams, R. W., M. J. Bastiani, B. Lia, and L. M. Chalupa (1986) Growth cones, dying axons, and developmental fluctuations in the fiber population of the cat's optic nerve. J. Comp. Neurol. *246*:32–69.

Wilson, P. D., M. H. Rowe, and J. Stone (1976) Properties of relay cells in the cat's lateral geniculate nucleus: A comparison of W-cells with X- and Y-cells. J. Neurophysiol. *39*:1193–1209.

Yamada, K. M., B. S. Spooner, and N. K. Wessells (1971) Ultrastructure and function of growth cones and axons of cultured nerve cells. J. Cell Biol. *49*:614–635.

Zimmerman, R. P., E. H. Polley, and R. L. Fortney (1985) Stages in the development of the inner plexiform layer of the cat retina. Soc. Neurosci. Abstr. *11*:14.

Chapter Two

POSTNATAL ANATOMICAL AND PHYSIOLOGICAL DEVELOPMENT OF THE VISUAL SYSTEM

MICHAEL J. FRIEDLANDER AND JOHN S. TOOTLE

Neurobiology Research Center and Department of Physiology and Biophysics
University of Alabama at Birmingham,
Birmingham, Alabama

I   INTRODUCTION

The visual system has served as a particularly useful model to study the development of the central nervous system. The retinotectal pathway of poikilothermic vertebrates has provided a focus for tests of specificity and development. Similarly, the retinotectal, retinothalamic, and thalamocortical pathways of homeothermic vertebrates have provided the basis for studying the ontogeny of neurophysiological processing and elaboration of functional circuitry in vision. Since this book is concerned with ontogeny of sensory systems in mammals and since other chapters (see Chapters 1 and 4) deal with prenatal development of structure and experiential factors, we have limited our discussion to the normal postnatal development of the mammalian visual system. Moreover, since space is limited, we have emphasized the cat visual system for which the most complete level of understanding of structural and functional development exists for pathways involving the retina, dorsal lateral geniculate (LGN_d) nucleus, superior colliculus, and visual cortex. Reference to related work in other mammals (e.g., rat, ferret, rabbit, monkey, and human) is made when applicable. Lest we give the mistaken impression that the ontogeny of the central visual pathways of the cat is fully understood, we have emphasized some of the gaps in our understanding and suggested some directions that future studies may take.

The mammalian visual system has received much attention from neurophysiologists and psychophysicists as an example of parallel processing. Considerable research suggests that the visual system not only performs sequential transformations of a signal as it moves through the neuraxis (Hubel and Weisel, 1963) but also uses functionally and anatomically separate parallel streams for simultaneously processing different aspects of a common stimulus (Stone, 1983). With attention to these two components of visual processing, we have examined ontogeny at each level of the visual pathway and discussed the identified parallel components (whenever the experimental design of the literature permits). However, it will become readily apparent to the reader that identification of the functional subclasses of neurons is more problematic in the neonate than the adult. Therein lies one of the challenges of future experiments on the developmental neurobiology of vision. The reader is referred to recent chapters for consideration of the functional and structural differences of the parallel visual pathways (W-, X-, and Y-cells) of adult mammals (Sherman and Spear, 1982; Stone, 1983).

II STRUCTURAL DEVELOPMENT OF THE EYE

During postnatal development changes occur in the structure of the mammalian eye that alter the information available for processing by the neural elements of the retina. In the cat, these changes include an increase in the overall size of the eye and an improvement in the quality of its optical media.

During the period from birth to adulthood, the axial length of the kitten eye increases by a factor of 2 from about 10 to 20 mm (Thorn et al., 1976). The growth of the eye results in a larger patch of retina viewing the same angular extent of visual space (Figure 1A). The larger retinal image makes easier the retina's task of extracting the fine spatial detail from the visual scene in the adult eye, as is illustrated in a simplified manner in Figure 1B. The same grating pattern is projected onto a kitten (left) and adult (right) retina and is sampled by a row of receptor cells of the same density in each. In order to resolve the grating, the retina must sample at twice its frequency, that is, two samples per grating period—the Nyquist frequency (Yellott, 1983). Because of the larger image, the sampling requirement is met by the adult eye, while the kitten retina with the same density of receptors fails to resolve the grating. Similar postnatal growth is observed in the eyes of other mammalian species [e.g., monkeys (Boothe, 1982; Blakemore and Vital-Durand, 1986) and humans (Larsen, 1971)].

During the first several postnatal weeks the optical quality of the kitten eye is severely compromised by the presence of a persistent pupillary membrane and a vascular network supplying the developing lens—the tunica vasculosa lentis (Thorn et al., 1976; Freeman and Lai, 1978). These translucent membranes scatter light (dashed arrows in Figure 1A) and dramatically reduce the transmission of patterned visual stimuli to the retina (Figure 1C) prior to 3 weeks of age (Bonds and Freeman, 1978) but have largely disappeared by 4 weeks postnatally as indicated by the modulation transfer functions (MTFs) of the kitten versus adult cat eye (Figure 1C). Specifically, the transmission of coarse to medium visual patterns (≤ 1 cycle per degree) is 80% or more of the adult value by the age of 4 postnatal weeks. When compared to the sensitivities of individual neurons in the visual pathways (see Figure 5), the slight decrease in transmittance at 4 or more postnatal weeks does not limit the capacity of the system for spatial visual processing. Similar opacities of the optics are observed in other species [e.g., rabbits (Rapisardi et al., 1975)]. However, the optics of lamb (Kennedy et al., 1980), human (Boettner and Walter, 1962), and monkey (Williams and Boothe, 1981) infants are much more adultlike by birth, showing only a slight improvement in optical quality postnatally.

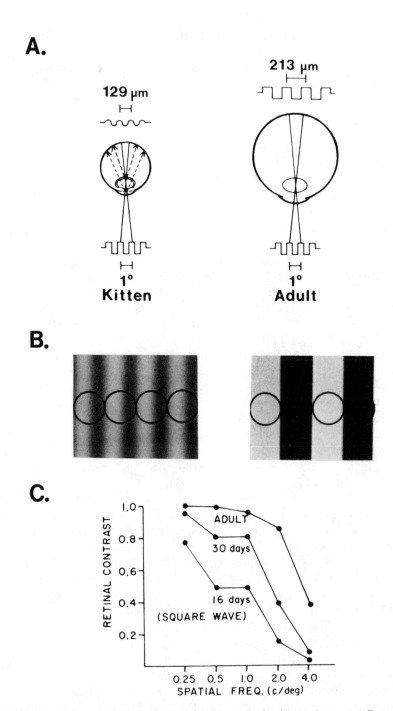

FIGURE 1. In (*A*) 2-week-old kitten and adult cat eyes are shown viewing a spatially periodic grating pattern consisting of alternating bars of high- and low-intensity light. Light rays from corresponding points on two bright bars are traced through the posterior nodal point and onto the retina of each eye. The linear distance between the two rays at the retina is about 1.5 times greater for the adult than the kitten [213 versus 129 μm (G. S. Tucker, personal commu-

The increase in contrast and size of the retinal image has important consequences for attempts to understand the development of visual function. Specifically, when one observes immaturities in the response properties of neurons in the visual pathways, for example, large receptive fields (RFs), poor contrast sensitivity, or reduced acuity, both optical and neural factors should be viewed as possible sources of the immaturities. For example, the very large receptive field center sizes reported for neonatal retinal ganglion cells (Rusoff and Dubin, 1977, 1978) may be due to both neural (increased convergence from more distal retinal neurons) and/or optical (light scatter by vascular membranes) immaturities and should not be attributed glibly to one or another source.

III   ANATOMICAL DEVELOPMENT OF THE RETINA

Visual information transmitted by the optics is transduced and encoded as patterns of electrochemical activity in the neural layers of the eye—the retina. At birth the retina of all mammalian species examined to date appears immature to inspection by both light and electron microscopy (Weidman and Kuwabara, 1969; Aguirre et al., 1972; Hendrickson and Kupfer, 1976; McArdle et al., 1977; Vogel, 1978; Hendrickson and Yuodelis, 1984). The immaturity is manifest in many features of retinal organization, including the density and distribution of retinal neurons, their laminar segregation, the density and ultrastructure of synapses, and the morphology of retinal cell types. These features determine the nature of the information that is extracted from the retinal image, and their maturation constitutes a structural basis for developmental changes in visual function. Interestingly, in nonprimate mammalian species, maturation of retinal structure proceeds

---

nication)] even though the angular subtense (1°) is the same for the two eyes. The dashed arrows indicate light rays scattered by the persistent pupillary membrane and tunica vasculosa lentis. In (B) the image of the grating pattern is projected onto the kitten (left) and adult (right) retinas, with assumption (for simplicity) that the density of receptor cells is the same in the two eyes. The spatial frequency (f) of the grating is defined as the inverse of its period (1/period). In order to resolve the grating, the retina must sample at twice its frequency ($2f$), the Nyquist frequency. Because of the larger image, the sampling requirement is met by the adult retina, while the kitten retina with the same density of receptors fails to resolve the grating. The actual situation in the retina is more complex, as the receptors (and some ganglion cells) are distributed approximately in a regular array and a two-dimensional analysis is required (Robson and Enroth-Cugell, 1978; Wassle and Riemann, 1978). (C) The optical quality of the eye is measured as a modulation transfer function (MTF) that plots the ratio of the contrast of the retinal image to the contrast of the stimulus as a function of spatial frequency. Contrast is defined as $I_{max} - I_{min}/I_{max} + I_{min}$, where I_{max} and I_{min} are, respectively, the maximum and minimum intensity of the light in the grating pattern. The MTFs show that the contrast of the retinal image of the kitten eye is reduced when compared to the adult at all spatial frequencies except the lowest tested. The magnitude of the reduction increases with increasing spatial frequency and causes the image of the square wave grating to appear blurred on the kitten retina as in (B).

in a central-to-peripheral direction, with maturation occurring first in the region near the area centralis and later near the retinal margin (Aguirre et al., 1972; Rusoff and Dubin, 1978; Rapaport and Stone, 1984). In primate species, including man, the converse appears true, that is, development of the foveal region lags behind that of the periphery (Mann, 1964; Samorajski et al., 1965; Abramov et al., 1982; Hendrickson and Yuodelis, 1984). Postnatal structural changes in the retina may also be contrasted with events occurring during prenatal development (Chapter 1).

A   Density and Distribution of Retinal Neurons

The density of retinal photoreceptors (along with patterns of convergence) sets the Nyquist frequency for the retina, and it is of interest to examine postnatal changes in density from a functional standpoint. The density of kitten receptor cells is initially higher than that of adult cats and decreases to adult values during the first 4 postnatal weeks (Tucker et al., 1979; Figure 2A). This apparently is due to changes in rod but not cone receptor density. The prenatal elimination of ganglion cells has produced adultlike densities by birth in the cat central retina (Stone et al., 1982; Figure 2A), suggesting that convergence of receptors onto ganglion cells is also initially higher for the neonate. This argument assumes, however, that the dendritic arbors of the ganglion cells (which determine in part the size of the receptor mosaic sampled) have reached their adult size. This is true for some (but not all) ganglion cell types by 2–3 weeks postnatally (Rusoff and Dubin, 1978; Dann et al., 1988). Increased receptor density and covergence might serve to "amplify" a weak signal from immature photoreceptors. No information is available for receptor densities in other developing mammalian species. The prenatal elimination of retinal ganglion cells to produce the density and distribution of the adult retina continues postnatally in several species including the cat (peripheral retina, Stone et al., 1982), hamster (Sengelaub and Finlay, 1982), and quokka (Dunlop and Beazley, 1985) but excluding monkeys and man (Rakic and Riley, 1983; Provis et al., 1985).

B   Lamination

All the nuclear and plexiform layers of the retina can be recognized at birth in some species, including rabbit and human (McArdle et al., 1977; Hendrickson and Yuodelis, 1984), but are less clear in others, for example, cat, dog, and mouse (Aguirre et al., 1972; Blanks et al., 1974; Vogel, 1978). In any case, the laminar pattern becomes more distinct during postnatal development largely as a result of the expanding neuropil as synapses are formed in the plexiform layers.

C   Synaptogenesis

Although a few synaptic contacts can be found prenatally in the cat retina (Cragg, 1975), synaptogenesis is overwhelmingly a postnatal occurrence in the cat as well as other mammalian species (Weidman and Kuwabara, 1969;

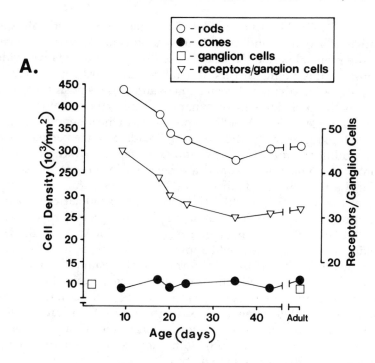

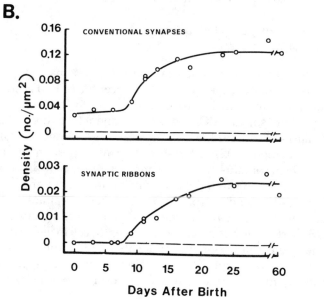

FIGURE 2. (A) Density of receptor and ganglion cells in developing kitten retina. (B) Synaptic density in the innerplexiform layer of rabbit retina. Receptor data in (A) are replotted from Tucker et al., 1979; ganglion cell data are from Stone et al., 1982; (B). (From McArdle et al., 1977.)

Blanks et al., 1974; McArdle et al., 1977; Vogel, 1978). In primate species qualitative observation indicates that synaptogenesis occurs principally during the prenatal period (Smelser et al., 1974), but quantitative evidence is lacking on this point. In cats and rabbits the most rapid increase in synapse formation occurs between about 8 and 20 days postnatally (Figure 2B). During this period the ribbon synapses made by the receptor cells in the outer plexiform layer (OPL) and by bipolar cells in the inner plexiform layer (IPL) develop, respectively, the triadic and diadic arrangement characteristic of the adult (Figure 3A). Conventional synapses, which are made by horizontal and amacrine cells and are believed to provide the structural basis for the receptive field surround (Dowling, 1970), are also maturing rapidly at this time (Figure 2B). The formation of bipolar cell ribbon synapses apparently lags behind that of the photoreceptors in several species [mouse (Olney, 1968); cat (Cragg, 1975); rabbit (McArdle et al., 1977)]. Interestingly, the converse would appear to be true regarding the development of conventional synapses. The formation of presumptive conventional synapses appears to precede those of ribbon synapses in the IPL and to follow the formation of ribbon synapses in the OPL. Synaptogenesis is substantially complete (Vogel, 1978) in the OPL of the cat by 30 days postnatally. Conventional synapse formation in the IPL was observed to end at the same time (Vogel, 1978), with ribbon synapses in the IPL requiring an additional 20 days or so to mature.

D   Morphology of Retinal Neurons

1   Receptor Cells

One of the most striking morphological features of postnatal development in the retina is the maturation of the photoreceptor cells (Figure 3A). At birth in nonprimate mammalian species, the receptor cell consists essentially of an immature somata (PC) and inner segment (Weidman and Kuwabara, 1969; Blanks et al., 1974; McArdle et al., 1977; Vogel, 1978). A primordial outer segment (OS) is present only as a portion of the inner segment (IS), which contains cytoplasm and a centriole with associated cilia and protrudes slightly through the external limiting membrane. At about 1 week postnatally the lamellae (photomembranous discs) are present but lack the characteristic orientation of the adult, that is, orthogonal to the long axis of the OS. Further development of the receptor cell includes addition of more lamellae to the outer segments and elaboration of the receptor terminal (RT) until adultlike morphology is attained at ages ranging from 2 to 9 weeks postnatally for nonprimate species. In primate species the receptor

---

FIGURE 3. (A) Development of photoreceptor morphology and vertical synaptic pathway through the rabbit retina. (B) Plot of the diameter of beta ganglion cell dendritic diameter for 3-week-old kittens and adult cats as a function of distance from the area centralis. (A) OS, outer segment. (From McArdle et al., 1977.) Inset in (B) shows drawings of example adult (left) and kitten (right) beta cells from near the area centralis. Scale bar is 50 μm. (From Rusoff and Dubin, 1978.)

A.

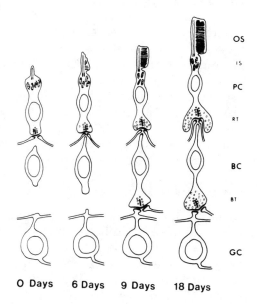

OS
IS
PC
RT

BC

BT

GC

O Days　6 Days　9 Days　18 Days

B.

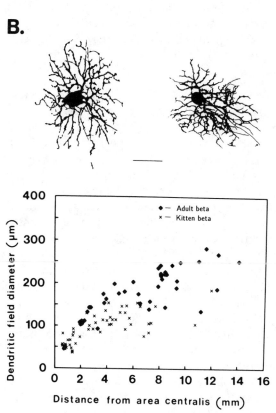

cells are present at birth and appear mature in the peripheral retina to light microscopic examination (Samorajski et al., 1965). In the foveal region, however, the cone outer segments are "stubby" and double in length by 8 weeks postnatally (Hendrickson and Kupfer, 1976). In humans, receptor maturation may not be complete until 15 months to 4 years postnatally (Hendrickson and Yuodelis, 1984). The appearance during development of ribbon synapses in both the OPL and IPL prior to formation of the outer segments has led to the suggestion that development of the photoreceptor cell is the limiting factor in the ontogenesis of visual function (Cragg, 1975).

2   Horizontal, Bipolar, and Amacrine Cells

Little is known about the morphological development of these cell types. The elaboration of horizontal cell morphology may precede that of bipolar cells. During synapse formation in the OPL, the lateral two postsynaptic elements in a triad, which consist of horizontal cell dendrites in the adult (Kolb, 1970), appear at the base of the cone cell pedicle prior to the central postsynaptic bipolar cell (BC) process (McArdle et al., 1977; Figure 3A, 0 days). Amacrine cell development may precede bipolar cell development if the late onset of ribbon synapse formation in the IPL can be taken as an index of bipolar cell morphological maturity (Dowling, 1970; McArdle et al., 1977).

3   Ganglion Cells

In the adult cat, retinal ganglion cells have been identified as belonging to several classes defined on morphological grounds. These include at least the alpha, beta, and gamma classes (Boycott and Wassle, 1974; Rodieck, 1979; Leventhal, 1982). Ganglion cells that resemble the alpha, beta, and gamma morphological types of the adult retina can be recognized by birth and appear qualitatively similar to those in the adult (Maslim et al., 1986; Dann et al., 1988). However, the neonatal ganglion cells express a number of transient, immature features including excessive axonal and dendritic branching (Ramoa et al., 1988), exuberant somatic and dendritic spines and bistratified ramifications of some alpha cell dendrites in the IPL (Dann et al., 1988). These features may represent a transient network of connectivity that could play an important role in the final determination of retinal ganglion cell function (Ramoa et al., 1988). The extent and structure of RGC dendritic arborizations is also affected by interaction with neighboring cells. However, factors intrinsic to an individual RGC such as genetic information and interaction with its own neurites is sufficient for attainment of adult morphology (Montague and Friedlander, 1989). This intrinsic growth strategy is independent of neighboring neurons, afferent input, or target tissue. The diameters of the somata and dendritic arbors of the beta cells in 2–4-week-old kittens (Figure 3B) do not differ significantly from the adult near the area centralis but are significantly smaller at greater eccentricities (Rusoff and Dubin, 1978; Dann et al., 1988; Figure 3B). This contrasts with the alpha cells whose somatic and dendritic sizes are already approaching adultlike dimensions by 15 days postnatally (Dann et al., 1988). The differential timing in the growth of the alpha and beta cell dendritic arbors indicates that the increased size of the arbors is not due to a passive stretching by the growth of the eye, but to active growth of the dendrites themselves.

IV PHYSIOLOGICAL DEVELOPMENT OF THE RETINA

A Electroretinographic Studies of the Distal Retina

Due to the formidable technical difficulty of obtaining single-neuron recordings from the photoreceptor, horizontal, bipolar, and amacrine cells in the *in vivo* mammalian retina, developmental studies have relied on recordings of the gross electrical potential evoked by homogeneous flashes of light—the electroretinogram (ERG)—to monitor development of function in these cell types. Two caveats must be kept in mind when interpreting the results of these studies. First, the origin of the different waves of the ERG remains a matter of controversy (Armington, 1974) despite recent advances (e.g. Sieving et al., 1986; Gottlob et al., 1988). However, it is probably reasonable to assume that the negative a-wave or late receptor potential (LRP) reflects the activity of the receptor cells and that the subsequent positive b-wave with its superimposed oscillatory potentials indicates the activity of both proximal and distal neurons and its effect on the retinal glial cells. Second, the ERG should be viewed as a relatively insensitive measure that will not indicate neural activity unless many neurons are responding in synchrony to a visual stimulus.

At birth no response to light can be evoked from the retinas of all non-primate species tested. These include cats, dogs, rabbits, mice, and rats (Olney, 1968; Weidman and Kuwabara, 1969; Masland, 1977; Tucker et al., 1979; Gunn et al., 1984). The first potential evoked by light is the a-wave, which appears at ages ranging from about 6 to 12 days postnatally. The appearance of the b-wave lags that of the a-wave from 1 to 7 days, depending on the species, suggesting that the photoreceptor may become functional before other neurons of the distal retina. Adultlike threshold intensities and intensity response functions for the different ERG components are attained much later during postnatal development. For example, in the cat adultlike thresholds and amplitudes for the a-wave (LRP) are not obtained until 2–3 weeks postnatally (Tucker et al., 1979). Rabbit b-wave thresholds mature at about 26–40 days postnatally (Masland, 1977), and adultlike canine ERGs are not observed until 5–8 weeks after birth (Gunn et al., 1984).

The onset of a measurable ERG can be loosely correlated with the development of the retinal anatomy. It occurs during a period when synaptogenesis is proceeding most rapidly and when the outer segments of the receptor cells are attaining adultlike morphology. The onset of visual function measured by the ERG also corresponds well with time of eye opening in different species. Two examples are cats, where eye opening occurs at 7–10 days postnatally and a measurable ERG is first recorded 9–10 days postnatally, and dogs, where both events occur at about 2 weeks postnatally. The ERG of pre-term human infants can be recorded as early as 30 weeks post-conception (Winkelman and Horsten, 1962; Mactier et al., 1988). On the day of birth both the a- and b-waves can be observed (Shipley and Anton, 1964) but adult-like latencies and amplitudes develop during a postnatal period that is not yet determined.

B   Ganglion Cells

The physiological development of the retinal ganglion cells has been described in several studies of rabbit (Bowe-Anders et al., 1975; Masland, 1977) and cat (Hamasaki and Flynn, 1977; Rusoff and Dubin, 1977; Hamasaki and Sutija, 1979) retina. Comparable data are not available for other mammalian species.

The onset of ganglion cell visual function has been best studied in peripheral retina of rabbit where (in the adult) most cells have center/surround receptive field (RF) organization and the complex RF types found in the visual streak are rare (Levick, 1967; Masland, 1977). Rabbit ganglion cells are electrically active at birth (Masland, 1977). They have spontaneous, periodic bursts of action potentials every 1–4 min and discharge continuously at 30–40 Hz following depolarization by high external K^+ concentrations. Interestingly, the earliest ganglion cell response to light occurs at 8 days postnatally (2 days after the appearance of a measurable ERG), suggesting an inability of more distal retinal neurons to drive synaptically the retinal ganglion cells prior to that time. The percentage of ganglion cells that respond to light increases from about 10% on day 8 to 100% by day 13. The receptive field organization of these cells is immature during this period. The immaturity is expressed as (1) a weak response to light (3–10 action potentials per stimulus); (2) rapid adaptation or fatigue to repeated stimulation; (3) the absence of an inhibitory receptive field surround for cells with very large RF centers; and (4) cells with "silent" suppressive surrounds, stimulation of which antagonizes the response to a stimulus presented in the RF center but does not excite the cell. By about postnatal day 20 cells with no surround effects become rare, the number of cells with only suppressive surrounds decreases, and ganglion cell responses are qualitatively indistinguishable from those of adults. It is likely, however, that quantitative tests of the RF properties would reveal differences from the adult beyond 20 days of age.

In the kitten retina, some ganglion cells must respond to light by 6–8 days postnatally, when visual responses can be recorded from neurons in the striate cortex (Hubel and Wiesel, 1963). At 3 weeks postnatally, the earliest age at which recordings from retinal ganglion cells have been reported, many kitten ganglion cells display immaturities just described for the rabbit retina. Some cells give weak responses to visual stimulation, have large RF centers, and have weak RF surround inhibition (Rusoff and Dubin, 1977). Cells with RF center sizes larger than any found in the adult (even after scaling for differences in size of the retinal image) are recorded in kittens up to 4 weeks postnatally, after which all kitten RF center sizes fall more nearly within the adult range (Figure 4, upper). It is possible that light scatter by the immature optics may account for the large RF centers observed in some studies of the younger animals. This would occur when bright spots of light are flashed on and off and the RF mapped by moving the spots from outside of the RF toward the center. Light would be scattered onto the RF center when the "true" image of the spot remains well outside the RF, resulting in an overestimation of the center diameter. Light scatter should be less of a problem for the area–threshold technique where a small flashing spot is placed in the center of the RF and center size is measured by

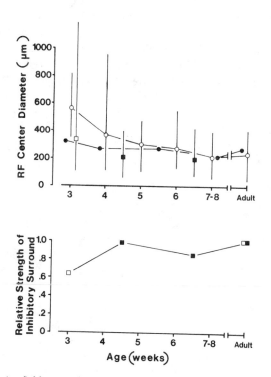

FIGURE 4. Receptive field center diameter of cat retinal ganglion cells (upper) and strength of the receptive field inhibitory surround (lower) both as a function of postnatal age. (upper) From Rusoff and Dubin (1977) (open circles); Hamasaki and Flynn (1977) (open squares); Hamasaki and Sutija (1979) (filled circles); and Tootle and Friedlander (1989) (filled squares). (lower) Average strength of kitten ganglion cell inhibitory surrounds normalized to an adult value of 1.

increasing the size of the spot until its threshold intensity no longer decreases. In this case, the use of low-threshold stimulus intensities reduces
the amount of scattered light. The light that is scattered falls on the less
sensitive noncentral region of the RF center. Since use of the area–threshold
technique yields very large RF center diameters in the young kittens (Figure
4, upper, open circles), it is likely they are not due to scattered light but
represent a neural immaturity.

Recently, we have used the technique of measuring the spatial contrast
sensitivity function (SCSF) of retinal ganglion cell axons in 4-week-old
kittens (Tootle and Friedlander, 1989). This method which employs randomly interleaved presentations of drifting sinusoidal grating patterns at
various contrast levels and spatial frequencies significantly minimizes the
effects of light scatter. It also permits a quantitative assessment of the size
and sensitivity of the receptive field center and surround mechanisms,
assuming a difference of the Gaussian functions model of the receptive field
(Rodieck, 1965; Enroth-Cugell and Robson, 1966). In this model, large RF
centers should produce lower spatial acuity (the highest spatial frequency to
which the neuron will respond) for the retinal ganglion cells of young
kittens, and this is found to be the case. In Figure 5, representative examples
of SCSFs obtained from retinal ganglion cell axons from 4-week-old kittens
are shown (Tootle and Friedlander, 1989); the receptive fields of the axons
were located more than 10° from the area centralis. The median acuity
(defined as the spatial frequency at which the contrast sensitivity falls to 1)

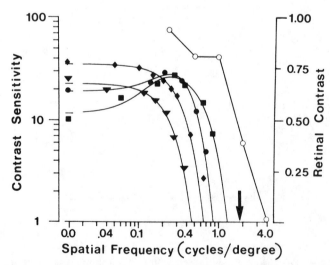

FIGURE 5. Example of spatial contrast sensitivity functions obtained from retinal ganglion
cells by axonal recordings in the optic tract of 4-week-old kittens. Median acuity of adult retinal
ganglion cells (arrow) and the modulation transfer function of the optics of a 30-day-old kitten
replotted from Figure 1. (From Tootle and Friedlander, 1989.)

of comparable adult ganglion cell axons is represented by the arrow in Figure 5. It can be seen that the acuity of the kitten cells is lower—about 1 cycle per degree versus about 2 cycles per degree for the adults. In order to assess the degree to which this difference may represent optical versus neural immaturity, we have replotted the MTF of the 30-day-old kitten optics from Figure 1A in Figure 5 (see right Y axis). The retinal contrast is reduced by only 20% (to 0.8) at 1 cycle per degree—the acuity of the kitten cells. This strongly supports the argument that the MTF of the immature optics does not limit the acuity of peripheral retinal ganglion cells at this age. The effect of ocular growth on estimates of neonatal RF center sizes using the SCSF technique are presented below (see section D.).

The strength of the inhibitory receptive field surround mechanism of kitten retinal ganglion cells has been measured quantitatively with two types of experimental approaches. In one, a suprathreshold intensity spot is flashed on and off in the RF center. Spot size is varied and the rate at which the response magnitude is reduced by progressive enlargement to cover more of the RF inhibitory surround is measured as the slope of the descending limb of the size response function (Figure 4, lower, open squares; Hamasaki and Flynn, 1977). In the second, spatial contrast sensitivity functions are measured and the volumes of the RF center and surround mechanisms are derived assuming a difference of Gaussian's model of the RF (the effect of the inhibitory surround on contrast sensitivity is seen as the decline in sensitivity at low spatial frequencies in Figure 5). In this case the strength of RF surround inhibition is quantified as the relative volumes of the surround and center Gaussians (Figure 4, lower, filled squares; Enroth-Cugell and Robson, 1966; Linsenmeier et al., 1982; Tootle and Friedlander, 1989). Application of these techniques indicates the RF inhibitory surround strength of kitten retinal ganglion cells is about two-thirds the adult value at 3 weeks postnatally and becomes adultlike during the next 1–2 weeks. In addition to the immaturities just described, the spontaneous and visually driven firing rates and temporal frequency resolving power of kitten ganglion cells are significantly lower than the adult (Hamasaki and Flynn, 1977; Tootle and Friedlander, unpublished).

C Physiological Classification of Ganglion Cells

In the retina of the adult cat, ganglion cells can be identified on the basis of a number of physiological properties as belonging to one of at least three functional groups: W, X, or Y [see Sherman and Spear (1982) and Stone (1983) for reviews]. Tests of three of these distinguishing properties are illustrated in Figure 6. The initial definition of X- and Y-cells was based on, respectively, linear or nonlinear summation of the visual input to the cells (Enroth-Cugell and Robson, 1966). Practically, linear spatial summation (as exhibited by X-cells) means that a position in the cells' RF can be found where the introduction and withdrawal of a contrast-modulated (grating) stimulus evokes no response from the cell (Figure 6A, left). Nonlinear (Y) cells (Figure 6A, right) respond at each introduction and withdrawal of the stimulus regardless of its position. The X- and Y-cells also have distinct response latencies to electrical stimulation of their axons in the optic chiasm (Figure 6B) and give, respectively, brisk-sustained and brisk-transient responses to a standing contrast stimulus (Figure 6C). The W-cells have longer response latencies to electrical stimulation of their axons, sluggish visual responses, and a variety of receptive field properties (Cleland and Levick, 1974). Correct classification of retinal ganglion cells depends critically on correlations between these and other properties. Two major questions are central to understanding the ontogeny of the functional classes: (1) To what extent are the different physiological types recognizable in the neonate? (2) What is the developmental sequence giving rise to the distinguishing physiological properties of the members of each class?

At 3 weeks postnatally the majority of kitten retinal ganglion cells cannot be placed into the adult classes by the application of one quantitative (Hamasaki and Flynn, 1977) or a few qualitative (Rusoff and Dubin, 1977) classificatory tests. Reasons cited are the lack of a clear "no response" or "null" position on a test of spatial summation and a sustained response by all cells tested. Moreover, since the conduction velocities of the ganglion cells are considerably slower in the neonate (primarily due to incomplete myelination), response latencies to electrical stimulation are greater than adult values used for classification purposes. Examples of cells putatively belonging to the three classes can be found as early as 4 weeks postnatally intermixed with cells that are clearly not classifiable by application of test criteria used for adult animals (Rusoff and Dubin, 1977; Hamasaki and Sutija, 1979). The age at which the proportion of cells that are putatively classifiable becomes adultlike is from 4 to 7 weeks postnatally (Rusoff and Dubin, 1977; Hamasaki and Sutija, 1979; Sur et al., 1984).

It is likely that application of a multivariate approach to cell classification would yield a higher rate of success in identifying ganglion cell types in very young kittens. For example, Tootle and Friedlander (1989) recently applied

FIGURE 6. Examples of three tests of physiological properties used to identify cat retinal ganglion cells as belonging to the W, X, or Y functional classes. (A) Responses of an off-center X-cell (left) and Y-cell (right) to the introduction and withdrawal of a sinusoidal grating stimulus into their receptive fields. The luminance profile of the grating relative to the RF center (circle) is illustrated to the right at the indicated phase angle. Upward and downward deflection of the trace at the bottom signals, respectively, introduction and withdrawal of the grating. (From Enroth-Cugell and Robson, 1966.) (B) Response latencies of intraocularly recorded adult cat retinal ganglion cells to electrical stimulation of the optic chiasm. The upper two histograms show the latencies of brisk-sustained (X) cells (filled bars) and brisk-transient (Y) cells (open bars). The latencies of sluggish (W) cells are illustrated in the lower histogram. (From Cleland and Levick, 1974.) (C) Sustained and transient responses to standing contrast presented to the RF center of cat retinal ganglion cells. The irregular line is a graph of the mean firing rate of the cell. (From Cleland et al., 1971.)

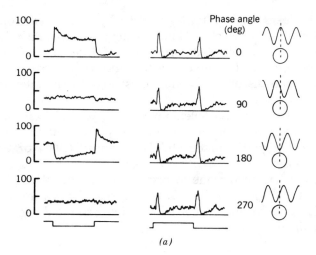

(a)

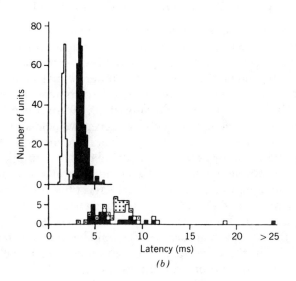

(b)

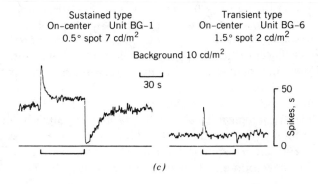

(c)

multivariate cluster analysis to classify retinal ganglion cell axons recorded in the optic tract of 4–5-week-old kittens. All the axons could be identified as belonging to two clusters that corresponded closely to the X- and Y-cell types. A more detailed treatment of this approach to cell classification is presented in the discussion of the physiology of the lateral geniculate nucleus.

Little is known about the development of the W retinal ganglion cells due to their small size and incomplete understanding of their functional and morphological properties in the adult [see Stanford (1987) for recent illumination of this issue].

No attempt has been made to place neonatal retinal ganglion cells of other species into the X-, Y-, and W-cell classes. Nor has any attempt been made to describe the ontogenetic events giving rise to the specific physiologically defined cell types.

D   Functional Synaptic Convergence onto Ganglion Cells

In the adult cat the mesopic receptive field center diameter of retinal ganglion cells is approximately the size of their dendritic arbors (Peichl and Wassle, 1983). This implies that the receptive field center mechanism of the ganglion cells receives synaptic inputs from outer retinal neurons lying immediately vitreal to the cells and receives little or no convergent input from more laterally placed neurons (Sterling et al., 1988). It is of interest, therefore, to examine the relationship between receptive field and dendritic diameters during development in order to seek evidence for changing patterns of convergence of input from more distal retinal neurons onto the ganglion cells. For example, if convergence is the same at 4 weeks postnatally as in adulthood, it may be predicted that the receptive field center sizes of beta cells (generally considered to be the morphological counterpart of physiological X-cells in the retina; see Boycott and Wassle, 1974; Saito, 1983; Stanford and Sherman, 1984; Stanford, 1987) would be similar near the area centralis but smaller in the peripheral retina in kittens versus adult cats. However, our recent work (Tootle and Friedlander, 1989) shows that the receptive field center sizes of peripheral X retinal ganglion cells remains constant during the period when beta cell dendritic arbors are growing. This suggests that there is an increased lateral convergence of functional synaptic input onto the beta cells in young kittens as compared to the adult. As the beta cell dendritic arbor grows, this convergent input is apparently rendered nonfunctional so as to maintain receptive field centers of constant retinal extent (Figure 7A,B).

Since the dendritic field diameters of alpha cells (the morphological correlate of physiological Y-cells in the retina) are already adultlike by 2 weeks postnatally (Dann et al., 1988), changes in the retinal extent of Y-cell receptive field centers should indicate changing patterns of convergent input during development. However, the receptive field center sizes of Y

Cluster 1 (χ-) Cells RF Eccentricity >10°

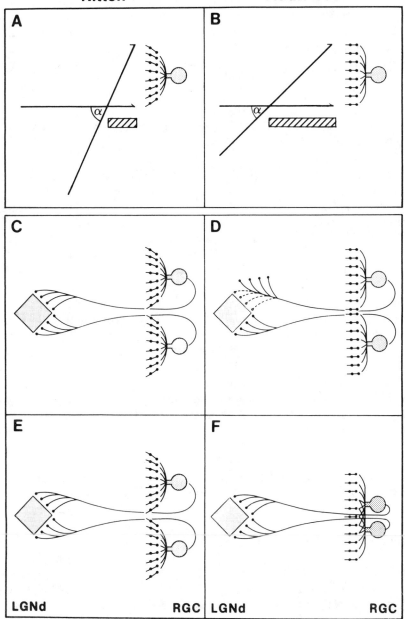

FIGURE 7. Proposed mechanism for constant retinal extent of receptive field diameter of peripheral X retinal ganglion cells in kittens (*A*) and adult cats (*B*) despite the smaller dendritic diameters in the kitten. Synaptic input from laterally placed neurons (black circles) serves to broaden the region of the photoreceptor matrix sampled in the kitten. (*C–F*) Possible mechanisms underlying the development increase the spatial resolution of peripheral X LGN_d neurons (stippled diamonds). Receptive field size shrinks due to reduced retinogeniculate convergence (*C, D*) or increased overlap of ganglion cell dendrites (*E, F*). (From Tootle and Friedlander, 1989.)

ganglion cells with peripheral receptive fields increase between 4–5 weeks postnatally and adulthood (Tootle and Fieldlander, 1989), indicating that there is an increase in laterally convergent synaptic input onto the Y-cells during postnatal development. Thus there appears to be a dynamic shaping of the synaptic input onto the ganglion cells during postnatal development with the specific pattern differing between the various ganglion cell types.

V ANATOMICAL DEVELOPMENT OF THE DORSAL LATERAL GENICULATE NUCLEUS

The mammalian dorsal lateral geniculate nucleus (LGN_d) undergoes considerable change in structure and circuitry during postnatal development. The individual LGN_d neurons of most species increase significantly in size during this period [cat (Garey et al., 1973; Kalil, 1978, 1980; Hickey, 1980; P. D. Wilson et al., 1984); rat (Parnevelas et al., 1977); human (Hickey, 1977, 1981; deCourten and Garey, 1982)] but apparently increase little in monkeys (Headon et al., 1985, but see Garey and Saini, 1981). The time for this process varies between species (from several weeks in rats to 6–24 months in human). The dendritic structure of the LGN_d neurons also changes during postnatal development. By comparing Golgi-stained neurons between neonates and adults, several authors have concluded that overall dendritic extent increases concomitantly with a reduction in the density of spinelike processes [rat (Parnevelas et al., 1977); cat (Mason, 1983); monkey (Garey and Saini, 1981)]. Others (Leuba and Garey, 1984) report that the extent of the dendritic arborizations of monkey LGN_d neurons decreases postnatally. However, due to the uncertainties associated with comparing samples of Golgi-impregnated material between age groups, this issue is not settled.

The neurons of the adult cat LGN_d can be divided into the same three types of functional classes as the retinal ganglion cells [W-, X-, and Y-cells (Cleland et al., 1971, 1976; Hoffman et al., 1972); see Sherman and Spear (1982) for a review]. The electrophysiological properties of the LGN_d neurons are largely determined by the type of ganglion cell that provides their dominant excitatory synaptic drive. The cat LGN_d is distinctly laminated with an alternation of inputs from contralateral and ipsilateral retinae to individual layers, with the most dorsal layer (layer A) receiving contralateral retinal input (Guillery, 1970). The LGN_d also has a separate medial division [the medial interlaminar nucleus (MIN); Rioch, 1929; Guillery et al., 1980]. In addition to the parcellation of contralateral and ipsilateral retinal input to alternating layers, the separation of functional parallel streams is reflected in the lamination (Figure 8A). The most dorsal layers (A and A_1) receive input from X- and Y-cells. The next ventral layer (C magnocellular) receives Y- and W-cell input and the more ventral layers (C_1 and C_2) are innervated predominantly by W-cells (Cleland et al., 1976). The MIN is primarily

A.

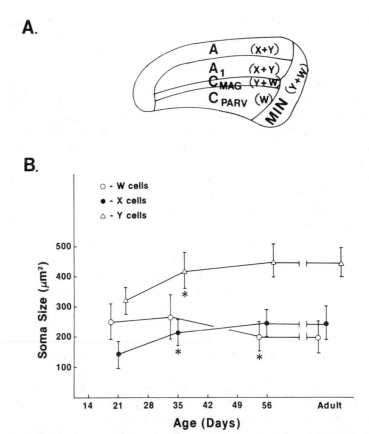

B.

FIGURE 8. (*A*) Schematic drawing of the cat dorsal lateral geniculate nucleus. Laminae receiving innervation from the contralateral eye are A, C magnocellular, part of C parvocellular (layer C_2, not illustrated), and part of the medial interlaminar nucleus (MIN). The laminae receiving innervation from the ipsilateral eye are A_1, part of C parvocellular (C_1), and part of MIN. The functional retinal ganglion cell types (W, X and Y) differentially innervate the various laminae, as illustrated. (*B*) Change in mean soma size $\pm$ S.D. of physiologically identified kitten LGN_d neurons [that have been filled with intracellular injection of horseradish peroxidase (HRP)]. Asterisks indicate age where the size is significantly different ($p < 0.05$, Mann-Whitney U-test) than the next earlier age. (From Friedlander, 1984.)

innervated by Y-cells (Kratz et al., 1978; Dreher and Sefton, 1979) via collateral branches of ganglion cell Y-axons that also innervate layers A and C magnocellular or A_1 of the LGN_d (Bowling and Michael, 1980, 1984; Sur and Sherman, 1982a) and by W-cells (Rowe and Dreher, 1982).

Based upon studies utilizing the intracellular HRP injection technique, both functional classes of cat LGN_d neurons in the dorsal layers of the nucleus (X- and Y-cells) were found to increase in soma size (Figure 8B) and elaborate dendritic structure (Figure 9) during the first 8 postnatal weeks

(Friedlander, 1982, 1984). Cells with physiological properties similar to the adult X class vary considerably in the degree of morphological maturity in the kitten. Some have patterns of dendritic arborizations with processes characteristic of adult X-cells; others have very restricted, simple dendrites with no processes. Cells with physiological properties similar to adult Y-cells have dendritic patterns similar to but more restricted than their adult counterparts. Some of these cells have a higher density of dendritic spines than those of the adult. This observation has been made with both the Golgi (Mason, 1983) and intracellular HRP injection (Friedlander, 1982) techniques. It is interesting to note that the predominant functional cell type in the ventral layers of the cat LGN_d (the W-cells that receive innervation from the class of W retinal ganglion cells that represent the plurality of ganglion cells) is already morphologically mature in terms of dendritic structure, extent, and soma size in the 3- to 4-postnatal-week kitten (Friedlander, 1982, 1984; P. D. Wilson et al., 1984; Figures 8B and 9). These cells decrease in size between 5 and 8 postnatal weeks. It has been suggested (Friedlander, 1982) that this early structural development of LGN_d W-cells along with their relatively mature visual responsiveness [as observed qualitatively in the studies of Daniels et al. (1978) and Friedlander (1982)] may result in a more dominant role for this system in neonatal versus adult vision. Moreover, several reports (Hickey, 1980; Leventhal and Hirsch, 1983; P. D. Wilson et al., 1984) suggest that the W-cells are considerably less sensitive (as evaluated by changes in their soma size) to the effects of visual deprivation than are the X- and Y-cell systems. This may be a consequence of the earlier postnatal development of their soma–dendritic structure. Several studies have also indicated that the W-cell projection to layer I of visual cortex is relatively mature in young kittens (LeVay et al., 1978; Kato et al., 1984). However, no direct data on the morphology of individual geniculocortical W-axon arborizations are available for kittens or adult cats.

The LGN_d circuitry as evaluated at the electron microscope level also undergoes considerable changes, postnatally. The adult cat LGN_d has a well-described (Guillery, 1969) synaptic circuitry that differs between the two major functional cell groups (X- and Y-cells) in the A layers of the cat LGN_d (J. R. Wilson et al., 1984; Figure 10A). The synapses made by retinal ganglion cell axons onto LGN_d neurons are primarily on dendritic appendages of X-cells (versus dendritic shafts of Y-cells). Moreover, these retinal inputs onto X-cell appendages tend to occur in triadic arrangements in glomeruli. The retinal axon terminal diverges to make an asymmetric synaptic contact on an LGN_d X-cells' dendrite and local circuit neurons, which in turn makes a symmetric synaptic contact on the LGN_d X-cells' dendrite. In the neonate, the number of synaptic profiles that appear to be morphologically similar to those that were shown to be of retinal origin in the adult slightly decreases in density per glomerulus, postnatally (Winfield et al., 1980; Figure 10B). During this same period, symmetric synaptic profiles [usually associated with the presence of gamma-aminobutyric acid

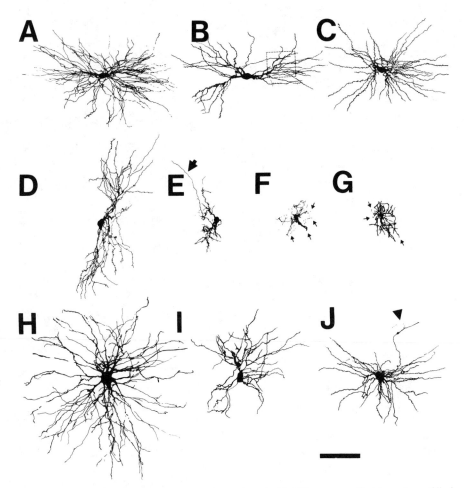

FIGURE 9. Line drawings of physiologically identified LGN$_d$ neurons that have been filled with HRP by intracellular iontophoresis. First column (A, D, H) are examples of a typical W-, X-, and Y-cells, respectively, from adult cats. All other cells are from kittens at 3–4 postnatal weeks. Rows indicate functional types [(A–C) are W-cells, (D–G) are X-cells, and (H)–(J) are Y-cells]. Scale bar = 100 μm. (From Friedlander, 1982.)

(GABA) activity in the adult] significantly increase in density per glomerulus (Figure 10B). GABA is thought to be the neurotransmitter of the interposed local circuit neuron that may provide additional circuitry for mediating both inhibitory (Sanderson et al., 1971; Tootle and Friedlander, 1986) and facilitatory responses (Sherman and Koch, 1986) of LGN$_d$ X-cells. Recent studies utilizing immunocytochemical localization of GABA (Kalil et al., 1985) or its synthetic enzyme [glutamic acid decarboxylase (GAD);

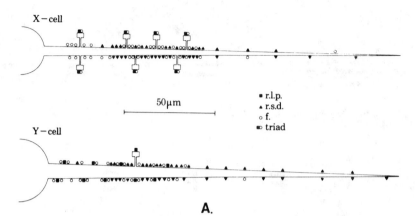

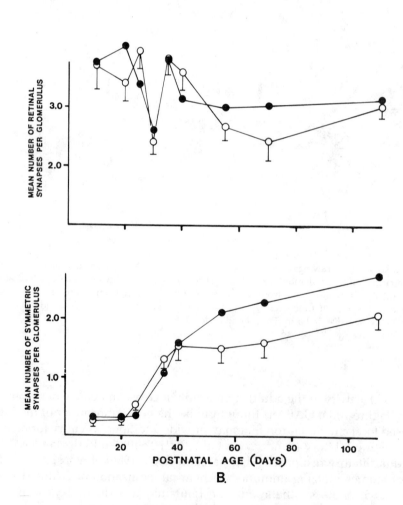

Shotwell et al., 1986] have shown reduced staining in neuropil of kitten LGN_d as compared to adult cat LGN_d. The relative immaturity of the putative inhibitory LGN_d circuitry may contribute to the immature spatial filtering properties of X-cells in the kitten LGN_d. LGN_d X-cells in adult cats behave as weak "bandpass" filters only allowing medium to relatively high-spatial-frequency components of a visual stimulus to pass. However, in the kitten LGN_d, many neurons with properties of X-cells behave more like low-pass filters (Lehmkuhle et al., 1980; Berardi and Morrone, 1984; Tootle and Friedlander, 1986, 1989). The following section contains a more detailed account of these functional changes.

The retinal axons that innervate the kitten LGN_d undergo changes in the structure and pattern of their terminal arborizations during the first 12 postnatal weeks. Using the technique of bulk filling of optic tract axons with HRP, Mason (1982a) reported immature terminal arborizations of ganglion cell axons in young kittens (up to 5 postnatal weeks) characterized by variably shaped endings with filopodia and growth cone-like tips. Many of these processes form synapses on dendrites and perikarya of LGN_d neurons (Mason, 1982b). With the application of the intracellular HRP injection technique to electrophysiologically classifed optic tract axons, the complete arborization of single retinogeniculate axons of adult cats (Bowling and Michael, 1980; Sur and Sherman, 1982a) and kittens (Friedlander et al., 1983; Sur et al., 1984; Friedlander et al., 1985) can be visualized. At 5 postnatal weeks, some retinal Y-axons still have very immature terminal arborizations with growth cone-like processes in the upper A layers of the LGN_d. However, most Y-axons have innervation patterns similar to their adult counterparts. The major difference is that the kitten Y-axons have smaller terminal arborizations with fewer boutons (Figure 11A,B). Therefore, the postnatal period from 4 weeks to adult is characterized by an expansion of the territory and density of innervation of the LGN_d by retinal Y-axons. We have estimated the change in density of synaptic boutons from all retinal Y-axons in the A-laminae of the kitten LGN_d as increasing from about 4.5×10^8 to 9.6×10^8 boutons per cm^3 between 4 and one-half

---

FIGURE 10. (A) Schematic drawing of distribution of synaptic profiles on physiologically identified individual X and Y LGN_d neurons from adult cat. Cells intracellularly filled with HRP via ionophoresis and subsequently examined with the electron microscope. The different symbols refer to synaptic profiles of various origin (r.l.p., retinal terminals; r.s.d., terminals from corticogeniculate axons or axon collaterals of geniculocortical axons; f., terminals with pleomorphic synaptic vesicles forming symmetric synapses and suggested to contain GABA). Triad refers to the particular synaptic arrangement described in the text. Note that X-cells tend to have more triadic synaptic structures. (From J. R. Wilson et al., 1984.) (B) Plots of mean values of numbers of synapses of probable retinal origin (upper) and symmetric synapses (lower) contained within encapsuled glomeruli in the LGN_d of kittens of various ages. Open circles are mean ($\pm$S.E.M.) for lamina A, closed circles for lamina A_1. Error bars and connecting lines are only drawn for A_1 values for clarity. Values are replotted from Winfield et al. (1980).

A.

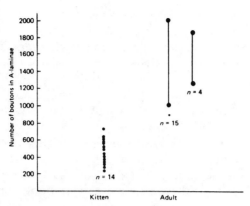

B.

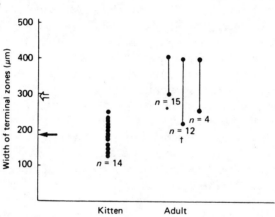

C.

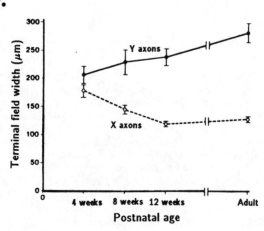

postnatal weeks and adult.[1] (The absolute number of synaptic boutons in the A layers from retinal Y-axons triples from approximately 4.3×10^6 to 13.9×10^6 during this same period; the difference in increased density is less profound due to the increased volume of the LGN_d during this same period of development).

In addition to the profound increase in retinal Y-cell innervation of the LGN_d during postnatal development, it has been suggested (Sur et al., 1984) that a concomitant reduction in the degree of X-cell innervation occurs during this same period (Figure 11C). These data suggest that the neurons of the A-layers of the kitten LGN_d are dominated by one particular functional class of retinal input (X-cells) in terms of numbers of retinal ganglion cells and the extent of innervation by each retinal ganglion cell, while the Y system comes to play a more dominant role in the adult. This is in fact the case (see Section VI). During development, a shift occurs (primarily due to the expansion of the terminal arborizations and elaborations of additional synaptic boutons) to increase the synaptic influence of Y-cells. Moreover, the LGN_d Y-cells expand their sphere of influence upon the visual cortex by increasing the size of their terminal arborizations and the number of synaptic contacts made by each bouton during this same period of develop-

---

[1] The calculation was made as follows: The mean number of synaptic boutons innervating an A layer of the LGN_d from a single, functionally identified retinal ganglion cell (rgc) Y-axon is 476 for the 4 and one-half-postnatal-week kitten and 1553 for the adult cat (Friedlander et al., 1985). The total number of rgcs per retina is estimated at $\approx 180,000$ at these two ages and the percentage of rgcs that belong to the Y functional class is taken as $\approx 5\%$. Since most rgc Y-axons innervate the LGN_d, it is calculated that ≈ 9000 rgc Y-axons innervate layer A or A_1 of the cat LGN_d. Therefore, the total number of Y synaptic boutons in either of these layers is the product of the number of Y-rgcs per retina and the average number of A laminae boutons per Y-rgc. The density calculation was obtained by calculating the ratio of total Y synaptic boutons from rgc's from a single retina by the approximate volume of the one of the A-laminae at each age. These estimates were derived by assuming that each of the A-laminae occupies approximately one-third of the total LGN_d volume and related to the actual measurements of total LGN_d volume of kittens and adult cats (Kalil, 1978).

FIGURE 11. (A) Comparison of numbers of boutons on the terminal arborizations of individual, physiologically identified Y retinogeniculate axons within the A-laminae. Each was filled with HRP by intracellular ionophoresis of the axon in the optic tract. All axons (in $4\frac{1}{2}$-postnatal-week kitten and adult cat) had their physiological property of nonlinear spatial summation (which assigns them to the Y category) rigorously determined with Fourier analysis of their averaged response to sinusoidally counterphased grating stimuli. ($\cdot$, Bowling and Michael, 1984.) (B) Width of terminal fields of Y retinogeniculate axons in kitten and adult cat A-laminae. Arrows indicate mean values of 192 μm for kittens and 293 μm for adult cats. (From Friedlander et al., 1985.) (*, Bowling and Michael, 1980; †, Sur and Sherman, 1982a.) (C) Summary of mean terminal field width of X and Y retinogeniculate axon arborizations from kittens of various ages and adult cats. (From Sur et al., 1984.)

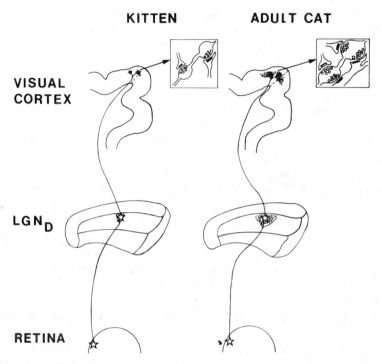

FIGURE 12. Schematic illustration of the expansion of the Y pathway that occurs in cats during postnatal development. The stars indicate retinal and LGN$_d$ Y-cells. Note the increasing width of the terminal arborizations of both retinogeniculate Y-axons projecting to the A-laminae and geniculocortical axons projecting to visual cortex area 18. Also note the additional expansion of the synaptic distribution of the geniculocortical Y-axons that occur during development as indicated by the individual boutons forming multiple versus single synaptic contacts in the adult cat versus the kitten (inset).

ment (Friedlander and Martin, 1989). The net result of these changes is illustrated in Figure 12. One function of the cat LGN$_d$ may be to amplify and distribute a small retinal Y-cell signal to a disproportionately large volume of visual cortex (Friedlander et al., 1981). This hypothesis has been further substantiated at the ultrastructural level by Freund et al. (1985a,b), who found that the boutons of axonal arborizations of adult LGN$_d$ Y-cells each contact several distinct postsynaptic targets in the visual cortex. This functional magnification develops postnatally (Sur et al., 1984; Friedlander et al., 1985; Friedlander and Martin, 1989) and may contribute to the sensitivity of the Y system to environmental factors (Sherman et al., 1972; Sur et al., 1982a; Friedlander et al., 1985, Friedlander and Stanford, 1984; McCarthy et al., 1989).

VI PHYSIOLOGICAL DEVELOPMENT OF THE DORSAL LATERAL GENICULATE NUCLEUS

A Receptive Field Properties

Neurons of the dorsal lateral geniculate nucleus can be activated synaptically by electrical stimulation of their retinal afferents prenatally in the cat (Shatz and Kirkwood, 1984) and as early as 2 days postnatally in the rabbit (Rapisardi et al., 1975). The earliest light-evoked activity of rabbit LGN_d neurons is obtained at 5–6 days postnatally (Rapisardi et al., 1975), indicating that in this species the maturation of the retinogeniculate synapse does not limit the onset of visual function in the LGN_d. The appearance of a visual response from the LGN_d neurons 2–3 days before the earliest recorded visually driven response from the retinal ganglion cells in another study (Masland, 1977) is unexplained but could be due to slight differences in rates of development between different strains or individual rabbits.

By 15 days postnatally 100% of rabbit retinal ganglion cells and LGN_d neurons respond to visual stimuli. In the kitten, 90% of the LGN_d neurons can be driven visually 6–13 days postnatally (Daniels et al., 1978). Immaturities in RF organization similar to those previously described for retinal ganglion cells are observed for LGN_d neurons during the first several postnatal weeks, including large RF centers, low spontaneous and visually driven firing rates, weak or absent RF surround inhibition and excitation, and fatiguible or labile response to repeated stimulation (Daniels et al., 1978; Wilson et al., 1982; Tootle and Friedlander, 1986; 1989). In Figure 13 the RF center sizes and strengths of the RF inhibitory surrounds of LGN_d neurons in 4–5-week-old kittens are compared to those of adult cats. Both data sets are scaled in terms of retinal extent eliminating differences in the size of the eye as a factor. The RF center areas of the kitten cells are on average significantly larger than those of the adult, although there is extensive overlap between the two groups. Similarly, the strength of the RF inhibitory surrounds of the kitten cells are, on average, considerably weaker than in the adult, the difference being somewhat more robust in this case. The weak inhibitory surrounds of kitten LGN_d neurons may be due to weak inhibitory surrounds of the retinal ganglion cells that provide their excitatory drive and/or from immature intrageniculate circuitry that contributes to the inhibitory receptive field surround of the LGN_d neurons. In adult cats, pharmacological and physiological evidence (Singer et al., 1972; Sillito and Kemp, 1983) suggests that such an intrageniculate component adds significantly to the inhibitory receptive field surround mechanism.

As is illustrated in Figure 14, both the spatial and temporal resolution of kitten LGN_d neurons improves during postnatal development. Acuity increases from about 1 cycle per degree at 3 weeks postnatally to about 3–4 cycles per degree in the adult for cells with linear spatial summation and RFs near the representation of the area centralis (Ikeda and Tremain, 1978;

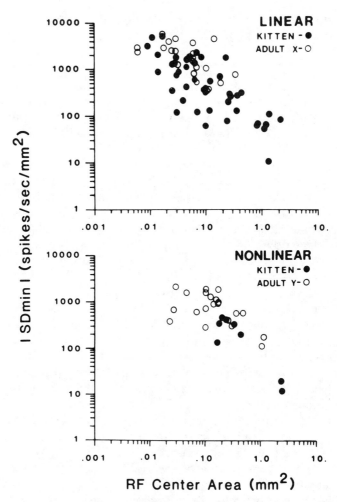

FIGURE 13. Scatter plots of a measure of strength of the receptive field, inhibitory surround ($|SD_{min}|$) as a function of RF center area expressed in terms of the area of retina subtended by a visual stimulus for LGN_d neurons of $4\frac{1}{2}$-postnatal-week kittens and adult cats. Values are plotted on log scales. (From Tootle and Friedlander, 1986.)

Mangel et al., 1983; Tootle and Friedlander, 1989). The improvement in acuity at the younger ages is greater than would be predicted on the basis of growth of the eye alone. This is illustrated in Figure 14A (diamond symbols) where the acuity predicted on the basis of eye size alone is plotted as a function of age (assuming an adult acuity of 4 cycles per degree). At ages younger than about 8 weeks the measured acuity is poorer than the predicted acuity, as is indicated by the shaded region on the graph. This difference between measured and predicted acuity is greatest in the youngest kittens, and it is tempting to conclude that it represents the magnitude of

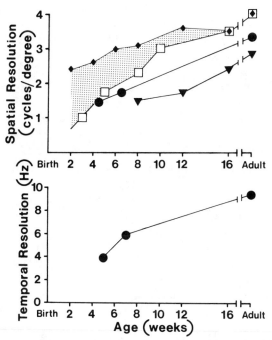

FIGURE 14. Average spatial and temporal frequency resolution of cat LGN$_d$ neurons as a function of postnatal age. Data are replotted from Ikeda and Tremain, 1978 and Ikeda and Wright, 1976 (squares), Mangel et al., 1983 (triangles), and Tootle and Friedlander, unpublished data (circles).

the neural component of the reduced acuity of the kittens. However, two important caveats must be born in mind before drawing this conclusion. The first is that it is probable that the transient vascular membranes of the eye contribute to the reduced acuity at ages younger than 4 weeks. The second is that there is an implicit assumption that the cells being compared in the kittens and adult cats (in the present case cells with linear spatial summation) belong to the same functional type. However, it is likely that the group of linear kitten cells at ages less than 8 postnatal weeks contains a significant number of immature Y-cells that have yet to develop their non-linear spatial summation property (Tootle and Friedlander, 1989). The poor acuity of these "linear Y-cells" probably contributes to the reduced acuity observed in the kittens.

In the more peripheral regions of the visual field (>10° eccentricity), a postnatal improvement in spatial resolving capacity of the LGN$_d$ X-type cells occurs in real terms as measured in retinal extent (Tootle and Friedlander, 1989). This improvement is not likely due to improvement in the real spatial resolution of the retinal ganglion cells but probably results from either (a) a reduction in functional retinogeniculate convergence or (b) increased overlap in the receptive fields of neighboring retinal ganglion cells that converge onto single LGN_d neurons (See Figure 7C–F). Support for the former hypothesis comes from studies on the extent of the terminal arborizations of the axons of kitten retinal ganglion cells (Sur et al., 1984; Friedlander et al., 1985). The hypertrophied arborizations of the kitten retinal X-axons and smaller arborizations of kitten retinal Y-axons provide an anatomical substrate for a transient increase in convergence of X retinal ganglion cells onto individual LGN_d neurons (both X and Y types). In order to test this hypothesis more directly, experiments that evaluate functional convergence utilizing intracellular recording from kitten LGN_d neurons and graded electrical stimulation of the retinal ganglion cell axons must be employed. The latter hypothesis of increasing overlap of receptive fields of neighboring retinal ganglion cells during development has no direct experimental support. Studies are needed to directly measure the extent of overlap of neighboring retinal ganglion cells at different postnatal ages.

The temporal resolving power of kitten LGN_d neurons (measured as the highest temporal frequency to which the cell responds to each cycle of a drifting sinusoidal grating pattern) also increases by a factor of about 2 during the same postnatal period (Figure 14B) from about four Hz to nine Hz (Tootle and Friedlander, unpublished).

In the LGN_d of Old World monkeys, X- and Y-type cells (as determined primarily by evaluating linearity of spatial summation) seem to be readily classifiable as early as the day of birth (Blakemore and Vital-Durand, 1986). Moreover, the relative proportion and distribution of these cell types appears similar in neonates and adults, suggesting that cell classification may not be an issue in young monkeys. These observations imply a fundamental difference in the postnatal elaboration of retinal and/or geniculate circuitry in monkeys versus cats. A considerable increase in the spatial resolving power of monkey LGN_d neurons occurs over the first postnatal year (Figure 15). This increase is greatest for X-cells located within the representation of the foveal area. It should be pointed out that even at the day of birth, the acuity of monkey foveal X-cells (≈ 5 cycles per degree) is better than that of most adult cat X-cells located at the representation of the area centralis. The most immature part of the neonatal primate retinogeniculate pathway is the region of central vision. This contrasts with the kitten where physiological and morphological evidence suggests a central-to-peripheral developmental gradient (see previous sections in this chapter). Overall, neonatal monkey LGN_d neurons appear to be relatively more mature than neurons of the kitten LGN_d including having more developed receptive field surrounds (Blakemore and Vital-Durand, 1986). However, these authors made no quantitative assessment of this property. Finally, the increased spatial resolving power of the monkey LGN_d neurons during postnatal development is not simply due to a change in eye size and other optical factors. A considerable portion of this change must be due to neural factors (as postulated for the cat retinogeniculate pathway). To date, no studies of the

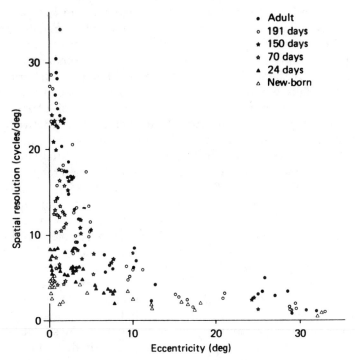

FIGURE 15. Spatial resolution as a function of receptive field eccentricity for X-cells in LGN$_d$ of several individual Old World monkeys of various postnatal ages. Ages are indicated in inset. Note the relative immaturity of the X-cells within 5° of the representation of central vision. (From Blakemore and Vital-Durand, 1986.)

postnatal development of monkey retinal ganglion cell properties have been reported to determine to what degree this change is due to intraretinal processing.

B   Physiological Classification of LGN$_d$ Neurons

In the adult cat, LGN$_d$ neurons, like the retinal ganglion cells that innervate them, can be placed into the X, Y, and W physiological classes. This is not surprising, since there is little convergence from ganglion cells belonging to different cell classes onto single LGN$_d$ neurons (Levick et al., 1972), and many of the properties determining class membership are simply "relayed" to the LGN$_d$ neurons. Additional functions are performed by a variety of intrageniculate circuits (Sherman and Koch, 1986; Sanderson et al., 1971; Lal and Friedlander, 1989). In the kitten, however, the possibility of differential development of retinogeniculate synaptic function for the various cell types makes it important to study the maturation of X-, Y-, and W-cell properties in physiologically identified neurons in the LGN$_d$.

There is general agreement that in kittens younger than 4 weeks postnatal, many LGN_d cells in the A layers cannot be identified as belonging to the X- or Y-cell class, typically due to "weak responses" or the absence of a "null," or no-response, position on a test for spatial summation properties (Daniels et al., 1978; Berardi and Morrone, 1984). This situation improves by 8 weeks postnatally when about 90% of A-layer (and medial interlaminar nucleus) neurons can be classified as X or Y types on the basis of one or a few classificatory tests (Wilson et al., 1982; Mangel et al., 1983). Between these two ages there is disagreement as to what percentage of cells can be classified with the null test as having linear or nonlinear spatial summation. Estimates of the percentage of cells that can be so classified range from 45% (Daniels et al., 1978) to about 95% (Tootle and Friedlander, unpublished). Among the cells that respond on a test for linearity of spatial summation, the incidence of those with nonlinear summation (Y-cells) increases with postnatal age (Tootle and Friedlander, 1986). For example, we find that about 17–20% of A-layer LGN_d neurons show nonlinear spatial summation at 4½ weeks [versus 33–36% in the adult (Friedlander et al., 1981; Friedlander and Stanford, 1984; Tootle and Friedlander, 1986, unpublished; Figure 16A)]. In their study of the MIN, Wilson et al. (1982) found that the proportions of electrophysiologically classified Y-cells increase fourfold during postnatal development (Figure 16A, squares). These data suggest that either many Y-cells are not physiologically active in the retina or LGN_d, the circuitry that mediates the nonlinear spatial summing property is immature at the retinal level, and/or the innervation of LGN_d neurons by axons of Y retinal ganglion cells is immature. There is some direct evidence for the latter suggestion (Friedlander et al., 1983, 1985; Sur et al., 1984; Tootle and Friedlander, 1986). Also, some features such as RF size vary with spatial summation properties in the neonate as in the adult while others [e.g., latency of response to stimulation of the retinal afferents (Daniels et al., 1978; Tootle and Friedlander, 1986; Figure 16B)] do not.

The application of a quantitative, multivariate approach to the classification issue would likely go a long way toward clarifying the maturational state of neonatal retinal ganglion and LGN_d neurons with regard to cell classification. This involves making quantitative measurements on several physiological properties of each neuron. The results are subjected to multivariate cluster analysis (Dixon and Brown, 1979; Engleman, 1980; Everitt, 1980), which assigns the cells into groups (clusters) on the basis of their similarity on all the properties considered together. The quantitative, multivariate nature of the approach minimizes the role of subjective judgment in classification, increases the likelihood of finding variables with significance for classification, and assumes no prior knowledge of cell class membership.

An example of the use of the multivariate approach we have employed is illustrated in Figure 17 for LGN_d neurons from the A layers of 4–7-week-old kittens and adult cats (Tootle and Friedlander, 1989). These plots show the

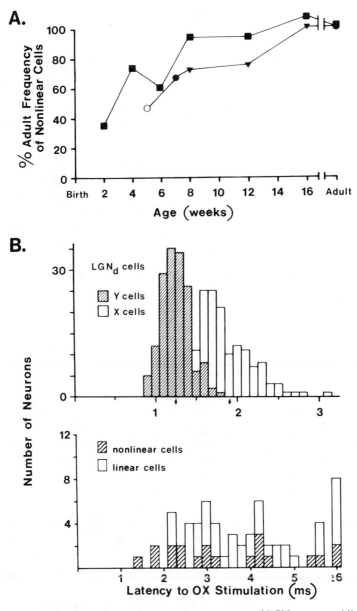

FIGURE 16. Development of spatial summation properties of LGN$_d$ neurons (*A*) and their latencies to electrical stimulation of the optic chiasm (*B*). (*A*) From Wilson et al. (1982) (squares), Tootle and Friedlander (1986) (open circle), Tootle and Friedlander (unpublished data) (filled circles), and Mangel et al. (1983) (triangles). (*B*) Latencies of 4½-week-old kitten (lower histogram) and adult (upper histogram) LGN$_d$ neurons to electrical stimulation of the optic chiasm. Open bars indicate X (linear) cells, hatched bars indicate Y (nonlinear) cells. The distribution of adult cells is bimodal with only slight overlap between cells belonging to the two classes. In the young kitten there is extensive overlap (no difference) between linear and nonlinear cell latencies. Notice also the longer latencies of the kitten neurons where latencies greater than 6 ms are observed. Kitten data are from the study of Tootle and Friedlander (1986). The adult data are reprinted from Hoffmann et al. (1972).

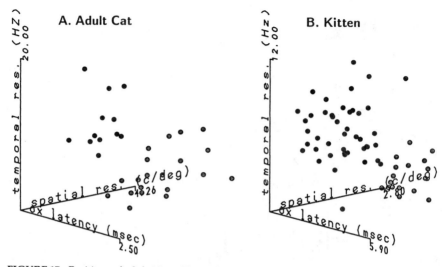

FIGURE 17. Positions of adult (*A*) and kitten (*B*) LGN$_d$ neurons on three of five variables used to identify cell types. Note the separations between the two clusters that contain X (stippled symbols) and Y (black symbols) cells. (From Tootle and Friedlander, 1989.)

position of each neuron in a three-dimensional coordinate system, where each axis represents the scores of the neurons on one of five classificatory tests. Variables used for clustering were spatial resolution, temporal resolution, probability of response to electrical stimulation of the optic chiasm (OX), response latency to OX stimulation, and a quantitative, continuously variable measure of degree of linearity of spatial summation. Using these variables, adult LGN$_d$ neurons form two distinct clusters, one containing X-cells, the other Y-cells as classified using conventional criteria. The kitten LGN$_d$ neurons also form two rather distinct clusters, and their relative positions on the classification variables indicate that the clusters correspond to the X and Y-types. Importantly, the two types can be identified even though many of the kitten cells fail to reach test criteria required for placing adult cells into the X and Y classes. For example, notice the long response latencies to OX stimulation of the kitten LGN$_d$ neurons in Figure 17*B*. These cells would be designated as unclassified in traditional approaches to identifying cell types and illustrate the advantage of the quantitative multivariate approach.

VII   ANATOMICAL DEVELOPMENT OF THE VISUAL CORTEX

The mammalian visual cortex undergoes considerable structural development, postnatally. This period varies between species (from weeks in rats to years in humans). Much of the development is a corollary of the increase in total cortical volume that occurs postnatally [e.g., the volume of striate cortex of monkey (*Macacca mulatta*) increases by 75% (Gottlieb et al., 1985) from birth and that of humans more than doubles (Huttenlocher, 1984)]. Consequently, neuronal and synapse packing density undergo significant changes in the neonate. In addition to these quantitative changes, recent studies suggest that transient expression of various chemicals that may serve as modulators of cortical circuitry occurs during the period of peak synaptogenesis.

Recent studies utilizing modern neuroanatomical tracing methods suggest that the basic patterns of afferent and efferent connectivity of the visual cortex are present at birth [rat (Olavarria and Van Sluyters, 1985); cat (Price and Blakemore, 1985; Kato et al., 1984; Henderson, 1982; Stein and Edwards, 1979); but see Laemle et al. (1972) and Anker and Cragg (1974)]. However, the precision of these projections is very immature. Using various combinations of anterograde and retrograde tracing methods, the following differences in connectivity have been observed: The neurons of the rat that contribute to interhemispheric projections of the corpus callosum are not restricted to the appropriate laminae in neonates (Olavarria and Van Sluyters, 1985); the LGN_d projection to the cat visual cortex is heavier to cortical layer I in the kitten (from large LGN_d neurons in the C and A layers versus only from small C-layer neurons in the adult; Kato et al., 1984); the corpus callosum projections are richer in kittens and involve neurons that in the adult cat only participate in ipsilateral corticocortical projections (Innocenti, 1981; Koppel and Innocenti, 1983; Innocenti et al., 1986); ocular dominance columns (representing the alternating LGN_d inputs from neurons innervated by the right and left eye) are less distinct in the kitten than in the adult cat (LeVay et al., 1978); corticotectal projections arise from more widely distributed and densely packed layer V neurons of visual cortex in kittens than in adult cats (Tsumoto et al., 1983); and the neurons that participate in association projections from area 17 to 18 become more restricted and patchy in their distribution during development (Price and Blakemore, 1985).

The morphology of individual cortical neurons and the extent of their axonal arborizations during development have been studied primarily with the technique of Golgi impregnation and retrograde filling of projection neurons after injection of various enzymes or fluorescent probes into their sites of axonal termination. The Golgi studies have yielded a similar picture of postnatal development; neurons generally have less extensive dendritic arborizations but greater densities of dendritic spines in neonates followed by a period of dendritic growth and spine elimination (Lund et al., 1977; Boothe et al., 1979; Becker et al., 1984; Michel and Garey, 1984; Muller et al., 1984).

The studies employing tracers have suggested that the extent of various projections to and from visual cortex is larger in the neonate, undergoing a period of retraction or pruning [LeVay et al., 1978; Kato et al., 1984; Innocenti, 1981 (but see Schoppmann, 1985).] However, it is difficult to infer the extent of a single neuron's axonal arborization based upon these studies. In experiments that directly visualize the entire terminal arborizations of individual, physiologically identified thalamocortical axons, the innervation density is greater but the overall extent of the arborization is less (Friedlander and Martin, 1989) in the kitten versus adult cat. Further work is needed to apply this method to the various cortical projection axons. Moreover, experiments that utilize the intracellular HRP method are needed in neonatal visual cortex (Friedlander and Martin, 1981) to complement and extend the Golgi studies of dendritic development of cortical neurons based on Golgi stains. This method has the advantage of fully staining the dendrites and axons of specific neuron classes in cortex (Gilbert and Wiesel, 1983; Martin and Whitteridge, 1984).

The ultrastructure of the visual cortex also changes extensively during postnatal development. Several studies have described the overall change in synaptic density during the postnatal period. The synaptic density initially increases and is then followed by a decrease [rat (Riccio and Mathews, 1985); cat (Cragg, 1975; O'Kusky, 1985); human (Garey, 1984; Huttenlocher, 1984)]. The peak synaptic density in visual cortex occurs in cats at about 5 postnatal weeks and in humans at 8 postnatal months (see Figure 18). The

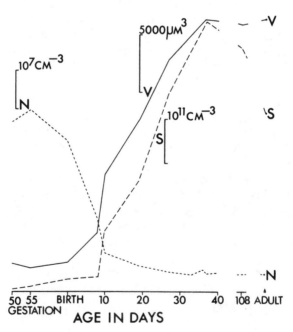

FIGURE 18. Plot of average cell density (N), volume of grey matter (V), and density of synapses (S) in cat visual cortex as a function of age. (From Cragg, 1975.)

synaptic density in cat area 17 (near the region that receives a projection representing central vision) continues to decline for 8 months (O'Kusky, 1985) while the synaptic density from regions of visual cortex representing the more peripheral parts of the visual field do not show a significant decline in synaptic density after 10 postnatal weeks. The decrease in synaptic density that occurs postnatally may correlate to the apparent reduction in available target sites (reduction in dendritic spines). This thinning process has been suggested to be the result of eliminating inappropriate connections or those that have been ineffective in driving the postsynaptic neuron during development.

The establishment of normally functioning circuitry in the visual cortex is known to be susceptible to environmental influences during the critical period of postnatal development (Hubel and Wiesel, 1963; Wiesel and Hubel, 1965; Hubel et al., 1977; see Chapter 4, this volume). Several substances [including norepinephrine, acetylcholine, and 5-hydroxytryptamine (5HT)] have been suggested to play a role in this plasticity (Kasamatsu, 1983; Bear and Singer, 1986). Therefore, the ontogeny of these chemicals' distributions, their synthetic and degradative enzymes, and their receptors has become a matter of considerable interest. The postnatal development of acetylcholinesterase (AchE) activity in visual cortex has been studied in rat (Robertson et al., 1985), cat (Bear et al., 1985), and monkey and human (Kostovic and Rakic, 1984). In rat, AchE levels first become noticeable at postnatal day 7 in layer IV. Staining intensity peaks at 2 postnatal weeks, then declines, and disappears by 3 postnatal weeks. This period of peaked AchE levels is thought to be associated with the time of establishment of functional geniculocortical circuitry. In cat, AchE levels do not become fully developed until 3 months postnatal. Levels in layers IV and VI peak at 1–2 months postnatal and then decline (see Figure 19). Layer VI cells transiently express AchE activity while layer V cells appear positive for AchE only later. Cholinesterase activity in monkey and human prestriate visual cortex develops with the pulvinar's projection to these areas. Ach binding sites can be labeled with a tritiated muscarinic antagonist (Shaw et al., 1984) at 3 postnatal days in layer IV of the visual cortex of the kitten. The number of binding sites peaked at 1 month and by 3 months layer IV had the lease dense binding.

Levels of 5HT in visual cortex have been studied during development in rat (Cano and Reinoso-Suarez, 1982) and monkey (Foote and Morrison, 1984). In both cases, a considerable increase occurs postnatally. In monkey, a strong 5HT projection to layer IV is apparent at birth. By 6 postnatal weeks, the adult patterns of heavy 5HT levels in layers IV_b and IV_c occur. Noradrenergic fibers also show an increase during this period in the monkey. Their density increases throughout the cortical layers over about 2 postnatal months (but remain less dense than the 5HT fibers).

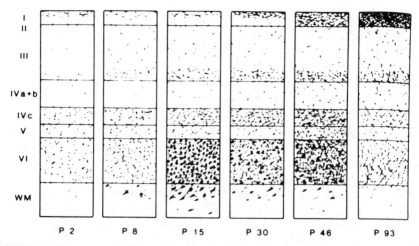

FIGURE 19. Summary drawing of the postnatal changes in the distribution of acetylcholinesterase staining in kitten striate cortex. Cortical layers are indicated as well as various postnatal ages (days) studied. (From Bear et al., 1985.)

VIII PHYSIOLOGICAL DEVELOPMENT OF THE VISUAL CORTEX

The development of the functional properties of visual cortical neurons has been evaluated in numerous studies. In addition to explaining the ontogeny of visual processing, many of these studies have sought to address the more general question: To what degree does the brain's functional circuitry depend on environmental cues versus innate factors? The more complete studies have been carried out in the cat, and these studies will provide the basis for discussion in most of this section.

Hubel and Wiesel (1963) initially suggested that many of the fundamental properties of the neurons in kitten visual cortex were already in place in neonates (1–3 postnatal weeks). These features include those characteristic of adult cat visual cortical neurons: orientation selectivity, direction selectivity, cell types with recognizable "simple" or "complex" receptive field organization (Hubel and Wiesel, 1963), and various levels of binocularity. However, they did note that there were also some considerable differences between the properties of neurons in neonates versus adults. These included difficulty in finding the appropriate visual stimulus to activate neurons, sluggish spontaneous activity, unusually large receptive fields, and a significant recovery time necessary for a neuron to become responsive to repeated visual stimulation. Other reports find varying degrees of mature responses in neurons of kitten visual cortex. For example, several investigators (Barlow and Pettigrew, 1971; Pettigrew, 1974; Buisseret and Imbert, 1976; Fregnac and Imbert, 1978) report that many properties of the kitten cortical neurons are immature (such as orientation selectivity). Blakemore and Van Sluyters (1975) found that some orientation-selective cells were present at the time of eye opening in the kitten, but this fraction increases during the first postnatal month [see Fregnac and Imbert (1984) for a detailed review of this subject].

In a more recent study (Albus and Wolf, 1984), the frequency of occurrence of visually responsive neurons was found to be adultlike at 1–3 postnatal weeks in cortical layers IV and VI. However, neurons in other layers (II, III, and V) were later to develop visual responses. The fraction of orientation-selective cells was significant (69%) in the 1-week kitten and increased to adult levels by 4 postnatal weeks (Figure 20). The fraction of neurons that could be classified as having adultlike receptive field properties ("simple" versus "complex" and flanking excitatory and suppressive zones) was, however, quite small in the 2-week kittens in this study (45%). Most receptive fields had only a single excitatory region that responded to decreased illumination alone. The postnatal development of the receptive field architecture has recently been described (Braastad and Heggelund, 1985). Using quantitative methods employing dual visual stimuli to separately evaluate the enhancement and suppressive zones of cortical neurons' receptive fields, these authors also report that most cells can be identified as having "simple" or "complex" receptive fields by 8 postnatal days (at the time of eye opening) in the kitten. In relative terms, the suppressive zones are as strong in the youngest kittens as in the adult cats. The sizes of the individual zones and the distance between zones in the receptive fields decrease during development. Overall, the orientation selectivity (both in terms of the fraction of neurons having this property and the degree of orientation selectivity by individual neurons) increases significantly between 2 and 5 postnatal weeks. By comparing these data on cortical neuron receptive field zones to the data on the postnatal development of retinal ganglion cell receptive field center sizes, the authors conclude that prior to 6 postnatal weeks, the larger sizes of receptive fields of cortical neurons are due to intrinsic neural factors, but after 6 weeks, the changes can be largely explained by growth of the eye alone. This result is similar to that which we have shown in Figure 14 for changes in LGN_d neuron receptive field size.

Derrington and Fuchs (1981) used drifting sinusoidal grating patterns to activate neurons in kitten visual (at ages 2–12 weeks postnatal) cortex. In this experiment, they derived the spatial frequency tuning curves for cortical neurons. At 2 weeks, most cells have poor contrast sensitivity with responses only at low spatial frequencies (see Figure 21). The spatial frequency selectivity increases significantly by 6 weeks postnatally. Both the number of neurons showing this selectivity and the degree of selectivity increase. An increase in the best spatial frequency occurs more gradually (over 12 weeks).

The degree of binocular interaction in kitten visual cortex has been considered normal (Hubel and Wiesel, 1963; Albus and Wolf, 1984; Freeman

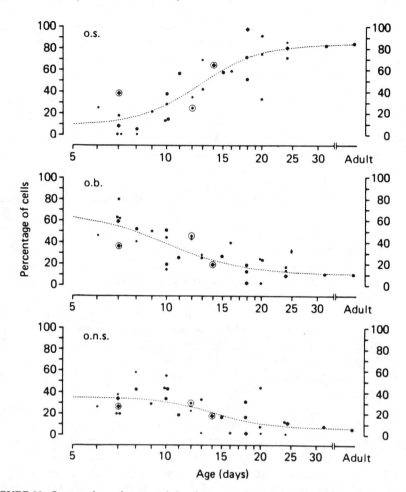

FIGURE 20. Scatter plots of postnatal development of orientation specificity in the kitten's visual cortex. The relative number of orientation-selective (o.s.), orientation-biased (o.b.), and orientation-nonspecific (o.n.s.) neurons are given for each kitten and plotted for each age kitten studied. Solid circles are from neurons with receptive fields located within 15° of the representation of the area centralis; diamonds are for those beyond 15°. Circles around symbols indicate samples from area 18. Curves are fitted by least-squares method. (From Albus and Wolf, 1984.)

and Ohzawa, 1986) or weighted toward greater binocular interactions than in the adult (LeVay et al., 1978). The latter suggestions has been related to the observation that ocular dominance columns (as measured anatomically) are less distinct in the neonate than in the adult (Figure 22). The less distinct nature of these columns in the neonate versus the adult cat is apparent in the horizontal sections through the striate cortex of kitten (Figures 22A,B) compared to adult cat (Figure 22C). By using the method of transynaptic

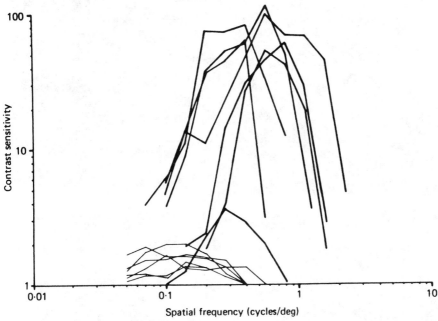

FIGURE 21. Spatial frequency tuning curves for area 17 neurons in a 2-postnatal-week (narrow lines) and 8-postnatal-week (wide lines) kitten. Each point represents the reciprocal of the geometric mean of four estimates of the contrast threshold. Receptive fields of all neurons are located within 2–10° of the representation of central vision. (From Derrington and Fuchs, 1981.)

anterograde transport of tritiated amino acids from the eye and correcting for "spillover" between the closely opposed LGN_d layers in the neonate, Levay et al. (1978) concluded that greater overlap between LGN_d afferents innervated by the right and left eyes occurs in the neonate. The consequences of increased overlap of the terminal arborizations of axons of LGN_d neurons or intracortical neurons in visual cortex may be a greater incidence of convergent excitatory binocular input. However, it should be recognized that while such a process may involve retraction of initially exuberant projections, a similar result would obtain if a rearrangement of the degree of overlap of axon arborizations from cells driven by the right or left eye occurred. More recent experiments (Friedlander and Martin, 1989) that directly evaluated the developmental changes that occur in one type of geniculocortical axon arborization (Y-axons projecting to visual cortical area 18 in kittens) found that the individual axon arborizations are not exuberant in terms of cortical coverage but slightly expand during the postnatal period (see Figure 23). The kitten geniculocortical Y-axons' terminal arborizations are therefore not "exuberant" in terms of cortical surface area innervated. However, quantitative analysis of the density of each axon's cortical innervation has revealed that the 5-week-old kitten geniculocortical Y-axons

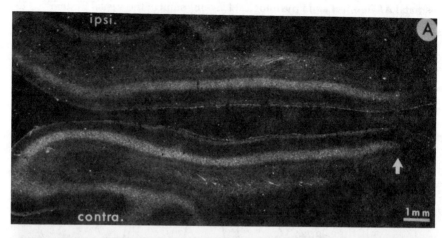

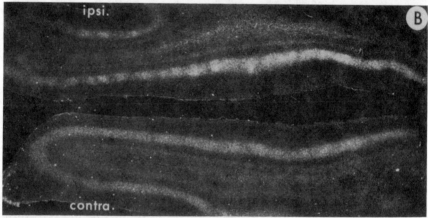

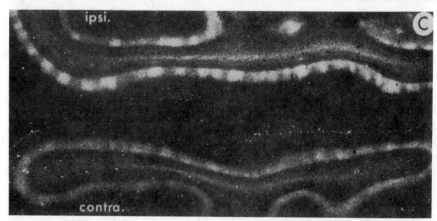

FIGURE 22. Dark-field autoradiographs of horizontal sections through the striate cortex of kittens at postnatal days (A) 15, (B) 22 and (C) 39 that received a unilateral injection of tritiated proline in the vitreas body of an eye 7 days prior to perfusion. The distribution of ocular dominance columns representing transsynaptic transport of the tracer from the retinal ganglion cells through the LGN$_d$ and to the visual cortex is visualized by the white areas representing

(particularly those projecting to cortical area 18) provide a greater concentration of synaptic boutons per unit volume of cerebral cortex (Friedlander and Martin, 1989). This finding is in agreement with Cragg's (1975) observation that the peak synaptic density in kitten visual cortex occurs at approximately 5 postnatal weeks with a subsequent 40% decline to adult values (see Figure 18). Future experiments using direct marking of individual axon arborizations in the neonate should be applied to X-axons as well. However, as discussed in Section VI, this type of study must employ a multivariate cluster analysis approach since some of the LGN$_d$ Y-cells in the neonate might otherwise be incorrectly classified as X if only a single classificatory test is used. In future studies, methods that can dynamically assess the size and structure of individual geniculocortical axon arborizations as they develop (as with time lapse video microscopy of individual neurons in cell culture) are necessary in order to more directly evaluate these changes.

Overall, it appears that some of the basic circuitry for mediating the responses of kitten visual cortical neurons is in place at the time of eye opening. However, in addition to an increase in the robustness of visual responses during postnatal development, it appears that considerable specificity is added to the system during this period. In the newborn monkey striate cortex, both anatomical (Hubel et al., 1977) and physiological (Wiesel and Hubel, 1974) evidence demonstrates a remarkable degree of maturity. While labeling of ocular dominance columns is slightly less distinct in the newborn monkey, by 3 postnatal weeks the pattern is very adultlike. Physiologically, a slightly higher incidence of binocular excitatory mixing occurs in layer IVc in the young animals. Moreover, the organization of orientation columns and the orientation tuning of individual neurons is remarkably developed in the newborn monkey.

The degree to which this increased specificity that occurs postnatally is due to the development of intracortical circuits is still unclear. Komatsu (1983) found that synaptic inhibition is reliably elicited in most neurons from kitten visual cortex (by age 15 days) in the *in vitro* slice preparation. Moreover, Braastad and Heggelund, (1985) evaluated the strengths of flanking suppressive zones of the cortical neurons' receptive fields to be relatively mature in the neonates. In a recent study (Wolf et al., 1986) the majority of neurons in 1- to 4-postnatal-week kitten striate cortex that showed orientation sensitivity (58%) had this property reduced or eliminated with the microiontophoretic administration of the GABA antagonist, bicuculline methiodide. This effect is similar to that for neurons in the adult cat visual cortex (Sillito et al., 1980). The implication of this experiment is

---

exposed silver grains in the overlying autoradiographic emulsion. Note that the separation of ocular dominance columns as represented by dark gaps between the label from the eye's projection is quite distinct in the older kitten, less so in the 22-postnatal-day kitten and hardly visible in the 15-postnatal-day kitten. The columns are more apparent in the visual cortex lateral to the side of the eye injection in kittens and adult cats. (From LeVay et al., 1978.)

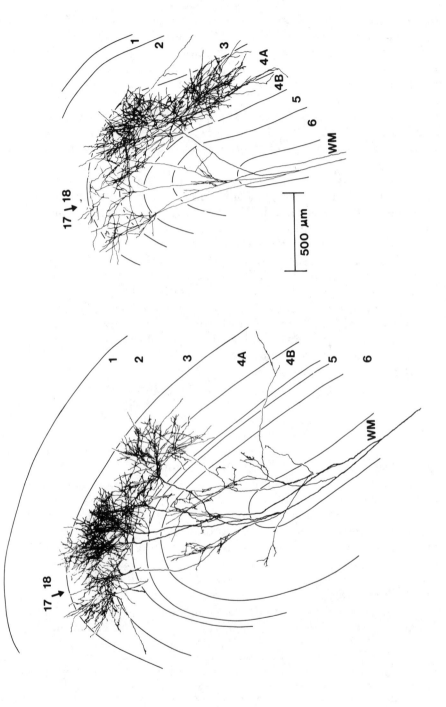

that local inhibitory circuits utilizing GABA in the visual cortex are mediating a considerable amount of the inhibition that confers orientation selectivity upon the cortical neurons. Immunocytochemical localization of glutamic acid decarboxylase (GAD) in kitten visual cortex also has an adultlike distribution at 5 postnatal weeks (Bear et al., 1985). However, in rats the number of GABA profiles shows a significant increase during postnatal development (Wolff et al., 1984). An alternative explanation for the considerable orientation selectivity in the neonate would be that this type of receptive field organization is constructed by convergent excitatory synaptic inputs from neighboring LGN_d neurons and that the increased orientation tuning that develops postnatally results from adding intracortical inhibitory effects to this. However, the bicuculline experiment suggests that the basic inhibitory circuit is in place in the neonate.

Finally, it is of interest to know to what degree the visual input is restricted to the visual cortex specifically during postnatal development. An emerging concept in developmental neurobiology holds that initial projections show "exuberance" or less specificity when compared to their adult counterparts. Early reports using surface recordings of evoked potentials (Ellingson and Wilcott, 1960) suggested that responses to visual stimuli in neonates resulted in activity over a variety of cortical areas beyond visual cortex. A more recent study (Kato et al., 1983) employed laminar analysis of field potentials with microelectrodes. These results showed that polarity reversals of the field potential in the depth of the cortex occurred only in visual cortex (areas 17, 18, and 19 and the lateral suprasylvian cortex) in response to visual stimuli in neonatal kittens. While other cortical areas showed a response when surface recordings were made with large electrodes, polarity reversal with depth indicative of a direct visual projection

---

FIGURE 23. Drawings of individual geniculocortical Y-axons in the adult cat (left) and 4½-postnatal-week kitten (right). In both cases, the axon was first identified by electrophysiological criteria including the property of nonlinear spatial summation by recording from the axon with a micropipette filled with 4% horseradish peroxidase (HRP). After recording from the axon intracellulary, the HRP was ionophoresed into the single axon. After appropriate histochemical processing, the axons' terminal arborizations were serially reconstructed from 25–50 serial sections each of 100 μm thickness. Both axons had similar receptive field locations and projected predominantly to visual cortical area 18. Both projected predominantly to the upper half of cortical layer 4 (layer 4A) and issued several thousand *en passant* boutons in this region (which were found to correlate to regions of presynaptic specialization in over 90% of the 200 sample boutons that were also studied at the electron microscope level). In the two-dimensional drawings of the terminal arborizations it appears that the adult axon more densely innervates layer IV than does the kitten axon. However, this is only apparent due to the adult axon spanning many more serial sections than the kitten axon. The surface area of cortical layer 4 occupied by the adult Y-axon is approximately 30% greater than that of the kitten axon. However, the kitten axon more densely innervates a smaller cortical area; that is, the kitten axon issues a greater number of boutons per unit area. These examples are typical of a larger sample of such physiologically and morphologically identified geniculocortical Y-axons projecting to cortical area 18 in kittens and adult cats (Friedlander and Martin, 1989.)

was not seen in these regions. Therefore, functional geniculocortical projections seem to be restricted to the appropriate cortical regions in the neonate. Moreover, geniculocortical afferents in the newborn kitten appear restricted to the region of presumptive visual cortex (Shatz and Luskin, 1986).

IX   DEVELOPMENT OF THE SUPERIOR COLLICULUS

The superior colliculus (SC) plays a central role in sensorimotor integration and control of eye and head movements. In addition to receiving a direct retinal projection, the SC is also a link in the geniculocortical system. The SC receives a projection from visual cortex as well as projecting to the LGN_d and pulvinar (Huerta and Harting, 1984). The mechanisms by which the SC controls eye movements in adult animals are discussed in a recent review (Sparks, 1986).

The neurons of the SC are arranged in several layers (Kanaseki and Sprague, 1974). Visually driven cells occur more predominantly in the superficial layers versus the deeper layers. The cells in the deeper layers generally have larger receptive fields than those in the superficial layers. In addition to receiving a direct retinal projection (predominantly from Y and W retinal ganglion cells in the cat), the neurons of the cat SC also receive a descending corticotectal projection from cells in layer V of visual cortex (Palmer and Rosenquist, 1974; Gilbert and Kelly, 1975) and require this projection for many of their receptive field properties (Wickelgren and Sterling, 1969). This pathway is largely composed of Y-afferents (the Y indirect pathway from retina to LGN_d to visual cortex to SC). The response properties of neurons in the SC differ from those of LGN_d neurons in several ways: they generally respond best to moving stimuli with characteristic direction and velocity; they have larger receptive fields; they are binocularly excited; and they tend to show a decremental response to regularly repeated visual stimulation. These properties vary between cells in layers and between layers.

The projections to the SC develop early. Both the retinotectal (Graybiel, 1975; Williams and Chalupa, 1982) and corticotectal (Stein and Edwards, 1979; Williams and Chalupa, 1982; Tsumoto et al., 1983) projections are in place on or before the day of birth in kitten. The cortical layer V cells that project to the SC are more widely distributed and densely packed in the newborn kitten than in the adult cat (Tsumoto et al., 1983). Using retrograde HRP filling of corticotectal cells, these authors concluded that the density of such cells declines in the second postnatal week as axon collaterals are eliminated. The trigeminal projection to the newborn kitten SC also appears mature in its distribution as evaluated with neuroanatomical tracing methods (McHaffie et al., 1986). Overall, the major afferentation of the kitten SC is established by birth. However, it is not known if the precision, synaptic efficacy, and ultrastructural development of these projections are also mature.

The efferent projections of the SC are also strikingly adultlike at birth. Collicular innervation of the parabigeminal nucleus, dorsal lateral pons, and inferior olive (Stein et al., 1984) and ventral central grey matter overlying the oculomotor nucleus (Stein et al., 1982) is present in the neonate. The projection to the paralemniscal zone shows some organizational changes during the postnatal period. The most striking difference in the efferent projections of the neonatal versus adult superior colliculus is from the SC to the LGN_d. In adult animals, this projection is from the cells of the superficial layers of the SC (in stratum griseum superficiale) to the ventral C layers of the LGN_d, which contain W-cells (Graham, 1977; Hughes and Mullikin, 1984). However, in neonatal kittens the projection from the same part of the SC, which itself receives a substantial W-cell projection from retina, is to all LGN_d layers in addition to the interlaminar zones and the MIN (Stein et al., 1985; Figure 24). These projections are lost between postnatal weeks 2 and

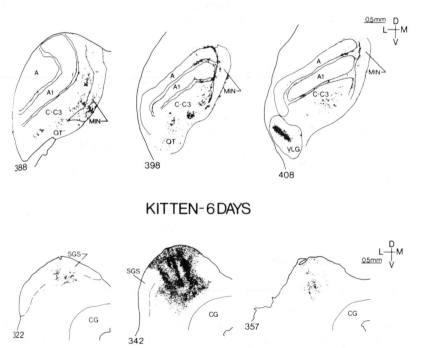

KITTEN-6 DAYS

FIGURE 24. Distribution of transported label to the LGN_d after injection of ^{3}H-leucine in the superior colliculus of a 6-day-old kitten. Dark dots represent the distribution of silver grains on an autoradiographic emulsion. Top row has three sections through kitten LGN_d (arranged rostral to caudal, left to right). Bottom row has three sections through the injection site in the superior colliculus. Note the presence of significant label across all layers, in the interlaminar zones, MIN, ventral lateral geniculate nucleus, and above the dorsal border of the LGN_d. The colliculogeniculate projection is much more extensive than in the adult cat where the projection to the LGN_d is confined to the lower C layers. (From Stein et al., 1985.)

3. This transient projection to regions of the LGN_d that contain cell types that do not receive SC input in the adult, particularly X-cells, suggests that the retinogeniculate pathway of neonates may be transmitting a substantially different signal to the striate cortex of neonates versus adults.

It is tempting to speculate that the kitten striate cortex is a W-cell-dominated system. We have already described (Section VII) the early development of the W-cells in the C layers of the kitten LGN_d and the rich projection to cortical layer I (which also includes a projection from cells of the A layers in kittens, Kato et al., 1984). This, coupled with a possible W indirect retinocolliculur–LGN_d–cortical projection potentially provides the visual cortex with a disproportionately large influence from this channel. The visual sensitivity of kittens as measured behaviorally (see Chapter 3) is quite low when compared to the adult. Similarly, the contrast sensitivity of adult cat LGN_d W-cells is very low (Sur and Sherman, 1982b). Therefore, the mature (anatomically) and exuberant W pathways of the neonate may provide the neurophysiological substrate that limits visual sensitivity. During postnatal development, the emerging X and Y systems would then provide the basis for increased visual performance. The exuberant W system thus serves as a functional pioneer pathway while the more dynamic X and Y systems are free to continue synaptic reorganization. Alternatively, the exuberant geniculocortical projection to cortical layer I may reflect the transfer of a chemical specificity signal. The "normal" LGN_d ventral C-layer projection to layer I may be the result of some signal that the LGN_d cells receive from W retinal ganglion cells and/or tectal W-cells. Likewise, the LGN_d neurons of the neonate's interlaminar zones and A layers that project transiently to cortical layer I may do so by virtue of their transient innervation by tectal W-cells.

The visual response properties of kitten SC cells are extremely immature when compared to those of adult cats. Visually elicited responses are not recorded until postnatal day 7 (Stein et al., 1973a,b). When responses do appear, they are immature with respect to a number of properties including strong monocular (contralateral) dominance, lack of directional selectivity, extreme response variability and habituation, reduced velocity preference, and large receptive fields without suppressive flanks [Stein et al., 1973a,b; Norton, 1974; Stein and Gallagher, 1981; see Stein (1984) for a review]. The development of these properties is illustrated in Figure 25. Note that the development of binocular responses occurs considerably later than the anatomical appearance of the corticotectal projection. This suggests that these synaptic circuits are functionally immature and/or the source of the binocular drive to the SC cells (the cortical layer V cells) are late to develop. It is an interesting contrast that most of the major pathways to and from the mammalian SC are present at birth, but a considerable period of postnatal development is necessary for the visual responses of the SC neurons to mature. Moreover, a variety of visual behaviors thought to be mediated through the SC are very poorly developed in the neonate (Norton, 1974).

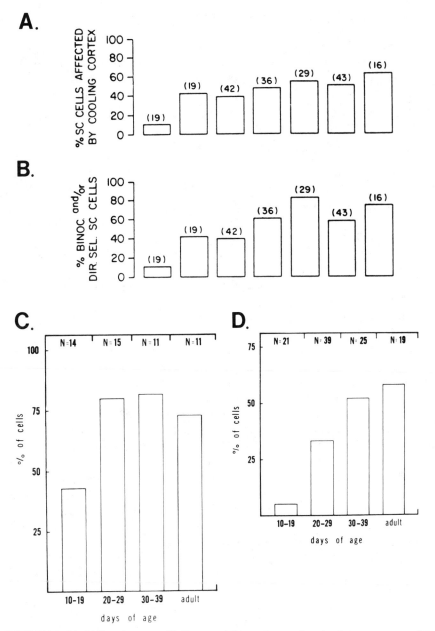

FIGURE 25. (*A, B*) Developmental influence of the corticotectal projection on neurons of the superior colliculus. In (*A*), the percentage of collicular cells affected by cooling of visual cortex is represented. A large increase in the cells so affected occurs in the third week. In (*B*), the percentage of collicular neurons with binocular visual responses and directional selectivity is represented as a function of postnatal age. Sample sizes are printed above each group. Panels represent, from left to right, groups at ages 8–12 days, 13–14 days, 3 weeks, 4 weeks, 5 weeks, 6–8 weeks, and adult. Reprinted from Stein and Gallagher, 1981. (*C*) Development of receptive field surround inhibition in the kitten superior colliculus. Bars indicate percentage of neurons that showed a minimum criteria of inhibition. (*D*) Development of direction selectivity in the kitten superior colliculus. Bars indicate proportion of neurons at each age that showed directional selectivity. (*C*) and (*D*) (From Norton, 1974.)

Much of the SC motor projections appear to be functional in the neonate (Stein et al., 1980), although some loci in the SC are incapable of generating eye movements in response to electrical stimulation. To what degree the immaturity of the integration of sensory inputs versus the motor transformations that occur in the SC contribute to the weak visual orienting of the neonate remains to be determined.

X CONCLUSIONS

The mammalian visual system undergoes a variety of profound changes in structure and function during postnatal development. However, what is most striking is the degree to which the basic functional circuits are in place at or near the time of parturition. The basic functional architecture of the receptive field of retinal ganglion cells, LGN_d, and visual cortical neurons develop very early. This specificity is largely under genetic control. One of the great challenges to students of development of sensory systems is to determine the genetic basis of this developmental program and how the microenvironment and spatio-temporal activity patterns of the nervous system contribute to cellular form and the establishment of specific synaptic circuitry.

The studies considered in this chapter point out some of the differences in the strategies of neural development between species. For example, the cat and monkey retinogeniculate pathways have different arrangements of the functional cell types. This may contribute to different modes of interactions between neighboring neurons during development (e.g., between X and Y retinal axons). Moreover, the optical quality and time of eye opening differs between these species. The optically delayed onset of patterned vision in the kitten may "permit" a more protracted period for the basic elaboration of the parallel circuits in this species. However, it appears that in all mammalian species studied, the spatial resolving capacity and briskness of visual responses require an extended period of postnatal maturation. It should also be emphasized that a significant fraction of this improvement is due to factors of neural maturation versus changes in the optical media and geometry. The mechanism of that reduction in receptive field size has not yet been elucidated for the mammalian retina, thalamus, or visual cortex. A major question that remains is to understand the functional and anatomical basis of these changes at the level of the neonatal retina. Studies employing quantitative analysis of the biophysical and neurophysiological properties of neonatal retinal ganglion cells (including intraocular recording from *in vivo* preparations and *in vitro* studies) and correlated morphology are necessary to directly evaluate the mechanisms underlying these changes. Finally, the recent appreciation of the postnatal development of various neurotransmitter systems in the visual cortex is an encouraging research direction that may provide an understanding of the basis for the dramatic sensitivity of the cerebral cortex to the sensory environment.

ACKNOWLEDGMENTS

The preparation of this chapter and the research of the authors considered in the text was supported by National Science Foundation grant BNS 8720069 and National Institutes of Health grant EY 05116. We also thank Ms. Judith L. Rodda for her expert assistance in preparation of the figures, Ms. Rhea McKinney and Diana Pullen for their superb word-processing skills, and Beverly La Borde Friedlander and Wendy Marsh-Tootle for their patience and support.

REFERENCES

Abramov, I., J. Gordon, A. Hendrickson, L. Hainline, V. Dobson, and E. Labossiere (1982) The retina of the newborn human infant. Science 217:265–267.

Aguirre, G. D., L. F. Rubin, and S. I. Bistner (1972) Development of the canine eye. Amer. J. Vet. Res. 33:2399–2414.

Albus, K., and W. Wolf (1984) Early postnatal development of neuronal functions in kitten's visual cortex: A laminar analysis. J. Physiol. (Lond.) 348:153–185.

Anker, R. L., and B. C. Cragg (1974) Development of the extrinsic connections of the visual cortex in the cat. J. Comp. Neurol. 154:29–42.

Armington, J. C. (1974) The electroretinogram. New York: Academic Press.

Barlow, H. B., and J. D. Pettigrew (1971) Lack of specificity of neurones in the visual cortex of young kittens. J. Physiol. (Lond.) 218:98–100.

Bear, M. F., and W. Singer (1986) Modulation of visual cortical plasticity by acetylcholine and noradrenaline. Nature 320:172.

Bear, M. F., D. G. Schmechel, and F. F. Ebner (1985) Glutamic acid decarboxylase in the striate cortex of normal and monocularly deprived kittens. J. Neurosci. 5:1262–1275.

Becker, L. E., D. L. Armstrong, F. Chan, and M. M. Wood (1984) Dendritic development in human occipital cortical neurons. Dev. Brain Res. 13:117–124.

Berardi, N., and M. C. Morrone (1984) Development of γ-aminobutyric acid mediated inhibition of X-cells in the cat lateral geniculate nucleus. J. Physiol. (Lond.) 357:505–523.

Blakemore, C., and R. C. Van Sluyters (1975) Innate and environmental factors in the development of kitten visual cortex. J. Physiol. (Lond.) 248:663–716.

Blakemore, C., and F. Vital-Durand (1986) Organizaiton and post-natal development of the monkey's lateral geniculate nucleus. J. Physiol. (Lond.) 380:453–491.

Blanks, J. C., A. M. Adinolfi, and R. N. Lolley (1974) Synaptogenesis of the photoreceptor terminal of the mouse retina. J. Comp. Neurol. 156:81–94.

Boettner, E. A., and J. R. Walter (1962) Transmission of the ocular media. Technical documentary report no. MRL-TDR-62-34. Wright-Patterson Air Force Base.

Bonds, A. B., and R. D. Freeman (1978) Development of the optical quality of the kitten eye. Vision Res. *18*:391–398.

Boothe, R. G. (1982) Optical and neural factors limiting acuity development: Evidence obtained from a monkey model. Curr. Eye Res. *2*:211–215.

Boothe, R. G., W. T. Greenough, J. S. Lund, and K. Wrege (1979) A quantitative investigation of spine and dendritic development of neurons in visual cortex (area 17) of Macaca nemestrina monkeys. J. Comp. Neurol. *186*:473–490.

Bowe-Anders, C., R. F. Miller, and R. Dacheux (1975) Developmental characteristics of receptive organization in the isolated retina-eyecup of the rabbit. Brain Res. *87*:61–65.

Bowling, D. B., and C. M. Michael (1980) Projection patterns of single physiologically identified optic tract fibres in the cat. Nature *286*:899–902.

Bowling, D. B., and C. R. Michael (1984) Terminal patterns of single, physiologically characterized optic tract fibers in the cat's lateral geniculate nucleus. J. Neurosci. *4*:198–216.

Boycott, B. B., and H. Wassle (1974) The morphological types of ganglion cells of the domestic cat's retina. J. Physiol. (Lond.) *240*:397–419.

Braastad, B. O., and P. Heggelund (1985) Development of spatial receptive-field organization and orientation selectivity in kitten striate cortex. J. Neurophysiol. *53*:1158–1178.

Buisseret, P., and M. Imbert (1976) Visual cortical cells: Their developmental processes in normal and dark reared kittens. J. Physiol. (Lond.) *255*:511–525.

Cano, J., and F. Reinoso-Suarez (1982) Postnatal development in the serotonin content of brain visual structures. Dev. Brain Res. *5*:199–201.

Cleland, B. G., and W. R. Levick (1974) Brisk and sluggish concentrically organized ganglion cells in the cat's retina. J. Physiol. (Lond.) *240*:421–456.

Cleland, B. G., M. W. Dubin, and W. R. Levick (1971) Sustained and transient neurones in the cat's retina and lateral geniculate nucleus. J. Physiol. (Lond.) *217*:473–496.

Cleland, B. G., W. R. Levick, R. Morstyn, and H. G. Wagner (1976) Lateral geniculate relay of slowly conducting retinal afferents to cat visual cortex. J. Physiol. (Lond.) *255*:299–320.

Cleland, B. G., W. R. Levick, R. Morstyn, and H. G. Wagner (1976) Lateral geniculate relay of slowly conducting retinal afferents to cat visual cortex. J. Physiol. (Lond.) *255*:299–320.

Cragg, B. G. (1975) The development of synapses in the visual system of the cat. J. Comp. Neurol. *160*:147–166.

Daniels, J. D., J. D. Pettigrew, and J. L. Norman (1978) Development of single-neuron responses in kitten's lateral geniculate nucleus. J. Neurophysiol. *41*:1373–1393.

Dann, J. F., E. H. Buhl, and L. Peichl (1988) Postnatal dendritic maturation of alpha and beta ganglion cells in cat retina. J. Neurosci. *8*:1485–1489.

deCourten, C., and L. J. Garey (1982) Morphology of the neurons in the human lateral geniculate nucleus and their normal development. Exp. Brain Res. *47*:159–171.

Derrington, A. M., and A. F. Fuchs (1981) The development of spatial-frequency selectivity in kitten striate cortex. J. Physiol. (Lond.) *316*:1–10.

Dixon, J. W., and M. B. Brown, eds. (1979) BMDP Biomedical Computer Programs. Berkeley: University of California Press.

Dowling, J. E. (1970) Organization of vertebrate retinas. Inv. Ophthalmol. *9*:655–680.

Dreher, B., and A. J. Sefton (1979) Properties of neurones in cat's dorsal lateral geniculate nucleus: A comparison between medial interlaminar and laminated parts of the nucleus. J. Comp. Neurol. *183*:47–63.

Dunlop, S. A., and L. D. Beazley (1985) Changing distribution of retinal ganglion cells during area centralis and visual streak formation in the marsupial *Setonix brachyurus*. Dev. Brain Res. *23*:81–90.

Ellingson, R. J., and R. C. Wilcott (1960) Development of evoked responses in visual and auditory cortices of kittens. J. Neurophysiol. *23*:363–375.

Engleman, L. (1980) Annotated computer output for BMDP K-means clustering. BMDP technical report #71. Los Angeles: BMDP Statistical Software.

Enroth-Cugell, C., and J. G. Robson (1966) The contrast sensitivity of retinal ganglion cells in the cat. J. Physiol. (Lond.) *187*:517–552.

Everitt, B. (1980) Cluster Analysis. New York: Halstead.

Foote, S. L., and J. H. Morrison (1984) Postnatal development of laminar innervation patterns by monoaminergic fibers in monkey (*Macaca fasicularis*) primary visual cortex. J. Neurosci. *11*:2667–2680.

Freeman, R. D., and C. E. Lai (1978) Development of the optical surfaces of the kitten eye. Vision Res. *18*:399–407.

Freeman, R. D., and I. Ohzawa (1986) Binocular interaction in young kittens. Soc. Neurosci. Abstr. *12*:784.

Fregnac, Y., and M. Imbert (1978) Early development of visual cortical cells in normal and dark-reared kittens. Relationship between orientation selectivity and ocular dominance. J. Physiol. (Lond.) *278*:27–44.

Fregnac, Y., and M. Imbert (1984) Development of neuronal selectivity in primary visual cortex of cat. Physiol. Rev. *64*:325–434.

Freund, T. F., K. A. C. Martin, and D. Whitteridge (1985a) Innervation of cat visual areas 17 and 18 by physiologically identified X- and Y-type thalamic afferents. I. Arborization patterns and quantitative distribution of postsynaptic elements. J. Comp. Neurol. *242*:263–274.

Freund, T. F., K. A. C. Martin, P. Somogyi, and D. Whitteridge (1985b) Innervation of cat visual areas 17 and 18 by physiologically identified X- and Y-type thalamic afferents. II. Identification of postsynaptic targets by GABA immunocytochemistry and Golgi impregnation. J. Comp. Neurol. *242*:275–291.

Friedlander, M. J. (1982) Structure of physiologically classified neurones in the kitten dorsal lateral geniculate nucleus. Nature *200*:180–183.

Friedlander, M. J. (1984) The postnatal development of the kitten dorsal lateral geniculate nucleus. In J. Stone, B. Dreher, and D. Rapaport (eds.): Development of Visual Pathways in Mammals. New York: Alan R. Liss. pp. 155–173.

Friedlander, M. J., and K. A. C. Martin (1981) An examination of the morphology and the response to visual and electrical stimulation of neurons in area 17 of kittens visual cortex. J. Physiol. (Lond.) *325*:79p.

Friedlander, M. J., and L. R. Stanford (1984) The effect of monocular deprivation on the distribution of cell types in the cat's dorsal lateral geniculate nucleus: A sampling study with fine-tipped micropipettes. Exp. Brain Res. 53:451–461.

Friedlander, M. J., C.-S. Lin, L. R. Stanford, and S. M. Sherman (1981) Morphology of functionally identified neurons in the dorsal lateral geniculate nucleus of cat. J. Neurophysiol. 46:80–129.

Friedlander, M. J., L. R. Stanford, and S. M. Sherman (1982) Effects of monocular deprivation on the structure-function relationship of individual neurons in the cat's lateral geniculate nucleus. J. Neurosci. 2:321–330.

Friedlander, M. J., K. A. C. Martin, and C. Vahle-Hinz (1983) The postnatal development of structure of physiologically identified retinal ganglion cell (r.g.c.) axons in the kitten. J. Physiol. (Lond.) 336:28p.

Friedlander, M. J. and K. A. C. Martin (1989) Development of Y-axon innervation of cortical area 18 in the cat. J. Physiol. (Lond.) 416:183–213.

Friedlander, M. J., K. A. C. Martin, and C. Vahle-Hinz (1985) The structure of the terminal arborizations of physiologically identified Y-retinal ganglion cell axons in the kitten. J. Physiol. (Lond.) 359:293–313.

Garey, L. J. (1984) Structural development of the visual system of man. Human Neurobiol. 3:75–80.

Garey, L. J., and K. D. Saini (1981) Golgi studies of the normal development of neurons in the lateral geniculate nucleus of the monkey. Exp. Brain Res. 44:117–128.

Garey, L. J., R. A. Fisken, and T. P. S. Powell (1973) Effects of experimental deafferentation on cells in the lateral geniculate nucleus of the cat. Brain Res. 52:363–369.

Gilbert, C. D., and J. P. Kelly (1975) The projection of cells in different layers of the cat's visual cortex. J. Comp. Neurol. 163:81–106.

Gilbert, C. D., and T. N. Wiesel (1983) Clustered intrinsic connections in cat visual cortex. J. Neurosci. 3:1116–1133.

Gottlieb, M. D., P. Pasik, and T. Pasik (1985) Early postnatal development of the monkey visual system. I. Growth of the lateral geniculate nucleus and striate cortex. Dev. Brain Res. 17:53–62.

Gottlob, I., L. Wundsch and F. K. Tuppy (1988) The rabbit electroretinogram: Effect of GABA and its antagonists. Vis. Res. 28:203–210.

Graham, J. (1977) An autoradiographic study of the efferent connections of the superior colliculus in the cat. J. Comp. Neurol. 173:629–654.

Graybiel, A. M. (1975) Anatomical organization of retinotectal afferents in the cat: An autoradiographic study. Brain Res. 96:1–23.

Guillery, R. W. (1969) A quantitative study of synaptic interconnections in the dorsal lateral geniculate nucleus of the cat. Z. Zellforsch. Mikrosk. Anat. 96:39–48.

Guillery, R. W. (1970) The laminar distribution of retinal fibres in the dorsal lateral geniculate nucleus of the cat. J. Comp. Neurol. 138:339–368.

Guillery, R. W., E. E. Geisert, E. H. Polley, and C. A. Mason (1980) An analysis of the retinal afferents to the cat's medial interlaminar nucleus and to its rostral thalamic extension, the "geniculate wing." J. Comp. Neurol. 194:117–142.

Gunn, G. G., K. N. Gelatt, and D. A. Samuelson (1984) Maturation of the retina of the canine neonate as determined by electroretinography and histology. Am. J. Vet. Res. 45:1166–1171.

Hamasaki, D. I., and J. J. Flynn (1977) Physiological properties of retinal ganglion cells of 3 week-old kittens. Vision Res. 17:275–284.

Hamasaki, D. I., and V. G. Sutija (1979) Development of X- and Y-cells in kittens. Exp. Brain Res. 35:9–23.

Headon, M. W., J. J. Sloper, R. W. Hiorns, and T. P. S. Powell (1985) Effect of monocular closure at different ages on deprived and undeprived cells in the primate lateral geniculate nucleus. Dev. Brain Res. 18:57–78.

Henderson, Z. (1982) An anatomical investigation of projections from lateral geniculate nucleus to visual cortical areas 17 and 18 in newborn kitten. Exp. Brain Res. 46:177–185.

Hendrickson, A., and C. Kupfer (1976) The histogenesis of the fovea in the macaque monkey. Inv. Ophthalmol. 15:746–756.

Hendrickson, A. E., and D. Yuodelis (1984) The morphological development of the human fovea. Ophthalmol. 6:603 612–.

Hickey, T. L. (1977) Postnatal development of the human lateral geniculate nucleus: Relationship to a critical period for the visual system. Science 198:836–838.

Hickey, T. L. (1980) Development of the dorsal lateral geniculate nucleus in normal and visually deprived cats. J. Comp. Neurol. 189:467–482.

Hickey, T. L. (1981) The developing visual system. Trends Neurosci. 4:42–44.

Hoffmann, K. P., J. Stone, and S. M. Sherman (1972) Relay of receptive-field properties in dorsal lateral geniculate nucleus of the cat. J. Neurophysiol. 35:518–531.

Hubel, D. H., and T. N. Wiesel (1963) Receptive fields of cells in striate cortex of very young, visually inexperienced kittens. J. Neurophysiol. 26:994–1002.

Hubel, D. H., T. N. Wiesel, and S. LeVay (1977) Plasticity of ocular dominance columns in macaque striate cortex. Phil. Trans. Roy. Soc. Lond. B. 278:377–410.

Huerta, M. F., and J. K. Harting (1984) The mammalian superior colliculus: Studies of its morphology and connections. In H. Vanegus (ed.): Comparative Neurology of the Optic Tectum. New York: Plenum, pp. 687–773.

Hughes, H. C., and W. H. Mullikin (1984) Brainstem afferents to the lateral geniculate of the cat. Exp. Brain Res. 54:253–258.

Huttenlocher, P. R. (1984) Synapse elimination and plasticity in developing human cerebral cortex. Am. J. Ment. Def. 88:488–496.

Ikeda, H., and K. E. Tremain (1978) The development of spatial resolving power of lateral geniculate neurons in kittens. Exp. Brain Res. 31:193–206.

Ikeda, H., and M. J. Wright (1976) Properties of LGN cells in kittens reared with convergent squint: A neurophysiological demonstration of amblyopia. Exp. Brain Res. 25:63–77.

Innocenti, G. M. (1981) Growth and reshaping of axons in the establishment of visual callosal connections. Science 212:824–827.

Innocenti, G. M., S. Clarke, and R. Kraftsik (1986) Interchange of callosal and association projections in the developing visual cortex. J. Neurosci. 6:1384–1409.

Kalil, R. E. (1978) A quantitative study of the effects of monocular enucleation and deprivation on cell growth in the dorsal lateral geniculate nucleus of the cat. J. Comp. Neurol. *189*:483–524.

Kalil, R. E. (1980) Development of the dorsal lateral geniculate nucleus of the cat. J. Comp. Neurol. *189*:483–524.

Kalil, R. E., R. J. Wenthold, and J. Zempel (1985) Postnatal development of neurons with GABA immunoreactivity in the lateral geniculate nucleus (LGN) and visual cortex of the cat. Soc. Neurosci. Abstr. *11*:806.

Kanaseki, T., and J. M. Sprague (1974) Anatomical organization of pretectal nuclei and tectal laminae in the cat. J. Comp. Neurol. *158*:319–338.

Kasamatsu, T. (1983) Neuronal plasticity maintained by the central norepinephrine system in the cat visual cortex. Prog. Psychobiol. *10*:1–12.

Kato, N., S. Kowaguchi, T. Yamamoto, A. Samejima, and H. Miyata (1983) Postnatal development of the geniculocortical projection in the cat: Electrophysiological and morphological studies. Exp. Brain Res. *51*:65–72.

Kato, N., S. Kowaguchi, and H. Miyata (1984) Geniculocortical projections to layer I of area 17 in kittens: Orthograde and retrograde HRP studies. J. Comp. Neurol. *225*:441–447.

Kennedy, H., K. A. C. Martin, V. M. Rao, and D. Whitteridge (1980) Neuronal plasticity in the visual system of the sheep. In F. Clifford, R. Behan, and P. O. Behan (eds.): Animal Models of Neurological Disease. Tunbridge Wells: Pitman Medical, pp. 249–265.

Kolb, H. (1970) Organization of the outer plexiform layer of the primate retina: Electron microscopy of Golgi-impregnated cells. Phil. Trans. Roy. Soc. Lond. B. *258*:261–283.

Komatsu, Y. (1983) Development of cortical inhibition in kitten striate cortex investigated by a slice preparation. Dev. Brain Res. *8*:136–139.

Koppel, H., and G. M. Innocenti (1983) Is there a genuine exuberancy of callosal projections in development? A quantitative electron microscopic study in the cat. Neurosci. Lett. *41*:33–40.

Kostovic, I., and P. Rakic (1984) Development of prestriate visual projections in the monkey and human fetal cerebrum revealed by transient cholinesterase staining. J. Neurosci. *4*:25–42.

Kratz, K. E., S. V. Webb, and S. M. Sherman (1978) Studies of the cat's medial interlaminar nucleus: A subdivision of the dorsal lateral geniculate nucleus. J. Comp. Neurol. *181*:601–614.

Laemle, L., C. Benhamida, and D. P. Purpura (1972) Laminar distribution of geniculocortical afferents in the visual cortex of the postnatal kitten. Brain Res. *41*:25–37.

Lal, R., and M. J. Friedlander (1989) Gating of retinal transmission by afferent eye position and movement signals. Science *243*:93–96.

Larsen, J. S. (1971) The saggital growth of the eye. IV. Ultrasonic measurement of the axial length of the eye from birth to puberty. Acta. Ophthalmol. *49*:873–886.

Lehmkuhle S., K. E. Kratz, S. C. Mangel, and S. M. Sherman (1980) Spatial and temporal sensitivity of X- and Y-cells in dorsal lateral geniculate nucleus of the cat. J. Neurophysiol. *43*:520–541.

Leuba, G., and L. J. Garey (1984) Development of dendritic patterns in the lateral geniculate nucleus of monkey: A quantitative Golgi study. Dev. Brain Res. *16*:285–299.

LeVay, S., M. P. Stryker, and C. J. Shatz (1978) Ocular dominance columns and their development in layer IV of the cat's visual cortex: A quantitative study. J. Comp. Neurol. 179:223–244.

Leventhal, A. G. (1982) Morphology and distribution of retinal ganglion cells projecting to different layers of the dorsal lateral geniculate nucleus in normal and siamese cats. J. Neurosci. 2:1024–1042.

Leventhal, A. G., and H. V. B. Hirsch (1983) Effects of visual deprivation upon the geniculocortical W-cell pathway in the cat: Area 19 and its afferent input. J. Comp. Neurol. 214:59–71.

Levick, W. R. (1967) Receptive fields and trigger features of ganglion cells in the visual streak of the rabbit retina. J. Physiol. (Lond.) 188:285–307.

Levick, W. R., B. G. Cleland, and M. W. Dubin (1972) Lateral geniculate neurons of cat: Retinal inputs and physiology. Inv. Ophthalmol. 11:302–311.

Linsenmeier, R. A., L. J. Frishman, H. G. Jakiela, and C. Enroth-Cugell (1982) Receptive-field properties of X- and Y-cells in the cat retina derived from contrast sensitivity measurements. Vision Res. 22:1173–1183.

Lund, J. S., R. G. Boothe, and R. D. Lund (1977) Development of neurons in the visual cortex (Area 17) of the monkey (*Macaca nemestrina*): A Golgi study from fetal day 127 to postnatal maturity. J. Comp. Neurol. 176:149–188.

Mactier, H., J. D. Dexter, J. E. Hewett, C. B. Latham and C. W. Woodruff (1988) The electroretinogram in preterm infants. J. Pediatr. 113:607–612.

Mangel, S. C., J. R. Wilson, and S. M. Sherman (1983) Development of neuronal response properties in the cat dorsal lateral geniculate nucleus during monocular deprivation. J. Neurophysiol. 50:240–264.

Mann, I. C. (1964) The Development of the Human Eye, 3rd ed. London: British Medical Association.

Martin, K. A. C., and D. Whitteridge (1984) Form, function and intracortical projections of spiny neurones in the striate visual cortex of the cat. J. Physiol. (Lond) 353:463–504.

Masland, R. (1977) Maturation of function in the developing rabbit retina. J. Comp. Neurol. 175:275–286.

Maslim, J. and J. Stone (1986) Synaptogenesis in the retina of the cat. Brain Res. 373:35–48.

Mason, C. A. (1982a) Development of terminal arbors of retinogeniculate axons in the kitten. I. Light microscopical observations. Neuroscience 7:541–559.

Mason, C. A. (1982b) Development of terminal arbors of retinogeniculate axons in the kitten. II. Electron microscopical observations. Neuroscience 7:561–587.

Mason, C. A. (1983) Postnatal maturation of neurons in the cat's lateral geniculate nucleus. J. Comp. Neurol. 217:458–469.

McArdle, C. B., J. E. Dowling, and R. H. Masland (1977) Development of outer segments and synapses in the rabbit retina. J. Comp. Neurol. 175:253–274.

McCarthy, D., L. A. Coleman, K. A. C. Martin and M. J. Friedlander (1989) Monocular deprivation affects Y-cell geniculocortical synapses in cat area 18. Invest. Ophthalmol. Vis. Sci. 30:30.

McHaffie, J. G., K. Ogasawara, and B. E. Stein (1986) Trigeminotectal and other trigeminofugal projectionsin neonatal kittens: An anatomical demonstration with horseradish peroxidase and tritiated leucine. J. Comp. Neurol. 249:411–427.

Michel, A. E., and L. J. Garey (1984) The development of dendritic spines in the human visual cortex. Human Neurobiol. *3*:223–227.

Montague, P. R., and M. J. Friedlander (1989) Expression of an intrinsic growth strategy by mammalian retinal neurons. Proc. Nat. Acad. Sci., U.S.A. *86*:7223–7227.

Muller, L. J., R. W. H. Verwer, B. Cardozo, and G. Vrensen (1984) Synaptic characteristics of identified pyramidal and multipolar non-pyramidal neurons in the visual cortex of young and adult rabbits. A quantitative Golgi–electron microscope study. Neuroscience *12*:1071–1087.

Nishimura, Y. and P. Rakic (1985) Development of the rhesus monkey retina. I Emergence of the inner plexiform layer and its synapses. J. Comp. Neurol. *241*:420–434.

Norton, T. T. (1974) Receptive-field properties of superior colliculus cells and development of visual behavior in kittens. J. Neurophysiol. *37*:674–690.

O'Kusky, J. R. (1985) Synapse elimination in the developing visual cortex: A morphometric analysis in normal and dark-reared cats. Dev. Brain Res. *22*:81–91.

Olavarria, J., and R. C. Van Sluyters (1985) Organization and postnatal development of callosal connections in the visual cortex of the rat. J. Comp. Neurol. *239*:1–26.

Olney, J. W. (1968) An electron microscopic study of synapse formation, outer segment development, and other aspects of developing mouse retina. Inv. Ophthalmol. *7*:250–268.

Palmer, L. A., and A. C. Rosenquist (1974) Visual receptive fields of single striate cortical units projecting to the superior colliculus in the cat. Brain Res. *67*:27–42.

Parnevalas, J. G., E. J. Mounty, R. Bradford, and A. R. Lieberman (1977) The postnatal development of neurons in the dorsal lateral geniculate nucleus of the rat: A Golgi study. J. Comp. Neurol. *171*:481–500.

Peichl, L., and H. Wassle (1983) The structural correlate of the receptive field centre of α ganglion cells in the cat retina. J. Physiol. (Lond.) *341*:309–324.

Pettigrew, J. D. (1974) The effect of visual experience on the development of stimulus specificity by kitten cortical neurones. J. Physiol. (Lond.) *237*:49–74.

Price, D. J., and C. Blakemore (1985) The postnatal development of the association projection from visual cortical area 17 to area 18 in the cat. J. Neurosci. *5*:2443–2452.

Provis, J. M., D. Van Driel, F. A. Billison, and P. Russell (1985) Development of the human retina: Patterns of cell distribution and redistribution in the ganglion cell layer. J. Comp. Neurol. *233*:429–451.

Rakic, P., and K. P. Riley (1983) Overproduction and elimination of retinal axons in the fetal rhesus monkey. Science *219*:1441–1444.

Ramoa, A. S., G. A. Campbell and C. J. Shatz (1988) Dendritic growth and remodeling of cat retinal ganglion cells during fetal and postnatal development. J. Neurosci. *8*:4239–4261.

Rapaport, D. H., and J. Stone (1984) The area centralis of the retina in the cat and other mammals: Focal point for function and development of the visual system. Vision Res. *11*:289–301.

Rapisardi, S. C., K. L. Chow, and L. H. Mathers (1975) Ontogenesis of receptive field characteristics in the dorsal lateral geniculate nucleus of the rabbit. Exp. Brain Res. *22*:295–305.

Riccio, R. V., and M. A. Mathews (1985) The postnatal development of the rat primary visual cortex during optic nerve impulse blockade by intraocular tetrodotoxin: A quantitative electron microscopic analysis. Dev. Brain Res. 20:55–68.

Rioch, D. M. (1929) Studies on the diencephalon of Carnivora. I. The nuclear configuration of the thalamus, epithalamus and hypothalamus of the dog and cat. J. Comp. Neurol. 49:1–119.

Robertson, R. T., A. A. Tijerina, and M. E. Gallivan (1985) Transient patterns of acetylcholinesterase activity in visual cortex of the rat: Normal development and the effects of neonatal monocular enucleation. Dev. Brain Res. 21:203–214.

Robson, J. G., and C. Enroth-Cugell (1978) Light distribution in the cat's retinal image. Vision Res. 18:159–173.

Rodieck, R. W. (1965) Quantitative analysis of cat retinal ganglion cell response to visual stimuli. Vision Res. 5:583–601.

Rodieck, R. W. (1979) Visual pathways. Ann. Rev. Neurosci. 2:193–225.

Rowe, M. J., and B. Dreher (1982) The W-cell projection to the medial interlaminar nucleus of the cat: Implications for ganglion cell classification. J. Comp. Neurol. 204:117–133.

Rusoff, A. C., and M. W. Dubin (1977) Development of receptive-field properties of retinal ganglion cells in kittens. J. Neurophysiol. 40:1188–1198.

Rusoff, A. C., and M. A. Dubin (1978) Kitten ganglion cells: Dendritic field size at 3 weeks of age and correlation with receptive field size. Inv. Ophthalmol. Vis. Sci. 17:819–821.

Saito, H.-A. (1983) Morphology of physiologically identified X-, Y- and W-type ganglion cells of the cat. J. Comp. Neurol. 221:279–388.

Samorajski, T., J. R. Keefe, and J. M. Ordy (1965) Morphogenesis of photoreceptor and retinal ultrastructure in a sub-human primate. Vision Res. 5:639–648.

Sanderson, K. J., P. O. Bishop, and I. Darian-Smith (1971) The properties of the binocular receptive fields of lateral geniculate neurons. Exp. Brain Res. 13:178–207.

Schoppmann, A. (1985) Functional and developmental analysis of a visual corticopretectal pathway in the cat: a neuroanatomical and electrophysiological study. Exp. Brain Res. 60:363–374.

Sengelaub, D. R., and B. L. Finlay (1982) Cell death in the mammalian visual system during normal development: I. Retinal ganglion cells. J. Comp. Neurol. 204:311–317.

Shatz, C. J., and P. A. Kirkwood (1984) Prenatal development of functional connections in the cat's retinogeniculate pathway. J. Neurosci. 4:1378–1397.

Shatz, C. J., and M. B. Luskin (1986) The relationship between the geniculocortical afferents and their cortical target cells during development of the cat's primary visual cortex. J. Neurosci. 6:3655–3668.

Shaw, C., M. C. Needler, and M. Cynader (1984) Ontogenesis of muscarinic acetylcholine binding sites in cat visual cortex: Reversal of specific laminar distribution during the critical period. Dev. Brain Res. 14:295–299.

Sherman, S. M., and C. Koch (1986) The control of retinogeniculate transmission in the mammalian lateral geniculate nucleus. Exp. Brain Res. 63:1–20.

Sherman, S. M., and P. D. Spear (1982) Organization of visual pathways in normal and visually deprived cats. Physiol. Rev. 62:738–855.

Sherman, S. M., K.-P. Hoffmann, and J. Stone (1972) Loss of a specific cell type from the dorsal lateral geniculate nucleus in visually deprived cats. J. Neurophysiol. 35:532–541.

Shipley, T. and M. T. Anton (1964) The human electroretinogram in the first day of life. J. Pediatr. 65:733–739.

Shotwell, S. L., C. J. Shatz, and M. B. Luskin (1986) Development of glutamic acid decarboxylase immunoreactivity in the cat's lateral geniculate nucleus. J. Neurosci. 6:1410–1423.

Sieving, P. A., L. J. Frishman and R. H. Steinberg (1986) M-wave of proximal retina in cat. J. Neurophysiol. 56:1039–1048.

Sillito, A. M., and J. A. Kemp (1983) The influence of GABAergic inhibitory processes on the receptive field structure of X- and Y-cells in cat dorsal lateral geniculate nucleus (dLGN). Brain Res. 277:63–77.

Sillito, A. M., J. A. Kemp, J. A. Milson, and N. Berardi (1980) A re-evaluation of the mechanisms underlying simple cell orientation selectivity. Brain Res. 194:517–520.

Singer, W., E. Poppel, and O. Creuztfeldt (1972) Inhibitory interaction in the cat's lateral geniculate nucleus. Exp. Brain Res. 14:210–226.

Smelser, G. K., V. Ozanics, M. Rayborn, and D. Sagun (1974) Retinal synaptogenesis in the primate. Inv. Ophthalmol. 13:340–361.

Sparks, D. L. (1986) Translation of sensory signals into commands for control of saccadic eye movements: Role of primate superior colliculus. Physiol. Rev. 66:118–171.

Stanford, L. R. (1987) Quantitative differences in morphology and physiology of W- and X-retinal ganglion cells. J. Neurophysiol. 57:1–21.

Stanford, L. R., and S. M. Sherman (1984) Structure/function relationships of retinal ganglion cells in the cat. Brain Res. 297:381–386.

Stein, B. E. (1984) Development of the superior colliculus. Ann. Rev. Neurosci. 7:95–125.

Stein, B. E., and S. B. Edwards (1979) Corticotectal and other corticofugal projections in neonatal cat. Brain Res. 161:399–409.

Stein, B. E., and H. Gallagher (1981) Maturation of cortical control over superior colliculus cells in cat. Brain Res. 223:429–435.

Stein, B. E., E. Labos, and L. Kruger (1973a) Sequence of changes in properties of neurons of superior colliculus of the kitten during maturation. J. Neurophysiol. 36:667–679.

Stein, B. E., E. Labos, and L. Kruger (1973b) Determinants of response latency in neurons of superior colliculus in kittens. J. Neurophysiol. 36:680–689

Stein, B. E., H. P. Clamann, and S. J. Goldbert (1980) Superior colliculus: Control of eye movements in neonatal kittens. Science 210:78–801.

Stein, B. E., R. F. Spencer, and S. B. Edwards (1982) Efferent projections of the neonatal superior colliculus: Extraoculomotor-related brain stem structures. Brain Res. 239:17–28.

Stein, B. E., R. F. Spencer, and S. B. Edwards (1984) Efferent projections of the neonatal cat superior colliculus: Facial and cerebellum-related brainstem structures. J. Comp. Neurol. 230:47–54.

Stein, B. E., J. G. McHaffie, J. K. Harting, M. F. Huerta, and T. Hashikawa (1985) Transient tectogeniculate projections in neonatal kittens: An autoradiographic study. J. Comp. Neurol. 239:402–412.

Sterling, P., M. A. Freed, and R. G. Smith (1988) Architecture of rod and cone circuits to the on-beta ganglion cells. J. Neurosci. 8:613–642.

Stone, J. (1983) Parallel processing in the visual system. In Colin Blakemore (ed.): Perspectives in Vision Research, New York. Plenum Press.

Stone, J., D. H. Rapaport, R. W. Williams, and L. Chalupa (1982) Uniformity of cell distribution in the ganglion cell layer of prenatal cat retina: Implication for mechanisms of retinal development. Dev. Brain Res. 2:231–242.

Sur, M., and S. M. Sherman (1982a) Retinogeniculate terminations in cat: Morphological differences between X- and Y-cell axons. Science 218:389–391.

Sur, M., and S. M. Sherman (1982b) Linear and nonlinear W-cells in C-laminae of the cat's lateral geniculate nucleus. J. Neurophysiol. 47:869–884.

Sur, M., R. E. Weller, and S. M. Sherman (1984) Development of X- and Y-cell retinogeniculate terminations in kittens. Nature 310:246–249.

Thorn, F., M. Gollender, and P. Erickson (1976) The development of the kitten's visual optics. Vision Res. 16:1145–1149.

Tootle, J. S., and M. J. Friedlander (1986) Postnatal development of receptive field surround inhibition in kitten dorsal lateral geniculate nucleus. J. Neurophysiol. 56:523–541.

Tootle, J. S., and M. J. Friedlander (1989) Postnatal development of the spatial contrast sensitivity of X- and Y-cells in the kitten retinogeniculate pathway. J. Neurosci. 9:1325–1340.

Tsumoto, T., K. Suda, and H. Sato (1983) Postnatal development of corticotectal neurons in the kitten striate cortex: A quantitative study with the horseradish peroxidase technique. J. Comp. Neurol. 219:88–99.

Tucker, G. S., D. I. Hamasaki, A. Labbie, and J. Muroff (1979) Anatomic and physiologic development of the photoreceptor in the kitten. Exp. Brain Res. 37:459–474.

Vogel, M. (1978) Postnatal development of the cat's retina. Adv. Anat. Embryol. Cell Biol. 54:1–65.

Wassle, H., and H. J. Riemann (1978) The mosaic of nerve cells in the mammalian retina. Proc. Roy. Soc. Lond. B. 200:441–461.

Weidman, T. A., and T. Kuwabara (1969) Development of the cat retina. Inv. Ophthalmol. 8:60–69.

Wickelgren, B. G., and P. Sterling (1969) Influence of visual cortex on receptive fields in cat superior colliculus. J. Neurophysiol. 32:16–23.

Wiesel, T. N., and D. H. Hubel (1965) Comparison of the effects of unilateral and bilateral eye closure on cortical unit responses in kittens. J. Neurophysiol. 28:1029–1040.

Wiesel, T. N., and D. H. Hubel (1974) Ordered arrangement of orientation columns in monkeys lacking visual experience. J. Comp. Neurol. 158:307–318.

Williams, R. A., and R. G. Boothe (1981) Development of optical quality in the infant monkey (Macaca nemestrina) eye. Inv. Ophthalmol. Vis. Sci. 21:728–730.

Williams, R. W., and L. M. Chalupa (1982) Prenatal development of retinocollicular projections in the cat: An anterograde tracer transport study. J. Neurosci. 2:604–622.

Wilson, J. R., D. E. Tessin, and S. M. Sherman (1982) Development of the electrophysiological properties of Y-cells in the kitten's medial interlaminar nucleus. J. Neurosci. 2:562–571.

Wilson, P. D., D. M. Murakami, and J. D. Parsons (1984) Cell growth in the lateral geniculate C-laminae of visually normal and monocularly deprived cats. In J. Stone, B. Dreher, and D. Rapaport (eds.): Development of Visual Pathways in Mammals. New York: Alan R. Liss, pp. 331–345.

Wilson, J. R., M. J. Friedlander, and S. M. Sherman (1984) Fine structural morphology of identified X- and Y-cells in the cat's lateral geniculate nucleus. Proc. Roy. Soc. Lond. B. 221:411–436.

Winfield, D. A., R. W. Hiorns, and T. P. S. Powell (1980) A quantitative electronmicroscopical study of the postnatal development of the lateral geniculate nucleus in normal kittens and kittens with eyelid suture. Proc. Roy. Soc. Lond. B. Biol. Sci. 210:211–234.

Winkelman, J. E. and G. P. M. Horsten (1962) The ERG of premature and full-term infants during their first days of life. Ophthalmologica 143:92–101.

Wolf, W., T. P. Hicks, and K. Albus (1986) The contribution of GABA-mediated inhibitory mechanisms to visual response properties of neurons in the kittens striate cortex. J. Neurosci. 6:2779–2795.

Wolff, J. R., H. Bottcher, T. Zetzsche, W. H. Oertel, and B. M. Chromwall (1984) Development of GABA-ergic neurons in rat visual cortex as identified by glutamate decarboxylase-like immunoreactivity. Neurosci. Lett. 47:207–212.

Yellott, J. I. (1983) Spectral consequences of photoreceptor sampling in the rhesus retina. Science 221:382–385.

Chapter Three

BEHAVIORAL ANALYSIS OF VISUAL DEVELOPMENT

LYNNE KIORPES AND J. ANTHONY MOVSHON

Department of Psychology and Center for Neural Science
New York University
New York, New York

I INTRODUCTION

The previous two chapters have described in detail the many anatomical and physiological changes that occur in the visual system during the prenatal and early postnatal weeks and months in several mammalian species.

125

In this chapter we describe the development of visual function as measured behaviorally. The majority of available data are from primates, both human and monkey; some data are also available for cats. Since the retina (Hendrickson and Kupfer, 1976; Abramov et al., 1982; Hendrickson and Yuodelis, 1984; Yuodelis and Hendrickson, 1986) and central visual pathways (LeVay et al., 1980; Blakemore and Vital-Durand, 1986) are immature in infant primates and undergo considerable postnatal development, it is not surprising that visual function as measured behaviorally undergoes substantial postnatal development. Although it is difficult to discern which level of the system underlies the development of any particular behaviorally measured visual function, there is some evidence to suggest that even the optical and early neural elements in the visual pathway undergo some postnatal development.

Our discussion begins with the development of the earliest elements in the visual system, that is, those that influence the quality of the visual image. Each subsequent visual function discussed reflects, as much as our present understanding permits, the maturation of successively higher levels of the visual pathway. We have excluded from this chapter a discussion of the development of color vision [a thorough recent review of the development of color vision in human infants is provided in Teller and Bornstein (1987)]; virtually nothing is known about the development of color vision in animals, either behaviorally or physiologically. It will become obvious that a great deal of work remains to be done to understand the development of visual behavior and the processes that underlie this development.

A   Methodology

Before beginning to discuss the development of visual behavior, it is important to gain a sense for how one measures visual sensitivity in a young animal or human. Most successful assessment techniques make use of some natural behavior of the organism, so that data can be obtained relatively quickly and without extended periods of training. This is particularly true of methods used with human infants, which are usually based on either natural pattern preferences or eye movements elicited by moving patterns. The preferential looking technique, now the most commonly used method for assessing visual sensitivity, is based on the natural tendency for infants to fixate a high contrast pattern (e.g., Fantz, 1965; Teller, 1979). Preferential looking was transformed into a robust psychophysical technique called forced-choice preferential looking (FPL) in Davida Teller's laboratory, initially for the testing of grating acuity in human infants (Teller et al., 1974). Subsequently, this method has been applied to assessment of a variety of visual functions such as color vision (e.g., Peeples and Teller, 1975), depth perception (e.g., Atkinson and Braddick, 1976), spatial contrast sensitivity (e.g., Atkinson, et al., 1977a,b), and light and dark adaptation (e.g., Dannemiller and Banks, 1983; Dannemiller, 1985).

The FPL technique requires a human observer to make forced-choice judgments about the location of a visual pattern given two choices. The choice is usually between a left or right position within an otherwise uniform field, and the pattern stimulus is generally presented opposite a stimulus that is matched in luminance to the pattern. The judgments are made on the basis of the infant's looking behavior, including eye movements, changes in pupil size, and other fixation cues, or differences in interest between the two stimulus fields. It is important to note that in the *forced-choice* version of this technique, the observer's task is to judge—using any available cues—the *location* of the pattern stimulus, not necessarily the side the infant "prefers" or the side of first fixation. The FPL technique has also been adapted for use with monkey infants (e.g., Teller et al., 1978) and, in one case, kittens (Sireteanu, 1985). The FPL technique can be used to test infant monkeys from birth until about 12 weeks, whereas human infants can be tested from birth until about 18 months. Beyond the ages over which FPL data can be collected—that is, when the patterns cease to attract the infants' attention reliably—operant techniques are used.

The performance of human infants on discrimination tasks is sometimes studied using an habituation method that relies on the infants' tendency to fixate novel displays. The infant is habituated to repeated presentations of a particular target, and a new one is then substituted. If the infant reliably shows renewed attention to the display, it is assumed that the two targets can be discriminated (Fantz, 1964).

In operant tasks, the subject makes the discrimination for itself in order to obtain a reward. These techniques require some period of training. The rewards are of course tailored to the species being studied. For example, a monkey may be rewarded with apple juice (Boothe et al., 1980) for correctly discriminating two stimuli, whereas a human infant may be rewarded with a Cheerio (Birch et al., 1983) or an attractive visual display (Mayer and Dobson, 1982). The tasks themselves must also be carefully chosen: a human infant can be asked to point to or touch the correct stimulus; a monkey infant can be trained to pull a grab-bar or touch one of several panels to indicate its choice; kittens are usually tested on a jumping stand (Mitchell et al., 1976). The jumping stand method requires the kitten to jump from a platform onto one of two surfaces; correct choices are rewarded with beef baby food or an equivalently palatable substance, while errors are punished by letting the animal fall a few inches through a trap door.

Most of the data discussed in this chapter were collected using one of these techniques. Absent from most of this discussion are data collected using the visual-evoked potential. The evoked potential provides an electrophysiological measure that, regrettably, does not have any clear quantitative relationship to behavioral data from individual infants (Sokol and Moskowitz, 1985). Furthermore, evoked potential data are available in quantity only for human infants and not for infants of nonhuman species. It is therefore difficult to correlate the origin of the evoked potential signal with specific neural function. We have included evoked potential data only in a few important cases where no behavioral measures of function are available.

II PHYSIOLOGICAL OPTICS

In cats and monkeys, the optical quality of the eye is suboptimal at birth and develops to adult levels postnatally. At the time of eye opening in kittens, the ocular media are cloudy, degrading light transmission by about 1 logarithmic unit. In addition, the *tunica vasculosa lentis*, a vascular network that supplies the developing lens, is still present during the early postnatal weeks, causing considerable scatter of the incoming light. The media clear and the vascular membrane breaks down progressively over the next 2–3 weeks, during which time the apparent quality of the optics also improves. Over the first 5–7 postnatal weeks, there is a factor of 2 improvement in the quality of optical imaging based on the width of the line spread function (Bonds and Freeman, 1978; see also Chapter 2). The optical modulation transfer function, which describes the contrast transfer properties of the optics, derived for 7-week-old kittens is similar to that derived for adult cats, although there is some evidence even at this age for a continuing high level of light scatter within the eye.

Although the ocular media are clear at birth in primates, there is measurable improvement in the quality of the retinal image in the early postnatal weeks (Williams and Boothe, 1981). During the first 13 postnatal weeks in monkeys, image quality as measured by the width of the line spread function shows nearly a factor of 2 improvement. Figure 1 shows line spread functions obtained from a single infant monkey at each of three ages. A progressive narrowing of the function from 1 to 13 weeks is evident, particularly at the level for which retinal illuminance is one-tenth that at the peak (tenth-height). The corresponding optical modulation transfer functions shown in Figure 2A demonstrate the improvement in contrast transmission between 1 and 13 weeks for this monkey. Optical modulation transfer functions for older monkeys are within the same range as those from 13-week-old monkeys; therefore it is assumed that the optical quality of the monkey eye is adultlike by 13 weeks. It is possible, though, as in the cat that there is greater light scatter in the young monkey eye than in the adult that is not revealed by the methods used by Williams and Boothe.

Although there is measurable improvement in retinal image quality during the early postnatal weeks in cats and monkeys, the condition of the optics in the newborn is probably not a major limiting factor for the development of visual sensitivity. In both cats and monkeys, the time course for the development of visual resolution extends well beyond the time period over which changes in optical quality have been demonstrated (see Section IV). Moreover, comparison between behaviorally measured contrast sensitivity

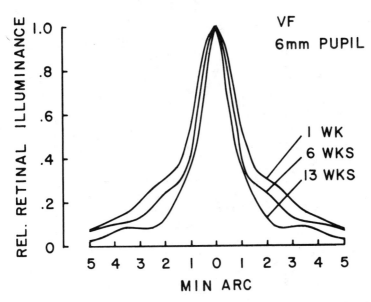

FIGURE 1. Retinal line spread functions for a single monkey infant measured at three ages. The three curves are normalized to 1 at 0 min arc. The data were collected using a double-pass optical technique. The line spread function is the distribution of light across the retinal image of a well focused thin bright line. (From Williams and Boothe, 1981.)

functions and derived optical modulation transfer functions in infant monkeys demonstrates that the behaviorally measured sensitivity is much poorer than the limit imposed by the optics. The data in Figure 2B show contrast sensitivity for an individual infant monkey at 5 and 13 weeks of age measured behaviorally (open squares; see Section IV for a more detailed consideration of contrast sensitivity measurements); the solid curves represent a numerical fit to these data. The dashed curves show—based on optical data from a different monkey taken at corresponding ages—the effect of correcting the fits for the contrast attenuation produced by the optics. The small differences at each age between the corrected and uncorrected curves are much less than the difference between the behavioral performance at the two ages, revealing that the development of the optics is not sufficient to account for more than a small part of the development of contrast sensitivity between 5 and 13 weeks. It is also obvious from a comparison of Figures 2A and 2B that the optics are capable of relaying information about spatial frequencies that the young monkey cannot resolve.

One aspect of optical development that is quantitatively important in considering the development of spatial properties in the visual system is the change in retinal image magnification that accompanies the growth of the eye. For example, the axial length of the eye in primates roughly doubles

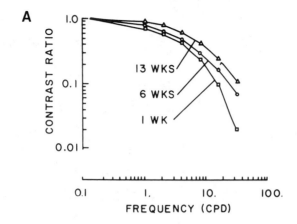

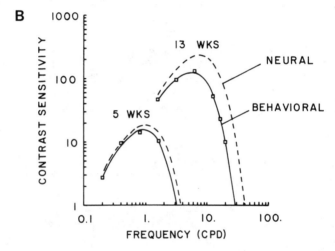

FIGURE 2. (A) Optical modulation transfer functions calculated by Fourier transformation of the line spread functions shown in Figure 1. (B) Behavioral contrast sensitivity functions obtained at two ages from a different infant monkey (solid curves and data points). The dashed curves show the theoretical effect of removing the spatial filtering produced by the optics of the eye measured at comparable ages [shown in (A)]. The improvement in contrast sensitivity produced by eliminating the optical contrast attenuation at either age is far less than the improvement in measured contrast sensitivity. (From Williams and Boothe, 1981.)

between birth and adulthood. This has no direct simple effect on the quality of the retinal image per se, but it alters the effect of that image on the subsequent neural elements of the visual system. All other things being equal, the visual resolution should double as the eye grows simply because the size of the retinal image doubles while the size of the neural elements used to analyze the image does not.

The determination of optical quality is accomplished experimentally by measuring the quality of the retinal image for a pattern that is in the best possible focus. Under natural viewing conditions, the accommodation control system is responsible for providing the retina with a well-focused image. The accommodation control system in primates is functionally immature at birth (see Aslin, 1987, for recent review). Human infants fail to accommodate accurately to targets presented at different distances (25–150 cm) prior to about 4 months postnatally. The closest distances measured correspond to four diopters (D) of accommodation for an emmetropic infant. Although younger infants often demonstrate the ability to accommodate correctly to a range of target distances, they do so less consistently than older infants. A similar trend is apparent in infant monkeys (Howland et al. 1982). Accommodative accuracy is poor in infant monkeys prior to about 5 postnatal weeks. Infants older than 5 weeks show consistently high accommodative accuracy over a range of target distances from 20 to 100 cm, corresponding to a 1–5-D range of accommodative power.

Although the degree of accommodative inaccuracy demonstrated by young primate infants would provide sufficient defocus in an adult eye to degrade visual performance, it is unlikely that this amount of defocus limits infant visual resolution. Green et al. (1980) have analyzed the relationship between eye size, visual acuity, and depth of focus. They show that in a small eye of low visual acuity (like that of a young infant) it is necessary to defocus an image substantially before the blur can be detected—the eye has a large depth of focus. This makes the accommodative inaccuracy of infants irrelevant to their vision. As the eye grows and visual acuity improves, the depth of focus decreases and accommodative accuracy improves concurrently. It therefore appears that accommodative control in infants is no worse than is needed to maintain an image of good apparent quality. It is also worth noting that, like optical quality, accommodative accuracy approaches adult levels much earlier than visual resolution and therefore probably does not impose a consistent limit to the development of visual resolution.

III EYE MOVEMENTS

It seems that the infant's visual system is provided with a reasonably clear and adequately focused retinal image. However, in order to make effective use of this image, the infant must have an oculomotor control system that is capable of positioning the image of the object of regard on the fovea with reliability and stability good enough to allow proper visual function. Fixational instability could effectively degrade visual resolution even in the presence of a clear and well-focused retinal image. It is therefore necessary to consider the development of eye movements and oculomotor control. Little is known about this development in any species. However, a recent quantitative study of human infants suggests that the oculomotor system can provide stable fixation and can produce rapid (saccadic) eye movements that are mature in speed, accuracy, and latency. Saccades are rapid, ballistically programmed movements that provide for the rapid foveation of visual targets. In a study of infants aged 2 weeks to 5 months, Hainline et al. (1984) found that under conditions of free viewing, infants produced many saccades that were adultlike in form and speed, along with two types of eye movements that were slower than any seen in the adult. The relative proportion of normal velocity to slow eye movements depended upon the type of visual stimulus presented to the infant; textured patterns elicited a higher proportion of adultlike eye movements than simple geometric forms. These results suggest that the attentional level of the infant is important for evaluating the form of the eye movements but that given appropriate stimuli, infants can produce rapid and well-controlled fixational eye movements.

Earlier studies of human infant eye movements suggested that saccades directed to targets in the peripheral visual field are less effective than in adults (Aslin and Salapatek, 1975; Salapatek et al., 1980; see also Aslin, 1987). Infants were presented with small targets at one of several distances away from the point of fixation, ranging from 10° to 30°. While adults would acquire the target in a single saccade or with one large saccade followed by a small corrective saccade, infants acquired the targets with a series of small saccades that were approximately equal in amplitude for a given target distance. This unusual pattern of eye movements was evident until about 2 months postnatally. In addition, the infants' latency for generating a saccadic eye movement was about five times longer than the latency for an adult saccade.

It is therefore not clear when saccadic eye movements actually become adultlike in both form and speed, although they appear to become at least grossly mature in humans between 2 and 5 months. Similarly, visual tracking behavior, or smooth pursuit, seems to become adultlike in the early postnatal months. Aslin (1981) studied smooth tracking behavior in young infants and found that newborns do not demonstrate smooth pursuit eye movements. Over the subsequent 2 months, infants gradually develop the ability to track smoothly moving targets, with characteristic accurate foveal pursuit for slowly moving targets developing before that for faster target movement. By 2 months, the infants tracked at a wide range of speeds, with a velocity gain of close to unity.

It is generally believed that the observed early development of infant oculomotor behavior reflects improvement in the visual control of eye movements rather than a purely mechanical or motor development. In this case, the development of oculomotor control would depend on calibration and integration of sensory and motor information during the first few postnatal months. Although sophisticated and elaborate methods exist for studying the basis of oculomotor control in nonhuman primates, no studies of the development of eye movement control in infant monkeys have been conducted.

The results of studies on the development of reflexive eye movements are consistent with the suggestion that sensory control of eye movements develops later than the motor aspects of oculomotor control. Optokinetic nystagmus (OKN) is a characteristic reflex pattern of eye movements elicited by large moving fields (see Figure 3A) and consists of slow phases in which the eye moves with a direction and speed roughly matching the stimulus interspersed with rapid saccadelike fast phases that bring the visual axis back in the opposite direction. Newborn infants (human, monkey, and cat) show a directional asymmetry in the production of monocular OKN (Atkinson, 1979; van Hof-van Duin, 1978). The asymmetry is characterized by a more vigorous optokinetic response to stimuli moving from the temporal visual field toward the nasal visual field as compared to that for stimuli moving from the nasal field toward the temporal field (Figure 3B). The asymmetry, as would be expected from a visual rather than a motor limit, is specific to the slow phase of the nystagmus. Naegele and Held (1982) demonstrated that the velocity of the slow phase component of OKN was higher for nasally directed stimuli than for temporally directed stimuli. This asymmetry gradually decreases in extent over the first 3–5 months in humans.

In monkeys and cats, the directional asymmetry is maintained only through the first 3–5 postnatal weeks. There is ample evidence from the cat to suggest that the following response for temporally directed stimuli depends on the integrity of the ipsilateral pathway from the retina to the nucleus of the optic tract via the striate cortex, which develops over a similar postnatal period (Cynader and Harris, 1980; Harris et al., 1980; Cynader and Hoffmann, 1981). Data from strabismic humans suggest further that the integrity of cortical binocularity is important for development and maintenance of symmetrical OKN (Atkinson, 1979; van Hof-van Duin and Mohn, 1986).

A possibly related asymmetry has been noted in the development of visual sensitivity in the nasal and temporal visual fields. Kittens (Sireteanu and Maurer, 1982) and human infants (Lewis, et al., 1985) younger than 8 weeks show poorer detection performance for stimuli presented in the nasal visual field than for stimuli presented in the temporal visual field. After 8 weeks, the ability to detect stimuli presented in the nasal and temporal fields appears to be similar. The delayed development of sensitivity in the nasal field is consistent with a relatively slow development of the ipsilateral pathway from the retina through the visual cortex to the superior colliculus, which is thought to contribute importantly to the process of orientation to visual stimuli. These data taken together suggest that the postnatal development of visual orienting behavior depends more on the maturation of sensory aspects of oculomotor control than on purely motor factors.

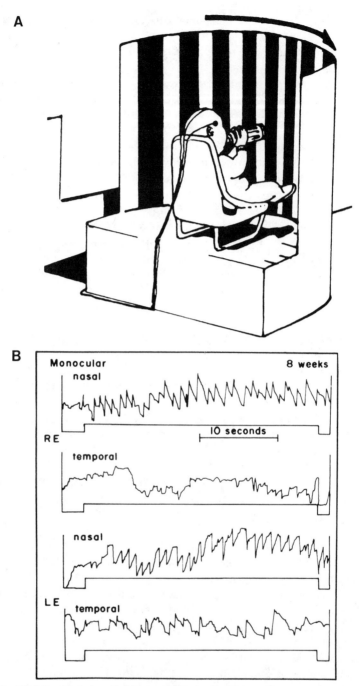

FIGURE 3. (*A*) A human infant (holding a bottle) positioned in front of an OKN target. The pattern is drifted across the infant's visual field at a constant speed while eye movements are recorded by electrooculography (EOG). (*B*) Sample EOG records from a single young human infant. The top two traces are records for the right eye; the bottom two traces are records for the left eye. The records show a more vigorous, consistent OKN response for nasalward target direction relative to temporalward target direction for each eye. (From Naegele and Held, 1982.)

IV   VISUAL SENSITIVITY AND RESOLUTION

It appears that the developing visual system has adequate optics to form a clear image and adequate oculomotor control to provide for the fixation and stabilization of that image. We now proceed to consider the development of the purely visual processes that determine sensitivity to light and to the spatial and temporal distribution of image contrast.

There are two distinct kinds of developmental change that contribute to changes in visual performance during development, which we can term changes of *scale* and changes of *sensitivity*. By changes of scale we mean changes in the spatial and/or temporal filtering or integration properties of elements of the visual system. The visual system of infants operates on a very much coarser scale than that of adults, at least spatially, and it may be that if allowance is made for this, the infant's visual capacity is otherwise more-or-less adultlike. We use the term "sensitivity" to describe the efficiency or accuracy with which the visual system can process targets adjusted for changes in spatial or temporal scale. Thus the sensitivity of an immature observer cannot be properly estimated if performance is only measured with targets selected for adults; it is often necessary to adapt the spatial or temporal characteristics of the display to the scale of the system under study. Regrettably, it is not always possible to distinguish the contributions of these two types of developmental change because it is often not possible to make the measurements of the spatial and temporal characteristics of vision that are needed to estimate or compensate effects of scale. The result is that some measurement that might appear to represent a development of sensitivity could in fact be the result of changes in the scale of visual processing that unknown to the experimenter, rendered the chosen test target inappropriate for the younger visual system.

A   Absolute Sensitivity and Light Adaptation

A good example of the influence of changes of scale on inferences about development arises in the consideration of the absolute sensitivity of infants to light. This is reliably found to be substantially poorer than in adults. Absolute threshold for the detection of light increments upon a dark background is elevated in 1–2 month old human infants by at least 1.2 logarithmic units relative to the adult (Powers et al., 1981; Brown, 1986; Hansen et al. 1986). Absolute sensitivity improves with age, although as late as 18 weeks postnatally sensitivity has not reached adult levels. Similarly, detection thresholds have been reported to be elevated under conditions of photopic illumination in young infants. Photopic sensitivity is reduced in infants aged 2–3 months by about 1.1 logarithmic units relative to the adult (Peeples and Teller, 1978; Pulos et al., 1980).

Initially, a number of studies suggested that the visual mechanisms underlying adaptation to changes in level of illumination are immature in young infants. Increment threshold functions that relate visual detection thresholds to the intensity of an adapting background light were found to be shallower for 1- and 2-month-old human infants than for older infants and adults for both scotopic and photopic levels of illumination (Hansen and Fulton, 1981; Dannemiller and Banks, 1983). Figure 4A and B show increment threshold functions for 7- and 12-week-old infants compared with average adult performance. The interpretation of this shallow slope is complicated, however, because adult observers have shallow increment threshold functions when small test targets are used (Barlow, 1972; illustrated in Figure 5). Because of the coarser scale of the infant's visual system, it may be that targets that are "large" for adults are functionally "small" for infants. Indeed, recent studies of light adaptation in infants, in which very large test fields were used, show that the slopes of increment threshold functions in infants are similar to those of adults if the larger spatial summation areas of the infant (Hamer and Schneck, 1984) are taken into account. Thus an apparent change in function related to sensitivity can in fact be attributed to the difference in spatial scale between infant and adult.

While adults and infants typically have increment threshold functions of the same shape for large test fields, the functions of infants are elevated by an amount that reflects their poorer sensitivity near absolute threshold. No simple effect of spatial scale can account for this difference between infants and adults. Brown (1986) showed that the lowest background intensity that elevates visual thresholds is similar in infants and adults. Because this measure of infants' sensitivity (the adapting effectiveness of background light) is apparently adultlike, she concludes that their reduced sensitivity for the *detection* of light must be due to incomplete development of mechanisms in the visual pathway that are central to the (probably retinal) mechanisms responsible for light adaptation.

B   Spatial Vision

The most useful basic measure of spatial visual function is now generally thought to be the *contrast sensitivity function*, which describes the performance of the visual system in terms of the minimal detectable contrast for sinusoidal grating patterns of varying spatial frequency (Campbell and Green, 1965). The inverse of the threshold at each spatial frequency is the contrast sensitivity, hence the name of the measure. Figure 6 shows typical contrast sensitivity functions for cat, monkey, and human observers obtained with stationary gratings. All these show a characteristic bandpass shape, with a range of intermediate spatial frequencies being detectable at lower contrasts than either lower or higher frequencies. More traditional measures of visual acuity, such as line resolution, are also captured by the contrast sensitivity function: the spatial frequency at which contrast sensitivity falls to 1 corresponds to the resolution limit for grating targets. These limits are about 3–6 cycles per degree for cats, and between 30 and 50 cycles per degree for macaque monkeys and humans.

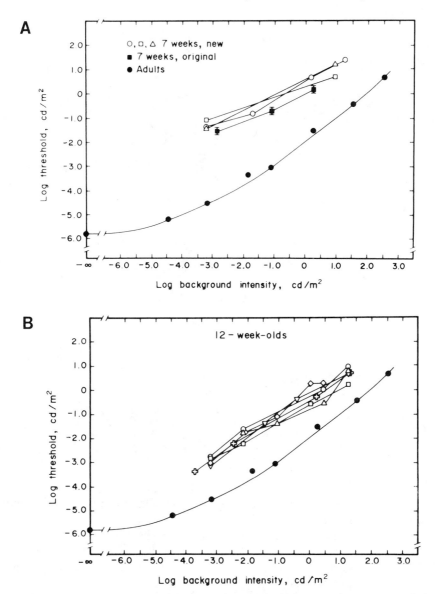

FIGURE 4. (*A*) Increment threshold functions for 7-week-old human infants (open symbols) compared with data from adults (filled symbols). The slopes of the infant functions are shallower than those for the adults. (*B*) Increment threshold functions for 12-week-old human infants (open symbols) compared with data from adults (filled symbols). By this age the slopes of the functions were adultlike. (From Dannemiller and Banks, 1983.)

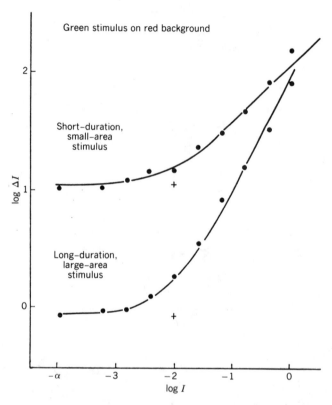

FIGURE 5. Increment threshold functions for adult observers with large, long-duration (bottom curve) and small, short-duration (top curve) test spots. The slope for the top curve is shallower than that for the bottom curve. (From Barlow, 1972.)

The development of sensitivity to spatially varying stimuli has been the subject of a great many studies in a variety of species, including cats as well as primates. The limit of spatial resolution, that is, the finest spatially periodic pattern that can be resolved, shows a similar developmental profile in all species examined. Spatial resolution in newborns is at least a factor of 10 poorer than in adults; it improves rapidly over the early weeks or months of life, then continues to develop at a slower rate to adult levels.

The interpretation of grating resolution measurements in neonatal kittens is hampered by the cloudy optic media that persist for several weeks after eye opening (see Section II and Chapter 2). However, it appears that in kittens, as in monkeys, these optical defects do not limit performance. The earliest behavioral measures of acuity in kittens can be obtained at about 1 month, at which time acuity is about 0.5 cycles per degree (Mitchell et al., 1976; Giffin and Mitchell, 1978; Sireteanu, 1985). During the next 2 months, resolution improves rapidly to near adult levels. By 4 months, resolution development is essentially complete at the level of 5–8 cycles per degree.

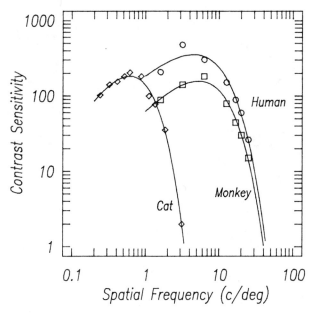

FIGURE 6. Contrast sensitivity functions for individual adult cat, monkey, and human subjects. All data were collected using stationary grating targets, operant two-alternative forced-choice psychophysical methods. Note that the peak sensitivity is similar for cats, monkeys, and humans; however, the range of spatial frequencies resolved is lower for the cat than for primates. [Primate data from Williams et al. (1981); cat data courtesy of T. Pasternak.]

Figure 7 (bottom) shows this developmental time course for the cat based on measurements made using the jumping stand technique.

The development of spatial resolution in primates is much slower than in cats. Whereas spatial resolution is adultlike by about 4 months in the cat, adult levels of resolution are not attained until near the end of the first year in monkeys (Boothe et al., 1988) and between 3 and 5 years in humans (Mayer and Dobson, 1982; Birch et al., 1983). The time courses for the development of resolution in monkeys and humans are shown in Figure 7 (middle and top, respectively). Comparison of the human and monkey data reveals several similarities. Spatial resolution is comparable in newborn human and monkey infants, both measuring between 1.0 and 2.0 cycles per degree. Although obscured by the use of a logarithmic scale for age in Figure 7, resolution improves rapidly for the first 6 postnatal weeks in monkeys (Teller et al., 1978; Lee and Boothe, 1981) and months in humans (reviewed by Dobson and Teller, 1978), followed by subsequent gradual development until adult levels of 30–50 cycles per degree are reached. The time courses for the development of resolution in monkeys and humans actually superimpose fairly well if human age is plotted in postnatal months and monkey age is plotted in postnatal weeks (Teller and Boothe, 1979)–a "four-to-one" rule that we will return to later.

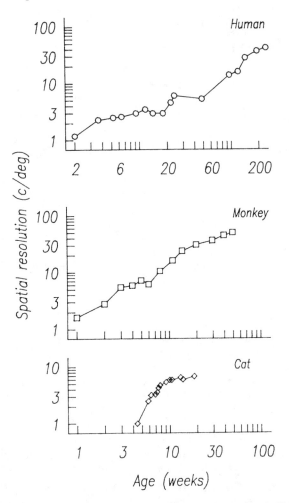

FIGURE 7. Development of spatial resolution for cat (bottom), monkey (middle), and human (top). Cat data were collected using the jumping stand technique (Mitchell et al., 1976; Giffin and Mitchell, 1978). Primate data were collected using a combination of FPL and operant techniques. Note that age is plotted on a logarithmic scale and that the age scale is different for human infants. This format creates the appearance that the developmental time course is roughly linear in primates. [Human infant data are from Mayer and Dobson (1982); monkey data are unpublished normative data of L. Kiorpes.]

The development of the whole contrast sensitivity function has been assessed in primate infants. Contrast sensitivity data are available for human infants and children from two age ranges: 1–3 months (Atkinson et al., 1977a; Banks and Salapatek, 1978) and 2½–8 years (Bradley and Freeman, 1982); one contrast sensitivity function for one 6-month-old infant has also been published (Harris et al., 1976). Macaque monkey data are available for ages ranging from 5 weeks to 1 year.

The contrast sensitivity function in human infants during the early postnatal months is strikingly different from that of the adult. Figure 8A shows data from young human infants, revealing a number of differences from the adult data shown in Figure 6. Most obvious is the restricted range of spatial frequencies resolved by the infant. Recall that the highest spatial frequency included by the envelope of the contrast sensitivity function represents the resolution limit. The poor spatial resolution of infants described above is directly reflected in the restricted range of resolvable spatial frequencies. Also obvious is the lower amplitude of the contrast sensitivity function in infants. Clearly, infants' sensitivity to contrast across the entire range of resolvable frequencies is reduced by at least a factor of 10 relative to the adult. Notice also that the reduced sensitivity is not uniform across spatial frequencies, meaning that the function must move not only upward but also to the right during development. This, of course, reflects a change in spatial scale as well as a change in sensitivity during development. The practical consequences for the infant is that its visual system can process only large, high-contrast stimuli.

Another important difference between the infant and adult contrast sensitivity function is the absence of a low-frequency falloff in the function obtained from an individual 1-month-old infant (open circles, Figure 8A). The drop-off of sensitivity at low frequencies in the adult contrast sensitivity function is usually attributed to lateral spatial antagonism in the visual system. Its absence in young infants suggests that the inhibitory mechanisms responsible may be immature at birth and develop sometime be-

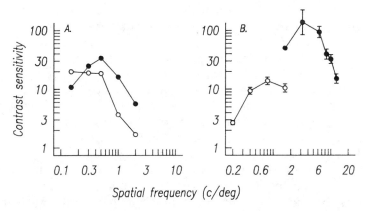

FIGURE 8. (A) Contrast sensitivity data from two young human infants (open symbols, 1-month-old; filled symbols, 3-month-old). Most 1-month human infants do not show attenuation of contrast sensitivity at low spatial frequencies, whereas older infants show the low-frequency falloff in sensitivity. (Data from Banks and Salapatek, 1981.) (B) Contrast sensitivity at two ages from one infant monkey (open symbols, 5 weeks; filled symbols, 9 weeks). Note the presence of the low-frequency falloff in the 5-week data and the combined upward and rightward shift of the function with age. (Data from Boothe et al., 1988.)

tween 1 and 3 months (filled circles, Figure 8A). However, a recent analysis suggests that at least some of this difference may be due to averaging of infant data (see Movshon and Kiorpes, 1988). Thereafter, it appears that the general form of the contrast sensitivity function is similar to that of the adult. Contrast sensitivity data from children reveal that development continues over the early childhood years. Bradley and Freeman (1982) found that the shape of the contrast sensitivity function in $2\frac{1}{2}$-year-old children was similar to that of adults but that sensitivity to contrast over most of the spatial frequency range continued to improve up to at least 5 years. Beyond 5 years, small residual differences in sensitivity between children and adults are generally ascribed to differences in response criterion rather than to immaturity of visual system function (Bradley and Freeman, 1982; Abramov et al., 1984).

The progression of contrast sensitivity development between the ages of 3 months and $2\frac{1}{2}$ years is not well-documented in human infants, largely because of methodological limitations. This gap can, however, be bridged by data from monkey infants if we use the four-to-one rule for relating monkey to human developmental time courses. Boothe et al. (1980, 1988) have studied the development of the contrast sensitivity function in individual monkey infants at ages ranging from 5 to 50 weeks. Similar to human infants, contrast sensitivity functions from monkeys at the earliest test ages were considerably reduced in overall amplitude as well as range of resolvable spatial frequencies (Figure 8B). Unlike data from human infants, though, the low-frequency falloff of sensitivity was present at the earliest tested ages in the monkey. However, based on the age correspondence of monkey weeks and human months established for the development of spatial resolution, the low-frequency falloff should be observable by 3 weeks in the monkey. Since the earliest age studied by Boothe et al. (1988) was 5 weeks, their data may not be relevant to this issue. If the four-to-one rule about developmental time course holds, it would be necessary to study contrast sensitivity in monkeys younger than 5 weeks to establish the absence of a low-frequency falloff in newborn monkeys.

Examination of the longitudinal development of contrast sensitivity in infant monkeys reveals that the observed changes in contrast sensitivity are the result of the function shifting upward in sensitivity and rightward toward higher spatial frequencies concurrently (compare open and filled symbols, Figure 8B). This process is evident from the plot of improvement in contrast sensitivity at the peak, peak spatial frequency, and cutoff frequency as a function of age for an individual infant monkey shown in Figure 9. In terms of the issues of scale and sensitivity we raised at the start of this section, the top panel in Figure 9, showing the development of peak contrast sensitivity, is a pure measure of sensitivity. The middle panel, showing the development of the spatial frequency at which peak sensitivity is observed, gives a good measure of the changes of scale. The bottom panel, showing the development of spatial resolution, shows a composite measure

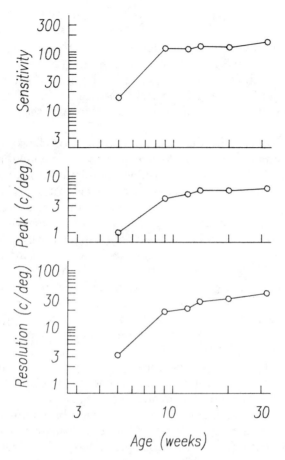

FIGURE 9. Development of the parameters of the contrast sensitivity curve for an individual monkey (the same monkey whose data appear in Figure 8*B*). The top graph shows development of sensitivity, that is, the height of the peak of the curve; the middle graph shows the development of the spatial frequency at which sensitivity is the highest; the bottom graph shows the development of spatial resolution, that is, the frequency at which the curve falls to a sensitivity of 1. Note that these features develop simultaneously, at similar rates within an individual. Development of contrast sensitivity for this monkey was essentially complete by 30 weeks (Data from Boothe et al., 1988.)

that is probably dominated by the change in the position of the peak but also depends on the contrast sensitivity. We have performed an analysis of the longitudinal data collected by Boothe et al. (1988), which reveals that the shape of the contrast sensitivity function does not change systematically during development, at least after the age of 1–2 months. This means that the changes plotted in Figure 9 adequately capture the phenomenon of contrast sensitivity development over the age range studied.

This pattern suggests that the development of contrast sensitivity cannot depend solely on one mechanism improving in sensitivity with age. Rather, it may be that an array of functional elements that vary in their spatial characteristics are simultaneously developing both higher sensitivity and finer spatial resolution. These data are consistent with the widely accepted notion that many different size-selective mechanisms ("spatial frequency channels") support spatial visual performance rather than simply one large filter through which visual information is processed (see, e.g., Graham, 1980).

More direct evidence for the existence of a range of size-selective mechanisms in the human infant visual system has been provided in a study by Banks et al. (1985), who used a masking paradigm to measure the bandwidths of spatial frequency selective mechanisms in 1.5- and 3-month-old infants. Using a narrow-band masking noise, they measured threshold elevation as a function of the center frequency of the masking noise. The results showed that threshold elevation occurs when the frequency content of the masking noise differs from the test frequency by less than two octaves (a factor of 4) in 3-month-olds, which is similar to the pattern seen in adult subjects. No masking effects were noted in the 1.5-month-olds. These data support the hypothesis that there are a number of different size-selective mechanisms operating in the visual system of infants as young as 3 months postnatal and that the bandwidth of these spatial frequency channels is at least roughly similar to those of adults.

It is likely that the time course for the development of spatial vision is limited by the development of neural elements at relatively peripheral stages of the visual system. Banks and Bennett (1988) suggest that spatial visual development during the early postnatal months in human infants can be accounted for by the maturation of foveal cone position and morphology. Thereafter, the maturation of response properties of visual neurons at the level of the ganglion cells or lateral geniculate nucleus may limit the developmental process (Blakemore and Vital-Durand, 1986). The notion that peripheral factors limit spatial contrast sensitivity is also generally accepted for adult observers. More central neural structures are, however, thought to limit performance on tasks such as vernier acuity that involve some kind of pattern discrimination (e.g., Levi et al., 1985). It is therefore of interest to study the development of pattern discrimination ability in infants as a possible behavioral method for analyzing cortical maturation.

Discrimination performance in infants has been measured to assess sensitivity to stimulus configuration. Braddick et al. (1986) used an habituation method to study the ability of young human infants to discriminate two patterns that were identical in spatial frequency content and contrast but differed in the phase relationship of the component spatial frequencies. As a group, infants in the 2–3-month age range were able to discriminate the patterns on the basis of the phase information, whereas younger infants failed to demonstrate this ability. A few studies in human infants (Shimojo et al., 1984; Shimojo and Held, 1987; Manny and Klein, 1984) and one study of macaque monkey infants (Kiorpes and Movshon, 1987, and in press) demonstrate that vernier acuity, as measured by discrimination of a grating stimulus from a grating with a vernier offset (see Figure 10), develops over a time course that is different from that of spatial resolution development. Figure 11 shows the relative rates of development of vernier acuity and grating acuity over the first 11 postnatal months in monkey infants. Grating acuity is relatively better than vernier acuity in newborns; however, vernier acuity develops faster than grating acuity so that in adults vernier performance is considerably better than grating resolution. It is generally believed

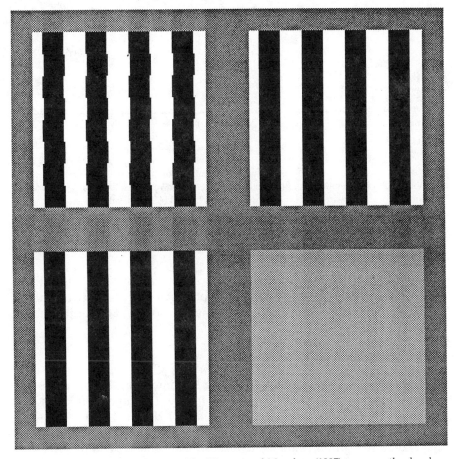

FIGURE 10. The stimulus pairs used by Kiorpes and Movshon (1987) to assess the developmental time courses for vernier acuity (top pair) and grating acuity (bottom pair) in infant monkeys. For grating acuity the grating target (bottom left), which is varied in spatial frequency, is paired with a homogeneous field of equal space average luminance (bottom right). For vernier acuity a grating target of low spatial frequency (top right) is paired with a grating containing offset regions (top left).

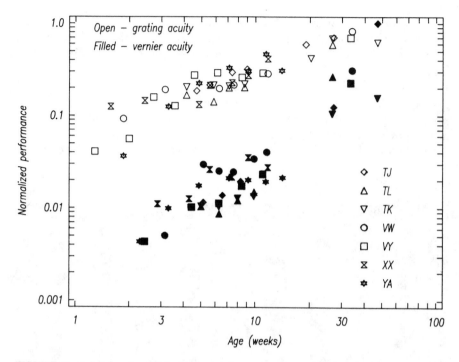

FIGURE 11. Relative rates of development for grating (open symbols) and vernier (filled symbols) acuity in individual infant monkeys. The data are normalized to the best performance obtained from the best animal at the oldest age tested (47 weeks). The values used are 0.14 min arc for vernier and 26.7 cycles per degree for grating acuity. Note that the scale for vernier acuity is the inverse of the usual one, so the normalization may be best considered to be 7.14 min arc^{-1}.

that vernier performance is dependent upon cortical function (Geisler, 1984; Levi et al., 1985; Wilson, 1986). Thus comparison of these two types of acuity may provide a means of relating the development of peripheral and central visual function.

C Temporal Aspects of Vision

The visual system's performance is limited in time as well as in space. One of the classically measured visual functions is the highest frequency at which the flicker of an unpatterned field can be detected, the *critical flicker frequency*. This bears the same relationship to temporal contrast sensitivity that spatial resolution bears to spatial contrast sensitivity; it describes the sensitivity of the visual system to flickering fields at frequencies lower than the resolution limit. The temporal contrast sensitivity function, like its spatial counterpart, is a powerful measure of basic visual performance (see, e.g., Kelly, 1972, for a review). In addition, the adult visual system's sensitivity to spatial patterns is not independent of their temporal characteristics:

the spatial contrast sensitivity function varies in shape and position according to the temporal pattern of presentation (Robson, 1966).

The postnatal development of sensitivity to temporally varying stimuli has been less intensively studied than spatial vision. A number of studies have been conducted to assess the upper limit of temporal resolution, the critical flicker frequency, for young infants. One systematic behavioral study of flicker perception in 1-, 2-, and 3-month-old infants using the FPL technique showed that an adultlike critical flicker frequency of about 50 Hz was present by about 2 months; a further slight improvement was found between 2 and 3 months (Regal, 1981). Similar results were found for longitudinal as well as cross-sectional data.

The development of sensitivity to temporal modulation at rates below the resolution limit, that is, the form of the temporal contrast sensitivity function, is virtually unexplored. However, there is some suggestion that there is further development of temporal contrast sensitivity beyond the age of 3 months. Electrophysiological studies of infant temporal vision (Hartmann et al., 1987) and spatiotemporal interactions (Moskowitz and Sokol, 1980) suggest that 3-month-olds are less sensitive relative to adults at flicker rates below the resolution limit, as measured by the amplitude of the visual-evoked potential. We are not aware of any behavioral measurements of the temporal contrast sensitivity function in infants of any species.

As would be expected from the shape of the spatial contrast sensitivity function, sensitivity to temporal modulation at low spatial frequencies appears to mature before sensitivity at middle and higher spatial frequencies. It is also the case that spatiotemporal interactions of the same character as those seen in adults are also apparent in 3-month-old infants. Atkinson et al. (1977b) showed that spatial contrast sensitivity is enhanced by temporal modulation of the contrast of grating stimuli, but only for relatively low spatial frequencies (cf. Robson, 1966). In adults, this pattern is thought to be due to the independent actions of two sets of visual channels. One set is optimally sensitive to flickering patterns of low spatial frequency, while the other responds best to stationary targets of higher spatial frequency (Graham, 1972). Because infants show a similar pattern of results, it seems reasonable to suppose that they possess both sets of functional channels, at least at the age of 3 months.

D   Binocular Vision

Because the two eyes have slightly different views of the world, the two retinal images are slightly disparate when an object is not in the plane of fixation. The adult visual system is exquisitely sensitive to this binocular disparity, which it analyzes to provide the sense of stereoscopic depth, or *stereopsis* (see Kaufman, 1975, for a review). The development of binocular vision has been studied in cats and human infants and has been shown to develop postnatally.

Only in kittens have studies of binocular function unambiguously tested stereopsis. Using the jumping stand technique, Mitchell and his colleagues (1979; Timney, 1981) have shown that kittens have superior performance on a depth discrimination task when tested binocularly relative to performance under monocular test conditions. This superiority of binocular performance develops rather abruptly between 4 to 6 postnatal weeks. By 6 weeks binocular thresholds are about a factor of 5 lower than monocular thresholds.

Binocular function in human infants has been measured by a variety of methods in a number of different laboratories (see Braddick and Atkinson, 1983). However, because none of these studies explicitly measured the discrimination of depth, none can be claimed to have studied stereoscopic vision. It is perfectly possible that an infant could detect the difference between the images in the two eyes and to use this difference to make perceptual judgments without having made any stereoscopic analysis of the pattern of differences. An example is provided by the study of Fox et al. (1980), who investigated the development of binocular function by studying fixational tracking behavior elicited by a disparate target created out of a dynamic random-dot display that lacked monocular cues to depth or form. In most infants, this tracking behavior emerged rather abruptly at an age between 3 and 6 months. Fox and his colleagues argue that their results reflect the development of stereopsis because the infants did not track all disparities equally well. But it seems equally likely that the infants detected the difference between the two retinal images and simply tracked this "zone of difference." There is no reason to imagine that the detectability of such a zone would be independent of disparity.

Another study that employed geometric bar stereograms and a preferential looking method also suggested that stereopsis in human infants develops around the age of 3–6-months (Birch, et al., 1982). Unfortunately, the use of geometric stereograms in this study makes it difficult to rule out some contribution of monocular cues to the results. And again, the study does not demonstrate that stereopsis, rather than the mere analysis of interocular image differences, is responsible. Shimojo et al. (1986) have also presented data that suggest that the nature of binocular vision in infants undergoes a fundamental change at around this same age. Their results appear to show that until the age of 3 months or so, the infant visual system combines the images from the two eyes but does not preserve information about the eye of origin of each feature. Neither stereopsis nor such other binocular process as rivalry can be evident until this "eye-of-origin" information is preserved by the visual system. Their results suggest that beyond about 3 months of age, binocular rivalry is present. Shimojo and his colleagues offer the intriguing speculation that the change in binocular function is related to the segregation of afferents from the two eyes into separate eye dominance columns in the visual cortex (see Chapter 4). This is broadly in agreement with the expected timing of this process in humans under the now-familiar four-to-one rule relating monkey to human development. It would be interesting to know more about the development of binocularity in monkeys, but we are aware of no studies on this topic.

V   SUMMARY AND CONCLUSIONS

In the past two decades, stimulated in part by new testing methods and in part by the renewed interest in the development of the nervous system, there has been a great deal of work on the development of visual performance in animals and humans. As we have seen in this chapter, the course of visual development is very dramatic, especially for most kinds of spatial visual performance. Moreover, most of this development appears to be limited by the development of the visual nervous system itself. Although such factors as the optical quality of the eye and the precision of accommodative and oculomotor control improve during early postnatal life, quantitative examination of these factors reveals that they cannot account for most of the changes in visual performance seen over the same period. There is, of course, a great deal of neural territory between the photoreceptors that register an image and the motoneurons that control the organism's behavioral response, and it is not immediately obvious where the most critical limiting stages lie. From the data that are presently available, however, it seems that in normal development most of the limits to the kinds of performance we have discussed are imposed relatively early in the visual pathway. For simple visual detection and resolution, the limits may be in the retina and are probably before the level of the visual cortex (Blakemore and Vital-Durand, 1986; Friedlander and Tootle, Chapter 2, this volume). Performance on more demanding visual discrimination tasks such as stereopsis or positional resolution may tap more central, cortical mechanisms. Interestingly, as we will see in the next chapter, most of the alterations in visual performance that can be produced by visual experience do not appear to result from changes in development in the peripheral visual nervous system but instead result from functional charges in the cortical structures involved in the higher processing of visual information.

ACKNOWLEDGMENTS

The preparation of this chapter was supported in part by grants from the National Institutes of Health (EY 02017 and EY 05864) and the National Science Foundation (BNS 82-16950).

REFERENCES

Abramov, I., J. Gordon, A. Hendrickson, L. Hainline, V. Dobson, and E. LaBossiere (1982) The retina of the newborn human infant. Science 217:265–267.

Abramov, I., L. Hainline, J. Turkel, E. Lemerise, H. Smith, J. Gordon, and S. Petry (1984) Rocket-ship psychophysics: Assessing visual functioning in young children. Invest. Ophthalmol. Vis. Sci. 25:1307–1315.

Aslin, R. N. (1981) Development of smooth pursuit in human infants. In D. F. Fisher, R. A. Monty, and J. W. Senders (eds.): Eye Movements: Cognition and Visual Perception. Hillsdale, NJ: Erlbaum.

Aslin, R. N. (1987) Motor aspects of visual development in infancy. In P. Salapatek and L. Cohen (eds.): Handbook of Infant Perception, Vol. 1, From Sensation to Perception. Orlando, FL: Academic Press.

Aslin, R. N., and P. Salapatek (1975) Saccadic localization of visual targets by the very young human infant. Percep. Psychophys. 17:293–302.

Atkinson, J. (1979) Development of optokinetic nystagmus in the human infant and monkey infant: An analogue to development in kittens. Developmental Neurobiology of Vision: NATO Advanced Study Institute, Series A 27A:277–287.

Atkinson, J., and O. Braddick (1976) Stereoscopic discrimination in infants. Perception 5:29–38.

Atkinson, J., O. Braddick, and K. Moar (1977a) Development of contrast sensitivity over the first 3 months of life in the human infant. Vision Res. 17:1037–1044.

Atkinson, J., O. Braddick, and K. Moar (1977b) Contrast sensitivity of the human infant for moving and static patterns. Vision Res. 17:1045–1047.

Banks, M. S. and P. J. Bennett (1988) Optical and photoreceptor immaturities limit the spatial and chromatic vision of human neonates. J. Opt. Soc. Amer. A. 5: 2059–2079.

Banks, M. S., and P. Salapatek (1978) Acuity and contrast sensitivity in 1-, 2-, 3-month-old human infants. Invest. Ophthalmol. Vis. Sci. 17:361–365.

Banks, M. S., and P. Salapatek (1981) Infant pattern vision: A new approach based on the contrast sensitivity function. J. Exp. Child Psych. 31:1–45.

Banks, M. S., B. R. Stephens, and E. E. Hartmann (1985) The development of basic mechanisms of pattern vision. Spatial frequency channels. J. Exp. Child Psych. 40:501–527.

Barlow, H. B. (1972) Dark and light adaptation: Psychophysics. In D. Jameson and L. M. Hurvich (eds.): Handbook of Sensory Physiology, Vol. VII/4, Visual Psychophysics. New York: Springer-Verlag.

Birch, E. E., J. Gwiazda, and R. Held (1982) Stereoacuity development for crossed and uncrossed disparities in human infants. Vision Res. 22:507–513.

Birch, E. E., J. Gwiazda, J. A. Bauer, Jr., J. Naegele, and R. Held (1983) Visual acuity and its meridional variations in children aged 7–60 months. Vision Res. 23:1019–1024.

Blakemore, C., and F. Vital-Durand (1986) Organization and postnatal development of the monkey's lateral geniculate nucleus. J. Physiol., Lond. 380:453–491.

Bonds, A. B., and R. D. Freeman (1978) Development of optical quality in the kitten eye. Vision Res. 18:391–398.

Boothe, R. G., R. A. Williams, L. Kiorpes, and D. Y. Teller (1980) Development of contrast sensitivity in infant *Macaca nemestrina* monkeys. Science *208*:1290–1292.

Boothe, R. G., L. Kiorpes, R. A. Williams, and D. Y. Teller (1988) Operant measurements of spatial contrast sensitivity in infant macaque monkeys during normal development. Vision Res. *28:* 387–396.

Braddick, O. J. and J. Atkinson (1983) Some recent findings on the development of human binocularity. Behav. Brain Res. *10*:141–150.

Braddick, O., J. Atkinson, and J. R. Wattam-Bell (1986) Development of the discrimination of spatial phase in infancy. Vision Res. 26:1223–1239.

Bradley, A., and R. D. Freeman (1982) Contrast sensitivity in children. Vision Res. 22:953–959.

Brown, A. M. (1986) Scotopic sensitivity of the two-month-old human infant. Vision Res. *26*:707–710.

Campbell, F. W., and D. G. Green (1965) Optical and retinal factors affecting visual resolution. J. Physiol., Lond. *181*:576–593.

Cynader, M., and L. Harris (1980) Eye movement in strabismic cats. Nature *286*: 64–65.

Cynader, M., and K. P. Hoffmann (1981) Strabismus disrupts convergence in the cat nucleus of the optic tract. Dev. Brain Res. *1*:132–136.

Dannemiller, J. L. (1985) The early phase of dark adaptation in human infants. Vision Res. 25:207–212.

Dannemiller, J. L., and M. S. Banks (1983) The development of light adaptation in human infants. Vision Res. 23:599–609.

Dobson, M. V., and D. Y. Teller (1978) Visual acuity in human infants: A review and comparison of behavioral and electrophysiological studies. Vision Res. *18*:1469–1483.

Fantz, R. (1964) Visual experience in infants: Decreased attention to familiar patterns relative to novel ones. Science *146*:668–670.

Fantz, R. (1965) Visual perception from birth as shown by pattern selectivity. Ann. N. Y. Acad. Sci. *118*:793–814.

Fox, R., R. N. Aslin, S. L. Shea, and S. T. Dumais (1980) Stereopsis in human infants. Science *207*:323–324.

Geisler, W. S. (1984) Physical limits of acuity and hyperacuity. J. Opt. Soc. Am. A. *1*:775–782.

Giffin, F., and D. E. Mitchell (1978) The rate of recovery of vision after monocular deprivation in kittens. J. Physiol., Lond. *274*:511–537.

Graham, N. (1972) Spatial frequency channels in the human visual system: Effects of luminance and pattern drift rate. Vision Res. *12*:53–68.

Graham, N. (1980) Spatial-frequency channels in human vision: Detecting edges without edge-detectors. In C. S. Harris (ed.): Visual Coding and Adaptability. Hillsdale, NJ: Erlbaum.

Green, D. G., M. K., Powers, and M. S. Banks (1980) Depth of focus, eye size, and visual acuity. Vision Res. *20*:827–835.

Hainline, L., J. Turkel, I. Abramov, E. Lemerise, and C. M. Harris (1984) Characteristics of saccades in human infants. Vision Res. *24*:1771–1780.

Hamer, R. D., and M. E. Schneck (1984) Spatial summation in dark-adapted infants. Vision Res. 24:77–85.

Hansen, R. M., and A. B. Fulton (1981) Behavioral measurement of background adaptation in human infants. Invest. Ophthalmol. Vis. Sci. 21:625–629.

Hansen, R. M., A. B. Fulton, and S. J. Harris (1986) Background adaptation in human infants. Vision Res. 26:771–779.

Harris L., J. Atkinson, and O. Braddick (1976) Visual contrast sensitivity of a 6-month-old infant measured by the evoked potential. Nature 264:570–571.

Harris, L. R., F. Lepore, J-P. Guillemot, and M. Cynader (1980) Abolition of optokinetic nystagmus in the cat. Science 210:91–92.

Hartmann, E. E., J. G. May, G. S. Ellis, Jr., and A. Love (1987) Infant temporal vision: A visual evoked potential (VEP) measure. Invest. Ophthalmol. Vis. Sci. 28:303.

Hendrickson, A. E., and C. Kupfer (1976) The histogenesis of the fovea in the macaque monkey. Invest. Opthalmol. 15:746–756.

Hendrickson, A. E., and C. Yuodelis (1984) The morphological development of the human fovea. Ophthalmology 91:603–612.

Howland, H. C., R. G. Boothe, and L. Kiorpes (1982) Accommodative defocus does not limit development of acuity in infant Macaca nemestrina monkeys. Science 215:1409–1411.

Kaufman, L. (1975) Sight and Mind. New York: Oxford University Press.

Kelly, D. H. (1972) Flicker. In D. Jameson and L. M. Hurvich (eds.): Handbook of Sensory Physiology, Vol. VII/4, Visual Psychophysics. New York: Springer-Verlag.

Kiorpes L., and J. A. Movshon (1987) Vernier acuity and spatial resolution in infant monkeys. Invest. Ophthalmol. Vis. Sci. 28:359.

Kiorpes, L., and J. A. Movshon (1989) Differential development of two visual functions in primates. Proc. Natl. Acad. Sci. USA 86: in press.

LeVay, S., T. N. Wiesel, and D. H. Hubel (1980) The development of ocular dominance columns in normal and visually deprived monkeys. J. Comp. Neurol. 191:1–51.

Lee, C. P., and R. G. Boothe (1981) Visual acuity development in infant monkeys (Macaca nemestrina) having known gestational ages. Vision Res. 21:805–809.

Levi, D. M., S. A. Klein, and A. P. Aitsebaomo (1985) Vernier acuity, crowding and cortical magnification. Vision Res. 25:963–977.

Lewis, T. L., D. Maurer, and K. Blackburn (1985) The development of the young infants' ability to detect stimuli in the nasal visual field. Vision Res. 25:943–950.

Manny, R. E., and S. A. Klein (1984a) The development of vernier acuity in infants. Curr. Eye Res. 3:453–462.

Manny, R. E., and S. A. Klein (1984b) A three alternative tracking paradigm to measure vernier acuity of older infants. Vision Res. 25:1245–1252.

Mayer, D. L., and M. V. Dobson (1982) Visual acuity development in infants and young children, as assessed by operant preferential looking. Vision Res. 22:1141–1151.

Mitchell, D. E., F. Giffin, F. Wilkinson, P. Anderson, and M. L. Smith (1976) Visual resolution in young kittens. Vision Res. 16:363–366.

Mitchell, D. E., M. Kaye, and B. Timney (1979) Assessment of depth perception in cats. Perception 8:389–396.

Mohn, G., R. Sireteanu, and J. van Hof-van Duin (1986) The relation of monocular optokinetic nystagmus to peripheral binocular interactions. Invest. Ophthalmol. Vis. Sci. 27:565–573.

Moskowitz, A., and S. Sokol (1980) Spatial and temporal interaction of pattern-evoked cortical potentials in human infants. Vision Res. 20:699–707.

Movshon, J. A., and L. Kiorpes (1988) Analysis of the development of spatial contrast sensitivity in monkey and human infants. J. Opt. Soc. Amer. A. 5: 2166–2172.

Naegele, J. R., and R. Held (1982) The postnatal development of monocular opto-kinetic nystagmus in infants. Vision Res. 22:341–346.

Peeples, D. R., and D. Y. Teller (1975) Color vision and brightness discrimination in two-month-old human infants. Science 189:1102–1103.

Peeples, D. R., and D. Y. Teller (1978) White-adapted photopic spectral sensitivity in human infants. Vision Res. 18:49–53.

Powers, M. K., M. E. Schneck, and D. Y. Teller (1981) Spectral sensitivity of human infants at absolute visual threshold. Vision Res. 21:1005–1016.

Pulos, E., D. Y. Teller, and S. L. Buck (1980) Infant color vision: A search for short-wavelength-sensitive mechanisms by means of chromatic adaptation. Vision Res. 20:485–493.

Regal, D. M. (1981) Development of critical flicker frequency in human infants. Vision Res. 21:549–555.

Robson, J. G. (1966) Spatial and temporal contrast sensitivity functions of the visual system. J. Opt. Soc. Am. 56:1141–1142.

Salapatek, P., R. N. Aslin, J. Simonson, and E. Pulos (1980) Infant saccadic eye movements to visible and previously visible targets. Child Develop. 51:1090–1094.

Shimojo, S., and R. Held (1987) Vernier acuity is less than grating acuity in 2- and 3-month-olds. Vision Res. 27:77–86.

Shimojo, S., E. E. Birch, J. Gwiazda, and R. Held (1984) Development of vernier acuity in human infants. Vision Res. 24:721–728.

Shimojo, S., J. Bauer, Jr., K. M. O'Connell, and R. Held (1986) Pre-stereoptic binocular vision in infants. Vision Res. 26:501–510.

Sireteanu, R. (1985) The development of visual acuity in very young kittens. A study with forced-choice preferential looking. Vision Res. 25:781–788.

Sireteanu, R., and D. Maurer (1982) The development of the kitten's visual field. Vision Res. 22:1105–1111.

Sokol, S., and A. Moskowitz (1985) Comparison of pattern VEP's are preferential-looking behavior in 3-month-old infants. Invest. Ophthalmol. Vis. Sci. 26: 359–365.

Teller, D. Y. (1979) The forced-choice preferential looking procedure: A psycho-physical technique for use with human infants. Infant Behav. Devel. 2:135–153.

Teller, D. Y., and R. G. Boothe (1979) The development of vision in infant primates. Trans. Ophthal. Soc. U.K. 99:333–337.

Teller, D. Y., and M. H. Bornstein (1987) Infant color vision and color perception. In

P. Salapatek and L. Cohen (eds.): Handbook of Infant Perception. Vol. 1, From Sensation to Perception. Orlando, FL: Academic Press.

Teller, D. Y., R. Morse, R. Borton, and D. Regal (1974) Visual acuity for vertical and diagonal gratings in human infants. Vision Res. *14*:1433–1439.

Teller, D. Y., D. Regal. T. Videen, and E. Pulos (1978) Development of visual acuity in infant monkeys (*Macaca nemestrina*) during the early postnatal weeks. Vision Res. *18*:561–566.

Timney, B. (1981) Development of binocular depth perception in kittens. Invest. Ophthalmol. Vis. Sci. *21*:493–496.

van Hof-van Duin, J. (1978) Direction preference of optokinetic responses in monocularly tested normal kittens and light deprived cats. Arch Ital. Biol. *116*:471–477.

van Hof-van Duin, J., and G. Mohn (1986) Monocular and binocular optokinetic nystagmus in humans with defective stereopsis. Invest. Ophthalmol. Vis. Sci. *27*:574–583.

Williams, R. A., and R. G. Boothe (1981) Development of optical quality in the infant monkey (*Macaca nemestrina*) eye. Invest. Ophthalmol. Vis. Sci. *21*:728–736.

Williams, R. A., R. G. Boothe, L. Kiorpes, and D. Y. Teller (1981) Oblique effects in normally reared monkeys (*Macaca nemestrina*): meridional variations in contrast sensitivity measured with operant techniques. Vision Res. *21*: 1253–1266.

Wilson, H. (1986) Responses of spatial mechanisms can explain hyperacuity. Vision Res. *26*:453–469.

Yuodelis, C., and A. E. Hendrickson (1986) A qualitative and quantitative analysis of the human fovea during development. Vision Res. *26*:847–855.

Chapter Four

THE ROLE OF EXPERIENCE IN VISUAL DEVELOPMENT

J. ANTHONY MOVSHON AND LYNNE KIORPES

Department of Psychology and Center for Neural Science
New York University
New York, New York

I INTRODUCTION

In the preceding chapters, we have seen how the development of the structure and function of the visual system proceeds in early pre- and postnatal life. In each previous chapter, the role of visual experience was alluded to in one context or another, and here we will examine this influence in more detail. Our emphasis will be on the role of experience in the development of neural *function*, and will consider structural issues only as they bear on functional development. We will also emphasize the role of experience in the development of visual *performance* and the development of the visual mechanisms that underly visual performance. In practice, this means that we will concentrate on the development of visual function in the cerebral cortex, especially the primary visual cortex, area 17. While there is growing evidence that experience has a role in the development of subcortical visual structures (e.g., Sherman and Spear, 1982), it is clear that most of the experiential influences that affect visual performance are expressed in the visual cortex. Because a chapter of this kind is necessarily selective, we refer the interested reader to other recent reviews for more comprehensive coverage of related issues (Movshon and Van Sluyters, 1981; Sherman and Spear, 1982; Mitchell and Timney, 1984; Boothe et al., 1985).

The prenatal development of the visual system, we now know, is extensive and complex and proceeds, of course, without influence from the visual environment (see Chapter 1, this volume). The early postnatal development of the visual system also proceeds largely independently of the visual environment so long as that environment is qualitatively adequate (see Chapter 2, this volume). Yet it is clear that disruption or limitation of the visual environment causes very dramatic changes in the pattern of development. This paradox leads to one of the major questions in current developmental research: Why is it that in the presence of normal visual experience, development proceeds largely according to an innate plan, while abnormal visual experience can disrupt this plan so thoroughly?

Several different roles have been ascribed to visual experience in development. The most conservative idea is that experience is necessary only so far as it acts to *maintain* innately specified functional characteristics. With normal visual input, the function and specificity of the visual system are merely extended but not refined beyond the state existing at birth. It is often argued that visual input does more than this and serves to *refine* the pattern of functional organization that was innately laid down. Finally, it may be that experience plays yet more active a role and can actually *specify* the functional connections and activity of portions of the visual pathways. Through this chapter we will consider this tripartite question—maintenance, refinement, or specification?—as we examine the ways that visual experience affects visual development.

II   EFFECTS OF FORM DEPRIVATION

The most direct and least subtle way to enquire about the role of experience in development is to deprive a growing animal of vision altogether. At the very least, this treatment shows what development the animal's visual system is capable of in the complete absence of visual stimulation. In some cases (e.g., the rabbit: Chow and Spear, 1974), this approach quickly reveals that the system under study develops in near-complete indifference to the visual environment. For other species, however, such as the cat and monkey, deprivation of form or light has a devastating effect on visual development.

A   Effects on Central Visual Processing

Although the issue has probably not been decisively laid to rest, it seems very likely that visual deprivation in mammals has no important effect on the development of retinal function. Despite scattered reports of anatomical changes in the retina, no one has reported a convincing change in the receptive field properties of retinal ganglion cells following deprivation; several reports suggest that ganglion cells are at least qualitatively normal in their responsiveness and organization (see Sherman and Spear, 1982). Deprivation–induced effects on the morphology of retinal ganglion cells have occasionally been reported in primates, but the reliability and significance of these observations is unclear (Chow et al., 1957; Hendrickson and Boothe, 1976; Von Noorden and Crawford, 1977).

Visual deprivation does, however, have substantial effects on the development of function in central visual structures. Several different forms of visual deprivation have been employed experimentally in studies of cortical development. The most common of these are eyelid suture, which deprives animals of form vision and attenuates the diffuse light entering the eye, and dark rearing, which removes all visual input. In many cases these two kinds of deprivation produce similar changes, although we will consider situations in which they seem to have different effects. The diligent may wish to seek out a recent exhaustive review of this topic (Sherman and Spear, 1982);

an earlier literature concentrating on the behavioral and anatomical effects of deprivation is reviewed in Riesen (1966).

In cats and monkeys, complete visual deprivation has rather striking effects on the development of central visual function, including profound alterations in the anatomy and physiology of the central visual pathways. There is some variation in the effects of complete deprivation that have been reported in the literature, but these vary only from the devastating (e.g., Watkins et al., 1978) to the merely severe (e.g., Hubel and Wiesel, 1965; Wiesel and Hubel, 1974). Most authors agree that visual deprivation in large part disrupts the development of the exquisitely organized visual receptive fields in cortical neurons, and this qualitative impression has received significant quantitative support (Derrington, 1984; Bonds, 1979; Ohzawa and Freeman, 1988). Compared to the normal cat or monkey cortex, where most cells have well-developed selectivity for orientation, direction of movement, spatial frequency, binocular disparity, and the like, the cortex of visually deprived animals is poorly equipped with stimulus selectivity. Visually unresponsive cells (which are practically never encountered in the cortex of normally reared animals) are common, forming as much as two-thirds of some samples of cortical neurons, although these cells' unresponsiveness may result from chronic inhibitory influences that do not operate in the same way in anesthetized and awake animals (Ramoa et al., 1987; Tsumoto and Freeman, 1987). Figure 1 summarizes these points using data replotted from Blakemore and Van Sluyters (1975). The upper panel of the figure shows data for seven normal kittens of various ages. The three curves plot the proportion of orientation selective (open circles), unselective (open triangles), and unresponsive (filled circles) neurons in these animals. By the age of 4 weeks in normal kittens, virtually all neurons are orientation selective. The lower panel plots data for seven binocularly deprived kittens using the same conventions. The proportions of cells in the three groups seem "frozen" at the proportions seen in newborn animals.

Qualitative assessments of visual behavior in dark-reared animals suggest that when they first emerge from the dark they are virtually blind. However, in cats and monkeys removed from the dark by 4 months of age, both visual responsiveness and visual acuity show recovery with time in the light (Timney et al., 1978; Regal et al., 1976). Most animals eventually recover nearly normal visual acuity and visual responsiveness, although the degree of recovery decreases with longer periods of dark rearing. Recovery can thus be quite extensive, even after the end of the period in development at which plasticity usually ends. The delayed period of visual experience may in fact represent a period of delayed plasticity, an issue to which we will return below in Section IIIA on regulation of visual cortical plasticity (see Cynader and Mitchell, 1980).

Finally, we should briefly consider whether deprivation of *light* (by dark rearing) and deprivation of *form* (by lid suture) have different effects. Early reports suggested that it was only deprivation of contoured visual stimula-

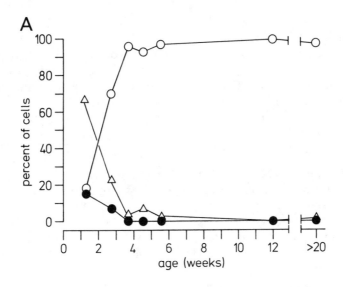

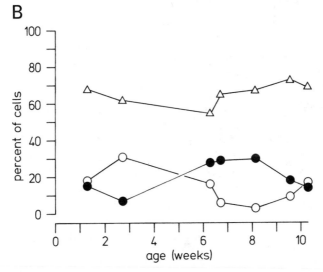

FIGURE 1. The development of response properties in striate cortex of normal and visually deprived kittens (*A*) Percentage of cells sampled in normal kittens that were normally selective (open circles; including orientation and direction selective cells), unselective (open triangles; including orientation-biased and nonoriented cells), or visually unresponsive (filled circles) as a function of age in weeks. (*B*) Percentage of cells sampled in visually deprived kittens that were normally selective, unselective, or unresponsive as a function of age [symbols same as (*A*)]. Visually deprived kittens show a reduction in normal, selective cells with a consequent increase in abnormal, unselective cells. (After Blakemore and Van Sluyters, 1975.)

tion that was significant (e.g., Wiesel and Hubel, 1963a,b, 1965a; Blakemore and Van Sluyters, 1975; Blakemore, 1976). More recently some evidence has appeared suggesting that there are differences between animals deprived of all light and animals deprived only of visual form in the degree to which subsequent visual experience can promote recovery from the effects of visual deprivation (e.g., Mower, et al., 1981). There may also be differential effects on the binocularity of cortical neurons (see Section III).

B Summary

In cats and monkeys (and probably also in humans: Von Senden, 1960), the preponderance of the evidence suggests that complete deprivation of the early experience of visual form arrests the development of central visual function and may even provoke some atrophy of the functional neural connections that exist near the time of birth. Thus visual experience is certainly necessary to *maintain* visual function. To establish whether experience has a more active role in refining or specifying the properties of central visual structures, it is necessary to use more subtle manipulations of the early visual environment.

III SELECTIVE EFFECTS OF VISUAL EXPERIENCE ON BINOCULAR INTERACTION

Binocular interaction in the central visual system has proved to be among the visual functions most susceptible to the effects of early visual experience. The modern era of enquiry into the effects of early experience was inaugurated by Wiesel and Hubel's (1963a,b) studies of the effects of monocular occlusion. Their subsequent work on this topic and on other manipulations of binocular visual experience remains their most enduring contribution to research in visual development.

A Organization and Development of Cortical Binocularity

The earliest recordings of receptive field properties from neurons in the striate cortex of cats revealed that some cortical neurons could be influenced by stimulation of either eye (Hubel and Wiesel, 1962). Hubel and Wiesel described a gradation of *ocular dominance* among striate cortical neurons. A few cells were strictly monocular (could be influenced by stimulation of one eye only); some were equally binocular (could be influenced equally well through either eye); the remainder could be influenced by both eyes, but one eye's influence was greater than that of the other eye. Figure 2A shows Hubel and Wiesel's data on the distribution of ocular dominance for large populations of neurons recorded from normally reared adult cats (A) and monkeys (B). Although the distributions are slightly different, with cats having more pronounced binocularity, it is clear that most cortical neurons in either species can be influenced by visual stimulation of either eye.

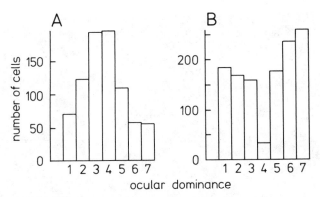

FIGURE 2. The distribution of ocular dominance in striate cortex of normal cats (*A*) and monkeys (*B*). The relative number of cells is shown for each ocular dominance group, where catagory 1 represents neurons responsive to the contralateral eye, category 7 represents neurons responsive to the ipsilateral eye, and category 4 represents neurons that are equally responsive to either eye. Categories 2, 3, 5, and 6 represent intermediate levels of influence from the two eyes; for example, category 2 represents neurons primarily driven by the contralateral eye with some influence by the ipsilateral eye. (From Hubel et al., 1977.)

Hubel and Wiesel noticed during some of the early developmental work in cats (1965) that cells of like ocular dominance were clustered together in the cortex. The clustering took the form of ordered columns comprised of cells with the same eye dominant; the left and right eyes alternated dominance across the cortex (Hubel and Wiesel, 1965, 1968). Our present understanding of the organization of ocular dominance in striate cortex differs only in detail from that originally described by Hubel and Wiesel. The columns extend through the depth of striate cortex, normal to the surface, and within each column the influence of one eye is dominant over the other. Throughout most layers of the cortex, cells within a column range from monocular, through several intermediate stages, to binocular. Layer 4 is an exception, however. The cells in layer 4, which receive their input from the lateral geniculate nucleus (LGN), are in macaques strictly monocular and in cats largely so (Hubel and Wiesel, 1968; LeVay, et al., 1978). The morphological basis of these eye dominance columns is a segregation, by eye of origin, of inputs to layer 4 from the LGN. Figure 3 shows two autoradiographs that reveal the distribution of input from the two eyes in the cortex of a macaque monkey. One of the animal's eyes was injected with a radioactively labeled amino acid tracer that was trans-synaptically transported to the visual cortex; the light regions in the dark-field autoradiographs show the location of transported radioactivity (Hubel et al., 1977). The upper panel (*A*) shows the cortex in cross section. The central light "stream" shows the fibers in the white matter underlying the cortex, while the patchy string of "beads" running through the middle layers of the cortex shows the alternating presence and absence of input from the injected eye in layer 4. The lower panel (*B*) shows a section that passed nearly

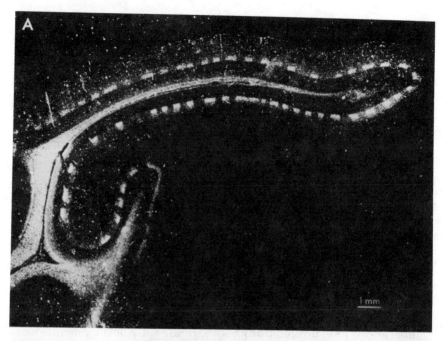

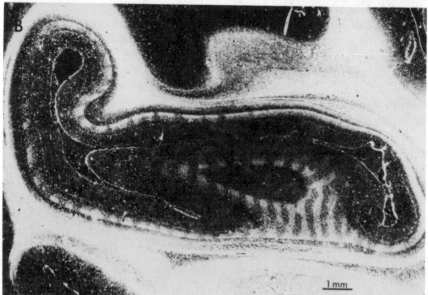

FIGURE 3. The alternating pattern of eye dominance in layer 4 of normal monkeys shown by injection of one eye with a radioactive tracer. The autoradiographs show the banding pattern in striate cortex ipsilateral in cross section (*A*) and contralateral, horizontally through layer 4 (*B*) to the injected eye. (From Hubel et al., 1977.)

parallel to layer 4. The parallel "striped" arrangement of the zones of input is clearly evident. Both panels show that input from the injected eye is present in roughly half of layer 4; other experiments show that the gaps are filled with input from the uninjected eye.

The development of the connections that subserve cortical binocularity begins well before birth in both cats and monkeys (see Chapter 1). Rakic and his collaborators have charted the prenatal generation and development of the macaque visual system using the technique of marking DNA replication with ³H-thymidine; he also extended the autoradiographic technique for tracing neuronal connections to fetal monkeys (see Rakic, 1977, for a review). Shatz and her colleagues have used similar techniques to study the prenatal development of the cat's visual system (Shatz, 1983; Luskin and Shatz, 1985).

All neurons that comprise the visual system are generated during the first and second trimester of gestation. Retinal ganglion cells and LGN cells are generated during the first trimester, while neurons destined for striate cortex are generated during the second trimester. When ganglion cell axons first arrive at the developing LGN, the terminals from the two eyes are completely intermixed—there is no laminar segregation apparent until the third trimester (recall that in the adult LGN the terminals from each eye are segregated into different layers within both the magnocellular and parvocellular divisions). Similarly, when the geniculate axons first arrive at their target layer in the cortex, there is no evidence of the clear segregation by eye shown in Figure 3. Late in the third trimester, segregation of geniculate afferents begins. At term, the divisions between the sublaminae of layer 4 are reasonably crisp; the segregation of ocular dominance in layer 4 is discernible but far from complete.

The remainder of the development of binocular organization occurs during the early postnatal weeks. LeVay, et al. (1980), in an extensive study of the postnatal development of ocular dominance in monkey striate cortex, determined that segregation of the geniculate afferents in layer 4 is complete by 6 weeks after birth. Figure 4 shows three representative autoradiographs taken from monkeys 6 days, 3 weeks, and 6 weeks old. It is evident that the crisp segregation of inputs into regions controlled by either eye is incomplete in the first week of life but basically finished 5 weeks later. Figure 5 shows in cartoon form a cross section of layer 4 during the process of segregation. The process of ocular dominance segregation is similar in the cat, although it appears to begin at about 3 weeks postnatally and end by about 6 weeks (LeVay et al., 1978). Information on the development of ocular dominance organization outside of layer 4 is curiously scarce. Two reports suggest that the overall distribution of ocular dominance in newborn monkeys is similar to that of the adult and that the grouping of cells resembles the columnar organization found for the adult (Wiesel and Hubel, 1974; Hubel et al., 1977). This segregation is curious in view of the immature anatomical segregation evident in Figure 4.

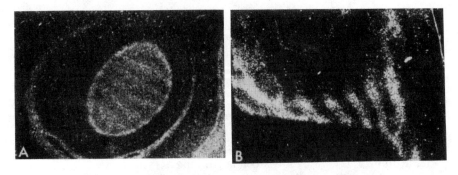

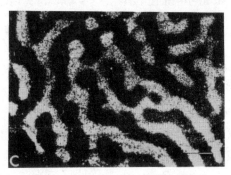

FIGURE 4. The process of segregation of geniculate afferents from each eye in layer 4 of normal monkeys. The pattern of ocular dominance development in striate cortex of young monkeys is shown in the series of autoradiographs. (A) The central oval area shows a mild degree of modulation of label in layer 4 ipsilateral to the injected eye in a 6-day-old monkey. (B) A section contralateral to the injected eye in a 3-week-old monkey shows sharper boundaries between the columns. (C) A montage of layer 4 ipsilateral to the injected eye in a 6-week-old monkey shows banding that is as sharply defined as in the adult. Thus there is a progressive sharpening of the banding pattern from the youngest to the oldest age. (From LeVay et al., 1980; Wiesel, 1982.)

B Prenatal "Visual Experience"

Clearly, the prenatal development of the visual system proceeds without influence from the visual environment. The organization of binocularity is therefore prespecified, and given normal gestation, development proceeds according to an innate plan. However, this innate plan can be disrupted if the normal constituents of the visual system are not present at the time that connections are formed. Rakic (1981) demonstrated that afferents from both eyes need to be present in the LGN at the time laminar segregation normally begins in order for the segregation process to occur. Removal of one eye prior to the time of segregation results in the complete failure of segregation; the LGN then has only two layers, corresponding to the magnocellular and parvocellular divisions, with a single interlaminar zone. The usual

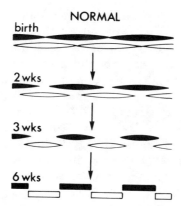

FIGURE 5. A cartoon representation of the presumed pattern of segregation of geniculate afferents after birth. Open and filled zones represent afferents from each eye; the width of the zone represents the presumed density of each set of terminations. In normal monkeys at birth the afferents from the two eyes are nearly completely overlapping. Between birth and 6 weeks the afferents from the two eyes gradually retract, leaving the sharp, alternating pattern of eye dominance shown at 6 weeks (From Hubel et al., 1977.)

pattern of cortical ocular dominance also fails to develop unless afferents from both eyes are present. Without input from both eyes, layer 4 shows continuous uninterrupted activity from the remaining eye.

The demonstration that the presence of both eyes is required for the initiation of segregation suggests that some kind of competitive interaction takes place between the terminals from each eye. This competitive interaction is required not only for the initiation of the process but also for its maintenance once begun. Removal of an eye during segregation causes the arrest of the process at the stage attained by the time of removal. It is worth noting that this disruption is selective for developmental functions that depend on binocular interaction; the segregation into magnocellular and parvocellular divisions proceeds normally.

An interesting question that arises in this context concerns the role of functional activity in regulating the development and segregation of binocular connections. In this context it is particularly interesting that Shatz and Kirkwood (1984) were able to demonstrate in a series of technically demanding experiments that individual geniculate neurons in fetal cats receive functional synaptic inputs from *both* eyes early in development. Later segregation of afferents eventually leads to the normal adult situation in which only one eye provides excitatory drive for each LGN neuron.

C   Effects of Binocular Deprivation on Binocular Interaction

We have seen that, given an anatomically complete visual system and an otherwise normal fetal environment, visual development proceeds essentially automatically until the end of the gestation period. It is worth considering whether or not visual experience in the immediate postnatal period is important for normal completion of the ocular dominance organization in striate cortex. If gestation were to continue beyond term, for example, or if the newborn were kept in the dark from the moment of birth, would ocular dominance development follow the same course? It appears that the segregation of ocular dominance columns in layer 4 proceeds normally in monkeys reared in the dark (LeVay et al., 1980). Physiological data from cats reared in complete darkness also suggest that a normal distribution of binocular connections develops (Frégnac and Imbert, 1978; Cynader and Mitchell, 1980; Mower et al., 1981). Thus, with normal visual experience or in the absence of all visual experience, the development of binocular organization proceeds to completion.

Binocular connections in binocularly deprived monkeys may be especially vulnerable to the effects of binocular deprivation by lid suture. Figure 6 shows distributions of ocular dominance for cats (A) and monkeys (B) deprived of vision early in life by binocular lid suture (Wiesel and Hubel, 1965a; Wiesel and Hubel, 1974). Comparison with Figure 2 reveals that a roughly normal proportion of binocularly driven neurons is evident in the cats but few remain in the deprived monkeys. Other reports have suggested that cats deprived in this way may also show a loss of binocular neurons (e.g., Kratz and Spear, 1976; Watkins et al., 1978; Mower et al., 1981), but most reports agree that binocularity is well preserved in animals deprived of vision by dark rearing. Curiously, bilateral lid suture may cause an increase in the proportion of abnormal neurons (those that are difficult to characterize or visually drive), compared to dark rearing (Wiesel and Hubel, 1965a, 1974; Blakemore and Van Sluyters, 1975; Mower et al., 1981). This may be a

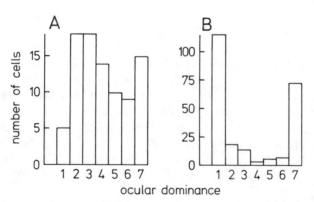

FIGURE 6. The distribution of ocular dominance in binocularly deprived cats (A) and monkeys (B). The distribution of binocularity in cats binocularly deprived by lid suture is similar to that found for dark-reared cats, whereas in binocularly deprived monkeys there is a dramatic reduction in the proportion of binocular cells. (Redrawn from Wiesel and Hubel, 1965a, 1974.)

result of the uncorrelated diffuse-light visual stimulation that passes even through the sutured eyelids of these animals (Loop and Sherman, 1977; Spear et al. 1978). Whether or not this is the reason, it appears that deprivation of patterned visual input has detrimental effects on the development of cortical binocularity in the early postnatal period.

However, even though binocular connections in deprived animals are crudely normal, the usual sensitivity of cortical neurons to the binocular disparity of visual stimuli is altogether lacking (Pettigrew, 1974), though Ohzawa and Freeman (1988) attribute this to abnormalities in the organization of *monocular* receptive fields. Extended periods of binocular deprivation, whatever the form, disrupt the binocular organization and specificity of cortical neurons and appear to cause a deterioration of these functions rather than a simple arrest of development (see also, Pettigrew, 1974). Since the development of cortical ocular dominance proceeds normally in the absence of visual experience, and deprivation of patterned visual input results in a deterioration of this organization, it is likely that the role of patterned visual experience in this respect is one of maintenance or refinement rather than of specification.

D   Effects of Monocular Deprivation

We saw that the presence of both eyes is required for the maintenance (indeed the initiation) of binocular organization prenatally. It is also the case that visual input from both eyes is required for the maintenance of cortical binocularity throughout the postnatal developmental period. The pioneering studies of Wiesel and Hubel first demonstrated the vulnerability of ocular dominance organization to imbalanced binocular input (see Wiesel, 1982). They discovered that closing one eyelid in a young kitten at or near the time of eye opening (age 3 weeks) resulted in the nearly complete shift of ocular dominance in striate cortex away from the closed eye. The effect seemed considerably more dramatic than that of closing both eyes. Wiesel and Hubel concluded that the imbalance of the visual input created competition between the afferents for the two eyes. Since the open eye provided stronger input than the closed eye, it came to dominate the available cortical territory. Figure 7A exemplifies this finding by showing the distribution of ocular dominance for neurons recorded from a monkey monocularly deprived from the age of 2 weeks. Compared with the usual pattern of ocular dominance in monkeys (Figure 2B), little influence of the deprived eye is evident in the cortex. Figures 7B and C show data obtained from two recording sessions in another monkey. The left-hand histogram (7B) shows the ocular dominance distribution for neurons recorded at the age of 3 weeks, before the beginning of deprivation. The right-hand histogram (7C) shows data obtained at the age of 7 months, after an intervening period of monocular deprivation. As one would expect from the previous discussion of the early development of cortical binocularity, monocular deprivation acts by disrupting a preexisting set of functional binocular connections.

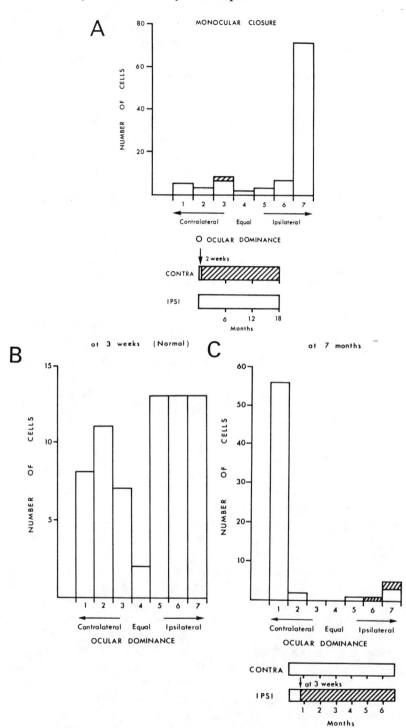

The effects of monocular deprivation can only be produced during a *sensitive period* early in life, a period during which the visual system can be modified by visual experience. In kittens, the sensitive period begins abruptly during the third week of life, reaches a peak of sensitivity between the ages of 4 and 5 weeks, and then gradually wanes until the age of 4–6 months, when visual experience can no longer cause a reliable change in cortical function (Hubel and Wiesel, 1970). The ability of reversed lid suture to promote recovery from the effects of monocular deprivation follows a similar time course (Blakemore and Van Sluyters, 1974; Movshon, 1976a). In monkeys, the sensitive period begins at or before birth and declines over the first year or two of life (LeVay et al., 1980; Blakemore et al., 1981).

Closer examination of the sensitive period for the effects of monocular deprivation in monkeys reveals that it can be divided into two distinct phases. In the first phase, deprivation produces changes in the anatomical organization of cortical afferents, which lead in turn to changes in cortical binocularity. In the second phase, deprivation produces changes in cortical binocularity, but these result from a rearrangement of intracortical connections. Early deprivation results in reduced width of the deprived eye columns in layer 4, with a complementary expansion of nondeprived eye columns. The morphological basis for this effect is shown in Figure 8A and 8B. Using methods like those used in Figure 4 Hubel et al. (1977) showed, in animals deprived from near the time of birth, that the representation of the nondeprived eye in layer 4 was greatly expanded (Figure 8A); labeling terminals from the deprived eye revealed a matching reduction in the extent of its input (Figure 8B). If the onset of deprivation is delayed beyond 6 weeks, however, no change in ocular dominance organization is evident anatomically, and labeling the deprived eye yields results like those shown for normal animals in Figure 4C. Figure 8C shows how Hubel and his colleagues explained this result in terms of the process of segregation of geniculocortical afferents. The left half of the figure (reproducing Figure 5) represents the pattern of ocular dominance segregation that occurs during the first 6 weeks of life in normally reared monkeys (see the preceding). The right half shows the pattern of ocular dominance organization revealed in cortex following deprivation beginning at each of the indicated ages. Input

---

FIGURE 7. The physiological effects of monocular deprivation on ocular dominance in striate cortex of monkeys. (A) Distribution of ocular dominance for a monkey monocularly deprived beginning at 2 weeks of age. The right eye was closed from 2 weeks to 18 months as indicated on the bar graph at the bottom of the figure; cells were recorded in the left hemisphere. Clearly, there is a dramatic shift of dominance away from the deprived eye. (B) Distribution of ocular dominance from a normal 3-week-old monkey just prior to closure of one eye. (C) Ocular dominance of the same monkey [as in (B)] following 7 months of monocular deprivation. The right eye was closed at 3 weeks; recordings were made from both hemispheres, however, ipsilateral refers to domination by the right eye. In all three histograms, the cross-hatched areas represent numbers of abnormal cells. (From Hubel et al., 1977.)

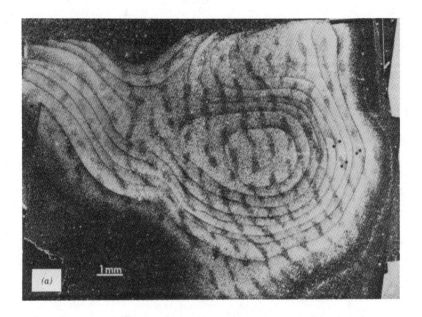

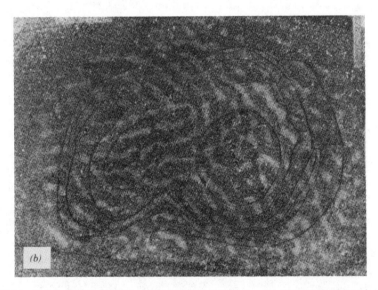

FIGURE 8. The anatomical effects of monocular deprivation on the pattern of ocular dominance in striate cortex. (A) An autoradiographic montage of layer 4 contralateral to the deprived eye of the monkey shown in Figure 7A, showing the reduction of column widths for the deprived eye represented by the dark stripes (the nondeprived eye was injected). (B) An autoradiographic montage of layer 4 ipsilateral to the deprived eye of the monkey shown in Figure 7B; the deprived eye is represented by the light stripes (the deprived eye was injected).

from the deprived eye survives only in regions of layer 4 from which input from the nondeprived eye has withdrawn before the onset of deprivation.

Outside layer 4, however, the effects of deprivation that does not begin until after the age of 6 weeks can be quite complete in that it remains difficult or impossible to detect the influence of the deprived eye. In layer 4, in regions receiving input from the deprived eye, visual signals from that eye can be readily detected. The intracortical connections that relay these signals to other layers, however, are radically weakened by deprivation. Detailed study reveals that these connections are not altogether abolished following deprivation of late onset because significant numbers of neurons retain functional—albeit weakened—connections with the deprived eye (e.g., Hubel and Wiesel, 1977; Shatz and Stryker, 1978; Blakemore, et al., 1978; Van Sluyters, 1978; Blakemore, et al., 1982; Freeman and Ohzawa, 1988). The later the onset of deprivation, the smaller the resulting change in cortical function. Some residual plasticity can be demonstrated as late as 4–6 months in cats and 1–1.5 years postnatally in monkeys, but this is entirely outside layer 4.

Wiesel and Hubel's original studies suggested that there was little effect of monocular deprivation on subcortical structures, especially the LGN, other than a pronounced shrinkage of the geniculate cells (Wiesel and Hubel, 1963a). Subsequently, Sherman, et al. (1972) found that Y-cells, a

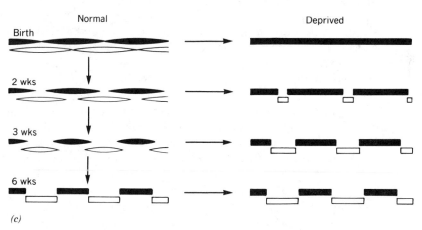

(c)

(C) A cartoon showing the presumed effects of monocular deprivation at different ages on the width of the columns in layer 4. Left: The same cartoon as shown in Figure 5. Right: Deprivation at birth (top) results in a complete takeover of layer 4 by the nondeprived eye. With later onset of deprivation, the deprived eye retains a greater proportion of territory in layer 4, the amount of which is related to the degree of segregation prior to the onset of deprivation. Monocular deprivation begun after 6 weeks fails to alter the pattern of ocular dominance in layer 4. (From Hubel et al., 1977; LeVay et al., 1980.)

particular functional class of geniculate neurons, seemed to be missing in deprived cats. Although this finding has been somewhat controversial, it now seems well established that deprivation affects the proportion of Y-cells in the deprived layers of the cat's LGN. A competitive interaction between X and Y retinal axons arriving in the geniculate seems to be a likely mechanism (Friedlander et al., 1982). In monkeys, however, Wiesel and Hubel's original observations seem to be borne out. Both Blakemore and Vital-Durand (1986) and Levitt et al., (1989) found that the deprived neurons in the LGN of Old World monkeys are quantitatively indistinguishable from nondeprived ones. Thus we may safely conclude that at least in the monkey, the effects of monocular deprivation on the functional characteristics of visual neurons are confined to the visual cortex.

Behavioral studies of the effects of monocular deprivation on visual performance unanimously find that visuomotor behavior (Dews and Wiesel, 1970; Movshon, 1976b; Cynader et al., 1980), visual acuity (von Noorden, et al., 1970; von Noorden, 1973; Mitchell et al., 1977; Giffin and Mitchell, 1978), contrast sensitivity (Harwerth et al., 1981, 1983a), and binocular vision (Harwerth et al., 1986) are all severely compromised. The deficits in visual performance are in fact greater than would be predicted on the basis of an arrest of normal development at the onset of deprivation. Therefore, it is likely that monocular deprivation leads to a deterioration of the neural elements underlying visual performance. As was found in the physiological studies of monocular deprivation, the earlier the onset of the deprivation (and the longer the period of deprivation), the greater are the deficits in visual performance. Studies of recovery from the effects of monocular deprivation reveal that the deficits can be reversed, depending on the age and duration of the initial deprivation, given enforced usage of the deprived eye (Dews and Wiesel, 1970; Movshon, 1976b; Mitchell et al., 1977; Giffin and Mitchell, 1978). Figure 9 shows behavioral data from a monocularly deprived cat whose rearing history is depicted by the bar graph at the bottom of the figure. The open portions of the bar indicate when each eye was open; the filled portions indicate when each eye was closed. Enforced usage of the deprived eye is usually accomplished by reversed lid suture: opening the deprived eye and closing the nondeprived eye. The acuity of the initially nondeprived eye develops normally until the time of reverse suture (open circle to the left of the shaded zone in Figure 9); the acuity of the initially deprived eye was essentially unmeasurable at the time of reverse suture (open arrow, filled symbols). Monocular deprivation during the first 2–3 months after eye opening in kittens followed by several weeks of reverse suture results in a virtually complete reversal of the deprivation effect as can be seen at the end of the shaded zone in Figure 9. The initially deprived eye comes to dominate in striate cortex and regains reasonable, though subnormal, levels of visual acuity while the initially nondeprived eye deteriorates to an extremely poor acuity level. Extended periods of deprivation beginning at very young ages result in large deficits that are

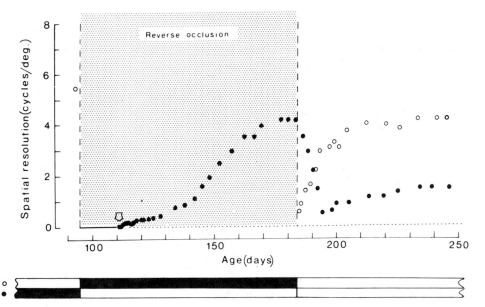

FIGURE 9. Behavioral data on the effects of monocular deprivation and reverse occlusion. Spatial resolution (acuity) is plotted as a function of age for each eye of a cat whose rearing history is depicted by the bar graph at the bottom of the figure. Data for the initally deprived and nondeprived eyes are represented by the filled and open symbols, respectively. The initially deprived eye was closed from 9 to 94 days of age, at which time it was opened and the originally nondeprived eye was closed; the acuity of the nondeprived eye at the time of reverse suture is shown as the single open circle to the left of the shaded zone. The shaded zone represents the period of reverse occlusion, during which the acuity of the initially deprived eye improved considerably (progression of filled circles). Following 89 days of reverse suture, the initially deprived eye had gained nearly normal acuity whereas the intially nondeprived eye deteriorated to a very low level. Thereafter, the cat was allowed normal binocular experience, during which time there was a reciprocal change in acuity for the two eyes. The initially nondeprived eye recovered (although not fully) and the initially deprived eye returned to a lower, poor level of acuity. (From Mitchell et al., 1984.)

difficult to reverse. Some recovery is also possible in the presence of binocular visual experience, at least in cats, although the degree of recovery is less dramatic than that following enforced usage of the deprived eye (Mitchell et al., 1977; Olson and Freeman, 1978; but see Wiesel and Hubel, 1965b, for a contradictory report). Binocular visual experience is apparently not sufficient to promote recovery from the effects of monocular deprivation in monkeys (LeVay et al., 1980; Blakemore et al., 1981).

While the nature of the recovery from monocular deprivation is such that the originally deprived eye regains influence over a substantial number of neurons in the cortex, the *binocular organization* does not recover. The cortex remains essentially monocular, and binocular visual function remains impaired. It is also important to realize that recovery following monocular deprivation is not necessarily permanent. Reopening the originally open eye (following reverse suture) results in the restoration of good visual acuity for the originally open eye and a complementary loss of visual acuity in the originally deprived eye, as shown in the right portion of Figure 9 (beyond the shaded zone) (Mitchell et al., 1984).

E   Artificial Strabismus and Other Forms of Interocular Decorrelation

The effects of monocular deprivation on binocular organization and visual performance are thought to be due to the lack of patterned visual input to the deprived eye, which creates a condition of imbalance between the eyes. While the deprivation of patterned input to one eye is sufficient to disrupt the binocular organization of the striate cortex, it is not a necessary condition. This is illustrated by studies employing rearing conditions that dissociate the input to the two eyes without depriving either eye of qualitatively good visual input. Strabismus, a misalignment of the visual axes, and alternating monocular occlusion both disrupt cortical ocular dominance when present during the early postnatal period; in both cases the quality of the visual input to each eye is similar. Hubel and Wiesel (1965) first documented the effects of artificial strabismus on binocular organization in cats. As illustrated in Figure 10A, which summarizes the ocular dominance distributions for their strabismic animals, they found that the condition produced a virtually complete breakdown of binocularity. Instead of the usual 80% of the neurons being influenced by both eyes, only 20% were binocular; the rest were monocular, with both eyes being equally represented. In spite of the breakdown of binocularity, the columnar structure of the cortex was preserved; indeed, the enhanced segregation of the two eyes' ocular dominance columns in these animals is what provoked Hubel and Wiesel to

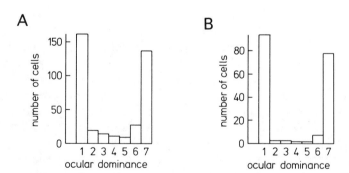

FIGURE 10. Ocular dominance distributions from cats raised with strabismus (A) and alternate monocular occlusion (B). There is a clear reduction in binocularity, with approximately equal representation of the two eyes, as a result of both forms of intervention. (Redrawn from Hubel and Wiesel, 1965.)

examine normal animals for signs of this sort of organization. Unlike the situation resulting from binocular deprivation, other properties of striate neurons (like overall responsiveness and orientation selectivity) appeared to be normal. Although the visual image in each eye is of good quality in strabismus, the two images are uncorrelated. Thus, like monocular deprivation, strabismus creates the conditions for competitive interaction between the two eyes. Hubel and Wiesel (1965) also investigated the possibility that the competitive interaction was responsible for the breakdown of binocularity by alternately occluding one eye each day. In this way, they allowed each eye equal visual experience without the possibility of competitive interaction between them. As is shown in Figure 10B, which plots ocular dominance data from these animals, cortical binocularity was disrupted by alternating monocular occlusion even more severely than by strabismus. Hirsch and Spinelli (1970) reared kittens wearing goggles that presented a vertical grating to one eye and a horizontal grating to the other; this form of binocular decorrelation also disrupted cortical binocularity completely. Therefore, elimination of simultaneous binocular competition is not sufficient to preserve cortical binocularity. It seems, then, that any condition that provides discordant input to the two eyes during the early postnatal period is sufficient to disrupt the organization of cortical binocularity.

Many subsequent investigations have replicated the physiological effects of discordant visual input reported by Hubel and Wiesel. However, an interesting species difference has emerged from these studies. While strabismic cats show an essentially equal representation of each eye in cortical ocular dominance (Hubel and Wiesel, 1965; Van Sluyters and Levitt, 1980; Kalil et al., 1984), artificial strabismus in the monkey results in a shift in ocular dominance away from the deviated eye as well as a breakdown in binocularity (Baker et al., 1974; Crawford and Von Noorden, 1979; Eggers et al., 1984). Figure 11 shows the distribution of ocular dominance from three monkeys made surgically strabismic by Eggers et al. (1984). It is evident that the deviating eye (D) controls far fewer cortical neurons than the nondeviating eye (N), unlike the situation in cats (Figure 10A). Binocularity in both cats and monkeys, however, is comparably reduced.

In many cases, the shift in ocular dominance correlated with the loss of visual capacity shown by the deviated eye (Baker et al., 1974; Wiesel, 1982; Eggers et al., 1984). However, it is unlikely that the number of neurons driven by the deprived eye by itself determines its level of visual function since kittens that showed deficits in visual performance with the deviated eye were found to have equal representation of the two eyes in striate cortex (Holopigian and Blake, 1983; Chino et al., 1983). Abnormalities in the spatial and temporal tuning properties of striate neurons have been reported in both strabismic cats and monkeys, which correlate well with the deficits in spatial vision exhibited by the animals (Chino et al., 1983; Eggers et al., 1984). These deficits are probably more closely related to those seen behaviorally (see Kiorpes et al., 1987; Movshon et al., 1987). The disruption of

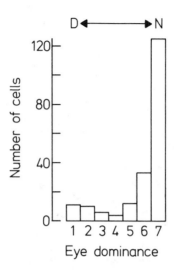

FIGURE 11. Ocular dominance from a group of strabismic monkeys. In this histogram, category 1 represents the deviated eyes and category 7 represents the nondeviated eyes. Monkeys show a similar loss of binocularity to strabismic kittens; however, in addition, there is a shift away from the deviated eye (From Eggers et al., 1984.)

binocularity in the cortex is probably more significant for binocular vision and stereopsis. Several studies have confirmed that interocular transfer of visual after effects, which depends on the function of binocular neurons, is impaired in strabismic humans (Movshon et al., 1972; Mitchell and Ware, 1974; Banks et al., 1975). Interocular transfer of visual discriminations is impaired in strabismic cats (Sherman, 1971). Also, cats raised with alternating monocular occlusion fail to demonstrate binocular summation (Von Grünau, 1979) or evidence of stereopsis (Packwood and Gordon, 1975; Blake and Hirsch, 1975). Crawford and von Noorden (1980) used the prism-rearing method developed by Van Sluyters and Levitt (1980) for optically producing strabismus in monkeys, leading to a breakdown of cortical binocularity but no shift in ocular dominance away from the deviated eye. The monkeys were raised wearing goggles that contained dissociating prisms that prevented simultaneous corresponding visual input to the two eyes. These monkeys showed no evidence of binocular summation or stereopsis (Crawford et al., 1983). Finally, children with strabismus typically fail to demonstrate evidence of stereopsis, at least in the central visual fields.

A curious effect of certain kinds of strabismus is to reduce the proportion of cortical neurons selectively sensitive to vertical orientations. This observation was first made in cats (Singer et al., 1979) and has been confirmed in monkeys (Eggers et al., 1984). Behavioral measurements of visual sensitivity as a function of orientation in primates correspond well with these physiological findings. Strabismic monkeys (Harwerth et al., 1983c) and humans (Sireteanu and Singer, 1980) show reduced sensitivity to vertical relative to other orientations. These findings are of particular interest in view of some other effects of early environment on cortical orientation preference (see below).

F   Summary

The effects of visual experience on binocularity provide the richest and most varied data on the role of the environment in determining cortical function. In addition to the effects of binocular deprivation on receptive field development (Section II), the prevention of patterned visual experience seems to have deleterious effects on cortical binocular organization. The effects of monocular deprivation, however, are altogether more striking and quite different from "half the effect of binocular deprivation." Monocular deprivation seems to act by means of a strong binocular competition mechanism that gives the advantaged eye the opportunity to control most or all of the neuronal machinery in the visual cortex. Monocular deprivation also provides the most extreme case in which visual experience actively *specifies* visual function: regions of cortex that would not normally receive signals from an eye become completely dominated by it after monocular deprivation. The effects of decorrelated binocular input also provide evidence on the adaptability of the visual system to abnormal inputs. It seems useful to think about the loss of cortical binocularity following strabismus or alternate occlusion as a *refinement* process that serves to adapt the visual system to its prevailing environment—in this case, one in which binocular connections have no functional utility. In general, much of the plasticity of the visual system seems to be related in some way to binocular function; Blakemore (1979) develops the hypothesis that the main purpose of visual plasticity is to guarantee the proper development of functional binocular vision.

IV   SELECTIVE EFFECTS OF EXPOSURE TO RESTRICTED VISUAL ENVIRONMENTS

The effects of deprivation on the cortex, as discussed in the previous section, appear to represent failure to maintain an organization and specialization that is probably present in very young animals. However, the methods used to produce the effects of deprivation are rather severe and leave open the possibility that less extreme forms of deprivation are more selective in their effects on the cortex. We will consider a number of types of restrictive rearing environments and their effects on specific properties of striate cortical neurons. The issue we will address is the extent to which the *selectivity* of cortical neurons is dependent on postnatal visual experience and whether the mechanisms involved in the modification of selectivity are similar to those involved in deprivation effects.

A   Restricted Experience of Visual Patterns

Orientation selectivity, like ocular dominance, is a highly ordered property of cortical organization. Cortical neurons are grouped by preferred orientation in a columnar pattern throughout area 17 in both cats and monkeys (Hubel and Wiesel, 1962, 1963b, 1968). Cells vertically arranged in the cortex tend to share a common preferred orientation. In addition, nearby columns tend to have similar orientation preferences, giving rise to local sequence regularity in the distribution of preferred orientations of neurons in different locations across the cortex (Hubel and Wiesel, 1974; Blasdel and Salama, 1986). Figure 12A shows an example of the regularity of this organization in data obtained from an adult macaque monkey by Hubel and Wiesel (1974). The inset tracing shows the position of the microelectrode penetration in the cortex, angled shallowly with respect to the surface so that it traversed many orientation columns. The graph shows the progression of preferred orientations across the cortex, which in this case shows great regularity for several millimeters.

Orientation specificity can be found in young kittens (Hubel and Wiesel, 1963a; Imbert and Buisseret, 1975; Blakemore and Van Sluyters, 1975) and monkeys (Wiesel and Hubel, 1974) and appears to have a cortical organization that is at least qualitatively similar to the adult shortly after birth in monkeys (Wiesel and Hubel, 1974). Figure 12B shows an example of this sort of data for a newborn monkey in a format similar to that used for adult data in Figure 12A. In this case two separate microelectrode penetrations were made; each gives rise to the data in one of the graphs, and each shows the characteristic sequence regularity seen in the adult.

Kittens are visually less mature than monkeys at birth, and there is less general agreement on the degree to which cortical orientation selectivity is adultlike in visually inexperienced kittens. Hubel and Wiesel (1963a) and later Sherk and Stryker (1976) found that cortical orientation selectivity was almost adultlike in young kittens. Barlow and Pettigrew (1971) found little or no orientation selectivity. Most others have found themselves in a middle ground between these two poles, finding some orientation selectivity but not an adultlike number or precision (e.g., Imbert and Buisseret, 1975; Blakemore and Van Sluyters, 1975). This controversy has been reviewed recently and will not be discussed further here (see Movshon and Van Sluyters, 1981; Mitchell and Timney, 1984; see also Chapter 2, this volume)

The state of orientation selectivity at birth is of particular importance to the interpretation of a long series of experiments beginning in 1970 that examined the degree to which the organization and specificity of visual cortical receptive fields could be modified by restricting the range of visual patterns experienced in early life. Following the initial reports of plasticity in ocular dominance organization during the early postnatal period, several groups of investigators set out to determine whether or not orientation selectivity could be similarly influenced by early visual experience.

Blakemore and Cooper (1970) and Hirsch and Spinelli (1970) raised kittens in environments in which visual experience was limited to contours of a single orientation. Although the rearing procedures were quite different (Hirsch and Spinelli used goggles to control visual stimulation, while Blakemore and Cooper gave their kittens visual experience in cylinders with patterns painted on the inner walls), both groups reported a bias in the distribution of orientation preferences in the cortex. They found more neurons with preferred orientations near the orientation experienced during rearing than other orientations. Figure 13A shows the rearing method adopted by Blakemore and his colleagues in which the kitten was given visual experience only in a cylinder whose inner walls were covered with specific visual patterns such as stripes. Figure 13B shows the results of subsequent recordings from the visual cortex of the first two kittens reared in this way, one in a vertical environment and one in a horizontal one. Each line represents the orientation preference of a single cortical neuron; the preferred orientations cluster around the orientations experienced in early life and tend to avoid those at right angles to the experienced orientation. Hirsch and Spinelli (1970) reported qualitatively similar results, although there were some critical differences between their procedures and those of Blakemore and Cooper. Unfortunately, these results have not gone unchallenged by subsequent experimenters. Figure 14 shows the results of very similar experiments conducted by Stryker and Sherk (1975), who reared their kittens in cylinders like those of Figure 13A, but found no association between the orientation experienced early in life and the preferred orientations of cortical neurons. The stark difference evident in these two sets of results provoked a series of experiments on this topic.

The important question that affects interpretation of these results is the original one we raised at the beginning of the chapter: does visual experience maintain, refine, or specify the pattern of cortical orientation selectivity? If the effect of restricted orientational experience is simply to permit normal development of orientation-selective neurons stimulated by the pattern used during rearing, then the notion of maintenance would seem most appropriate. Possibly, if orientation selectivity is only partly evident, the refinement model would be best. Finally, if the state of the cortex at birth is something like a *tabula rasa*, then perhaps the early visual environment actually specifies the pattern of cortical function. To choose among these views, one must know both the initial conditions of the cortex (see the preceding) and the detailed effects of rearing in restricted environments. In particular, it is crucial to know whether large numbers of nonorientation-selective neurons are found or whether extended zones of cortex exist that contain visually unresponsive neurons that might be "atrophied" ones having the undesired orientation preference (see Movshon and Van Sluyters, 1981).

The neural basis of the modification may depend on the severity of the visual restriction during rearing. Hirsch and Spinelli (1970) used goggles

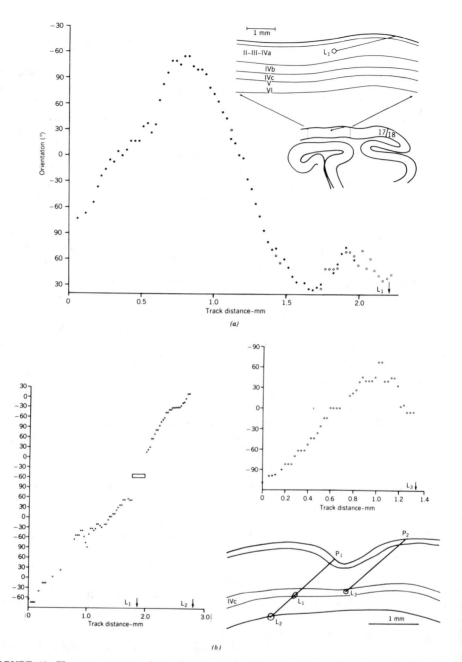

FIGURE 12. The organization of orientation selectivity in monkey striate cortex. (*A*) Graph of receptive field orientation as a function of electrode track distance for a single oblique penetration through striate cortex of a normal adult monkey. A schematic diagram of the location of the track and marking lesion (L_1) is shown in the upper right. There is a regular progression of preferred orientations with track distance, including several reversals in the direction of the orientation shifts. (From Hubel and Wiesel, 1974.) (*B*) Graphs show receptive field orientation as a function of electrode track distance for two oblique penetrations through striate cortex of a young, visually naive monkey. A schematic diagram of the penetrations (P_1 and P_2) and locations of marking lesions (L_1, L_2, and L_3) appears in the bottom right of the figure. The regular progression of preferred orientations with track distance through the cortex is apparent in both graphs; the open box near L_1 (left graph) represents the unoriented cells of layer 4. (From Wiesel and Hubel, 1974.)

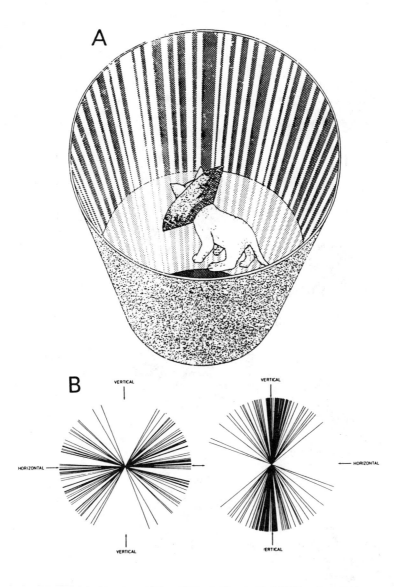

FIGURE 13. The effects of selective exposure to striped patterns during development in kittens. (*A*) Blakemore and Cooper (1970) reared kittens with exposure to either horizontal or vertical stripes by placing them in striped cylinders as shown for a specific period of time each day; the kittens were otherwise kept in darkness. (*B*) Preferred orientations of cortical neurons in kittens exposed to horizontal (left) or vertical (right) stripes. Each line represents the preferred orientation of a single neuron. In each case, there was a lack of neurons tuned to the orientation not present during rearing. (From Blakemore and Cooper, 1970.)

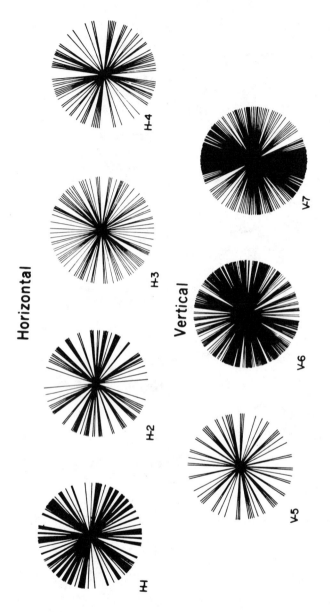

FIGURE 14. Preferred orientations of cells from a series of cats reared by Stryker and Sherk (1975), showing a failure to obtain orientation bias in kittens reared with exposure only to horizontal (top) or vertical (bottom) stripes using the rearing methods of Blakemore and Cooper. (From Stryker and Sherk, 1975.)

containing high-contrast stripes of a single orientation—vertical in one eye and horizontal in the other—to restrict the visual environment of their kittens; this procedure sharply restricted the visual field and removed all opportunity for visuomotor integration as well as restricting the form of the visual input. These goggle-reared kittens had an inordinately large number of nonresponsive and abnormal cells, suggesting partial maintenance—or a preservation of selectivity—only of neurons with preferred orientations present during rearing. Neurons preferring other orientations would be in effect binocularly deprived [see also Stryker et al. (1978) who replicated the results of Hirsch and Spinelli (1970) using the methods of Stryker and Sherk (1975)]. Blakemore and Cooper (1970) reared kittens in patterned cylinders, providing a less restrictive environment than that of the goggle-reared kittens as well as permitting some visuomotor integration. Kittens reared in this manner have a lower proportion of abnormal cells than the goggle-reared kittens (Blakemore, 1976; Blasdel et al. 1977), but they also have a less dramatic bias of orientation preference, perhaps because mobility of the animal can produce retinal stimulation at orientations quite different from the canonical one.

Several more recent studies have investigated the effects of early orientation bias using cylindrical lenses to restrict the range of contours experienced; the lenses blur contours of one orientation while permitting correct focus of orthogonal contours (see Figure 18A in Section VC.; Freeman and Pettigrew, 1973; Cynader and Mitchell, 1977; Rauschecker and Singer, 1981; Singer et al., 1981; Boothe and Teller, 1982). These studies generally support the conclusion that orientation preference can be biased by early rearing, but the mechanism by which the bias occurs may be refinement rather than selective maintenance. Rauschecker and Singer (1981) and Singer et al. (1981) found that columns devoted to the experienced orientation were expanded relative to the nonexperienced orientations. They suggested that a competitive interaction near the borders of the columns devoted to the experienced orientation between the "experienced" cells and the neighboring "nonexperienced" cells is responsible for the expansion, similar to the proposed mechanism for the expansion of ocular dominance columns (Hubel et al., 1977; LeVay et al., 1980). The result of these experiments suggest that local modifications of orientation selectivity may be induced by early experience.

The most extreme evidence concerning the development of neuronal specificity suggests an active role of visual experience in the specification of orientation selectivity. Some evidence (e.g., Hirsch and Spinelli, 1970; Pettigrew and Garey, 1974) suggests that the receptive fields of some cortical neurons in stripe-reared kittens may actually come to resemble in shape the stimulus pattern presented during rearing. Other evidence in support of this view comes from experiments in which animals were raised in environments containing no extended contours (Van Sluyters and Blakemore, 1973; Pettigrew and Freeman, 1973). Some neurons in these animals apparently acquire unusual properties, though the power and generality of this finding may not be sufficient to support a strong theory of instructional specificity by the visual environment (see Blakemore and Van Sluyters, 1975; Movshon and Van Sluyters, 1981).

Finally, it is worth considering some recent experiments that revive the spirit of the Hirsch and Spinelli variant of the stripe-rearing paradigm by combining orientationally biased visual experience with a difference in visual inputs between the eyes. Carlson et al. (1986) raised monkeys under conditions in which they received monocular visual experience of contours of a single orientation. As expected, the eye receiving visual experience controlled more cortical neurons than its unstimulated fellow. The deprivation effect was restricted, however, to neurons whose preferred orientations matched the orientation seen during rearing; neurons having orthogonal orientation preference were dominated equally often by either eye. Similar results have been reported in cats (Cynader and Mitchell, 1977). These results can be interpreted with equal validity as demonstrating orientation-selective effects of monocular deprivation or eye-selective effects of restricted orientational experience. Those inclined to favor maintenance and refinement as explanations of stripe-rearing results tend to favor the first explanation; those inclined to favor specification favor the second.

B   Restricted Experience of Visual Motion

In addition to orientation selectivity, striate cortical cells in cats and to a somewhat lesser extent in monkeys often exhibit *directional selectivity*, which gives them a preference for one of the two directions of motion of an optimally oriented contour. Directional selectivity, like orientation selectivity, can be modified by early visual experience. Two methods have been used to show this effect: rearing animals under conditions that provide only one direction of motion or rearing them under conditions that deprive them of smooth motion altogether by rearing in a stroboscopic environment.

Cynader et al. (1975) reared kittens in a visual environment in which the only visual stimuli were inchoate "blobs" that always moved to the left. The effects of this rearing on the direction and orientation preferences of cortical neurons is shown in Figure 15, which contains polar histograms representing the numbers of cells preferring particular orientations and directions of motion. The left-hand figure reveals a strong tendency for cortical neurons to prefer directions experienced during rearing. The right-hand figure shows that there was also an effect on the orientation preferences of cortical neurons, which tend to cluster at right angles to the preferred direction of motion. This tendency is also evident in other studies in which directional rearing was done with moving oriented targets (e.g., Tretter et al., 1975; Daw and Wyatt, 1976). These studies found biases both in the direction and orientation of preferences of cortical neurons in cats. Interestingly, Berman and Daw (1977) provided evidence that the period during

direction preference

orientation preference

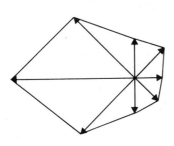
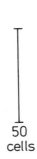
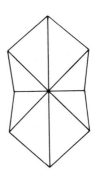

50
cells

FIGURE 15. The effect on cortical direction and orientation selectivity produced by rearing kittens in a unidirectional environment. The two polar histograms represent the distributions reported by Cynader et al. (1975) following rearing in an environment of leftward-moving "blobs." The left-hand panel shows the resulting preferred directions of cortical neurons; the right-hand panel shows the distribution of preferred orientations. The length of each line in the polar histogram represents the number of neurons having direction or orientation preferences within 22.5° of the indicated angle.

which the visual system is susceptible to environmental modification by directional motion ends sooner than the sensitive period for the effects of monocular deprivation.

Deprivation of effective visual stimulation by smooth motion can be achieved by rearing animals in a stroboscopically illuminated environment. This experiment was first done using illumination at a low rate (less than 1 Hz) by Cynader et al. (1973) and by Olson and Pettigrew (1974); both reports describe a loss of directional selectivity combined with a collection of defects reminiscent of those seen following binocular deprivation. Subsequent experiments have revealed the similarity between cats raised under low-rate stroboscopic illumination and dark-reared cats (Pasternak et al., 1981). A more interesting effect occurs if the animals are raised under illumination at higher rates (e.g., 8 Hz). Under these conditions, cortical receptive field properties are generally preserved but directional selectivity is altogether absent (Cynader and Chernenko, 1976). Figure 16 shows the results of an analysis of cortical directional selectivity in several animals of this kind by Pasternak et al. (1985). The upper histogram shows the distribution of directional biases (described in the legend) for a population of cortical neurons from normal cats. The lower histogram shows the distribution of the same measure for neurons from strobe-reared cats. Neurons whose direction indices exceed 0.5 are directionally selective; such neurons are very common in normal cats and all but absent from strobe-reared ones. Pasternak et al. (1985) were also able to show that the contrast detection performance of these animals was roughly normal but their performance on directional discrimination tasks was very poor.

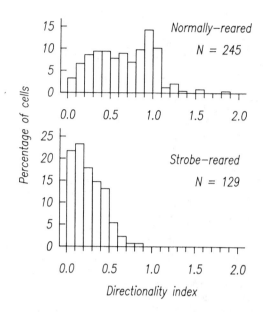

FIGURE 16. The distributions of directional selectivity for populations of neurons recorded from the striate cortex of normal cats (top) and cats reared in an environment illuminated stroboscopically at 8 Hz (bottom). The directionality index is calculated as $1 - np/p$, where np is the response in the nonpreferred direction, and p is the response in the preferred direction. An index of 0.5 or more indicates directional selectivity, while an index of zero indicates non-directionality. Two-thirds of neurons from normal cats are directionally selective, while barely one-tenth of neurons from strobe-reared cats are. (From Pasternak et al., 1985.)

Thus it seems that normal experience of moving contours is required to maintain the normal property of cortical directional selectivity. The generally positive reports on the effects of unidirectional rearing suggest also that some refinement of innately specified preferences for direction can be provided by visual experience. There seems to be little evidence suggesting the still more active role of specification by the visual environment in this case.

C   Summary

Experiments on the effect of raising animals under conditions of abnormal visual pattern stimulation have provoked some of the most exciting—and least reproducible—experimental results in modern visual neuroscience. In the past few years, the dust surrounding this area seems to have settled somewhat. It now seems that the most radical claims of environmental modifiability were overstated, as were the most radical claims of immunity to environmental influence. The effects of binocular deprivation (Section II) show that visual experience is needed to *maintain* normal pattern specificity. If we neglect the most extreme of the claims that visual experience *specifies* neuronal pattern specificity, we are left with the view that the main effect of abnormal early visual experience of patterns is to promote the *refinement*—in some cases the pathological refinement—of functional connections to which the visual system is innately predisposed.

V MODIFICATION OF THE HUMAN VISUAL SYSTEM BY EARLY EXPERIENCE

There is ample evidence that the human visual system is susceptible to abnormal early visual experience in the same way as in kittens and monkeys. Indeed, the abnormalities of vision that follow early strabismus provoked Hubel and Wiesel's early exploration of this area of research. Two kinds of evidence strongly suggest the similarity between animal models and human vision: abnormalities of binocular visual experience leading to *amblyopia,* and abnormalities of patterned visual experience leading to other forms of visual pattern deficits.

A Amblyopia

The most compelling evidence that the development of the human visual system can be influenced by early visual experience comes from studies of amblyopia. Amblyopia is most generally defined as a deficit in visual acuity that cannot be corrected optically and appears in the absence of any obvious trauma or ocular pathology. Amblyopia is associated with the presence of disorders such as anisometropia (unequal refractive errors for the two eyes), cataracts (opacities of the lens), and strabismus (misalignment of the visual axes) during infancy and early childhood. These disorders, when present in adults, do not lead to the development of amblyopia. The sensitive period for the development of amblyopia in humans may extend over the first 8 postnatal years (Von Noorden, 1980). Most studies of the development of amblyopia in humans are unfortunately compromised both by their retrospective nature and the intervention that becomes necessary once the condition is discovered. However, there is enough evidence to conclude that permanent deficits in visual function often follow the abnormal visual experience produced by these conditions during early life.

Approximately 2.5% of human infants and children develop amblyopia. The conditions most commonly associated with amblyopia are anisometropia and strabismus, either separately or in combination. The causal nature of these conditions is not established with certainty but is emphasized by data from a few prospective studies documenting the development of amblyopia subsequent to the appearance of high refractive errors and/or strabismus (Ingram and Walker, 1979; Ingram et al. 1979; Thomas et al., 1979; Jacobson et al., 1981a; Birch and Stager, 1985). In addition, several studies have documented changes in visual acuity as a result of patching therapy (occlusion of the "normal" eye) that demonstrate the susceptibility of the human infant visual system to visual deprivation (Thomas et al., 1979; Mohindra et al., 1979, 1983). This susceptibility appears to persist for at least the first 6–8 postnatal years, although there are reports that amblyopia can be treated up to the teenage years (Lennerstrand and Lundh, 1980; see Birnbaum et al., 1977).

Data from studies of human infants with unilateral cataracts confirm the relevance of the animal studies to human vision. Human infants show extremely poor vision following removal of unilateral congenital cataracts. Electrophysiological studies suggest abnormalities in the visual cortex of human infants who had even short periods of monocular deprivation (Awaya et al., 1973, 1979). Visual performance improves with enforced usage of the deprived eye provided therapy is begun at an early age (Enoch and Rabinowicz, 1976; Beller et al., 1981; Jacobson et al., 1981b, 1983). However, full-time patching therapy can result in reversal of the deprivation effects; the acuity of each eye remains labile throughout the sensitive period (Von Noorden, 1973; Jacobson et al., 1981b, 1983).

B   Animal Models of Amblyopia

Additional evidence that strabismus and anisometropia are sufficient to cause the development of amblyopia comes from studies of primate models. Generally these studies are done by experimentally creating a strabismus or anisometropia in an infant monkey whose visual development is then followed (e.g., Kiorpes and Boothe, 1980; Kiorpes et al., 1987, 1989); in some cases visual function is evaluated only after the developmental period is completed (e.g., Harwerth et al., 1983a,b; Smith et al., 1985). Figure 17 shows the time course for the development of visual acuity in each eye of an experimentally strabismic monkey. Acuity, which is within the normal range prior to intervention, continues to develop normally for some weeks after intervention in both eyes of this monkey; thereafter the development of acuity for the operated eye lagged behind that of the nonoperated eye, representing the development of strabismic amblyopia. This pattern of acuity development is common among experimentally strabismic monkeys (Kiorpes et al., 1989).

It should be noted that only 60–70% of experimentally strabismic monkeys (Kiorpes et al., 1989) and 40–70% of naturally strabismic humans (Costenbader et al., 1948; Von Noorden, 1980; Birch and Stager, 1985) actually develop amblyopia. Animals and humans who adopt an alternating pattern of fixation tend not to develop amblyopia, suggesting that equal use of each eye prevents amblyopia development. The development of anisometropic amblyopia also appears to be somewhat dependent on the extent of clear visual input through the anisometropic eye. The extent of anisometropic amblyopia is correlated with the degree of anisometropia in humans (Sen, 1980) and is related to the degree of defocus of the treated eye in experimental animals (Kiorpes et al., 1987).

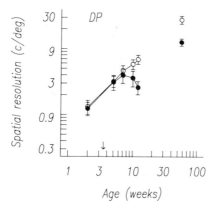

FIGURE 17. Behavioral data on the development of spatial resolution in an experimentally strabismic monkey. Spatial resolution is plotted as a function of age in weeks for the nondeviated (open symbols) and deviated (closed symbols) eye; the age at esotropia induction is indicated by the arrow on the abscissa. The development of acuity for the deviated eye proceeded in parallel with that of the nondeviated eye for several weeks after the strabismus was created. Thereafter, the development of the deviated eye lagged behind that of the nondeviated eye, resulting in an amblyopia. (From Kiorpes et al., 1989.)

C   Restricted Pattern Experience in Humans: Meridional Amblyopia

An interesting observation bearing on the role of visual experience on the human visual system was reported by Mitchell et al. (1973). Inspired by the animal work on stripe rearing (see the preceding), they examined data on the variation in visual acuity with orientation among individuals having astigmatic refractive errors. Astigmatism leads to an orientation-selective pattern of defocus like that illustrated in Figure 18*A*. Contours of the properly focused orientation are clearly imaged, while contours of other orientations are blurred. Mitchell and his colleagues reasoned that if astigmatic refractive errors occurred early in life, the resulting visual image abnormality might provoke developmental changes like those seen in kittens. Reexamining data from an earlier study (Mitchell et al., 1967) led them to the view that this hypothesis was tenable, and they collected visual acuity measurements for a large sample of optically corrected astigmatic and emmetropic adult observers. Their results are summarized in Figure 18*B*, which shows the relative visual acuities measured at the best and worst meridians for emmetropes and astigmats. As expected, the ratio of acuities for emmetropes tends to be near 1 (top). In the astigmatic population, however, there is a larger spread of acuity ratios, and most of the ratios are significantly below 1, meaning that acuity was significantly worse at the blurred meridian than at the correctly focused one. This retrospective study thus provided evidence consistent with the hypothesis that orientation-selective effects of early visual experience could be seen in humans as well

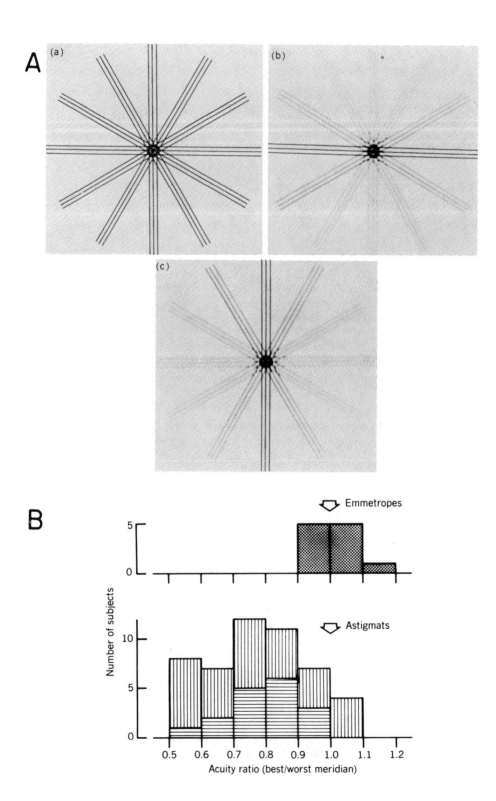

as in animals, although the detailed correlation between the degree of defocus and the magnitude of the acuity difference was not as close as expected. These measurements have subsequently been confirmed and extended to measurements of spatial contrast sensitivity (Freeman and Thibos, 1975; Mitchell and Wilkinson, 1977).

As in other kinds of amblyopia, definitive evidence that the abnormal visual experience is a *causal* factor—rather than a merely associated one—is difficult to obtain. Finding astigmatism in an adult does not guarantee that the same refractive error was present in early life, when one presumes that visual experience could have modified the visual system. Indeed, there is evidence that astigmatism present in young children often disappears during childhood (Atkinson et al., 1980). Even if the refractive error were known to be stable, the accommodative behavior of astigmats can vary, meaning that the correctly focused meridian at one time might be defocused at other times. It is difficult to rule out the possibility that the ocular factors leading to astigmatism might also lead to other meridional variations in ocular or retinal structure that could cause meridional variations in acuity.

Boothe and Teller (1982) showed that externally applied cylindrical lenses could provoke a condition resembling meridional amblyopia in monkeys, providing additional evidence that abnormal early visual experience could provoke this kind of deficit. Held and his colleagues (Held, 1978; Gwiazda et al., 1985, 1986) have tried to associate the pattern of refractive errors with the development of meridional variations in visual acuity in human infants. Their results provide some support for the relationship between these factors but do not rule out the possibility that some separate factor might provoke *both* the refractive changes and the changes in relative visual acuity. Others (Atkinson and French, 1979) have found the relationship between infant refraction and meridional variations in acuity to be more elusive.

D Summary

In summary, data on amblyopia (both meridional and otherwise) in humans provides evidence that suggests but does not prove that the human visual system can be modified by early visual experience in several ways that all

---

FIGURE 18. (*A*). The effects of astigmatism on the visibility of oriented contours. A target (*a*) consisting of lines at different orientations spaced at 30° intervals is represented as it would appear to an astigmatic eye with either vertical (*b*) or horizontal (*c*) astigmatism. (From Mitchell et al., 1973.) (*B*). Visual acuity deficits in humans with "meridional amblyopia." The ratio of visual acuity for grating targets at the best and worst meridians for 11 emmetropic observers and 49 observers who had significant astigmatism oriented at or near a primary meridian in early life. Measurements were made with full optical correction. Visual acuity is expressed as a resolution distance, so an acuity ratio of 0.5 indicates that performance at the best meridian was double that at the worst meridian. Vertically hatched portions of the lower distribution indicate astigmats for whom vertical was the orientation of best focus; horizontally hatched portions indicate cases in which horizontal was the orientation of best focus. (Redrawn from Mitchell et al., 1973.)

have counterparts in the animal literature. Certainly it seems parsimonious to assume that similar mechanisms operate during the development of human and animal visual function. But it is prudent to recall that many factors that are well controlled in laboratory studies may be both uncontrolled and important during human visual development and that there are a number of differences between the human and animal literature.

VI CONCLUSIONS

Throughout this chapter, we have considered the question of whether visual experience serves only to *maintain* innately specified connections, *refine* a pattern more or less crudely prepared by innate factors, or *specify* the detailed form of the neuronal architecture of vision. Considering the whole range of experimental observations available, it seems that the notion of maintenance is too limited to explain the variety and diversity of the visual system's responses to the visual environment. The effects of monocular deprivation, strabismus, and rearing in patterned environments all show a shaping influence of the visual world on the visual system, an influence too great to be considered merely a maintenance device. On the other hand, the argument that the visual environment specifies the form of the visual system, freely shaping it to suit the particular quirks and vagaries of the visual environment present in early life, seems to be ill-founded. In many cases alluded to in this chapter, the most extreme claims for visual system modifiability have been contested or shown to be excessive. We are left, then, with the general principle that the role of the visual environment during visual development is to refine a developmental plan broadly laid out by innate factors. This interpretation seems to put the role of phylogenetic and ontogenetic factors into a cooperative and balanced relationship and offers a guidepost for future experiments on the mechanisms that underly both genetic and environmental specification of visual function.

A critical fact of visual development that has been touched on several times throughout this chapter is the existence of the early sensitive period within which environmental alterations may influence the course of visual development (Hubel and Wiesel, 1970). The existence of this defined and limited period of plasticity is both a mystery and a challenge to developmental neurobiology. What aspects of the developmental process govern the sensitive period? How are its duration and sensitivity regulated? Why does it vary from species to species? It is in the answers to many of these questions about the *regulation* of visual system plasticity that much current work is invested. The role of specific monoamine systems in the regulation of cortical plasticity first proposed by Kasamatsu and Pettigrew (1976) has received an increasing amount of attention in recent years, and there is increasing evidence that some of these play a critical role in controlling the course of early development (see Gordon et al., 1988, for a recent review of this literature). Singer (1979) and his colleagues have come to emphasize more general aspects of the control of forebrain development by central core projection systems of several kinds. Shaw et al. (1985) have begun an exhaustive examination of the distribution and modification of neurotransmitter receptors in developing cortex, and Aoki and Siekevitz (1985) have introduced the notion that developmentally significant cortical protein molecules can be identified and tracked during development. All these groups and approaches are homing in on the issue of how cortical plasticity is regulated. In the next few years, there is little doubt that these approaches will reveal much about the process and control of cortical development and perhaps change altogether the way we think about developmental processes today.

The final issue to consider in this chapter is the deceptively simple, yet unanswered question at the root of all this work: why is the visual system susceptible at all to modification of the visual environment? In many ways, the studies described in this chapter document the fact that, if left alone, the visual system proceeds neatly and smoothly through its normal course of development. Disrupted by deprivation of various forms and extents, the pattern of neuronal development is altered, sometimes disastrously. The answer to this question must lie in an analysis of the kinds of information that the environment of a *particular* individual can supply but that general knowledge about the developmental process of the whole species cannot. The most likely sort of information is that which characterizes and differentiates an individual's visual system. Establishing the basic geometric parameters of binocular stereopsis may require considerable flexibility and adaptability (Blakemore, 1979). Dealing with such basic calibration issues as the location and irregularity of the distribution of photoreceptors and the particular physical, optical, and oculomotor characteristics of the visual system present a formidable challenge to a visual system as refined as the primate's (Maloney, 1989). The role of visual system development may therefore be to take the *general* principles that lead to the evolution of a species' visual capacity and style and refine them to work effectively for each *specific* individual.

ACKNOWLEDGMENTS

The preparation of this chapter was supported in part by grants from the National Institutes of Health (EY 02017 and EY 05864) and the National Science Foundation (BNS 82-16950).

REFERENCES

Aoki, C., and P. Siekevitz (1985) Ontogenetic changes in the cyclic adenosine 3′,5′–monophosphate-stimulatable phosphorylation of cat visual cortex proteins, particularly of microtubule-associated protein 2 (MAP2): Effects of normal and dark rearing, and of the expsure to light. J. Neurosci. 5:2465–2483.

Atkinson, J., and J. French (1979) Astigmatism and orientation preference in human infants. Vision Res. 19:1315–1317.

Atkinson, J., O. Braddick, and J. French (1980) Infant astigmatism: Its disappearance with age. Vision Res. 20:891–893.

Awaya, A., Y. Miyake, Y. Imaizumi, Y. Shiose, T. Kandu, and K. Komuro (1973) Amblyopia in man, suggestive of stimulus deprivation amblyopia. Jap. J. Ophthalmol. 17:69–82.

Awaya, S., M. Suguwara, and S. Miyake (1979) Observations in patients with occlusion amblyopia. Trans. Ophthalmol. Soc. UK 99:447–454.

Baker, F. H., P. Grigg, and G. K. Von Noorden (1974) Effects of visual deprivation and strabismus on the responses of neurons in the visual cortex of the monkey, including studies on the striate and prestriate cortex in the normal animal. Brain Res. 66:185–208.

Banks, M. S., R. N. Aslin, and R. D. Letson (1975) Sensitive period for the development of human binocular vision. Science 190:675–677.

Barlow, H. B., and J. D. Pettigrew (1971) Lack of specificity of neurons in the visual cortex of young kittens. J. Physiol. Lond. 218:98P–101P.

Beller, R., C. S. Hoyt, E. Marg, and J. V. Odom (1981) Good visual function after neonatal surgery for congenital monocular cataracts. Amer. J. Ophthalmol. 91:559–565.

Berman, N., and N. W. Daw (1977) Comparison of the critical periods for monocular and directional deprivation in cats. J. Physiol. Lond. 265:249–259.

Birch, E. E., and D. R. Stager (1985) Monocular acuity and stereopsis in infantile esotropia. Invest. Ophthalmol. Vis. Sci. 26:1624–1630.

Birnbaum, M. H., K. Koslowe, and R. Sanet (1977) Success in amblyopia therapy as a function of age: A literature survey. Amer. J. Optom. Physiol. Opt. 54:269–275.

Blake, R., and H. V. B. Hirsch (1975) Deficits in binocular depth perception in cats after alternating monocular deprivation. Science 190:1114–1116.

Blakemore, C. (1976) The conditions required for the maintenance of binocularity in the kitten's visual cortex. J. Physiol. Lond. 261:423–444.

Blakemore, C. (1979) The development of stereoscopic mechanisms in the visual cortex of the cat. Proc. Roy. Soc. Lond. B 204:477–484.

Blakemore, C., and G.F. Cooper (1970) Development of the brain depends on the visual environment. Nature 228:477–478.

Blakemore, C., and R. C. Van Sluyters (1974) Reversal of the physiological effects of monocular deprivation in kittens: Further evidence for a sensitive period. J. Physiol. Lond. 237:195–216.

Blakemore, C., and R. C. Van Sluyters (1975) Innate and environmental factors in the development of the kitten's visual cortex. J. Physiol. Lond. 248:663–716.

Blakemore, C., and F. Vital-Durand (1986) Effects of visual deprivation on the development of the monkey's lateral geniculate nucleus. J. Physiol. Lond. 380:493–511.

Blakemore, C., L. J. Garey, and F. Vital-Durand (1978) The physiological effects of monocular deprivation and their reversal in the monkey's visual cortex. J. Physiol. Lond. *283*:223–262.

Blakemore, C. F. Vital-Durand, and L. J. Garey (1981) Recovery from monocular deprivation in the monkey. I. Recovery of physiological effects in the visual cortex. Proc. R. Soc. Lond. Ser. B *213*:399–423.

Blakemore, C., M. J. Hawken, and R. F. Mark (1982) Brief monocular deprivation leaves subthreshold synaptic input on neurones of the cat's visual cortex. J. Physiol. Lond. *327*:489–505.

Blasdel, G. G., and G. Salama (1986) Voltage-sensitive dyes reveal a modular organization in monkey striate cortex. Nature *321*:579–585.

Blasdel, G. G., D. E. Mitchell, D. W. Muir, and J. D. Pettigrew (1977) A physiological and behavioural study in cats of the effect of early visual experience with contours of a single orientation. J. Physiol. Lond. *265*:615–636.

Bonds, A. B. (1979) Development of orientation tuning in the visual cortex of kittens. In R. D. Freeman (ed.): Developmental Neurobiology of Vision. New York: Plenum, pp. 31–41.

Boothe, R. G., and D. Y. Teller (1982) Meridional variations in acuity and CSFs in monkeys (*Macaca nemestrina*) reared with externally applied astigmatism. Vision Res. *22*:801–810.

Boothe, R. G., V. Dobson, and D. Y. Teller (1985) Postnatal development of vision in human and nonhuman primates. Ann. Rev. Neurosci. *8*:495–545.

Carlson, M., D. H. Hubel, and T. N. Wiesel. (1986) Effects of monocular exposure to oriented lines on monkey striate cortex. Dev. Brain Res. *25*:71–81.

Chino, Y. M., M. S. Shansky, W. L. Jankowski, and F. A. Banser (1983) Effects of rearing kittens with convergent strabismus on development of receptive-field properties in striate cortex neurons. J. Neurophysiol. *50*:265–286.

Chow, K. L., and P. D. Spear (1974) Morphological and functional effects of visual deprivation on the rabbit visual system. Exp. Neurol. *42*:429–477.

Chow, K. L., A. H. Riesen, and F. W. Newell (1957) Degeneration of retinal ganglion cells in infant chimpanzees reared in darkness. J. Comp. Neurol. *107*:27–42.

Costenbader, F., D. Bair, and A. McPhail (1948) Vision in strabismus. Arch. Ophthalmol. *40*:438–453.

Crawford, M. L. J., and G. K. Von Noorden (1979) The effects of short-term experimental strabismus on the visual system in *Macaca mulatta*. Inv. Opthalmol. Vis. Sci. *18*:496–505.

Crawford, M. L. J., and G. K. Von Noorden (1980) Optically induced comitant strabismus in monkeys. Invest. Ophthalmol. Vis. Sci. *19*:1105–1109.

Crawford, M. L. J., G. K. Von Noorden, L. S. Meharg, J. W. Rhodes, and R. S. Harwerth (1983) Binocular neurons and binocular function in monkeys and children. Invest. Ophthalmol. Vis. Sci. *24*:491–495.

Cynader, M., and G. Chernenko (1976) Abolition of directional selectivity in the visual cortex of the cat. Science *193*:504–505.

Cynader, M., and D. E. Mitchell (1977) Monocular astigmatism effects on kitten visual cortex development. Nature *270*:177–178.

Cynader, M., and D. E. Mitchell (1980) Prolonged sensitivity to monocular deprivation in dark-reared cats. J. Neurophysiol. *43*:1026–1040.

Cynader, M., N. Berman, and A. Hein (1973) Cats reared in stroboscopic illumination: Effects on receptive fields in visual cortex. Proc. Natl. Acad. Sci. USA 70:1353–1354.

Cynader, M., N. Berman, and A. Hein (1975) Cats raised in a one-directional world: Effects on receptive fields in visual cortex and superior colliculus. Exp. Brain Res. 22:267–280.

Cynader, M., B. N. Timney, and D. E. Mitchell (1980) Period of susceptibility of kitten visual cortex to the effects of monocular deprivation extends beyond six months of age. Brain Res. 191:515–550.

Daw, N. W., and H. J. Wyatt (1976) Kittens reared in a unidirectional environment: Evidence for a critical period. J. Physiol. Lond. 257:155–170.

Derrington, A. M. (1984) Development of spatial frequency selectivity in striate cortex of vision-deprived cats. Exp. Brain Res. 55:431–437.

Dews, P. B., and T. N. Wiesel (1970) Consequences of monocular deprivation on visual behaviour in kittens. J. Physiol. Lond. 206:437–455.

Eggers, H. M., M. S. Gizzi, and J. A. Movshon (1984) Spatial properties of striate cortical neurons in esotropic macaques. Invest. Ophthalmol. Vis. Sci. Suppl. 25:278.

Enoch, J. M., and I. M. Rabinowicz (1976) Early surgery and visual correction of an infant born with unilateral lens opacity. Doc. Ophthalmol. 41:371–382.

Freeman, R. D., and I. Ohzawa (1988) Monocularly deprived cats: Binocular tests of cortical cells reveal functional connections from the deprived eye. J. Neurosci. 8:2491–2506.

Freeman, R. D., and J. D. Pettigrew (1973) Alteration of visual cortex from environmental asymmetries. Nature 246:359–360.

Freeman, R. D., and L. N. Thibos (1975) Visual evoked responses in humans with abnormal visual experience. J. Physiol. Lond. 247:711–724.

Frégnac, Y., and M. Imbert (1978) Early development of visual cortical cells in normal and dark-reared kittens: Relationship between orientation selectivity and ocular dominance. J. Physiol. Lond. 278:27–44.

Friedlander, M. J., L. R. Stanford, and S. M. Sherman (1982) Effects of monocular deprivation on the structure-function relationship of individual neurons in the cat's lateral geniculate nucleus. J. Neurosci. 2:321–330.

Giffin, F., and D. E. Mitchell (1978) The rate of recovery of vision after early monocular deprivation in kittens. J. Physiol. Lond. 274:511–537.

Gordon, B., E. E. Allen, and P. Q. Trombley (1988) The role of norepinephrine in plasticity of visual cortex. Prog. Neurobiol. 30:171–191.

Gwiazda, J., I. Mohindra, S. Brill, and R. Held (1985) Infant astigmatism and meridional amblyopia. Vision Res. 25:1269–1276.

Gwiazda, J., J. Bauer, F. Thorn, and R. Held (1986) Meridional amblyopia does result from astigmatism in early childhood. Clin. Vision Sci. 1:145–152.

Harwerth, R. S., M. L. J. Crawford, E. L. Smith III, and R. L. Boltz (1981) Behavioral studies of stimulus deprivation amblyopia in monkeys. Vision Res. 21:779–789.

Harwerth, R. S., E. L. Smith III, R. L. Boltz, M. L. J. Crawford, and G. K. von Noorden (1983a) Behavioral studies on the effect of abnormal early visual experience in monkeys; Spatial modulation sensitivity. Vision Res. 23:1501–1510.

Harwerth, R. S., E. L. Smith III, R. L. Boltz, M. L. J. Crawford, and G. K. von Noorden (1983b) Behavioral studies on the effect of abnormal early visual experience in monkeys: temporal modulation sensitivity. Vision Res. 23:1511–1517.

Harwerth, R. S., E. L. Smith III, and O. J. Okundaye (1983c) Oblique effects, vertical effects and meridional amblyopia in monkeys. Exp. Brain Res. 53: 142–150.

Harwerth, R. S., E. L. Smith III, G. C. Duncan, M. L. J. Crawford, and G. K. von Noorden (1986) Multiple sensitive periods in the development of the primate visual system. Science 232:235–238.

Held, R. (1978) Development of visual acuity in normal and astigmatic infants. In S. J. Cool and E. L. Smith III (eds.): Frontiers in Visual Science. Berlin: Springer.

Hendrickson, A. E., and R. Boothe (1976) Morphology of the retina and lateral geniculate nucleus in dark-reared monkeys (*Macaca nemestrina*). Vision Res. 16:517–521.

Hirsch, H. V. B., and D. N. Spinelli (1970) Visual experience modifies distribution of horizontally and vertically oriented receptive fields in cats. Science 168:869–871.

Holopigian, K., and R. Blake (1983) Spatial vision in strabismic cats. J. Neurophysiol. 50:287–296.

Hubel, D. H., and T. N. Wiesel (1962) Receptive fields, binocular interaction and functional architecture in the cat's visual cortex. J. Physiol. Lond. 160:106–154.

Hubel, D. H., and T. N. Wiesel (1963a) Receptive fields of cells in striate cortex of very young, visually inexperienced kittens. J. Neurophysiol. 26:994–1002.

Hubel, D. H., and T. N. Wiesel (1963b) Shape and arrangement of columns in cat's striate cortex. J. Physiol. Lond. 165:559–568.

Hubel, D. H., and T. N. Wiesel (1965) Binocular interaction in striate cortex of kittens reared with artificial squint. J. Neurophysiol. 28:1041–1059.

Hubel, D. H., and T. N. Wiesel (1968) Receptive fields and functional architecture of monkey striate cortex. J. Physiol. Lond. 195:215–243.

Hubel, D. H., and T. N. Wiesel (1970) The period of susceptibility to the physiological effects of unilateral eye closure in kittens. J. Physiol. Lond. 206:419–436.

Hubel, D. H., and T. N. Wiesel (1974) Sequence regularity and geometry of orientation columns in the monkey striate cortex. J. Comp. Neurol. 158:267–294.

Hubel, D. H., and T. N. Wiesel (1977) Functional architecture of macaque monkey visual cortex. Proc. R. Soc. Lond. Ser. B 198:1–59.

Hubel, D. H., T. N. Wiesel, and S. LeVay (1977) Plasticity of ocular dominance columns in monkey striate cortex. Philos. Trans. R. Soc. Lond. Ser. B 278:377–409.

Imbert, M., and P. Buisseret (1975) Receptive field characteristics and plastic properties of visual cortical cells in kittens reared with or without visual experience. Exp. Brain Res. 22:25–36.

Ingram, R. M., and C. Walker (1979) Refraction as a means of predicting squint or amblyopia in preschool siblings of children known to have these defects. Brit. J. Ophthalmol. 63:238–242.

Ingram, R. M., M. J. Traynar, C. Walker, and J. M. Wilson (1979) Screening for refractive errors at age 1 year: A pilot study. Brit. J. Ophthalmol. 63:243–250.

Jacobson, S. G., I. Mohindra, and R. Held (1981a) Age of onset of amblyopia in infants with esotropia. Doc. Ophthalmol. Proc. Ser. 30:210–216.

Jacobson, S. G., I. Mohindra, and R. Held (1981b) Development of visual acuity in infants with congenital cataracts. Brit. J. Ophthalmol. 65:727–735.

Jacobson, S. G., I. Mohindra, and R. Held (1983) Monocular visual form deprivation in human infants. Doc. Ophthalmol. 55:199–211.

Kalil, R. E., P. D. Spear, and A. Langsetmo (1984) Response properties of striate cortex neurons in cats raised with divergent or convergent strabismus. J. Neurophysiol. 52:514–537.

Kasamatsu, T., and J. D. Pettigrew (1976) Depletion of brain catecholamines: Failure of ocular dominance shift after monocular occlusion in kittens. Science 194:206–209.

Kiorpes, L., and R. G. Boothe (1980) The time course for the development of strabismic amblyopia in infant monkeys (Macaca nemestrina). Invest. Ophthalmol. Vis. Sci. 19:841–845.

Kiorpes, L., R. G. Boothe, A. E. Hendrickson, J. A. Movshon, H. M. Eggers, and M. S. Gizzi (1987) Effects of early unilateral blur on the macaque's visual system: I. Behavioral observations. J. Neurosci. 7:1318–1326.

Kiorpes, L., M. R. Carlson, and D. Alfi (1989) Development of visual acuity in experimentally strabismic monkeys. Clin. Vision Sci. 4:95–106.

Kratz, K. E., and P. D. Spear (1976) Effects of visual deprivation and alterations of binocular competition on responses of striate cortex neurons in the cat. J. Comp. Neurol. 170:141–151.

Lennerstrand, G., and B. L. Lundh (1980) Improvement of contrast sensitivity from treatment for amblyopia. Acta Ophthalmol. 58:292–294.

LeVay, S., M. P. Stryker, and C. J. Shatz (1978) Ocular dominance columns and their development in layer IV of the cat's visual cortex: A quantitative study. J. Comp. Neurol. 179:223–244.

LeVay, S., T. N. Wiesel, and D. H. Hubel (1980) The development of ocular dominance columns in normal and visually deprived monkeys. J. Comp. Neurol. 191:1–51.

Levitt, J. B., J. A. Movshon, S. M. Sherman, and P. D. Spear (1989) Effects of monocular deprivation on macaque LGN. Invest. Ophthalmol. Vis. Sci. Suppl. 30:296.

Loop, M. S., and S. M. Sherman (1977) Visual discriminations during eyelid closure in the cat. Brain Res. 128:329–339.

Luskin, M. B., and C. J. Shatz (1985) Neurogenesis of the cat's primary visual cortex. J. Comp. Neurol. 242:611–631.

Maloney, L. T. (1989) Learning by assertion: A method for calibrating a simple visual system. Neural Computation 1: 387–395.

Mitchell, D. E., and B. Timney (1984) Postnatal development of function in the mammalian visual system. In I. Darian-Smith (eds.): Nervous System. III. Handbook of Physiology, Vol. 3, Sect. 1. Washington, D.C.: American Physiological Society, pp. 507–555.

Mitchell, D. E., and C. Ware (1974) Interocular transfer of a visual aftereffect in normal and stereoblind humans. J. Physiol. Lond. 236:707–721.

Mitchell, D. E., and F. Wilkinson (1977) The effect of early astigmatism on the visual resolution of gratings. J. Physiol. Lond. 243:739–756.

Mitchell, D. E., R. D. Freeman, and G. Westheimer (1967) Effect of orientation on the modulation sensitivity for interference fringes on the retina. J. Opt. Soc. Amer. 57:246–249.

Mitchell, D. E., M. Cynader, and J. A. Movshon (1977) Recovery from the effects of monocular deprivation in kittens. J. Comp. Neurol. 176:53–64.

Mitchell, D. E., K. M. Murphy, and M. G. Kaye (1984) Labile nature of the visual recovery promoted by reverse occlusion in monocularly deprived kittens. Proc. Natl. Acad. Sci. USA 81:286–288.

Mitchell, D. E., R. D. Freeman, M. Millodot, and G. Haegerstrom (1973) Meridional amblyopia: Evidence for modification of the human visual system by early visual experience. Vision Res. 13:535–558.

Mohindra, I., S. G. Jacobson, J. Thomas, and R. Held (1979) Development of amblyopia in infants. Trans Ophthalmol. Soc. UK 99:344–346.

Mohindra, I. S. G. Jacobson, J. Zwann, and R. Held (1983) Psychophysical assessment of visual acuity in infants with visual disorders. Behav. Brain Res. 10:51–58.

Movshon, J. A. (1976a) Reversal of the physiological effects of monocular deprivation in the kitten's visual cortex. J. Physiol. Lond. 261:125–174.

Movshon, J. A. (1976b) Reversal of the behavioural effects of monocular deprivation in the kitten. J. Physiol. Lond.261:175–187.

Movshon, J. A., and R. C. Van Sluyters (1981) Visual neural development. Ann. Rev. Psychol. 32:477–522

Movshon, J. A., B. E. I. Chambers, and C. Blakemore (1972) Interocular transfer in normal humans, and those who lack stereopsis. Perception. 1:483–490.

Movshon, J. A., H. M. Eggers, M. S. Gizzi, A. E. Hendrickson, L. Kiorpes, and R. G. Boothe (1987) Effects of early unilateral blur on the macaque's visual system. III. Physiological observations. J. Neurosci. 7:1340–1351.

Mower, G. D., D. Berry, J. L. Burchfiel, and F. H. Duffy (1981) Comparison of the effects of dark-rearing and binocular suture on development and plasticity of cat visual cortex. Brain Res. 220:255–267.

Ohzawa, I., and R. D. Freeman (1988) Binocularly deprived cats: Binocular tests of cortical cells show regular patterns of interaction. J. Neurosci. 8:2507–2516.

Olson, C. R., and R. D. Freeman (1978) Monocular deprivation and recovery during sensitive period in kittens. J. Neurophysiol. 41:65–74.

Olson C. R., and J. D. Pettigrew (1974) Single units in visual cortex of kittens reared in stroboscopic illumination. Brain Res. 70:189–204.

Packwood, J., and B. Gordon. (1975) Stereopsis in normal domestic cat, Siamese cat, and cat raised with alternating monocular occlusion. J. Neurophysiol. 38:1485–1499.

Pasternak, T., W. H. Merigan, and J. A. Movshon (1981) Motion mechanisms in strobe-reared cats: Psychophysical and electrophysiological measures. Acta Psychologica 48:321–332.

Pasternak, T., R. A. Schumer, M. S. Gizzi, and J. A. Movshon (1985) Abolition of cortical directional selectivity affects visual behavior in cats. Exp. Brain Res. 61:214–217.

Pettigrew, J. D. (1974) The effect of visual experience on the development of stimulus specificity by kitten cortical neurons. J. Physiol. Lond. *237*:49–74.

Pettigrew, J. D., and R. D. Freeman (1973) Visual experience without lines: Effect on developing cortical neurons. Science *182*:599–601.

Pettigrew, J. D., and L. J. Garey (1974) Selective modification of single neuron properties in the visual cortex of kittens. Brain Res. *66*:160–164.

Rakic, P. (1977) Prenatal development of the visual system in rhesus monkey. Phil. Trans. R. Soc. Lond. Ser. B. *278*:245–260.

Rakic, P. (1981) Development of visual centers in the primate brain depends on binocular competition before birth. Science *214*:928–931.

Ramoa, A. S., M. Shadlen, and R. D. Freeman (1987) Dark-reared cats: Unresponsive cells become visually responsive with microiontophoresis of an excitatory amino acid. Exp. Brain Res. *65*:658–665.

Rauschecker, J. P., and W. Singer (1981) The effects of early visual experience on the cat's visual cortex and their possible explanation by Hebb synapses. J. Physiol. Lond. *310*:215–239.

Regal, D. M., R. Boothe, D. Y. Teller, and G. B. Sackett (1976) Visual acuity and visual responsiveness in dark-reared monkeys (*Macaca nemestrina*). Vision Res. *16*:523–530.

Riesen, A. H. (1966) Sensory deprivation. Prog. Physiol. Psychol. *1*:117–147.

Sen, D. K. (1980) Anisometropic amblyopia. J. Ped. Ophthalmol. Strab. *17*:180–184.

Shatz, C. J. (1983) The prenatal development of the cat's retinogeniculate pathway. J. Neurosci. *3*:482–499.

Shatz, C. J., and P. A. Kirkwood (1984) Prenatal development of functional connections in the cat's retinogeniculate pathway. J. Neurosci. *4*:1378–1397.

Shatz, C. J., and M. P. Stryker (1978) Ocular dominance in layer IV of the cat's visual cortex and the effects of monocular deprivation. J. Physiol. Lond. *281*:267–283.

Shaw, C., M. C. Needler, M. Wilkinson, C. Aoki, and M. Cynader (1985) Modification of neurotransmitter receptor sensitivity in cat visual cortex during the critical period. Devel. Brain Res. *22*:67–73.

Sherk, H., and M. P. Stryker (1976) Quantitative study of cortical orientation selectivity in visually inexperienced kitten. J. Neurophysiol. *39*:63–70.

Sherman, S. M. (1971) Role of visual cortex in interocular transfer in the cat. Exp. Neurol. *30*:34–45.

Sherman, S. M., and P. D. Spear (1982) Organization of visual pathways in normal and visually deprived cats. Physiol. Rev. *62*:738–855.

Sherman, S. M., K. P. Hoffmann, and J. Stone (1972) Loss of a specific cell type from the dorsal lateral geniculate nucleus in visually deprived cats. J. Neurophysiol. *35*:532–541.

Singer, W. (1979) Central core control of visual cortex functions. In F. O. Schmitt and F. G. Worden. (eds.): The Neurosciences: Fourth Study Program. Cambridge, MA: MIT Press, pp. 1093–1109.

Singer, W., J. P. Rauschecker, and M. W. von Grünau (1979) Squint affects striate cortex cells encoding horizontal image movements. Brain Res. *170*:182–186.

Singer, W., B. Freeman, and J. P. Rauschecker (1981) Restriction of visual experience to a single orientation affects the organization of orientation columns in cat visual cortex: A study with deoxyglucose. Exp. Brain Res. 41:199–215.

Sireteanu, R., and W. Singer (1980) The "vertical effect" in human squint amblyopia. Exp. Brain Res. 40:354–357.

Smith, E. L. III, R. Harwerth, and M. L. J. Crawford (1985) Spatial contrast sensitivity deficits in monkeys produced by optically induced anisometropia. Invest. Ophthalmol. Vis. Sci. 26:330–342.

Spear, P. D., L. Tong, and A. Langsetmo (1978) Striate cortex neurons of binocularly deprived kittens respond to visual stimuli through closed eyelids. Brain Res. 155141–146.

Stryker, M. P., and Sherk (1975) Modification of cortical orientation selectivity in the cat by restricted visual experience: a reexamination. Science 190:904–906.

Stryker, M. P., H. Sherk, A. G. Leventhal, and H. V. B. Hirsch (1978) Physiological consequences for the cat's visual cortex of effectively restricting early visual experience with oriented contours. J. Neurophysiol. 41:896–909.

Thomas, J., I. Mohindra, and R. Held (1979) Strabismic amblyopia in infants. Amer. J. Optom. Physiol. Opt. 56:197–201.

Timney, B., D. E. Mitchell, and F. Giffin (1978) The development of vision in cats after extended periods of dark-rearing. Exp. Brain Res. 31:547–560.

Tretter, F., M. Cynader, and W. Singer (1975) Modification of direction selectivity in neurons in the visual cortex of kittens. Brain Res. 84:143–149.

Tsumoto, T., and R. D. Freeman (1987) Dark-reared cats: Responsivity of cortical cells influenced pharmacologically by an inhibitory antagonist. Exp. Brain Res. 65:666–672.

Van Sluyters, R. C. (1978) Reversal of the physiological effects of brief periods of monocular deprivation in the kitten. J. Physiol. Lond. 284:1–17.

Van Sluyters, R. C., and C. Blakemore (1973) Experimental creation of unusual neuronal properties in visual cortex of kittens. Nature 246:506–508.

Van Sluyters, R. C., and F. B. Levitt (1980) Experimental strabismus in the kitten. J. Neurophysiol. 43:686–699.

Von Grünau, M. (1979) Binocular summation and the binocularity of cat visual cortex. Vision Res. 19:813–816.

Von Noorden, G. K. (1973) Experimental amblyopia in monkeys. Further behavioral observations and clinical correlations. Invest. Ophthalmol. 12:721–726.

Von Noorden, G. K. (1980) Burian and Von Noorden's Binocular Vision and Ocular Motility: Theory and Management of Strabismus. St. Louis: C. V. Mosby.

Von Noorden, G. K., and M. L. J. Crawford (1977) Form deprivation without light deprivation produces the visual deprivation syndrome in Macaca mulatta. Brain Res. 129:37–44.

Von Noorden, G. K., J. E. Dowling, and D. C. Ferguson (1970) Experimental amblyopia in monkeys. I. Behavioral studies of stimulus deprivation amblyopia. Arch. Ophthalmol. 84:206–214.

Von Senden, M. (1960) Space and Sight. Trans. P. Heath. Methuen: London.

Watkins, D. W., J. R. Wilson, and S. M. Sherman (1978) Receptive field properties of neurons in binocular and moncular segments of striate cortex in cats raised with binocular lid suture. J. Neurophysiol. 41:322–337.

Wiesel, T. N. (1982) Postnatal development of the visual cortex and the influence of environment. Nature 299:583–591.

Wiesel, T. N., and D. H. Hubel (1963a) Effects of visual deprivation on morphology and physiology of cells in the cat's lateral geniculate body. J. Neurophysiol. 26:978–993.

Wiesel, T. N., and D. H. Hubel (1963b) Single-cell responses in striate cortex of kittens deprived of vision in one eye. J. Neurophysiol. 26:1003–1017.

Wiesel, T. N., and D. H. Hubel (1965a) Comparison of the effects of unilateral and bilateral eye closure on cortical unit responses in kittens. J. Neurophysiol. 28:1029–1040.

Wiesel. T. N., and D. H. Hubel (1965b) Extent of recovery from the effects of visual deprivation in the kitten. J. Neurophysiol. 28:1060–1072.

Wiesel, T. N., and D. H. Hubel (1974) Ordered arrangement of orientation columns in monkeys lacking visual experience. J. Comp. Neurol. 158:307–318.

Part Two

THE AUDITORY SYSTEM

Chapter Five

DEVELOPMENT OF AUDITORY SYSTEM STRUCTURES

JAMES R. COLEMAN

Departments of Psychology and Physiology
University of South Carolina
Columbia, South Carolina

I INTRODUCTION

The auditory system is organized in an intricate yet ordered arrangement to provide the organism with the ability to detect, locate, and evaluate sound energy from the environment. In humans, the auditory system provides a means for acquiring language skills. Understanding the mechanisms for auditory function requires an appreciation of underlying neuroanatomical and neurophysiological processes as well as behavioral manifestations. Studies of underlying neuroanatomical structures during prenatal and postnatal development of the organism show that formation of the auditory system is the result of a sequelae of changes, many occurring in parallel, the first of which results from the expression of genetic programming. The acoustic environment further interacts with the system through generated functional activity as peripheral and central structures develop toward adult capacity. The structural features of the auditory system during early development, maturation, and adulthood have been studied in a variety of mammals and are the target for discussion in this chapter. The reader may find further detail in previous reviews of neuroanatomical organization of the auditory system by Harrison and Howe (1974), Willard and Ryugo (1983), and Cant and Morest (1984) and on its development by Rubel (1978) and the volumes edited by Romand (1983) and Eggermont and Bock (1985).

II ANATOMICAL OVERVIEW OF THE AUDITORY SYSTEM

A Ear Structures

Acoustic energy first encounters the external ear, which consists of the pinna (ear flap) and a tube, the external auditory meatus (ear canal), which leads to the paper-thin tympanic membrane or ear drum (see Figure 1). The outer ear plays a role in sound localization, which may be emphasized by head and pinna movements. Because of the resonant characteristics of the external meatus, which is essentially a tube closed at one end, certain frequencies may become emphasized. The resonant energy is dependent upon the length of the meatus and therefore varies among mammals. In humans with an ear canal length of about 2.5 cm, the peak resonance is around 3000 Hz.

The tympanic membrane is set into motion by acoustic energy, and the pressure is transformed to the ossicles of the middle ear: the malleus, incus, and stapes. These ossicles are phylogenetically derived from the articular, quadrate, and hyomandibular skeletal structures of lower vertebrates. In mammals, the middle ear ossicles, which normally reside in an air-filled cavity, serve to reduce the impedance differences between the tympanic membrane and the fluid-filled cochlea. Energy is focused upon the oval window primarily by exertion of force over a much smaller stapes area than

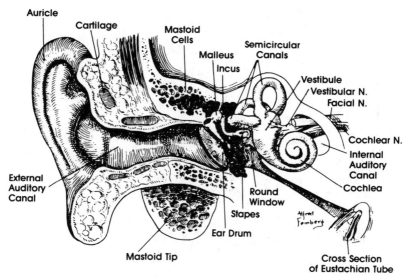

FIGURE 1. Schematic of human ear structures. The ear is divided into external (auricle pinna; external canal/meatus; ear drum or tympanic membrane), middle (malleus, incus and stapes ossicles), and inner components (cochlea and vestibular apparatus). (Adapted from Davis, 1947.)

that of the tympanic membrane and also by a lever action of the ossicular chain. The middle ear also contains two muscle groups, the tensor tympani, which attaches to the malleus, and the stapedius muscle, which attaches to the stapes. These muscles serve to protect inner ear mechanisms from very intense sounds by altering the means of vibration of the auditory ossicles.

The inner ear contains a coiled tube called the cochlea, which is snail-like in appearance (Figure 1). The cochlea actually contains two thin membranes that divide this structure into chambers. It is the cochlear duct, which is separated from the remaining chambers by Reissner's membrane and the basilar membrane, that contains the receptor elements for hearing. Specifically, the organ of Corti is the site of transduction of mechanical energy. The organ of Corti rests upon the basilar membrane and contains the inner and outer hair cells, which are innervated by fibers of the eighth cranial nerve (Figure 2). Mammals typically have one row of inner hair cells and three rows of outer hair cells. A rather rigid tectorial membrane lies just above the fine cilia of hair cells. The layout of the hair cells from the base of the cochlea to its apex provides a substrate for coding of sound frequency. This is the place theory originally advanced by Helmholtz (1863) and supported by the work of Bekesy (1960). Compression waves from high-frequency stimuli displace the basilar membrane, which widens near the base of the cochlea at the stapes end. The stereocilia of hair cells at the focus of maximal wave motion are mechanically activated because of the overhanging tectorial membrane. The place of maximal displacement is the site of chemical trans-

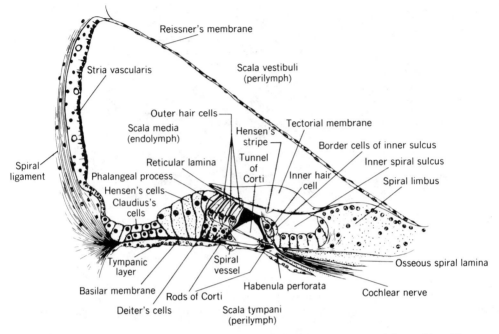

FIGURE 2. Drawing representing the organ of Corti in a cross section of the cochlea. The organ of Corti is located in the scala media on the basilar membrane and is bathed in endolymph. (From Yost and Nielsen, 1977.)

mitter release by hair cells and the source of greatest activation of auditory nerve fibers. In essence, the simplest interpretation of this model is that the cochlea acts as a mechanical frequency analyzer to convert tonal information into neural action potentials. The fibers from the spiral ganglion then convey activity to the central auditory system. Inner hair cells generate activity through radial afferent fibers and outer hair cells via spiral afferent fibers. In addition to this afferent activity, there are efferent fibers from the brainstem that innervate cochlear hair cells and radial afferent fibers.

B Central Auditory Pathways

Numerous methods have been applied to the study of the morphology and connections of brain auditory neurons. Important information has been provided by Golgi, Nissl, and anterograde degeneration methods as well as by anterograde and retrograde transport of neural tracers (horseradish peroxidase) and other approaches. Description of cells and connections described below are far from exhaustive and are oriented toward discussion of structures most studied during development. The general ascending pathways are summarized in Figure 3.

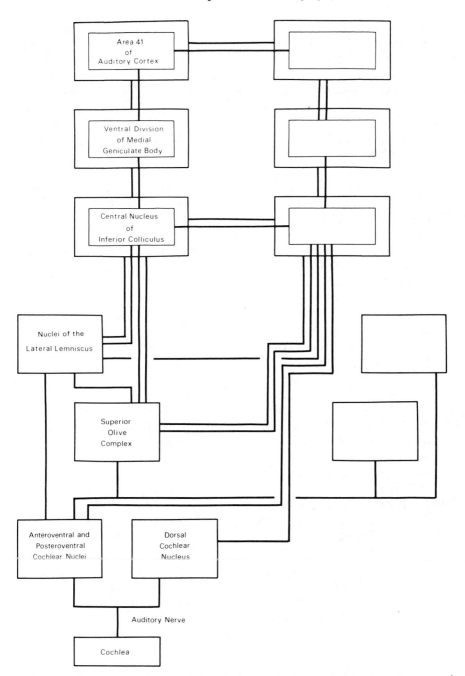

FIGURE 3. Diagram of major ascending and crossing projections to important structures of the central auditory pathways. Subnuclei of several structures are not shown.

Axons of the eighth nerve innervate cells of the dorsal and ventral cochlear nuclei. The distribution of rostrally and caudally branching afferent fibers retains the tonotopic order observed in the cochlea. In cat, cells located more dorsally in each of these nuclei are tuned to higher frequencies with low frequencies represented along a more ventral continuum. These cells usually receive monaural input. The ventral cochlear nucleus has been divided into the anteroventral and posteroventral cochlear nuclei since the time of Ramon y Cajal (1909); more recent work has further subdivided the anteroventral and posteroventral cochlear nuclei (Brawer et al., 1974; see Cant and Morest, 1984). Based upon cytoarchitectonic criteria, the anteroventral cochlear nucleus contains many spherical cells and the posteroventral cochlear nucleus has so-called octopus cells. The spherical cells are identified as bushy cells in Golgi material, and they are recipients of large axosomatic endbulbs of Held from auditory nerve fibers (Ryugo and Fekete, 1982). Other cell types, including globular and multipolar cells, are found in both subdivisions. The dorsal cochlear nucleus shows a laminar arrangement particularly characterized by a layer containing many granule cells and multipolar or fusiform cells.

The superior olivary complex consists of several cell groups located in the medulla and pons that provide the first sites for binaural interactions in the auditory system. Prominent among these are the lateral and medial superior olivary nuclei and the medial nucleus of the trapezoid body (Harrison and Feldman, 1970). The lateral superior olive is a convoluted structure containing principal cells that are often ovoid, as well as elongated cells. It derives ipsilateral input from spherical cells of the anteroventral cochlear nucleus and from the medial nucleus of the trapezoid body. The medial superior olive consists of a column of cells with dendrites positioned medially and laterally. Large spherical cells of the anteroventral cochlear nucleus innervate proximal halves of each medial superior olive, which provide substrates for alteration of neuronal discharge dependent upon timing and intensity differences of the acoustic signal reaching each ear. The medial nucleus of the trapezoid body contains mainly principal cells that are often ovoid shaped. These cells receive a single large calyx of Held that is derived from globular cells of the contralateral cochlear nucleus. Other groups of the superior olivary complex include preolivary or periolivary nuclei and lateral and ventral nuclei of the trapezoid body.

The inferior colliculus is a conspicuous midbrain structure that receives converging input from ascending and descending sources. It largely consists of a central nucleus and dorsal and external cortices as described by Ramon y Cajal (1909). The central nucleus is characterized by principal cells with disc-shaped dendritic fields organized into laminae (Oliver and Morest, 1984). This arrangement with similarly oriented incoming afferents from the lateral lemniscus forms the substrate for tonotopic organization in the inferior colliculus. The central nucleus receives particularly heavy input bilaterally from the lateral and medial superior olives and the contralateral cochlear nuclei. The distribution of this input is not uniform for each source, and thus a nucleotopic arrangement is evident (Brunso-Bechtold et al., 1981). In contrast, the dorsal and external cortices receive substantial input from auditory cortex (Coleman and Clerici, 1987). All subdivisions receive commissural afferents from the contralateral inferior colliculus. Located in the tegmentum below the inferior colliculus are the nuclei of the lateral lemniscus. These may be divided into dorsal, intermediate, and ventral nuclei. All lemniscal nuclei appear to project to the ipsilateral inferior colliculus, while contralateral projections are also evident.

Finally, the auditory forebrain consists of the medial geniculate body and auditory cortex. Situated in the caudolateral thalamus, the medial geniculate body is traditionally divided into ventral, dorsal, and medial subdivisions (Ramon y Cajal, 1909; Morest and Winer, 1986; Clerici and Coleman, 1990). The ventral division is characterized by cells with tufted dendrites. This region is the primary recipient of fibers from the central nucleus of the inferior colliculus (Figure 3) and is tonotopically arranged. The dorsal division contains many cells with radiate dendritic patterns, while cells of the medial division show the greatest diversity in neuronal architecture. The auditory cortex is the prime recipient of efferents from the medial geniculate body. Primary auditory cortex, area AI of the cat, receives an orderly projection from the ventral division of the geniculate, whereas cells of the dorsal division have a separate cortical target; AI has reciprocal connections with the ventral division of the medial geniculate body as well as with ipsilateral and contralateral auditory cortical fields (Andersen et al., 1980; Imig and Reale, 1980).

III   FORMATION OF THE CONDUCTIVE APPARATUS

Development of structures of the external and middle ears are of interest partly to examine the contributions and interactions of primordial tissues as well as to understand patterns of malformation. A detailed description of development of these structures in mouse, and amniotes generally, is provided by Van De Water et al. (1980). A lateral growth of the hyoid pouch ventral to the developing otocyst becomes the first sign of external and middle ear differentiation. At the time of formation of the early otic capsule (which later will include the cochlea), the primordial ossicles appear as chondroblasts. With continued chondrification of ossicular elements the pouches from the tubotympanic sulcus grow dorsally around the ossicles. These spaces become the middle ear cavities as they meet dorsal to the ossicles. The middle ear is permeated by mesenchyme residuals until about postnatal day 16 in mouse. Formation of the external meatus begins as a depression laterally by 13 days of gestation in mouse (Van De Water et al., 1980). As with the adjacent body surface, the meatus consists of a single layer of peridermal cells and germinal epithelium at this stage. The downward growth of the developing pinna covers the lateral depression of the meatal plate (Figure 4). The ependymal surfaces may also be compressed by growth patterns of mesenchymal tissue from presumptive pinna cartilage. By postnatal day 9, the peridermal cells of the meatal plate contain keratohyalin granules. At this age, cornification is accompanied by opening of the meatus, while a multilayered periderm covers the outer meatal surface. Following this, the meatus completely opens to expose the maturing tympanic membrane. Opening of the meatus occurs at 12–14 days postpartum in rat (Silverman and Clopton, 1977; Coleman and O'Connor, 1979; Brunjes and Albert, 1981). In mouse, the tympanic membrane achieves maturity by postnatal day 18, whereas the oval window is of mature size by postnatal day 7 (Huangfu and Saunders, 1983).

The developmental features of the external and middle ears clearly impact on early maturation of functional activity in the cochlea. The development of the external meatus, ossicles, and middle ear cavity parallels that of

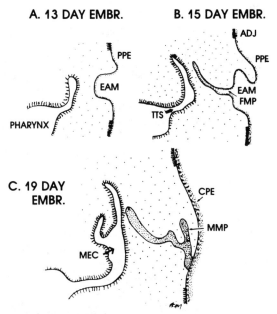

FIGURE 4. Diagram representing development of the external auditory meatus and meatal plate at three embryonic ages in mouse. (A) At embryonic day 13 the lining of the external auditory meatus (EAM) appears similar to that of the nonotic skin (ADJ) and presumptive pinnal tissues (PPE). (B) The tubotympanic sulcus (TTS) grows dorsal from the pharynx by the 15th day to approach the presumptive meatal plate (FMP). The lumen of the FMP contains only a single layer of periderm cells, unlike presumptive pinnal tissue (PPE) and adjacent skin that has several layers of peridermal cells. (C) Occlusion of the external meatus and enlarged meatal plate (MMP) is complete by embryonic day 19. The pinna epiderm (CPE) now shows some cornification below layers of peroderm. In contrast, epidermal cells of the meatal plate remain apposed at this stage and do not contain kerotohyalin. The developing middle ear cavity (MEC) has enlarged. (Adapted from Van De Water et al., 1980.)

the cochlea, gradually providing more efficient substrates for sound transmission. For example, ear canals are smaller and shorter in immature mammals, including humans, which results in a higher resonance frequency and lower gain (see Saunders et al., 1983). Of further interest is the improved performance of middle ear mechanisms with age, which enhances sound transmission to the developing cochlea, thus contributing to reduction of auditory thresholds. In the hamster, middle ear admittance levels (inverse of impedance) increase monotonically from birth and then negatively accelerate to a constant level (Relkin et al., 1979). Obvious morphological changes include growth and ossification of the auditory ossicles and clearance of mesenchyme (Anson and Donaldson, 1981). However, the period of cavity enlargement is more protracted to include growth of air sinuses and expansion of the temporal bone. In addition, growth of the tympanic ring encircling the tympanic membrane continues postnatally after initial fusion during fetal life in humans (Anson and Donaldson, 1981); tympanic ring development occurs postnatally in many mammals, such as the rabbit (Hoyte, 1961). In rabbit, Hoyte (1961) showed that the tympanic membrane is adultlike in size at birth but becomes rotated toward the vertical until about postnatal day 22. All these morphological changes combine to alter the stiffness, resistance, and mass characteristics of the middle ear (Saunders et al., 1983).

IV ONTOGENESIS OF THE INNER EAR

Important issues arise concerning the emergence of cochlear structures. One involves the order of appearance of sensory hair cells and spiral ganglion cells. Another question concerns the role of neural input on survival and organization of the sensory receptive cells. Structural development and functional activity in the cochlea may also have significant impact on later organization of central auditory pathways, even as distant from the end organ as auditory cortex (Brugge et al., 1985; Reale et al., 1987; see Chapter 8, this volume).

The otic placode forms as an ectodermal thickening. There is an invagination of this tissue that subsequently separates to form the otic cup and then the otocyst, which remains surprisingly close to the neural folds at this stage (Bast and Anson, 1949; Anson and Donaldson, 1981). This process is dependent upon inductive effects from underlying mesoderm as well as from the developing nervous system (Li et al., 1978). Van De Water and Ruben (1976) show that abnormal formation of the rhombencephalon in mutant mice leads to anomalous development of the adjacent inner ear. Most current data suggests that all components of the organ of Corti, as well as the spiral ganglion, are derived from the otic placode. During embryonic development there appears to be a remarkable synchrony in the generation of cells at a given position in the cochlea of mouse (Ruben, 1967). Terminal mitosis in mouse occurs on gestational day 14 for inner and outer hair cells, spiral ganglion cells, pillar cells, and various other supporting cells including Deiter's and Hensen's cells. However, it has been known for decades that maturation of different cochlear cells takes various lengths of time (Wada, 1923; see below). Unfortunately, there is also little data available on the sequence of proliferation of cochlear structures, including hair cells as a function of position along the length of the cochlea. In one study on mouse, mitotic division of cells are reported to begin at the apex and then proceed successively toward the base of the cochlea (Ruben, 1967). This observation is not supported by the maturational gradient in the cochlea (e.g., Rubel et al., 1984; Burda, 1985). More studies of proliferation patterns of the developing cochlea are needed to clarify important issues concerning the base-to-apex continuum.

The question of the integrity of the spiral ganglion input for development of structures of the organ of Corti is addressed in organ culture experiments. Removal of the presumptive statoacoustic ganglion in fetal mice to eliminate its trophic effect does not impair development of sensory structures of the organ of Corti including hair cells (Van De Water, 1976, 1986). The cultured cochleas develop normally in a base-to-apex manner. These and other results (Hirokawa, 1977; Sobkowicz et al., 1983; Anniko, 1986; Corwin and Cotanche, 1989) suggest that neural elements associated with the acoustic ganglion do not play a major trophic role in early morphological development of receptor components of the cochlea. However, early ingrowth of neuronal processes that precede cytodifferentiation of hair cells (Sher, 1961; Pujol and Lavigne-Rebillard, 1985; Whitehead and Morest, 1985b) may still influence aspects of hair cell development.

V NEURAL GENERATION PATTERNS IN CENTRAL AUDITORY STRUCTURES

The timing and pattern of proliferation of central auditory cells has been most thoroughly studied in rat. Neurons of the anteroventral and posteroventral cochlear nuclei are generated during a period between embryonic days 13 and 17 (Altman and Bayer, 1980). These cell proliferation times overlap the generation times of hair cells and spiral ganglion cells of the auditory periphery. Furthermore, cells of the dorsal cochlear nucleus may be generated as early as embryonic day 12 but may also still proliferate into the postnatal period (Altman and Bayer, 1980). As is true of proliferation in neocortex and other brain structures, the largest cells (pyramidal) of the dorsal cochlear nucleus are mainly generated first, beginning on embryonic day 12. Proliferation of the small granule cells begins later and continues into postnatal life. Observations on proliferation times of the mouse cochlear nuclei confirm this result (Taber-Pierce, 1967; Martin and Rickets, 1981). Such data on rat and mouse also demonstrate no orderly generation gradient across these structures, such as that related to future tonotopicity. Corresponding data in developing chick magnocellular nucleus suggests that there is a gradient of cell death that can be related to the adult tonotopic order (Rubel et al., 1976). One study in the opossum by Willard and Martin (1986) demonstrates that a cellular band can be identified medial to the presumptive cochlear nuclei at birth and that this band migrates laterally to reach adult locations (Figure 5); these cells mainly correspond to the large

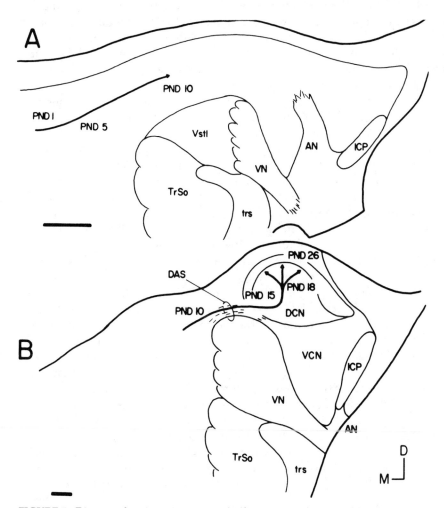

FIGURE 5. Diagram showing migratory path of neurons in the precochlear band from postnatal day (PND) 1 to 26 in opossum illustrated in drawing at PND 5 (A) and PND 35 (B). Note that the bulk of these cells later differentiate in the dorsal cochlear nucleus (DCN). Abbreviations: AN, auditory nerve; ICP, inferior cerebellar peduncle; trs, tract of descending spinal trigeminal nucleus; TrSo, spinal trigeminal nucleus, pars oralis; VCN, ventral cochlear nucleus; VN, vestibular nerve; Vstl, lateral vestibular nucleus. Scale bars 100 μm each. (From Willard and Martin, 1986.)

multipolar and giant cells of the dorsal cochlear nucleus and large multipolar neurons of the ventral cochlear nucleus. An interesting observation of this study was that an injection of horseradish peroxidase into the inferior colliculus as early as 17 days postconception resulted in retrograde labeling of cells at an intermediate position. This work suggests that while neurons are migrating they can send out axons to distant targets of the auditory pathway (Willard and Martin, 1986).

Cells of the inferior colliculus in rat are produced between embryonic day 14 and the perinatal period (Altman and Bayer, 1981). Generally, cells of the inferior colliculus are generated in an outside-in fashion. Cells located rostral, lateral, and ventral in the central nucleus are generated first, and those of the caudal portion of dorsal cortex are generated last. Only very grossly can this be construed as corresponding to the tonotopic arrangement observed in the adult (Coleman et al., 1982; Clerici and Coleman, 1986, 1987). Cells of the medial geniculate body of rat show a proliferation gradient from lateral to medial that corresponds to the adult tonotopic order observed in cat (Altman and Bayer, 1989). The tonotopic organization of the rat medial geniculate body has not yet been firmly established, so that a direct comparison of cytogenetic gradient and adult functional activity has yet to be determined for the rat (or any mammal). In addition, there are no apparent centripetal cytogenetic effects upon the medial geniculate body or auditory cortex by newly generated cells of the inferior colliculus. Although cortical cells in general proliferate between embryonic days 15 and 21 in rat (Berry and Rogers, 1965; Hicks and D'Amato, 1968; Bisconte and Marty, 1975), cells of the medial geniculate body proliferate during embryonic days 13–15 when a recognizable structure is produced. Therefore, most cells of the medial geniculate body are generated prior to those of inferior colliculus so that the geniculate cytogenesis gradient must be independent of ascending influences. Although these data do not preclude the possibility that geniculocortical fibers can influence generation or migration of cells in auditory cortex, current evidence (Maxwell et al., 1988) suggests that geniculocortical fibers do not invade auditory cortex in rat until about postnatal day 3—clearly past the main period for neural genesis of neocortex. Because the cochlear nuclei show no cytogenesis gradient corresponding to a tonotopic arrangement, it is likely that central gradients of proliferation are independent of related influences by the cochlea. As a consequence, it is probable that most, if not all, cytogenesis gradients in the central auditory pathways are each free from influence of other auditory structures.

VI   MATURATION OF THE INNER EAR

A   Organ of Corti

Innervation of the cochlea and maturation of its structural components have implications for continued development of central auditory pathways.

Functional activity initiated at the cochlea produces physiological changes in neurons of widespread auditory regions. Therefore, how the cochlea develops becomes a major factor in how the central auditory system becomes organized.

The major sensory elements of the organ of Corti, known in primordial form as Kollicker's organ, are the inner and outer hair cells, which show differential maturation sequences. Inner hair cells exhibit earlier adultlike features than do outer hair cells (Sobin and Anniko, 1984; Pujol, 1985; Pujol and Lavigne-Rebillard, 1985; Lavigne-Rebillard and Pujol, 1986). Dendritic components of the spiral ganglion cells invade the inner hair cell region to form synapses. Growth cones of fibers invade the wall of the otocyst where the basement membrane is absent (Carney and Silver, 1983). There is also likely a limited period of chemotaxis for attraction of eighth nerve fibers to receptor cells (Van De Water and Ruben, 1983; Van De Water, 1986). However, hair cell differentiation is apparently intrinsic as demonstrated by *in vivo* and *in vitro* experiments (Van De Water, 1986; Corwin and Cotanche, 1989) and by a study that added aminoglycoside antibiotics to suppress chemical interactions between nerve fibers and hair cells (Anniko, 1986). The inner hair cells form presynaptic specializations that include groups of vesicles. During development there may be a slight reduction in the number of afferent fibers and possibly a decline in number of these presynaptic specializations (Pujol, 1985). Efferent endings on inner hair cells appear during the same time span as afferent endings (Figure 6). The latter results, observed in rodents and cat, are also consistent with findings from the fetal organ of Corti in humans (Pujol and Lavigne-Rebillard, 1985). The most apparent change in innervation patterns on developing inner hair cells concerns the reduction of efferent endings directly on the receptor cell and a clear increment in efferent synapses upon afferent endings (Figure 6). As a result, efferent endings in adult mammals synapse almost solely on these afferent structures, which then synapse on inner hair cells.

Ontogenetic changes involving outer hair cells are even more profound (Pujol, 1985). Approximately 10 days prior to onset of function, at the time of invasion of fibers below the inner hair cells, there is a stage exemplified by multiple incursion of afferent fibers in the region of the outer hair cells. At this time, presynaptic specializations are observed in the outer hair cells. The innervation pattern at this stage resembles that of inner hair cells. Within a few days there is a rapid decline in presynaptic bodies. Efferent fibers then appear, first forming axodendritic synapses upon afferents, then direct synapses form on the outer hair cells through apparent competition with the afferent endings (Figure 6). Postsynaptic cisternae are now observed in outer hair cells, which gradually acquire more elongated shape. As the outer hair cells take on adult form, the characteristic large efferent endings appear, with relatively few afferent endings remaining. These structural changes in outer hair cell morphology and efferent innervation are correlated with physiological maturation of the cochlea in mammals (see

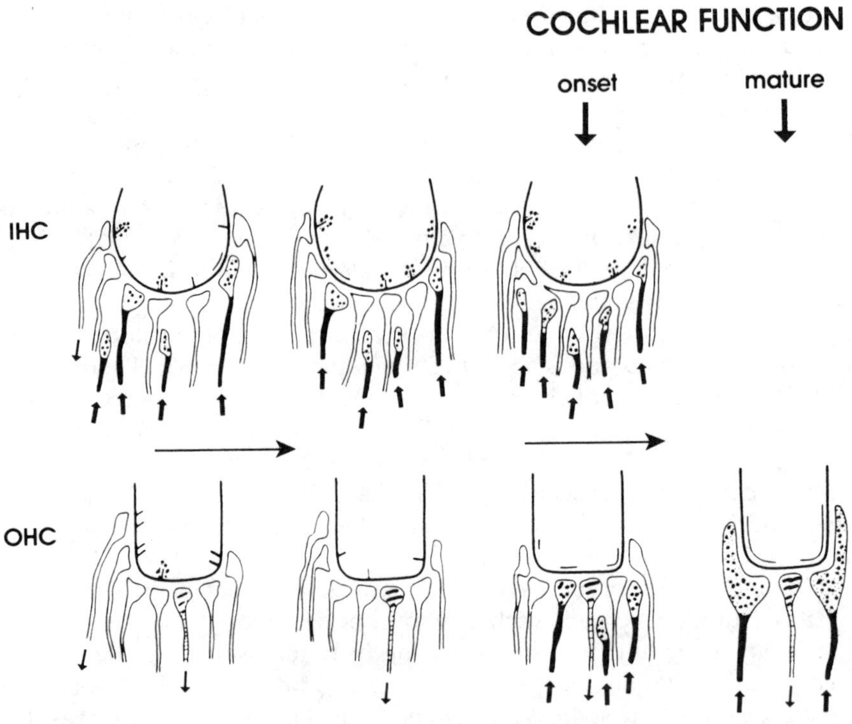

FIGURE 6. Diagram showing sequence of synaptogenesis on cochlear hair cells in mammals. In contrast to the development of innervation of inner hair cells (IHC), there are substantive alterations in the patterns of endings on outer hair cells (OHC). These changes are characterized by gradual replacement of most afferent endings (white or dashed) with efferent endings that are large at maturity (black and dotted). (Adapted from Pujol, 1985.)

Pujol, 1985). Of further interest is the observation that mouse neuron-specific enolase activity appears in nerve endings of inner hair cells at birth, but comparable activity does not develop in nerve endings of outer hair cells until after postnatal day 3 (Whitlon and Sobkowicz, 1988). It is tempting to speculate that neuron-specific enolase activity may represent the differentiation process of the efferent fibers that predominate on the surface of outer hair cells. Parallels of this process extend beyond mammals, as similar anatomical changes are observed in developing chick cochlea (Whitehead and Morest, 1985a,b). The latter studies showed that hair cell development is characterized by loss of basal trailing processes and transitory overproduction of synaptic bodies. It is also noteworthy that in preparations with vestibular nerve section prior to arrival of efferents, the outer hair cells still assume normal morphology but now are surrounded exclusively by afferent endings (Pujol and Carlier, 1982).

Other important structural changes are observed in developing cochlea. Maturation of cochlear elements at a given position along the length of cochlea occurs in parallel. In rat, this process includes hair cells and various supporting cells that can be identified on the day of birth (Wada, 1923; see Figure 7). The greater and lesser epithelial ridges, prominent at birth in rat (Figure 7), first appear in the basal turn of mouse cochlea on embryonic day 16 (Lim and Anniko, 1985). Due to the position and angulation of hair cells, it appears that inner hair cells are derived from the greater epithelial ridge and the outer hair cells from the lesser (Figure 7). Observations in mouse show that associated with the onset of cochlear function, hair cells and supporting cells that transiently have a kinocilium lose this structure (Kikuchi and Hilding, 1965; Lim and Anniko, 1985; see Figure 8). Tall stereocilia continue to grow, while microvilli on hair cells recede with age (Figure 8). Supporting cells also lose abundant cilia during this time. Such data also confirm the phylogenetic source of these cells as mechanoreceptors (Lim and Anniko, 1985). The tectorial membrane, a vital component of the transduction process that covers the sensory epithelium, consists of major and minor membrane portions. The major portion is initially secreted by greater epithelial ridge cells and the minor portion by lesser epithelial ridge cells (Lim and Anniko, 1985; Lim, 1987). In the mouse, the tectorial membrane incompletely covers hair cells in the basal turn; by 3 days after birth the hair cells are nearly covered, although the hair cells in the apical part of the cochlea are not enveloped at all. The apical portion is only partly covered at 6 days, but by 14 days the tectorial membrane shows adult form (Lim and Anniko, 1985; Lim, 1987). The basilar membrane is derived from epithelial cells and is created from radially oriented fibers and radially oriented cells (i.e., along the cochlear coils; Lim and Anniko, 1985). Substantial changes in cochlear development ensue behavioral responses to sound. In mouse, the filaments of the basilar membrane and pillar cells stain more intensively after this period, the tympanic cover layer on the basilar membrane is reduced in thickness, the cross-sectional area of the tunnel of Corti expands, and hook-shaped connections between the tectorial membrane and reticular membrane disappear (Krause and Aulbach-Kraus, 1981). Some of these changes may have functional consequences for the micromechanics of the cochlea and augmentation of hearing sensitivity.

A major feature of cochlear development, which is reflected in a surprising way by developing auditory sensitivity, is that development and maturation proceeds from basal regions toward the apex. This observation is well documented in rat (Wada, 1923; Lenoir et al., 1980; Burda, 1985), which may serve as typical of other mammalian species (see Lim and Anniko, 1985). In the adult cochlea high-frequency stimulation maximally displaces the basilar membrane near the oval window, while progressively lower frequencies displace the basilar membrane toward the apex of cochlea. These observations would lead one to conclude that the first electrophysiological and behavioral responses would be to relatively high-frequency stimulation. However, just the opposite is observed. In rat, responses are recorded to lower frequency stimuli first, and this is followed within a few days by the

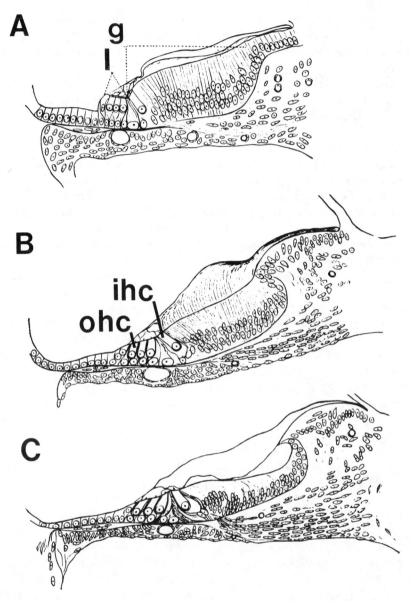

FIGURE 7. Drawings of morphological changes in the developing rat cochlea in radial section. (A) Day of birth. Two days (B) and five days (C) subsequent to birth. Both inner and outer hair cells (ihc, ohc) are present at birth but increase in size during early postnatal life. Abbreviations: g, greater epithelial ridge; l, lesser epithelial ridge. (Adapted from Wada, 1923.)

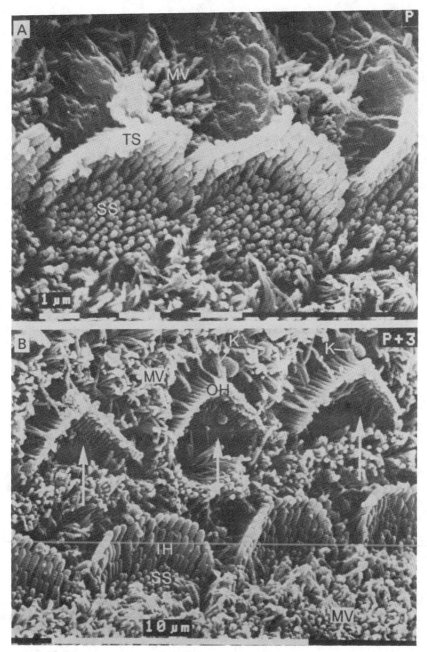

FIGURE 8. (*A*) To show inner hair cell ciliary bundles in the newborn mouse. Tall stereocilia (TS) are largely retained and transitional short stereocilia (SS) later recede. Other microvilli (MV) are also present at birth. (*B*) At 3 days of age the mouse inner hair cells (IH) show distinct bundles of sensory stereocilia with short stereocilia also present. Sensory stereocilia are observed on outer hair cells (OH) although the short stereocilia have apparently regressed by this age, and the kinocilia (K) disappear by postnatal day 21. (From Lim and Anniko, 1985).

appearance of responses to high frequencies (Carlier et al., 1979; Clerici and Coleman, 1986; Blatchley et al., 1987; Ryan and Woolf, 1988). These observations are confirmed by behavioral measures in rat (Brunjes and Albert, 1981). The results in rat may be generalized to other mammals as well as to birds (Rubel, 1978; Rubel et al., 1984). The explanation for this paradoxical result is that the basal cochlea is structurally incapable of processing high frequencies early on. This portion of the cochlea instead is activated by lower frequencies, and with age there is a systematic shift in the frequency representation so that processing of low frequencies moves apically and high-frequency capability is achieved at the cochlear base (Rubel and Ryals, 1983; Harris and Dallos, 1984; Rubel et al., 1984; but see Manley et al., 1987 and Arjmand et al., 1988). Changes in central auditory representations of tonotopic order conform to these modifications (e.g., Rubel et al., 1984).

B   Spiral Ganglion and Auditory Nerve

Development of the spiral ganglion and its processes are coextensive with developmental changes occuring in the cochlea and cochlear nuclei. Tissue development in these structures shows a base-to-apex progression corresponding to that observed in the cochlea. Work by Anniko (1983) in mouse shows that the spiral ganglion can be identified at birth and that unmyelinated axons are readily observed during the first 3 days after birth. At the ultrastructural level spiral ganglion cells are distinguishable from developing Schwann cells on the third postnatal day as the processes of Schwann cells ensheath the spiral ganglion cell body. At this age, even in the same sector of the ganglion, there is substantial variation in the stage of myelination (Figure 9). By 7 days Anniko reports that most nerves between the spiral ganglion and habenula perforata have a thick myelin sheath, and by the end of the second postnatal week all neurons have some form of myelination. These results are consistent with observations in other mammals (Romand et al., 1976; Pujol and Abonnenc, 1977; Romand et al., 1980; Schwartz et al., 1983; Romand and Romand, 1985). In cat (Romand et al., 1976; Romand, 1983), the cross-sectional area of individual cochlear nerve fibers more than triples from birth to adulthood; this is partly due to increased myelination of axons, which contributes to the maturation of action potential conductance and other physiological features.

The spiral ganglion contains two morphologically distinct cell types referred to as type 1 (the most common) and type 2. During development in rat, myelinated laminae appear in both cell types between postnatal days 4 and 6. The two cell types are discriminable by day 8 when type 2 cells show densely packed neurofilamentous structures (Schwartz et al., 1983; Romand and Romand, 1985). These studies show that morphological maturity of the cells is achieved by day 14 and that the myelin sheath of fibers contains more laminae that the soma. No comprehensive studies of cell counts of age-graded developing spiral ganglion are available for mammals. In chick there

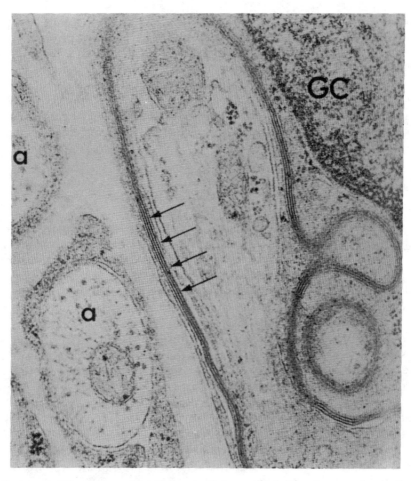

FIGURE 9. Electron micrograph of the spiral ganglion in the basal coil region of mouse at 5 days after birth. An axon leaving the ganglion cell (GC) has five layers of myelin (arrows). In contrast, axons (a) from nearby ganglion cells are enclosed by only a single layer of Scwann cell cytoplasm. ×11,200. (From Anniko, 1983.)

is a 25% reduction in the number of spiral ganglion neurons between embryonic days 8 and 14 (Ard and Morest, 1984). These changes correspond to the period of contact with the sensory epithelium and central auditory cells and presumably reflect fiber interactions at these levels. A study of the waltzing guinea pig, which has a genetically induced postnatal loss of all hair cells, shows that 43% of the spiral ganglion cells degenerate between postnatal days 30 and 60; after 90 days the spiral ganglion cell population stabilizes (Gulley et al., 1978). This work suggests that the hair cell synapse is a critical variable for survival of many cells of the spiral ganglion. This hypothesis is born out in recent work by Zhou and Van De Water (1987), who studied ganglion cell growth in mouse embryo explants after 14 days *in vitro*. Only 18.5% of statoacoustic neurons survived when grown in isolation as compared to much higher survival in explants grown with peripheral or central targets or both. Other evidence suggests that a nerve growth factor, present only during early postnatal life in hair cells of the rat, may be a vital contributor to survival of cochlear nerve fibers (Despres et al., 1988). These results suggest that hair cells of the cochlea and neurons of the cochlear nuclei play a trophic role in survival and differentiation of ganglion neurons.

VII   DEVELOPMENT OF COCHLEAR NUCLEI

The cochlear nuclei are a mandatory central processing station for auditory information originating in the cochlea. Volumetric observations of the dorsal and ventral cochlear nuclei of rat show that structural growth patterns are not a monotonic function of age (Coleman et al., 1982a; see Figure 10). The rat ventral cochlear nucleus dramatically increases in size (42%) between postnatal days 10 and 16. As the animal matures further, the increments in tissue volume minimize; changes between 16 and 24 days (25%) are greater than from 24 to 36 days, after which only modest growth is observed. A similar pattern appears for the dorsal cochlear nucleus except the growth gradient is not so sharp and essentially no change is observed after 36 days (Coleman et al., 1982; Figure 10). These relative growth patterns are also reflected in the greater sensitivity of the ventral cochlear nucleus than the dorsal cochlear nucleus to the effects of acoustic deprivation (Coleman et al., 1982) or cochlear ablation (Moore and Kowalchuk, 1988). In humans, a more than twofold increase in ventral cochlear nucleus volume occurs from birth to adulthood (Konigsmark and Murphy, 1972).

Systematic patterns of somal growth are observed in the cochlear nuclei of mouse and cat. Webster and Webster (1980) report somal growth in multipolar cells, octopus cells, globular cells, and small and large spherical cells, all of the mouse ventral cochlear nucleus. Their results show that each of these cell types increment in area until 12 days when adult size is reached. The gradient for cells of the central region of the dorsal cochlear nucleus is more abrupt, with no significant increase in somal size after postnatal day 6 in mouse. A comprehensive study in cat by Larsen (1985) indicates that cytoplasmic areas in small spherical and octopus cells increase about 50% during the first postnatal month. Large spherical cells are no more than 75% of adult size by 12 weeks of age, whereas cells of the central region of dorsal cochlear nucleus reach adult size at 4 weeks. The large fusiform cells of the dorsal cochlear nucleus are somewhat intermediate in growth pattern. These results in various species suggest that the most marked somal growth in cells of the cochlear nuclei occur during earlier phases of postnatal life and that cells of the ventral cochlear nucleus, particularly large ones in the

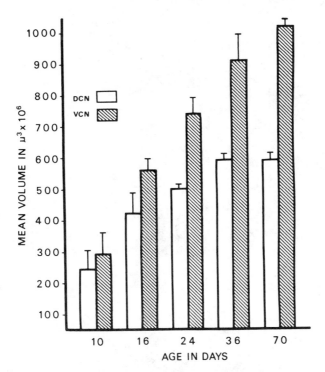

FIGURE 10. Postnatal development of volume of the cochlear nuclei in rat. The ventral cochlear nucleus (VCN) shows a rapid increase in volume between postnatal days 10 and 16, which encompasses the time of opening of the external meatus and the onset of hearing. This period also marks rapid growth in the dorsal cochlear nucleus (DCN), although overall growth patterns level off earlier in the DCN than the VCN. (From Coleman et al., 1982).

anterior division, mature at a slower rate than those of the dorsal cochlear nucleus. In this context, cells of the ventral cochlear nucleus are the ones that show the greatest reduction in somal size following acoustic deprivation by conduction blockade, particularly when initiated prior to the onset of hearing function (Coleman and O'Connor, 1979; Webster and Webster, 1979; Blatchley et al., 1983; see Chapter 8 of this volume). Neuron survival in the ventral cochlear nucleus is clearly dependent upon neural input from the cochlea in mammals (e.g., Trune, 1982; Moore and Kitzes, 1985; Moore and Kowalchuk, 1988; Hashisaki and Rubel, 1989) as are projections from the cochlear nuclei to inferior colliculus (Trune, 1983; Moore and Kitzes, 1985; Moore and Kowalchuk, 1988).

A major synaptic configuration of the anteroventral cochlear nucleus is the endbulb of Held. Ryugo and Fekete (1982) demonstrate differential stages of formation of this synapse in kitten (Figure 11). As the soma of the postsynaptic neuron reaches full size, the presynaptic element extends across the surface to form a single endbulb. By increasing the functional

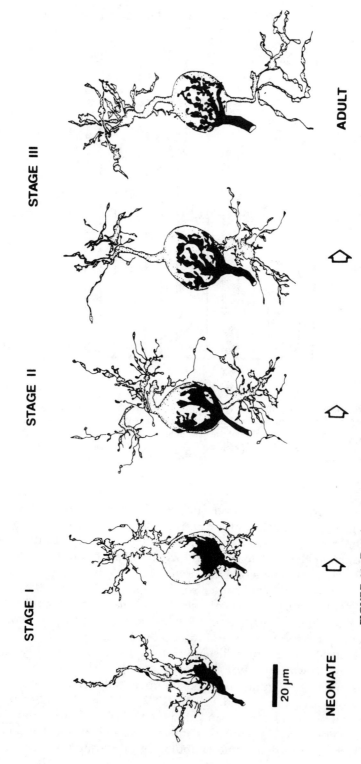

FIGURE 11. Drawings representing hypothetical stages of development and maturation of the endbulb of Held in cat. Growth of terminal space in the endbulb enhances efficacy of auditory nerve fibers. (From Ryugo and Fekete, 1982.)

STAGE I   STAGE II   STAGE III

ADULT

NEONATE

20 µm

surface for synaptic contacts, this developmental change may contribute to reduction in response latency and threshold. Similarly, from about 6 days of age in rat the incoming endbulb processes gradually cover somal appendages around the major dendrite of the spherical cell to form multiple synapses (Neises et al., 1982). By 16 days this configuration resembles that of the adult rat. The spherical cell membrane of rat shows particle aggregates opposite presynaptic zones; the distribution of particle aggregates shifts from dendritic processes at 6 days to the soma and somal appendages after 8 days of age (Mattox et al., 1982). The number of active vesicle sites located in the endbulb appear to be a function of the level of environmental acoustic stimulation encountered following the onset of hearing (Gulley, 1978). Furthermore, the developing waltzing guinea pig with genetic hair cell loss shows a reduction in number of endbulbs of Held and fewer synaptic vesicles in remaining endbulbs (Gulley et al., 1978). The presence of a large endbulb from the eighth nerve is not unique to mammals, as it develops on cells of the chick nucleus magnocellularis after retraction of postsynaptic somal processes (Jhaveri and Morest, 1982a,b). Formation of this connection apparently involves a reduction in the number of branching cochlear nerve fibers (Jackson and Parks, 1982); however, the normal reduction of dendritic processes of the postsynaptic neurons in chick is not dependent on cochlear nerve input, as cochlear ablation prior to target innervation fails to alter the pattern of dendritic retraction (see Jackson and Parks, 1982).

Further information on development of the dorsal cochlear nucleus is revealed by studies using the Golgi preparation and electron microscopy. Kane and Habib (1978) show that fusiform cells of the newborn kitten are covered with multiform projections and filled with large Golgi complexes and Nissl bodies. During the second postnatal week several adult synaptic types appear; this and subsequent periods are characterized by decline in somatic contacts. Fusiform cells become separated by growth of the neuropil at 4–6 weeks. Data from 45–95-day-old animals reveal the presence of glomeruli and synaptic nests that mature after 120 days in cat (Kane and Habib, 1978). Schweitzer and Cant (1984) show that in hamster the cochlear fibers invade the neonatal ventral but not dorsal cochlear nucleus. Fibers enter the hamster dorsal cochlear nucleus over the first week and a half of postnatal life and infiltrate layers containing giant and fusiform cells (Figure 12). Typical afferent terminals (of apparent cochlear origin) on these cells appear about 2 days after fiber growth into the appropriate layer. The period of ingrowth of cochlear fibers and of subsequent synapse formation appears to be of significance for dendritic growth of neurons in the dorsal cochlear nucleus (e.g., giant cells). After birth, the large cells are morphologically similar (Figure 12), but coincident with fiber ingrowth there is further dendritic development so that by postnatal day 5 in hamster the neurons begin to show some adultlike structural characteristics. The specific influence of afferent fibers on dendritic development of cells of the

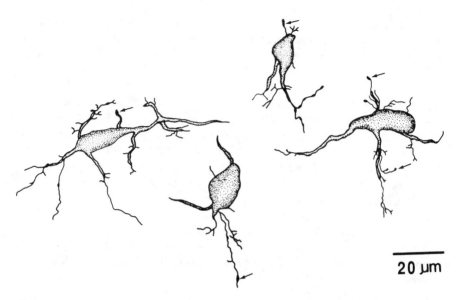

FIGURE 12. Drawings of Golgi-impregnated large cells of the dorsal cochlear nucleus of the hamster on postnatal day 1. Hairlike neurites that extend from these cells often show expansions at the tips (arrows), which likely represent growth cones. (From Schweitzer and Cant, 1984.)

dorsal cochlear nucleus is unclear, although the temporal synchrony of growth in presynaptic and postsynaptic elements is a remarkable one. This issue is made more difficult by the observation that only one type of terminal on these cells is of cochlear origin (at least in hamster). Furthermore, as predicted from cochlear maturation, the fibers from the basal turns are first to invade the dorsal cochlear nucleus where they grow into the dorsomedial portion. These data also suggest that there are maturation gradients in the cochlear nuclei that parallel cochlear development. Neurons are organized into middle and deep laminae by postnatal day 15; these neurons show several mature features except that the apical dendrites of fusiform cells have not yet acquired the spines observed in the adult (Schweitzer and Cant, 1985). Finally, the dorsal cochlear nucleus is a major binding site for muscimol and strychnine, suggesting that GABA and glycine are important transmitters here (Glendenning and Baker, 1988). Development of transmitter activity and receptor characteristics in the cochlear nuclei of mammals merits considerable intensive study. In chick, GABA immunoreactive terminals appear in the nucleus magnocellularis around EI5 when endbulbs of Held normally form (Code et al., 1989). These authors also demonstrated that the reactive terminals display a gradient of increasing density from rostromedial to caudolateral in this nucleus.

VIII   DEVELOPMENT OF HIGHER BRAINSTEM STRUCTURES

According to Webster and Webster (1980), somal growth patterns of cells in the superior olivary complex mirror those of cells in the cochlear nuclei.

Somal size of neurons in the lateral superior olive and medial nucleus of the trapezoid body in mouse increments until about 12 days when the neurons are of adult magnitude. These results may be compared with growth patterns of cells of the medial superior olive in rat (Rogowski and Feng, 1981) where somal size increases from the day of birth to about postnatal day 8; after a period of stabilization there is a modest decline in cell size to adult values (Figure 13). Somal growth is accompanied by thickening and branching of dendrites and appearance of appendages, growth cones, and filopodia on dendrites. In the stabilizing phase that occurs after onset of hearing there is a decrease in the number of dendritic branches as well as a decrement in appendages, growth cones, and filopodia of dendrites (Figure 13). How these processes are influenced by or influence incoming afferents is unclear in the rat and in other mammals. Recent work (Kil et al., 1989) shows that unilateral cochlear ablation of neonatal gerbils results in the formation of efferent projections to both sides of each medial superior olive. In the developing chick the formation of the gradient of dendritic length in third-order neurons is not impaired by bilateral removal of the embryonic otocysts (Parks et al., 1987). In the latter study, total dendritic length is nonetheless reduced by otocyst removal. Direct deafferentation of these neurons results in rapid decreases in microtubule and neurofilament densities (Deitch and Rubel, 1989). Normally observed changes in mammals are also occurring during a period of rapid electrophysiological development of the auditory brainstem (Blatchley et al., 1987). Electrophysiological changes including reductions in response latencies, which continue after stabilization of the morphological parameters just described, may reflect further myelinization and synaptic efficiency. Of final significance is that development of tonotopic organization of third order neurons parallels changes observed in the cochlea. Sanes et al. (1989) showed that the tonotopic map of neurons of the gerbil lateral superior olive is altered during postnatal development resulting in particular sectors of this nucleus coding successively higher frequencies with age.

The central nucleus receives convergent input from a variety of sources in the adult, including cells of the cochlear nuclei and superior olivary complex. Cells of the inferior colliculus of rat are generated from embryonic day 14 to around birth. Our research (Maxwell et al., 1988) shows that by birth fibers from neurons of the cochlear nuclei and superior olive complex have

FIGURE 13. Drawings of Golgi-impregnated neurons of the rat medial superior olive on postnatal days 12 (left) and 30 (right). The more mature neuron shows a reduction in thick dendritic branches and a modest decrease in somal size. (From Rogowski and Feng, 1981.)

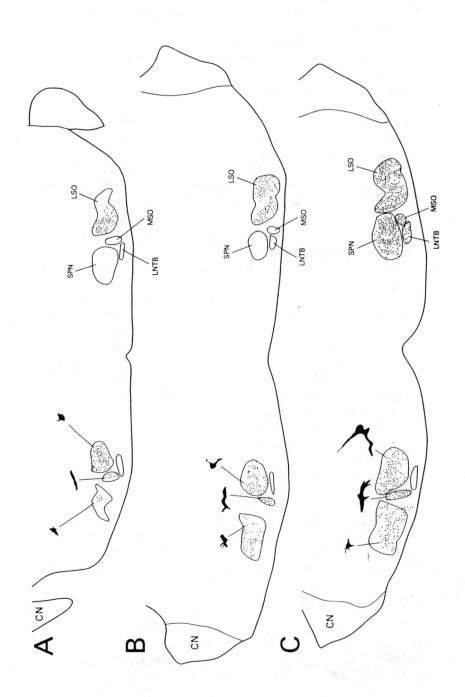

already invaded the region containing the central nucleus of the inferior colliculus in rat. Furthermore, many of the projecting neurons, although small, have acquired morphological features recognizable in the adult (Figure 14). These results imply that there is a massive afferent input from lower brainstem auditory structures while neurons may still be migrating in the inferior colliculus and possibly still being generated there. In contrast, there is no input to the inferior colliculus from pyramidal cells of auditory cortex at birth in the rat and none until at least postnatal day 3 (Maxwell et al., 1988). This work demonstrates that retrograde transport of horseradish peroxidase appears in pyramidal cells of auditory cortex of rat after collicular injection of horseradish peroxidase on postnatal day 5.

The preferred orientation of dendrites of cells in the inferior colliculus of rat changes between postnatal days 8 and 20 (Dardennes et al., 1984). There is a lengthening of proximal and intermediate dendritic segments from postnatal day 8 to 16. The most distal segments increment in length from postnatal day 16 to 20 (Dardennes et al., 1984). These alterations in dendritic length are accompanied by reabsorption of dendritic spines in each segment. The phase of changes in the proximal and intermediate segments appears to correlate with the maturation of brainstem afferent fibers as well as a decrement in the extracellular space of the rat inferior colliculus (Pysh, 1969). Parallels of spatial reorientation and dendritic growth patterns of rat are also observed in the cat (Meininger and Baudrimant, 1981). In opossum, dendritic differentiation of central nucleus neurons generally begins before neurons of the dorsal cortex (Morest, 1969). Somal size changes studied in mouse colliculus indicate a peak in growth by postnatal day 12, a modest decline in size by the 24th day, and again a further increment afterward (Webster and Webster, 1980). Finally, the lipid content of the inferior colliculus, including levels of cerebrosides, increases through postnatal day 30 in rat (Shah et al., 1978); these changes are reflected in latency shifts of auditory brainstem potentials (Shah et al., 1978; Blatchley et al., 1987). Although there is growing evidence that the central nucleus of inferior colliculus contains considerable glutamate and aspartate (Eyerly et al., 1989) and this region contains receptors for glycine, GABA, and acetylcholine (Glendenning and Baker, 1988), there remains a need for characterizing transmitter and receptor properties of this structure during prenatal and postnatal development.

FIGURE 14. Distribution of retrograde label in sections of the superior olive complex after injections of horseradish peroxidase into the inferior colliculus. (A) After a unilateral injection on postnatal day 1 there is substantial retrograde label in neurons of each major nucleus that is labeled at 5 days (B) or older. Even at postnatal day 1 the labeled neurons show some of the basic morphology that will be elaborated in cells of older animals, as in those observed in (C) at postnatal day 7 following bilateral injection of inferior colliculus. Labeled neurons of the cochlear nuclei are not illustrated. Key: CN, cochlear nuclei; LNTB, lateral nucleus of the trapezoid body; LSO, lateral superior olive; MSO, medial superior olive; SPN, superior paraolivary nucleus.

The cell generation and morphological data suggest that many aspects of neural development within the auditory system are occurring in parallel. However, there is also a clear trend for neural differentiation from lower order to higher order auditory structures. Morest (1969) used Golgi material from several mammalian species to show that dendritic differentiation in the cochlear nuclei begins prior to that in the superior olivary complex and inferior colliculus. Dendritic differentiation then begins in the medial geniculate body and, lastly, in the auditory cortex. Furthermore, there is evidence for a centripetal trend in maturation of functional responsiveness to acoustic stimulation as determined by methods that evaluate different levels of the neuraxis in the same preparation (Ryan et al., 1982; Clerici and Coleman, 1986; Blatchley et al., 1987; Ryan and Woolf, 1988). Using pure tone stimulation, Blatchley et al. (1987) demonstrated a sequential appearance of auditory brainstem response components in rat. A response component of nonneural origin is prominent on postnatal day 12; this response appears to be a summating potential representing hair cell activity. By postnatal day 14 two waves are routinely recorded to lower or intermediate-frequency presentation. However, waves 3 and 4 are not consistently observed at this age, nor are neural responses to high-frequency stimulation. A fifth wave is sometimes recorded in rat on postnatal day 20 but not at 16 days (Blatchley et al., 1987). Therefore, the rat auditory system shows centripetal maturation patterns, and earlier response components appear to lower frequency stimuli. In the Mongolian gerbil, Ryan et al. (1982) demonstrate that wide-band noise increases 2-deoxyglucose uptake in the anteroventral and posteroventral cochlear nuclei but not in higher order auditory structures on postnatal day 12. There is more stimulus-driven uptake in the cochlear nuclei on day 14, when uptake now also appears in the superior olive complex and ventral nucleus of the lateral lemniscus; not until postnatal day 16 does noise stimulation increase uptake in the gerbil inferior colliculus, and by postnatal day 18 stimulus-related uptake is visible in the medial geniculate body and auditory cortex. In a later study in gerbil using pure tone stimulation, Ryan and Woolf (1988) found no enhancement of 2-deoxyglucose uptake in the inferior colliculus until postnatal day 18 and not until after day 20 in the medial geniculate and auditory cortex. In the rat inferior colliculus, a weak band of 2-deoxyglucose uptake is observed on postnatal day 17 but not at earlier ages (Clerici and Coleman, 1986). Behavioral evidence in rat also suggests that lower auditory nuclei mature earlier than upper auditory structures (Hyson and Rudy, 1983).

IX   AUDITORY FOREBRAIN DEVELOPMENT

Structural studies focused on development of the medial geniculate body have provided insight on the somal and dendritic growth of constituent neurons. The medial geniculate body of mammals is divided into ventral, dorsal, and medial divisions, each with component nuclei (see Section IIB). In the newborn rat, the ventral division is well formed and readily discernable from the dorsal division, which is relatively small at this stage (Clerici et al., 1987a,b; Coleman et al., 1989). Cells of the ventral and ovoid nuclei of the ventral division, the dorsal and deep dorsal nuclei of the dorsal division, and cells of the medial division all show synchronously sharp increases in somal growth from postnatal days 3 to 7 in rat (Clerici et al, 1987b; Coleman et al., 1989; see Figure 15A). During the same period there is also an expotential reduction in somal density in all geniculate nuclei (Clerici et al., 1987b; Coleman et al., 1989; see Figure 15B). In Golgi-stained material the principal tufted neuron of the ventral nucleus is recognized on postnatal day 1 in rat; this cell shows apparent growth cones and needlelike appendages on cell processes with the appendages also appearing on the soma (Figure 16). The ovoid nucleus, which also contains tufted cells, shows the most distinct double spiral between postnatal days 7 and 11 in rat (Clerici et al., 1987b; Coleman et al., 1989). This work also demonstrates that fusiform-shaped cells are more characteristically observed in the deep dorsal nucleus in early postnatal life as they align with the afferent fibers of the midgeniculate bundle. In rat, the medial geniculate body is invaded by fibers from the inferior colliculus at birth (Asanuma et al., 1988); however, these fibers become unequally distributed in density to the geniculate subnuclei over the first postnatal days (Maxwell et al., 1988).

In a study of dendritic growth patterns of neurons from Golgi stains of many brain regions, Morest (1969) made observations on development of the medial geniculate body of cat and opossum. First, the principal (tufted) neurons of the ventral nucleus show dendritic differentiation before cells of the dorsal nucleus. Second, the dendrites of the small Golgi Type II neurons differentiate later than principal neurons of various subnuclei. Morest also draws parallels between growth patterns of principal neurons in the medial geniculate body and those of the dorsal nucleus of the lateral geniculate body—among similar features he notes the forked sprouts at the ends of the growing dendrites.

The auditory cortex, including the primary area (41) and secondary regions, is the recipient of afferents from the medial geniculate body and provides corticogeniculate and corticocollicular output. In rat, the auditory cortex increases greatly in thickness between the day of birth to postnatal day 7, with the sharpest growth increment between postnatal days 5 and 7 (Coleman et al., 1987; see Figure 17). Essentially all layers of cortex show expansion during this period; increments between postnatal days 11 and 14 (the external meatus opens on days 11–12) are largely due to enlargement of laminae III and IV (Coleman et al., 1987). Golgi observations show that in lamina V pyramidal cells of rat auditory cortex, the emergence of the apical dendrite and axon precede that of basal dendrites (Coleman et al., 1987). Although basal dendrites have begun to form in these neurons at birth, the shape of the soma has not attained the characteristic pyramidal shape that

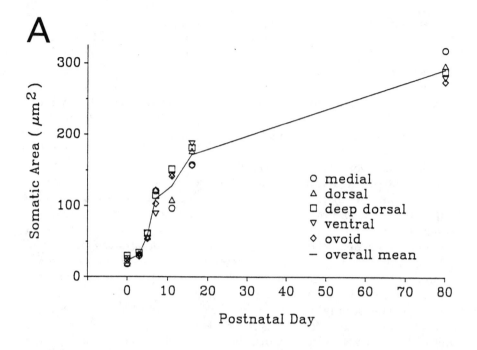

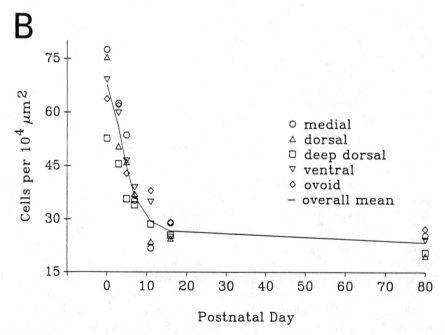

FIGURE 15. (*A*) Summary curve of somatic areas of cells in subdivisions of the rat medial geniculate body from birth to postnatal day 80. Symbols each represent the mean of 100 measurements taken from five animals. Note the particularly sharp growth slope for all geniculate cells between postnatal days 3 and 7. (*B*) Somatic density of geniculate subdivisions from birth to postnatal day 80.

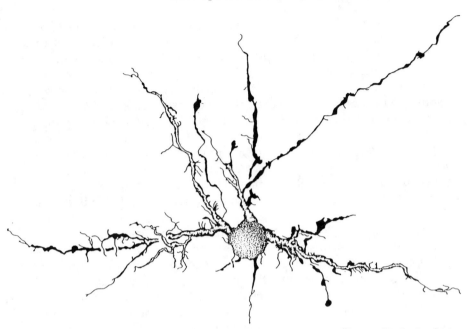

FIGURE 16. Drawing of a tufted cell of the ventral nucleus of the medial geniculate body of rat on postnatal day 1. Needlelike appendages and apparent growth cones are characteristic of neurons at this stage. Scale bar 25 μm.

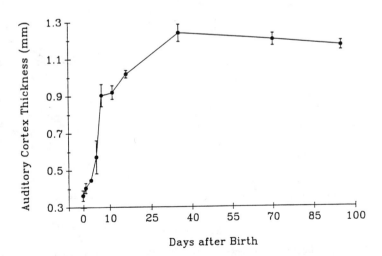

FIGURE 17. Graph representing thickness of the six laminae of area 41 in the postnatal rat. Note particularly large increment from postnatal days 5 to 7.

develops along with the arborization of basal dendrites. In rat, the second-ary and tertiary branches of basal dendrites increase in number until about postnatal day 11 (Figure 18). Typically, large varicosities appear in the apical dendrite during the first few postnatal days; in 7–11-day-old animals these varicosities are more associated with secondary branches off the apical dendrite. The numbers of spines on the apical dendrite of layer V pyramidal cells measured at the level of lamina IV increments gradually from postnatal days 5–11, then more acutely from postnatal days 11–16 (Coleman et al., 1987). There is a further slow increase to reach a maximum spine density around postnatal day 35. In rabbit, unilateral deafening at birth decreases spine numbers in the basal dendrites of layer III/IV pyramidal cells without influencing radial growth and branching patterns (McMullen and Glaser, 1988).

The chandelier cells of cortex, which contact initial segments of pyra-midal neurons, are considered inhibitory neurons, and terminals of these cells are immunoreactive for glutamic acid decarboxylase. In auditory cortex of cat, these cells can be identified by 9 days of age and are developing elongated vertical axon complexes during the period from postnatal days 15–23 (De Carlos et al., 1985). Chandelier cells then show adult morphology by postnatal day 42 in cat. Further work on the development of neural morphology in auditory cortex is clearly required to describe features of other neurons.

Another approach to the study of development in the auditory cortex is reported by Feng and Brugge (1983). They show that the cellular and afferent columnar organization observed in the callosal projection systems

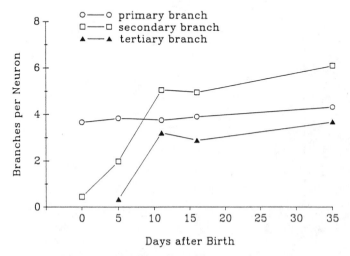

FIGURE 18. Graph showing age-related changes in basal branching of lamina V pyramidal cells of area 41 in rat. Note that the primary branches are retained from birth, but secondary and tertiary branches increment to about postnatal day 11.

of the adult cat are not observed in kittens during the first postnatal week. From an initial diffuse pattern the afferent columns from neurons of the opposite hemisphere emerge after the first postnatal week and are clearly defined by postnatal day 18. Soma of callosally projecting neurons, on the other hand, may not segregate into discrete columns until the third month of postnatal life. One additional study concerns the development of acetylcholinesterase activity in fetal human thalamocortical systems (Krmpotic-Nemanic et al., 1983). Activity of this enzyme is present in fetuses at about 10.5 weeks as part of the initial outgrowth of thalamic fibers but is not yet observed in auditory neocortex. By fetal age 16–18 weeks there are acetylcholinesterase-positive fibers in the subplate layer, and by 22–28 weeks such fibers have penetrated the auditory region of the developing cortical plate.

X   SUMMARY AND CONCLUSIONS

The auditory system is a complex of peripheral and central tissues that serve to process information from the acoustic environment. The external and middle ear structures are formed in parallel with the developing otocyst. Opening of the external meatus and conduction through the middle ear are vital for the inception of hearing. However, even at the time when the cochlea and auditory pathways permit high threshold hearing, tympanic compliance and displacement properties of the ossicles are not mature due in part to retention of primordial mesenchyme, and therefore the sensorineural apparatus is still receiving an attenuated signal.

The otocyst, including the future cochlea, forms from the otic placode, which in turn is derived from an ectodermal thickening. Development of a normal inner ear is dependent upon contact with the emerging rhombencephalon, which provides vital inductive factors. Substantial evidence also suggests that several structural elements at a given position of the growing inner ear are generated in relative synchrony. It was Wada (1923) who was astonished by the relative synchrony in development of hair cells and various supporting cells (Deiters, Henson's, etc.) at a given turn in the infant rat cochlea. Although there are likely many interactions between such cells, concurrent structural development of an orchestral nature brings together the necessary cohesion to acquire cochlear function. In addition, evidence from several mammals shows that cells near the base of the cochlea are generated and mature first, while cells more apical and those at the very base show later development gradients. However, the region near the base of the cochlea appears incapable of processing high-frequency information at the time of onset of hearing as it does in the adult. Functional processing of lower frequencies occurs at progressively more apical portions of cochlea with further development.

In vitro studies have demonstrated that the spiral ganglion apparently plays no major role as a trophic influence on hair cell development. Inner hair cell maturation tends to precede that of outer hair cells and is characterized by a reduction of efferent fibers directly on the receptor cell and an increment of efferents onto afferent endings. The efferent fibers are in apparent competition for outer hair cells; the efferent fibers eventually form the large endings observed on outer hair cells characteristic of adults. These changes in innervation and elongation of the outer hair cells are associated with the period of onset of auditory function. Survival and growth of cell populations in the spiral ganglion and associated fibers is, at least in part, dependent upon hair cell integrity.

Neurons of the cochlear nuclei are not generated in a manner related to tonotopicity in the adult, and central auditory structures do not depend on the cochlea for their proliferation patterns. Except for the inferior colliculus and auditory cortex, cells in most central auditory structures are generated during clearly overlapping periods of development. As a result, newly generated neurons have little time to have any influence on the generation and early development of neurons at other levels of the auditory system neuraxis. In fact, the events of neurogenesis and initial migration and growth of neurons are simply another example of parallel or synchronous mechanisms actuated by genetic programming in the developing nervous system. It is also obvious that the entire developmental sequence (to biological maturation) is really a continuous process in which major events are rarely abrupt. In the cochlear nuclei, maturation is nonmonotonic with most major changes occurring during the period that encompasses several days prior to and following the onset of auditory function. Increments in somal size of central auditory neurons generally precede opening of the external meatus and auditory function. Therefore, much of the growth of neurons does not rely on external stimulation.

A major synapse in the anteroventral cochlear nucleus, the endbulb of Held on spherical cells, increases its surface contacts across the soma to form a single element. The number of endbulbs are contingent upon normal hair cell development and innervation of these cells by the developing spiral ganglion. The influx of afferent fibers and subsequent synapses, such as the endbulb of Held, provides the substrate for biochemical interactions which have functional consequences that precede the impact of external sensory stimulation. In the dorsal cochlear nucleus, various synaptic types emerge at different stages of development. Formation of the first terminals of the dorsal cochlear nucleus ensues initial fiber ingrowth to the dorsal cochlear nucleus by about 2 days. Innervation of the anteroventral and posteroventral cochlear nuclei precedes that of the dorsal cochlear nucleus, and fibers from the basal portion of cochlea are the first to invade these structures. Neurons of more rostral brainstem auditory structures show systematic changes involving increases in somal size, reorientation of dendrites and alterations of dendritic surface. Fiber invasion into one structure, the inferior colliculus, is not simultaneous. Input to the central nucleus from lower brainstem groups, which provides the foundation for a tonotopic map in the inferior colliculus, antecedes by days the influx of fibers from the auditory neocortex to the dorsal cortex of the colliculus.

Development of structural features of the auditory forebrain are least understood and should be the target of future study. We know, for example, that in the newborn rat afferent collicular fibers have invaded the medial geniculate body when considerable dendritic growth of neurons of the dorsal and ventral divisions of the geniculate already exists. We also know that growth of principal neurons of geniculate subdivisions precedes that of interneuron components. Because geniculate cells are mainly generated before those of the colliculus, initial development of geniculate cells must be independent of collicular influence; however, the relative contributions of afferent and intrinsic components on further development of geniculate organization remains unexplored. The auditory cortex is another structure in which cells are generated and start growth without ascending or contralateral input. The pyramidal cells of deeper layers differentiate earlier than those of upper layers, and growth of apical dendrites and axons of these cells precedes that of basal dendrites. Spine formation occurs after most of the dendritic branching of apical and basal dendrites is complete.

There is clear evidence that although some differences in neural generation times exist at various levels of the auditory neuraxis, there are also striking parallels in early neural development of these structures. For example, somal growth patterns in the medial geniculate body largely mimic (at a modest delay) cell enlargement in the cochlear nuclei. Nevertheless, functional evidence suggests a trend toward centripetal maturation in the auditory system, and it is likely that the cochlea is the first component to mature. The present data also suggest that the span of early development to maturity is a continuous one, not marked by abrupt changes but characterized by gradual alterations in structural and physiological features that ultimately lead to optimal hearing sensitivity for the animal. A myriad of questions remain, many concerning unexplored structural development along central auditory pathways of mammals. What are the morphological transformations that mediate changes in frequency coding and synaptic efficacy from the cochlear nuclei to auditory cortex? There is special need for understanding patterns of development and neuroplasticity during prenatal life of mammals and how the groundwork established during prenatal and early postnatal life is modulated by further genetically programmed events as well as by later influences from acoustic stimulation. The role of neural activity before and after responsiveness to external stimulation on the development of structural features merits careful study. As we slowly achieve knowledge of the transmitter agents underlying coding of auditory information in neurons, it will be necessary to understand what role these transmitters and other modulatory ions and molecules play in development of auditory function.

ACKNOWLEDGMENTS

I wish to thank William Clerici, Sonia Johnson and Mark Zrull for helpful comments. I am also grateful for the assistance of Andrea Lahti and Ivy Oxendine. This work was supported by grant NS-20785 from the National Institutes of Health and by a grant from the Deafness Research Foundation.

REFERENCES

Altman, J., and S. A. Bayer (1980) Development of the brain stem in the rat. III. Thymidine-radiographic study of the time of origin of neurons of the vestibular and auditory nuclei of the upper medulla. J. Comp. Neurol. 194:877–904.

Altman, J., and S. A. Bayer (1981) Time and origin of neurons of the rat inferior colliculus and the relations between cytogenesis and tonotopic order in the auditory pathway. Exp. Brain Res. 42:411–423.

Altman, J., and S. A. Bayer (1989) Development of the rat thalamus. V. The posterior lobule of the thalamic neuroepithelium and the time and site of origin and settling pattern of neurons of the medial geniculate body. J. Comp. Neurol. 284:567–580.

Andersen, R. A., P. L. Knight, and M. M. Merzenich (1980) The thalamocortical and corticothalamic connections of AI, AII, and the anterior auditory field (AAF) in the cat: Evidence for two largely segregated systems of connections. J. Comp. Neurol. 194:663–701.

Anniko, M. (1983) Early development and maturation of the spiral ganglion. Acta Otolaryngol. 95:263–276.

Anniko, M. (1986) Antibiotics and sensorineural interactions. In vitro studies. Acta Otolaryngol (Suppl.) 429:17–21.

Anson, B. J., and J. A. Donaldson (1981) Surgical Anatomy of the Temporal Bone. Philadelphia: Saunders.

Ard, M. D., and D. K. Morest (1984) Cell death during development of the cochlear and vestibular ganglia of the chick. Int. J. Dev. Neurosci. 2:535–547.

Arjmand, E., D. Harris, and P. Dallos (1988) Developmental changes in frequency mapping of the gerbil cochlea: Comparison of two cochlear locations. Hear. Res. 32:93–96.

Asanuma, C., R. Ohkawa, B. B. Stanfield, and W. M. Cowan (1988) Observations on the development of certain ascending inputs to the thalamus in rats. I. Postnatal development. Dev. Brain Res. 41:159–170.

Bast, T. H., and B. J. Anson (1949) The Temporal Bone and the Ear. Springfield, IL: Thomas.

Bekesy, G. V. (1960) Experiments in Hearing. New York: McGraw.

Berry, M., and A. W. Rogers (1965) The migration of neuroblasts in the developing cerebral cortex. J. Anat. 99:691–709.

Bisconte, J.-C., and R. Marty (1975) Etude quantitative du marquage radioautographique dans le systeme nerveux du rat. II. Characteristiques finale dans le cerveau de l'animal adulte. Exp. Brain Res. 22:37–56.

Blatchley, B. J., W. A. Cooper, and J. R. Coleman (1987) Development of auditory brainstem response to tone pip stimuli in the rat. Dev. Brain Res. 32:75–84.

Blatchley, B., Williams, J., and J. Coleman (1983) Age-dependent effects of acoustic deprivation on spherical cells in the rat anteroventral cochlear nucleus. Exp. Neurol. 80:81–93.

Brawer, J. R., D. K. Morest, and E. C. Kane (1974) The neuronal architecture of the cochlear nucleus of the cat. J. Comp. Neurol. 155:251–300.

Brugge, J. F., S. S. Orman, J. Coleman, J. C. K. Chan, and D. P. Phillips (1985) Binaural interactions in cortical area AI of cats reared with unilateral atresia of the external ear canal. Hear. Res. 20:275–287.

Brunjes, P. C., and J. R. Albert (1981) Early auditory and visual function in normal and hyperthyroid rats. Behav. Neurol. Biol. 31:393–412.

Brunso-Bechtold, J. K., G. C. Thompson, and R. B. Masterton (1981) HRP study of the organization of auditory afferents ascending to central nucleus of inferior colliculus in cat. J. Comp. Neurol. 197:705–722.

Burda, H. (1985) Qualitative assessment of postnatal maturation of the organ of Corti in two rat strains. Hear. Res. 17:201–208.

Cant, N. B., and D. K. Morest (1984) The structural basis for stimulus coding in the cochlear nucleus of the cat. In C. I. Berlin (ed.): Recent Developments in Hearing Science. San Diego: College-Hill Press.

Carlier, E., M. Lenoir, and R. Pujol (1979) Development of cochlear frequency selectivity tested by compound action potential tuning curves. Hear. Res. 1:197–201.

Carney, P. R., and J. Silver (1983) Studies on cell migration and axon guidance in the developing distal auditory system of the mouse. J. Comp. Neurol. 215:359–369.

Clerici, W. J., and J. R. Coleman (1986) Resting and high-frequency evoked 2-deoxyglucose uptake in the rat inferior colliculus: Developmental changes and effects of short-term conduction blockade. Dev. Brain Res. 27:127–137.

Clerici, W. J., and J. R. Coleman (1987) Resting and pure tone evoked metabolic responses in the inferior colliculus of young adult and senescent rats. Neurobiol. Aging 8:171–178.

Clerici, W. J., and J. R. Coleman (1990) Anatomy of the rat medial geniculate body. I. Cytoarchitecture, myeloarchitecture and neocortical connectivity. J. Comp. Neurol, in press.

Clerici, W. J., B. Maxwell, and J. R. Coleman (1987a) Cytoarchitecture of the medial geniculate body of adult and infant rats. Anat. Rec. 218:23A–24A.

Clerici, W. J., B. Maxwell, D. R. Byrd, and J. R. Coleman (1987b) Development of the rat medial geniculate body: Quantification of neurons in the ventral division. Soc. Neurosci. Abstr. 13:325.

Code, R. A., G. D. Burd, and E. W. Rubel (1989) Development of GABA immunoreactivity in brainstem auditory nuclei of the chick: Ontogeny of gradients in terminal staining. J Comp. Neurol. 284:504–518.

Coleman, J. R., and W. J. Clerici (1987) Sources of projections to subdivisions of the inferior colliculus in the rat. J. Comp. Neurol. 262:215–226.

Coleman, J. R., and P. O'Connor (1979) Effects of monaural and binaural sound deprivation on cell development in the anteroventral cochlear nucleus of rats. Exp. Neurol. *64*:553–566.

Coleman, J., B. J. Blatchley, and J. E. Williams (1982a) Development of the dorsal and ventral cochlear nuclei in rat and effects of acoustic deprivation. Dev. Brain Res. *4*:119–123.

Coleman, J. R., M. Campbell, and W. J. Clerici (1982b) Observations on tonotopic organization within the rat inferior colliculus using 2-deoxy-D[1-^3H] glucose. Otolaryngol. Head Neck Surg. *90*:795–800.

Coleman, J. R., J.-M. Ding. A. Wei, and H. Dorn (1987) Postnatal development of cortical cytoarchitecture and lamina V pyramidal cells in area 41 of rat. Soc. Neurosci. Abstr. *13*:325.

Coleman, J. R., W. J. Clerici, B. Maxwell, and M. C. Zrull (1989) Organization and postnatal development of the rat medial geniculate body. Soc. Neurosci. Abstr. 747.

Corwin, J. T., and D. A. Cotanche (1989) Development of location-specific hair cell stereocilia in denervated embryonic ears. J. Comp. Neurol. *288*:529–537.

Dardennes, R., P. H. Jarreau, and V. Meininger (1984) A quantitative Golgi analysis of the postnatal maturation of dendrites in the central nucleus of the inferior colliculus of the rat. Dev. Brain Res. *16*:159–169.

Davis, H. (1947) Hearing and Deafness. New York: Murray Hill Books.

DeCarlos, J. A., L. Lopez-Mascaraque, and F. Valverde (1985) Development, morphology and topography of chandelier cells in the auditory cortex of the cat. Dev. Brain Res. 22:293–300.

Deitch, J. S., and E. W. Rubel (1989) Rapid changes in ultrastructure during deafferentation-induced dendritic atrophy. J. Comp. Neurol. *281*:234–258.

Despres, G., N. Giry, and R. Romand (1988) Immunohistochemical localisation of nerve growth factor-like protein in the organ of Corti of the developing rat. Neurosci. Lett. *85*:5–8.

Eggermont, J. J., and G. R. Bock (1985) Normal and abnormal development of hearing and its clinical applications. Acta Otolaryngol. (Suppl.) *421*:1–128.

Eyerly, M. R., J. R. Coleman, M. C. Zrull, and A. J. McDonald (1989) Glutamate and aspartate: Localization and colocalization in the rat inferior colliculus. Soc. Neurosci. Abstr. *15*:747.

Feng, J. Z., and J. F. Brugge (1983) Postnatal development of auditory callosal connections in the kitten. J. Comp. Neurol. *214*:416–426.

Glendenning, K. K., and B. N. Baker (1988) Neuroanatomical distribution of receptors for three potential inhibitory neurotransmitters in the brainstem auditory nuclei of the cat. J. Comp. Neurol. 275:288–308.

Gulley, R. L. (1978) Changes in the presynaptic membrane of the synapses of the anteroventral cochlear nucleus with different levels of acoustic stimulation. Brain Res. *146*:373–379.

Gulley, R. L., R. J. Wenthold, and G. R. Nieses (1978) Changes in the synapses of spiral ganglion cells in the rostral anteroventral cochlear nucleus of the waltzing guinea pig following hair cell loss. Brain Res. *158*:279–294.

Harris, D. M., and P. Dallos (1984) Ontogenic changes in frequency mapping of a mammalian ear. Science 225:741–743.

Harrison, J. M., and M. L. Feldman (1970) Anatomical aspects of cochlear nucleus and superior olivary complex. In W. D. Neff (ed.): Contributions to Sensory Physiology, Vol. 4. New York: Academic Press, pp. 95–142.

Harrison, J. M., and M. E. Howe (1974) Anatomy of the afferent auditory nervous system of mammals. In W. D. Keidel and W. D. Neff (eds.): Handbook of Sensory Physiogy, Vol. V, Pt. 1, Auditory System Anatomy Physiology (Ear). Berlin: Springer-Verlag, pp. 283–336.

Hashisaki, G. T., and E. W. Rubel (1989) Effects of unilateral cochlea removal on anteroventral cochlear nucleus neurons in developing gerbils. J. Comp. Neurol. 283:465–473.

Helmholtz, H. L. F. (1863) Die Lehre von den Tenepfindungen als Physiologische Grundlage Furdie Theorie der Musik. New York: Dover Reprint, 1954.

Hicks, S. P., and C. J. D'Amato (1968) Cell migrations to the isocortex in the rat. Anat. Rec. 160:619–634.

Hirokawa, N. (1977) Disappearance of afferent and efferent nerve terminals in the inner ear of the chick embryo after chronic treatment with B-bungarotoxin. J. Cell Biol. 73:27–46.

Hoyte, D. A. N. (1961) The postnatal growth of the ear capsule in the rabbit. Amer. J. Anat. 108:1–16.

Huangfu, M., and J. C. Saunders (1983) Auditory development in the mouse: Structural maturation of the middle ear. J. Morphol. 176:249–259.

Hyson, R. L., and J. W. Rudy (1983) Ontogenesis of learning: II. Variation in the rat's reflexive and learned responses to acoustic stimulation. Dev. Psychobiol. 17:263–283.

Imig, T. J., and R. A. Reale (1980) Patterns of cortico-cortical connections related to tonotopic maps in cat auditory cortex. J. Comp. Neurol. 192:293–332.

Jackson, H., and T. N. Parks (1982) Functional synapse elimination in the developing avian cochlear nucleus with simultaneous reduction in cochlear nerve axon branching. J. Neurosci. 2:1736–1743.

Jhaveri, S., and D. K. Morest (1982a) Sequential alterations of neuronal architecture in nucleus magnocellularis of the developing chicken: A Golgi study. Neuroscience 7:837–853.

Jhaveri, S., and D. K. Morest (1982b) Sequential alterations of neuronal architecture in nucleus magnocellularis of the developing chicken: An electron microscopic study. Neuroscience 7:855–870.

Kane, E. S., and C. P. Habib (1978) Development of the dorsal cochlear nucleus of the cat: An electron microscopic study. Amer. J. Anat. 153:321–344.

Kikuchi, K., and D. Hilding (1965) The development of the organ of Corti in the mouse. Acta Otolaryngol. 60:207–222.

Kil, J., F. A. Russell, and L. M. Kitzes (1989) Experimentally induced projections from the ventral cochlear nucleus occur before the onset of hearing. Soc. Neurosci. Abstr. 15:745.

Konigsmark, B. W., and E. A. Murphy (1972) Volume of the ventral cochlear nucleus in man: Its relationship to neuronal population and age. J. Neuropathol. Exp. Neurol. 31:304–316.

Krause, H-J., and K. Aulbach-Kraus (1981) Morphological changes in the cochlea of the mouse after the onset of hearing. Hear. Res. *4*:89–102.

Krmpotic-Nemanic, J., I. Kostovic, Z. Kelovic, D. Nemanic, and L. Mrzljak (1983) Development of the human fetal auditory cortex: Growth of afferent fibres. Acta Anat. *116*:69–73.

Larsen, S. A. (1985) Postnatal maturation of the cat cochlear nucleus complex. Acta Otolaryngol. (Suppl.) *417*:1–43.

Lavigne-Rebillard, M., and R. Pujol (1986) Development of the auditory hair cell surface in human fetuses: A scanning electron microscopy study. Anat. Embryol. *174*:369–377.

Lenoir, M., A. Shnerson, and R. Pujol (1980) Cochlear receptor development in the rat with emphasis on synaptogenesis. Anat. Embryol. *160*:253–262.

Li, C. W., T. R. Van De Water, and R. J. Ruben (1978) The fate of mapping of the eleventh and twelfth day mouse otocyst: An "in vitro" study of the sites of origin of the embryonic inner ear sensory structures. J. Morphol. *157*:249–268.

Lim, D. J. (1987) Development of the tectorial membrane. Hear. Res. *28*:9–21.

Lim, D. J., and M. Anniko (1985) Developmental morphology of the mouse inner ear: A scanning electron microscopic observation. Acta Otolaryngol. (Suppl.) *422*:1–69.

Manley, G. A., J. Brix, and A. Kaiser (1987) Developmental stability of the tonotopic organization of the chick's basilar papilla. Science *237*:655–656.

Martin, M. R., and C. Rickets (1981) Histogenesis of the cochlear nucleus of the mouse. J. Comp. Neurol. *197*:169–184.

Mattox, D. E., G. R. Neises, and R. L. Gulley (1982) Species differences in the synaptic membranes of the end bulb of Held revealed with the freeze-fracture technique. Anat. Rec. *204*:271–279.

Maxwell, B. W., W. J. Clerici, J. Brady, A. J. McDonald, and J. R. Coleman (1988) Sources of connections to the inferior colliculus in the immature rat. Anat. Rec. *220*:62A.

McMullen, N. T., and E. M. Glaser (1988) Auditory cortical responses to neonatal deafening: Pyramidal neuron spine loss without changes in growth or orientation. Exp. Brain Res. *72*:195–200.

Meininger, V., and M. Baudrimont (1981) Postnatal modifications of the dendritic tree of cells of the inferior colliculus of the cat. A quantitative Golgi analysis. J. Comp. Neurol. *200*:339–355.

Moore, D. R., and L. M. Kitzes (1985) Projections from the cochlear nucleus to the inferior colliculus in normal and neonatally cochlea-ablated gerbils. J. Comp. Neurol. *240*:180–195.

Moore, D. R., and N. E. Kowalchuk (1988) Auditory brainstem of the ferret: Effects of unilateral cochlear lesions on cochlear nucleus volume and projections to the inferior colliculus. J. Comp. Neurol. *272*:503–515.

Morest, D. K. (1969) The growth of dendrites in the mammalian brain. Z. Anat. Entwickl.-Gesch. *128*:290–316.

Morest, D. K., and J. A. Winer (1986) The comparative anatomy of neurons: Homologous neurons in the medial geniculate body of the opossum and cat. Adv. Anat. Embryol. Cell Biol. *97*:1–96.

Neises, G. R., D. E. Mattox, and R. L. Gulley (1982) The maturation of the end bulb of Held in the rat anteroventral cochlear nucleus. Anat. Rec. 204:271–279.

Oliver, D. L., and D. K. Morest (1984) The central nucleus of the inferior colliculus in the cat. J. Comp. Neurol. 222:237–264.

Parks, T. N., and H. Jackson (1984) A developmental gradient of dendritic loss in the avian cochlear nucleus occurring independently of primary afferents. J. Comp. Neurol. 277:459–466.

Parks, T. N., S. S. Gill, and H. Jackson (1987) Experience-independent development of dendritic organization in the avian nucleus laminaris. J. Comp. Neurol. 260:312–319.

Pujol, R. (1985) Morphology, synaptology and electrophysiology of the developing cochlea. Acta Otolaryngol. (Suppl.) 421:5–9.

Pujol, R., and M. Abonnenc (1977) Receptor maturation and synaptogenesis in the golden hamster cochlea. Arch. Oto-Rhino-Laryngol. 217:1–12.

Pujol, R., and E. Carlier (1982) Cochlear synaptogenesis after sectioning the efferent bundle. Dev. Brain Res. 3:151–154.

Pujol, R., and M Lavigne-Rebillard (1985) Early stages of innervation and sensory cell differentiation in the human fetal organ. Acta Otolaryngol. (Suppl.) 423:43–50.

Pysh, J. J. (1969) The development of the extracellular space in neonatal rat inferior colliculus: An electron microscopy study. Amer. J. Anat. 124:411–430.

Ramon y Cajal, S. (1909). Histologie du Systeme Nerveux de l'Homme et des Vertebres. Madrid: Instit. Ramon y Cajal.

Reale, R. A., J. F. Brugge, and J. C. K. Chan (1987) Maps of auditory cortex in cats reared after unilateral cochlear ablation in the neonatal period. Dev. Brain Res. 34:281–290.

Relkin, E. M., J. C. Saunders, and D. F. Konkle (1979) Development of middle ear admittance in the hamster. J. Acoust. Soc. Amer. 136:133–139.

Rogowski, B. A., and A. S. Feng (1981) Normal postnatal development of medial superior olivary neurons in the albino rat: A Golgi and Nissl study. J. Comp. Neurol. 196:85–97.

Romand, R. (1983) Development of Auditory and Vestibular Systems. New York: Academic Press.

Romand, R., and M-R. Romand (1985) Qualitative and quantitative observations of spiral ganglion development in the rat. Hear. Res. 18:11–20.

Romand, R., A. Sans, M-R. Romand, and R. Marty (1976) The structural maturation of the stato-acoustic nerve in the cat. J. Comp. Neurol. 170:1–16.

Romand, R., M-R. Romand, Ch. Mulle, and R. Marty (1980) Early stages of myelination in the spiral ganglion cells of the kitten during development. Acta Otolaryngol. 90:391–397.

Rose, J. E. (1942) The ontogenetic development of the rabbit's diencephalon. J. Comp. Neurol. 77:61–130.

Rubel, E. W. (1978) Ontogeny of structure and function in the vertebrate auditory system. In M. Jacobson (ed.): Handbook of Sensory Physiology, Vol. IX, Development of Sensory Systems. New York: Springer-Verlag.

Rubel, E. W., D. J. Smith, and L. C. Miller (1976) Organization and development of brain stem auditory nuclei of the chicken: Ontogeny of *N. magnocellularis* and *N. laminaris*. J. Comp. Neurol. *166*:469–490.

Rubel, E. W., W. R. Lippe, and B. M. Ryals (1984) Development of the place principle. Ann. Otol. Rhinol. Laryngol. *93*:609–615.

Ruben, R. J. (1967) Development of the inner ear of the mouse: A radiographic study of terminal mitosis. Acta Oto-Laryngol. (Suppl.) *220*:1–44.

Ryan, A. F., and N. K. Woolf (1988) Development of tonotopic representation in the Mongolian gerbil: A 2-deoxyglucose study. Dev. Brain Brain Res. *41*:61–70.

Ryan, A. F., N. K. Woolf, and F. R. Sharp (1982) Functional ontogeny in the central auditory pathway of the mongolian gerbil: A deoxyglucose study. Exp. Brain Res. *47*:428–436.

Ryugo, D. K., and D. M. Fekete (1982) Morphology of primary axosomatic endings in the anteroventral cochlear nucleus of the cat: A study of the endbulbs of Held. J. Comp. Neurol. *210*:239–257.

Sanes, D. H., M. Merickel, and E. W. Rubel (1989) Evidence for an alteration of the tonotopic map in the gerbil cochlea during development. J. Comp. Neurol. *279*:436–444.

Saunders, J. C., J. A. Kaltenbach, and E. M. Relkin (1983) The structural and functional development of the outer and middle ear. In R. Romand (ed.): Development of Auditory and Vestibular Systems. New York: Academic Press.

Schwartz, A. M., M. Parakkal, and R. L. Gulley (1983) Postnatal development of spiral ganglion cells in the rat. Amer. J. Anat. *167*:33–41.

Schweitzer, L., and N. B. Cant (1984) Development of the cochlear innervation of the dorsal cochlear nucleus of the hamster. J. Comp. Neurol. *225*:228–243.

Schweitzer, L., and N. B. Cant (1985) Differentiation of the giant and fusiform cells in the dorsal cochlear nucleus of the hamster. Dev. Brain Res. *20*:69–82.

Shah, S. N., V. K. Bhargava, and C. M. McKean (1978) Maturational changes in early auditory evoked potentials and myelination of the inferior colliculus in rats. Neuroscience *3*:561–563.

Sher, A. (1971) Embryonic and postnatal development of the inner ear of the mouse. Acta Otolaryngol. (Suppl.) *285*:1–77.

Silverman, M. S., and B. M. Clopton (1977) Plasticity of binaural interaction. I. Effect of early auditory deprivation. J. Neurophysiol. *40*:1266–1274.

Sobin, A., and M. Anniko (1984) Early development of cochlear hair cell stereociliary surface morphology. Arch. Oto-Rhino-Laryngol. *241*:53–64.

Sobkowicz, H. M., J. E. Rose, G. E. Scott, and S. M. Slapnick (1983) Ribbon synapses in the developing intact and cultured organ of Corti in the mouse. J. Neurosci. *2*:942–957.

Taber-Pierce, E. (1967) Histogenesis of the dorsal and ventral cochlear nuclei of the mouse. An autoradiographic study. J. Comp. Neurol. *131*:27–54.

Trune, D. R. (1982) Influence of neonatal cochlear removal on the development of mouse cochlear nucleus. I. Number, size and density of its neurons. J. Comp. Neurol. *209*: 409–424.

Trune, D. R. (1983) Influence of neonatal cochlear removal on the development of mouse cochlear nucleus. III. Its efferent projections to inferior colliculus. Dev. Brain Res. 9:1–12.

Van De Water, T. R. (1976) Effects of removal of the statoacoustic ganglion complex upon the growing otocyst. Ann. Otol. Rhinol. Laryngol. (Suppl.) 85:1–32.

Van De Water, T. R. (1986) Determinants of neuron-sensory receptor cell interaction during development of the inner ear. Hear. Res. 22:265–277.

Van De Water, T. R., and R. J. Ruben (1976) Organogenesis of the ear. In R. Hinchcliffe and D. Harrison (eds.): Scientific Foundations of Otolaryngology. London: William Heinemann Medical Books, pp. 173–184.

Van De Water, T. R., and R. J. Ruben (1983) A possible embryonic mechanism for the establishment of innervation of inner ear sensory structures. Acta Oto-Laryngol. 95:470–479.

Van De Water, T. R., and R. J. Ruben (1984) Neurotrophic interactions during in vitro development of the inner ear. Ann. Otol. Rhinol. Laryngol. 93:558–564.

Van De Water, T. R., P. F. A. Maderson, and T. K. Jaskoll (1980) The morphogenesis of the middle and external ear. In R. J. Gorlin (ed.): Morphogenesis and Malformation of the Ear. Birth Defects: Original Article Series, Vol. XVI, pp. 147–180.

Wada, T. (1923) Anatomical and physiological studies on the growth of the inner ear of the albino rat. Mem. Wistar Inst. Anat. Biol. 10:1–174.

Webster, D. B., and M. Webster (1979) Effects of neonatal conduction hearing loss on brain stem auditory nuclei. Ann. Otol. Rhinol. Laryngol. 88:684–688.

Webster, D., and M. Webster (1980) Mouse brainstem auditory nuclei development. Ann. Otol. Rhinol. Laryngol. (Suppl.) 89:254–256.

Whitehead, M. C., and D. K. Morest (1985a) The development of innervation patterns in the avian cochlea. Neuroscience 14:255–276.

Whitehead, M. C., and D. K. Morest (1985b) The growth of cochlear fibers and the formation of their synaptic endings in the avian inner ear: A study with the electron microscope. Neuroscience 14:277–300.

Whitlon, D. S., and H. M. Sobkowicz (1988) Neuron-specific enolase during the development of the organ of Corti. Int. J. Dev. Neurosci. 6:77–87.

Willard, F. H., and G. F. Martin (1986) The development and migration of large multipolar neurons into the cochlear nucleus of the North American opossum. J. Comp. Neurol. 248:119–132.

Willard, F. H., and D. K. Ryugo (1983) Anatomy of the central auditory system. In J. F. Willott (ed.) The Auditory Psychobiology of the Mouse. Springfield, Il: Thomas.

Yost, William A., and D. W. Nielsen (1977) Fundamentals of Hearing: An Introduction. New York: Holt, Rinehart and Winston.

Zhou, X-N., and T. R. Van De Water (1987) The effect of target tissues on survival and differentiation of mammalian statoacoustic ganglion neurons in organ culture. Acta Otolaryngol. 104:90–98.

Chapter Six

DEVELOPMENT OF AUDITORY SYSTEM PHYSIOLOGY

LEONARD M. KITZES

Department of Anatomy and Neurobiology
University of California, Irvine, California

I INTRODUCTION

Activation of the central auditory system must await the functional development of outer, middle, and inner ear structures. Since several structures mature concurrently, it is impossible to identify the maturation of any particular one as being the critical event that allows the central auditory system to begin functioning. The purpose of this chapter is to discuss these structural and functional variables and their interactions, which determine the ontogeny of auditory system physiology.

Understanding the developing auditory system is limited by our understanding of the mature auditory system. For example, the functional significance of certain aspects of its structural organization are not well understood. Brugge and O'Conner (1984) have demonstrated that several response properties of the dorsal and posteroventral portions of the cochlear nuclear complex appear to be mature prior to the time when certain synaptic arrangements in these structures attain their adult configuration. Clearly, analysis of the functional development of these synaptic arrangements cannot proceed until their functional significance in the adult has been fully characterized.

Both excitatory and inhibitory systems develop within the central auditory system seemingly without the need of acoustically driven cochlear function. The lack of spontaneous activity in the auditory nerve until the time when the cochlea is able to transduce sounds suggests that afferent neuronal activity from the periphery might actually play a very minor role in determining the primary function and connectivity of the auditory neuroaxis. Nevertheless, as discussed by Clopton and Snead (Chapter 8), experimental manipulations in the neonate, such as occlusion of one acoustic meatus or destruction of one cochlea, will lead to rather dramatic distortions of both the physiology and anatomy of the auditory system. The form of the growing auditory system, therefore, is susceptible to modification, depending largely upon the local structural and functional environment of the constituent neurons.

A complete description of the physiology and anatomy of the mature auditory system is beyond the scope of this chapter. While explanations of the pertinent response functions will be presented, the reader is advised to consult the referenced articles and books for a more detailed presentation of the adult physiology. Similarly, knowledge of the anatomy of the peripheral structures and central auditory system will be beneficial, as will a firm understanding of the development of these systems as described by Coleman in Chapter 5.

II   INFORMATION PROCESSING BY THE NEONATAL AUDITORY SYSTEM

Studying *how* the auditory system functions is greatly facilitated by understanding *what* the auditory system does, what it accomplishes as the animal interacts with its acoustic environment. What it accomplishes, manifested in the behavior of the animal, provides the fundamental questions of auditory neurobiology. For example, a click sound presented directly in front of an animal arrives at the two ears at the same time. A trained human observer can distinguish such a click from a second one delivered from a source displaced slightly laterally such that the sound arrives at the proximal ear some microseconds earlier than at the distal ear. This behavior raises the question of how the auditory system is able to deal with acoustic cues in the range of microseconds, considering the fact that the central nervous system operates in the range of milliseconds. In this chapter we shall attempt to summarize what is known about how such precision develops.

The approach often used to study the physiological development of the auditory system is to track the maturation of a particular response function to the adult level. The value of this approach depends in large part upon the state of knowledge of the physiology of the mature auditory system, for it assumes that the response function being measured indicates how the auditory system actually does process acoustic stimuli. However, the task of relating electrophysiologically defined auditory system function to perceptual and behavioral measures of auditory system function is enormous and, to a very great extent, remains to be accomplished. The task of understanding the significance of immature response functions is made more difficult by insufficient information regarding the perceptual and behavioral capabilities of the immature animal.

The postnatal development of behavioral thresholds in cat, an animal used frequently in the study of the adult and developing auditory system is illustrated in Figure 1 (Ehret and Romand, 1981). During the first week of postnatal life, behavioral thresholds exceed 100 dB and there is no indication of a preferential sensitivity to any of the stimulus frequencies to which the animal responds. Three changes in the behavioral audiogram are apparent subsequent to the first week. First, there is an overall diminution of thresholds, particularly between days 6 and 10 and, second, a preferential decrease around 4 kHz. The human is most sensitive to frequencies around 3 kHz while cat is most sensitive to frequencies around 8–12 kHz. Third, these behavioral functions demonstrate that the range of frequencies to which the kitten is responsive broadens during development. The effective frequency range widened from 0.5–3.0 kHz on days 2 and 4 to 0.2–6.0 kHz on the sixth postnatal day, the first day during which all the tested kittens responded to tonal stimuli. The upper limit of the effective stimulus frequency continued to increase over the first month of postnatal life, extending to 15 kHz at day 12, 25 kHz at day 15, 40 kHz at day 22, and 50 kHz at day 30. These observations are consistent with those made in rather diverse species, including man, dog, mink, rabbit, rat, mouse, bat, and chicken (Rubel, 1978; Rubel et al., 1984), that sensitivity is initially restricted to lower stimulus frequencies and subsequently spreads to higher frequencies as the animal matures.

The time course of the development of responsiveness to acoustic stimuli varies across species. Guinea pigs, for example, not only respond to the occurrence of acoustic stimuli during the first 4 days of postnatal life; they also are capable of making directional movements toward the source of a sound during this time period (Clements and Kelly, 1978). The ability to localize the source of a sound in space requires the integration, at least at the

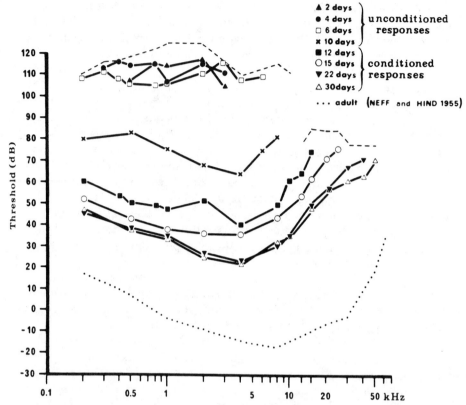

FIGURE 1. Postnatal development of absolute auditory thresholds in the kitten. Thresholds were obtained by unconditioned responses for kittens 2–10 days old and by conditioned responses at the older ages. The lower dotted line shows the absolute auditory thresholds of the adult cat. The upper dashed lines indicate the maximum sound pressure level produced by the equipment without distortion. (From Ehret and Romand, 1981.)

level of the superior olivary complex, of acoustic information impinging upon the two ears. The utilization of binaural information by guinea pigs 4 days of age or younger was demonstrated by changing artificially the relative strength of the stimulus at the two ears. Beginning 4–18 h after birth, one or both ears were blocked with wax, and the accuracy of approach responses to a sound source located at random positions within a circular field was determined. Blocking of one ear reduced the probability of correct approach responses to chance. However, the approach responses of animals with both ears blocked, which reduces the overall stimulus level but leaves the relative intensity of the stimulus to the two ears unchanged, were indistinguishable from those of control animals with no ear plugs. Using very similar procedures, Kelly and Potash (1986) demonstrated that gerbil pups 16–19 days of age made appropriate approach responses significantly above chance levels, whereas the responses of pups 12–15 days of age were essentially at chance levels. The utilization of binaural information by gerbil pups 16–23 days of age was demonstrated using the monaural and binaural ear plug procedure. Again, animals with both ears blocked approached the sound source with the same precision as did the unblocked control animals, whereas animals with one ear blocked performed at chance levels. The difference between the monaurally blocked animals on the one hand and the binaurally blocked and unblocked control animals on the other hand could arise only if the behavior depended upon the integration of binaural information by these very young animals.

These studies demonstrate that the anatomical and physiological systems that enable an animal to localize a sound source in space are operative at the same time or very shortly after the time when the animal first becomes responsive to acoustic stimuli. Very high levels of acoustic stimulation are required to evoke behavioral and, as will be discussed later, physiological responses in very young animals, particularly in very young gerbils. Since such intense stimuli occur only very rarely in the environment, these data indicate that the structural and functional systems that integrate acoustic information impinging upon the two ears normally develop independent of environmental stimulation.

III   THE AUDITORY PERIPHERY

The ontogeny of auditory system physiology depends largely upon the development of the cochlea. An appreciation of the structure and function of the cochlea is valuable, therefore, in order to understand some of the primary determinants of auditory system physiology in the developing animal. A cross section of the mammalian cochlea is depicted in Figure 2 of Chapter 5 in this volume. Scala vestibuli terminates at the oval window and communicates through the helicotrema at the apex of the cochlea with scala tympani. Scala tympani terminates at the round window. Waves of air pressure, such as are produced by sound, are funneled through the external ear to the tympanic membrane and are then transmitted by the bones of the middle ear, the ossicular chain, to the oval window. Movement of the oval window establishes a pressure gradient across scala media, causing the basilar membrane to be displaced into or out of scala media. Since the basilar and tectorial membranes are hinged at different points, this movement results in a sheering motion of one structure relative to the other. This relative movement of the basilar and tectorial membranes causes the stereocilia of the hair cells, which are embedded in the tectorial membrane, to deflect radially toward the internal limbus or toward the cells of Hensen, depending upon the direction of basilar membrane movement. The deflection of the stereocilia toward the cells of Hensen results in the release of a

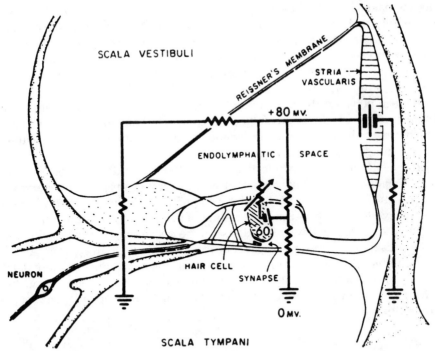

FIGURE 2. Electrophysiological model for excitation in the organ of Corti. The +80-mV endocochlear potential and −60-mV intracellular potential of the hair cell act in series to polarize strongly the stereocilia-bearing surface of the hair cell membrane. Deflection of the stereocilia modulates the resistance of this surface and, thereby, the current flowing through the hair cell. (From Davis, 1968.)

currently unknown transmitter that excites the afferent terminals of auditory nerve fibers located at the base of the hair cells.

Figure 2 depicts an electrophysiological model of the cochlea proposed originally by Davis (1959). The model emphasizes the large potential difference that exists across the hair cell membrane, the sum of the positive endocochlear potential (EP) and the negative intracellular resting membrane potential. Davis hypothesized that the electrical resistance of the hair cell membrane, and therefore the amount of current allowed to flow through the hair cell, is modulated by the position of the stereocilia. This modulatory control exerted by the stereocilia has been confirmed by intracellular recordings of hair cell preparations: deflection of the stereocilia in the excitatory direction results in the reduction of the membrane resistance and the depolarization of the hair cell (see Pickles, 1985, for a review). The depolarization of the hair cell is presumably involved in the release of transmitter at the base of the hair cell and the consequent excitation of the afferent terminals of the auditory nerve.

The ontogeny of the passive electrical properties of the hair cell membrane, which to a very great extent determine the operation of the hair cell, is presently unknown. Similarly, the development of the molecular configuration of the stereocilia, for example, the formation of actin and appropriate ion channels, that is crucial for the modulation of membrane resistance is presently unknown. Whereas the contribution of these and other micromechanical variables to the ontogeny of cochlear function have not yet been investigated, much information has been adduced from the study of the developing cochlea and from the study of cochlear function as reflected in its output, that is, the activity of individual auditory nerve fibers.

The amplitude of the EP is assessed by measuring the direct current (DC) potential recorded by a microelectrode as it is moved through scala tympani into scala media. In each of the several species in which it has been measured, the EP is minimal at birth and increases to adult levels within a few weeks of age. Data obtained in cat are illustrated in Figure 3 (Fernandez and Hinojosa, 1974). The mean value of the EP was 8.8 mV during the first postnatal day and increased in a regular fashion to 75.7 mV at postnatal day

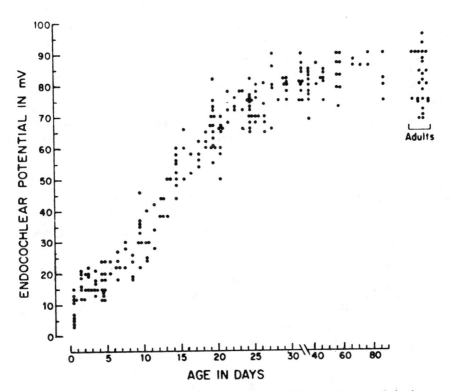

FIGURE 3. Development of endocochlear potential in cat. Note that the recorded values are well within the adult range by the beginning of the fourth week. (From Fernandez and Hinojosa, 1974.)

27. The mean value of the EP in the adult cat was 80.4 mV. The growth of the EP was shown by these authors to correlate very well with the anatomical development of the stria vascularis, which is known to be the source of the EP. This structure reaches its mature form by approximately postnatal day 25. Development of the EP varies across species. In the rat, for example, the increase in EP amplitude does not begin until 1 week after birth but attains its asymptotic value when the animal is approximately only 16 days of age (Bosher and Warren, 1971).

Development of the EP parallels the ontogenetic functions of several parameters of auditory nerve activity, including the reduction in response threshold, increase in number of evoked discharges, and increase in spontaneous discharge rate. The spontaneous discharge rate of auditory nerve fibers in cat, for example, increases from essentially zero at postnatal day 6 to adult levels by day 20 (Walsh and McGee, 1987). Such correlations suggest the hypothesis that the rate at which EP develops determines the functional development of cochlear output. Indeed, Sewell (1984a) described experimental data that support this hypothesis. Intravenous injections of furosemide reduced synchronously the EP and spontaneous discharge rates of auditory nerve fibers in adult cats. However, other factors have been shown to influence the same response parameters. For example, Liberman and his colleagues (Liberman and Dodds, 1984; Liberman and Kiang, 1984) have demonstrated severely reduced spontaneous discharge rates and increased response thresholds of auditory nerve fibers that innervate hair cells located at a focus of cochlear damage. The structural correlate of the altered activity was a selective loss of the tallest row of stereocilia on the inner hair cells. These kinds of data emphasize the fact that the proper functioning of the cochlea depends upon the appropriate action of and interaction between multiple delicate systems.

IV   THE REPRESENTATION OF STIMULUS FREQUENCY

Scala media and the sensory epithelium of the organ of Corti extend from the base to the apex of the cochlea. Rather than maturing at the same time throughout its longitudinal extent, development of the organ of Corti progresses from the base to the apex (see Chapter 5). The basilar membrane is said to be "tuned" in that low stimulus frequencies will cause maximal oscillations near the apex of the cochlea and progressively higher stimulus frequencies will cause maximal oscillations at progressively more basal loci of the cochlea. It thus acts as sort of a mechanical Fourier analyzer, providing a spatial representation along the organ of Corti of the spectral components of a complex sound.

Recent evidence indicates that the resonant properties of the basilar membrane, which provide this spatial representation of stimulus frequency, change progressively as the structure and micromechanics of the organ of Corti mature. Rubel and Ryals (1983) took advantage of the fact that a prolonged, very intense, pure tone will severely damage or destroy the hair cells located at the locus on the basilar membrane that is tuned to the frequency of the tonal stimulus. They demonstrated in perinatal chickens that an intense tone caused localized damage to increasingly more apical regions of the sensory epithelium as a function of developmental age. That is, with increasing developmental age the damage produced by a given stimulus frequency occurred more distant from the cochlear base. The three frequencies used in this experiment, that is, 0.5, 1.5, and 3.0 kHz, essentially cover the spectrum of sound to which a chicken is sensitive. The slopes of the change in the location of damage as a function of developmental age were parallel for the three stimulus frequencies.

Dallos and his colleagues (Harris and Dallos, 1984; Yancey and Dallos, 1985) used the gerbil to examine the tonotopic organization of the developing mammalian cochlea. The cochlea in the gerbil is approximately full size at birth and easily accessible from the middle ear cavity. In this species the cochlea is cartilaginous at birth, and the first sound-evoked responses appear at postnatal day 12–13 (Finck et al., 1972; Woolf and Ryan, 1984; Harris and Dallos, 1984). The two studies by Dallos and his colleagues were specifically designed to exclude possible contamination by any change in the transmission of acoustic energy to the cochlea by external and middle ear structures that might occur during development, such as an initially reduced transmission of high frequencies (Relkin and Saunders, 1980). A response recorded at a specific location within the cochlea was compared with the same type of response recorded at the round window. Responses recorded at the round window reflect activity evoked by the highest frequencies to which the organ of Corti is sensitive. The amplitude of responses recorded at these two loci would be influenced similarly by the characteristics of the middle ear transfer function. Consequently, any differences between the two responses that occur as a function of developmental age would most likely be the result of developmental changes occurring within the cochlea.

In the first study, Harris and Dallos compared the cochlear microphonic measured at the round window with the cochlear microphonic measured by a microelectrode located in the scala tympani at a midbasal location of the cochlea. The data were the sound pressure levels necessary to evoke a criterion amplitude (1 μV) cochlear microphonic at the two locations in an age-graded series of gerbils. The sensitivity of the intracochlear response relative to that of the round window response for stimulus frequencies between 1 and 20 kHz is illustrated in Figure 4A. A negative value indicates that the intracochlear response was more sensitive, that is, required a lower sound pressure level, than the response measured at the round window. It is clear that the highest stimulus frequency at which the intracochlear response was more sensitive than the round window response increased progressively from 14 days of age to 19 days of age, at which time the

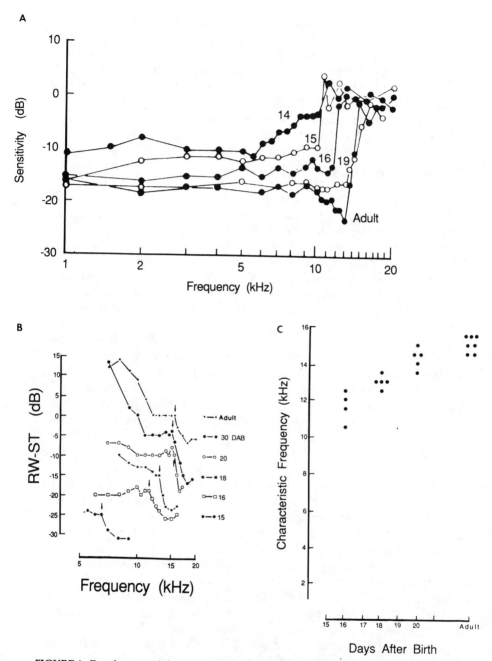

FIGURE 4. Developmental changes in the representation of stimulus frequency in the cochlea. (A) Difference in decibels between stimuli required to evoke 1-μV-amplitude cochlear microphonic repsonses within the first turn of the cochlea and the round window as a function of frequency and age (in days). Note that the highest frequency at which the intracochlear response is more sensitive than the round window response increases with developmental age. (B) Difference in decibels between stimuli required to evoke a 25-μV-amplitude summating potential within the first turn of the cochlea and the round window as a function of frequency and age. Curves are normalized to 0 dB at the sound level where they fall (at CF).

frequency response of that location of the cochlea was essentially equal to that seen in the adult. In animals 12 and 13 days of age, the upper frequency limit of the intracochlear response was approximately 5 kHz, but the upper "cutoff" frequency was impossible to determine.

Using the same electrode configuration and stimulating procedure in an age-graded series of gerbils, Yancey and Dallos (1985) compared the amplitude of the summating potential at a point within the cochlea and at the round window. The summating potential is a DC potential produced by nonlinearities of the basilar membrane response that is largest at the region of maximal stimulation of the hair cells, that is, at the region of maximal displacement of the basilar membrane. The stimulus frequency that requires the least intensity to evoke the criterion amplitude summating potential is thus taken to define the best, or "characteristic," frequency (CF) of that point on the basilar membrane. The data obtained at the round window were again subtracted from those obtained at the intracochlear electrode in order to remove the influence of the transfer function of the middle ear. The highest frequencies at which the summating potential recorded at the intracochlear electrode was more sensitive than the potential recorded at the round window is indicated by the arrows for an age-graded series of animals in Figure 4B. The increase in characteristic frequency for the midbasal portion of the cochlea as a function of developmental age for the sample of animals is shown in Figure 4C. Echteler, et al. (1989) demonstrated in a definitive study of an age graded series of gerbils that the CF of individual auditory nerve cells located at the same longitudinal position within the modiolus increases with developmental age. At postnatal day 14 the tips of individual tuning curves were centered between 5 and 7 kHz. The CFs of the tuning curves increased by one octave by postnatal day 15 and by an additional half octave to mature levels only two days later.

It is thus clear that the characteristic frequency of a point on the basilar membrane increases by more than one octave over the time period between the onset of cochlear function and the maturation of adult levels of performance. Since development progresses from the base toward the apex, we may summarize the development of the tonotopic organization of the organ of Corti by saying that the spatial representation of stimulus frequency expands progressively from the base to the apex and that a given locus will initially be more sensitive to lower frequencies than it will after the cochlea has reached the adult stage of development.

Lippe (Lippe and Rubel, 1985; Lippe, 1987) demonstrated that the spatial shift of best frequency in the developing cochlea is apparent in the physiol-

Each curve displaced by 5 dB for purposes of display. Arrows point to CF for each curve. (C) Scatter plot of CFs for all animals derived from summating potential data as shown in (B) showing increase of CF at intracochlear electrode as function of age. Age of the animals is indicated for each curve. (A) Reproduced from Harris and Dallos (1984). (B,C) From Yancey and Dallos (1985).

ogy of second- and third-order neural structures of the auditory system. He compared the spatial distribution of best frequencies in nucleus magnocellularis, homologous to the anteroventral cochlear nucleus, and nucleus laminaris, homologous to the medial superior olive, across an age-graded series of chickens. The data illustrated in Figure 5 demonstrate that the tonotopic organization of these two neural structures shifts progressively in accordance with the development of the chicken cochlea. More recently, Sanes et al. (1989) demonstrated a very similar phenomenon in the LSO of the gerbil. The CFs of neurons at a given locus within LSO increased significantly during development. Since this neural representation of cochlear function is transmitted throughout the auditory neuroaxis, it appears that each neural structure in the auditory system is most sensitive to progressively higher stimulus frequencies as the cochlea matures to its adult form. The predicted increase in the high-frequency limits of neuronal responses has been described in the central nucleus of the inferior colliculus (ICC) in cat (Pujol, 1972; Aitkin and Reynolds, 1975; Aitkin and Moore, 1975) and mouse (Shnerson and Willott, 1979) and in auditory cortex of cat (Pujol, 1972). The developmental progression from low to high frequencies has also been demonstrated using the auditory brainstem responses recorded in an age-graded series of rats (Blatchley et al., 1987).

The tuning of a neuron or the basilar membrane to a band of stimulus frequencies is typically demonstrated by assessing the level of tonal stimuli required to evoke either a threshold response or a criterion amplitude response. The set of derived stimulus level values constitutes the "tuning curve" for the structure being studied. Three tuning curves obtained by

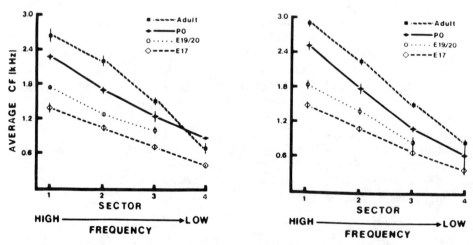

FIGURE 5. Change in represented stimulus frequency in nucleus magnocellularis (left) and nucleus laminaris (right) as a function of developmental age in chicken. The longitudinal extent of each nucleus was divided into equal-length sectors. Note that for both nuclei the average CF for each sector increases with developmental age. (After Lippe, 1987.)

Robles et al. (1986) in adult chinchilla are illustrated in Figure 6. The stimulus levels required to evoke a specified velocity (open circles) and amplitude (closed circles) of basilar membrane displacement and an average threshold response for auditory nerve fibers are shown. These functions demonstrate the typical form of tuning curves: a CF that requires the least intensity to evoke the criterion response, a high-frequency slope of several hundred decibels per octave, and a less steep low-frequency skirt. The consistency of the mechanical and neural tuning curves suggest that the form of the neural curve is determined completely by the mechanical properties of the basilar membrane. It is reasonable to assume, therefore, that the form of the neural

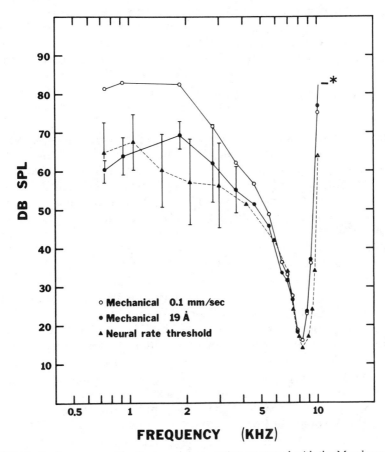

FIGURE 6. Tuning curves of basilar membrane motion measured with the Mossbauer technique and auditory nerve fibers. Function with open circles represents composite isovelocity (0.1 mm/s) curve from five cochleas. Function with closed circles represents composite isoamplitude values for 19 Å, the amplitude of vibration corresponding to 0.1 mm/s at a mean CF of 8.35 kHz. Mean auditory nerve tuning curves (triangles) for fibers with CF between 7 and 10 kHz. (From Robles et al., 1986.)

tuning curve is probably a good reflection of the form of the basilar membrane displacement.

The development of sensitivity to a restricted band of stimulus frequencies is indicated by the progressive change in the shape of tuning curves of auditory nerve fibers. Tuning curves of auditory nerve fibers obtained from an age-graded series of kittens are shown in Figure 7 (Romand, 1983). Examples of fibers with best frequencies around 700 Hz and around 7 kHz were selected to show the progressive changes in the typically more broadly tuned low-frequency sensitivity and the typically more acutely tuned higher frequency sensitivity. During the first postnatal week the frequency response of auditory nerve fibers in the cat is essentially flat, with little indication of a discernible CF or high- and low-frequency slopes. Frequency selectivity develops rapidly over the succeeding 3 weeks. There is a progressive decrease in threshold of about 80 dB or more for a restricted band of frequencies and the formation of asymmetrical slopes around the most effective frequency. While the age at which tone-evoked responses can first be recorded and the age at which they assume an adult profile varies across species, such changes in the shape of tuning curves as a function of developmental age have been found in every species in which they have been examined.

The data discussed in the preceding concerning the spatial representation of stimulus frequency on the basilar membrane as a function of developmental age (Rubel and Ryals, 1983; Harris and Dallos, 1984; Yancey and Dallos, 1985; Lippe and Rubel, 1985; Lippe, 1987; Sanes and Rubel, 1988; Echteler et al, 1989; Sanes et al, 1989) suggest that the CF of an auditory nerve fiber identified in a tuning curve obtained during an early period of cochlear development might be significantly lower than that defined for the same fiber after the sensory epithelium has fully matured. Indeed, the changing tonotopic organization of the second- and third-order auditory nuclei during development (Figure 4) seems to require that the CF of auditory nerve fibers must increase as the sensory epithelium matures. Thus, rather than indicating the maturation of frequency selectivity at a single longitudinal position along the organ of Corti, a collection of tuning curves focused on the same stimulus frequency, as in the bottom panel of Figure 7, might actually reflect the frequency response during development of progressively more apical positions along a longitudinal segment of the organ of Corti. After the sensory epithelium has matured, the maximal response to a given tone would arise at the apical limit of that initially responsive segment of the organ of Corti.

Thresholds of cat auditory nerve fiber responses to their CF stimuli as a function of CF and age are indicated in Figure 8 (Kettner et al., 1985). Minimum thresholds fall from values greater than 100 dB at birth to nearly adult levels by the end of the third week. The decrease in threshold that occurs during the first 2 weeks in cat is due largely to increasingly effective transmission of energy to the cochlea. The pinna is initially folded over the

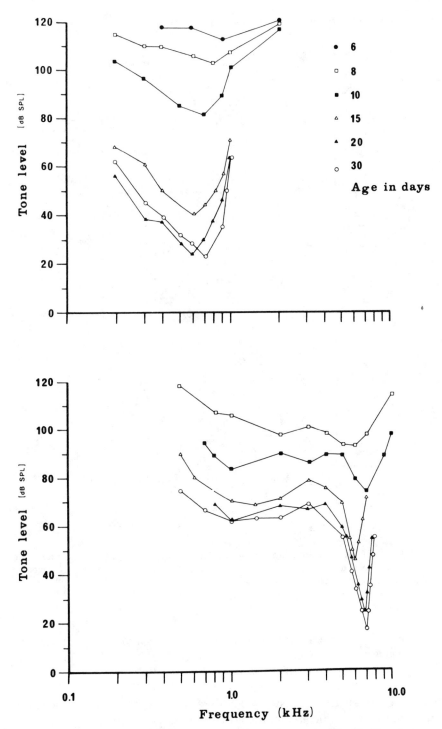

FIGURE 7. Comparison of shapes and values of cat auditory nerve threshold tuning curves centered at about 700 Hz (upper panel) and 7.0 kHz (lower panel) as a function of age. Note the overall diminution in threshold and the relatively greater diminution at CF. (From Romand, 1983.)

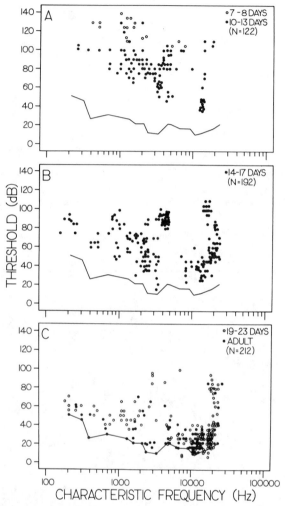

FIGURE 8. Thresholds at CFs as a function of CF for auditory nerve fibers in young kittens and adult cats. The solid line indicates the lowest thresholds obtained in adult cat. Number of threshold values in each panel denoted by N. Note the increasing high-frequency limit as a function of developmental age. (From Kettner et al., 1985.)

entrance to the external acoustic meatus and opens a few days after birth. The external acoustic meatus, in turn, is collapsed and effectively closed until postnatal day 9 or 10 (Aitkin and Moore, 1975; see also Coleman, Chapter 5). Furthermore, the middle ear cavity is initially filled with undifferentiated mesenchymal tissue that adheres to the ossicles and to the inner surface of the tympanic membrane. The mesenchyme is gradually resorbed over the first or second week postpartum. In the kitten the ossicles are not fully calcified at birth while in the gerbil both the ossicular chain and the cochlea itself are cartilaginous during at least the initial week of postnatal life. These differences between the kitten and gerbil are reflected in the observations that single unit responses can be recorded from auditory nerve fibers and cochlear nucleus cells of 4- and 5-day old kittens (Brugge et al., 1978, 1981; Brugge and O'Conner, 1984; Romand, 1984; Dolan et al., 1985), while the first signs of auditory nerve fiber responses in the gerbil occur at day 12 and do not become reliable until day 14 (Woolf and Ryan, 1985). These electrophysiological data are remarkably consistent with the results of the behavioral experiments of Ehret and Romand (1981) with cat and Kelly and Potash (1986) with gerbil described at the beginning of this chapter.

The diminution of response thresholds evident in Figures 7 and 8 is probably not due entirely to the removal of mechanical obstructions and improved transmission of energy by the middle ear to the cochlea. The tuning curves shown in Figure 7 demonstrate both the development of a CF and a reduced threshold for any stimulus to which the fiber is sensitive. The threshold reduction at CF is approximately 30–40 dB greater than the reduction at the extremes of the tuning curve. This suggests the development of micromechanical or physiological systems within the cochlea that provide nonlinear sensitivity to CF stimuli (Rhode, 1971). The existence of such special systems in the adult is supported by the observation that the threshold at the tip of a tuning curve, in contrast to its lower and higher frequency tails, is selectively increased as a result of damage to the cochlea. That is, damage to the cochlea as a result of excessive acoustic stimulation, a large opening of the osseous spiral lamina, or ototoxic drug administration will often result in elevated thresholds at the tip of a tuning curve with no apparent change in threshold at the tails of a tuning curve. This is true for measurements of the frequency sensitivity of the basilar membrane (e.g., Rhode, 1971, 1973; Robles et al., 1986) and auditory nerve fibers (e.g., Dallos and Harris, 1978; Schmiedt et al., 1980; Liberman and Kiang, 1984). Further discussion of the nature of these micromechanical or physiological systems that might develop or become functional during this time period is beyond the scope of this chapter. Suffice it to say that they might be involved in the contribution made by active mechanical processes to the acute resolution of stimulus frequency in the cochlea [see Pickles (1985) for an excellent review of this material].

The data in Figure 8 also indicate the common observation referred to earlier (Rubel, 1978; Rubel et al., 1984; Harris and Dallos, 1984; Yancey and Dallos, 1985) that sensitivity is initially restricted to lower stimulus frequencies and subsequently spreads to higher frequencies as the animal matures. Thus, at 7–8 days of age the highest CF encountered was approximately 8 kHz while the average CF was between 1 and 2 kHz. The adult frequency range obtained by Kettner et al. (1985) was not attained until the animals were 14–17 days of age, approximately 9–12 days after evoked single-unit activity could be recorded in the auditory nerve. Such physiological data appear paradoxical in light of the well-established anatomical observations that cochlear maturation begins at or very near the base, which in the adult is most sensitive to *high*-frequency stimuli, and proceeds toward the apex, which in the adult is most sensitive to *low*-frequency stimuli (Rubel, 1978). Fortunately, the apparent discrepancy between these anatomical and physiological data seems to be resolved by the studies discussed above on the progressive change in the spatial representation of stimulus frequency on the basilar membrane during development.

V   RESPONSIVENESS TO SUPRATHRESHOLD STIMULI

Responses of single neurons to suprathreshold stimuli undergo significant changes during development. One way of assessing such responses is to tally the number of discharges evoked by each of a set of stimulus frequencies delivered at intensities that increase from subthreshold values to levels that evoke maximal discharge rates. Six "response areas" of cells in the anteroventral cochlear nucleus (AVCN) obtained in this manner from kittens between 7 and 29 days of age are shown in Figure 9. Each response area demonstrates a CF and, aside from the extended response to very intense, higher frequency stimuli of the cell shown in Figure 9B (which is not seen in adult), a limited band of effective frequencies.

The response area obtained in a 7-day-old kitten shown in Figure 9A is typical for animals during the first postnatal week. Thresholds for CF stimuli almost invariably exceed 100 dB. Second, the dynamic range, that is, the intensity range over which discharge rate increases, is severely limited. For example, the discharge rate at CF for the unit shown in Figure 9A asymptotes at stimulus levels within 10–15 dB of threshold while the discharge rate of the unit from a 29-day-old animal shown in Figure 9E asymptotes at the stimulus level 25 dB above threshold. Brugge et al. (1981) assessed the dynamic range of responses to CF tones of cells in the AVCN by measuring the difference between the stimulus levels that evoked 10 and 90% of the maximal discharge rate. The median intensity increment required to produce the 80% increase in discharge rate was 13 dB during the first week and 17 dB during the second week. By the third week the median value, 32 dB, exceeded the lower limit of the dynamic ranges of auditory nerve fibers and AVCN cells studied in adult animals. Third, as is evident in the response areas shown in Figure 9, the maximal evoked discharge rate is severely limited during the first week of postnatal life in the cat. The maximal discharge rates at CF, converted to spikes per second in order to partial out differences among stimulus conditions, for response areas in Figures 9A–E are 28, 144, 250, 350, and 370, respectively. This progressive increase in maximal discharge rate is representative of populations of AVCN cells recorded over the first 3–4 weeks of postnatal life (Brugge et al., 1978). Adult levels are attained during the third or fourth week postpartum.

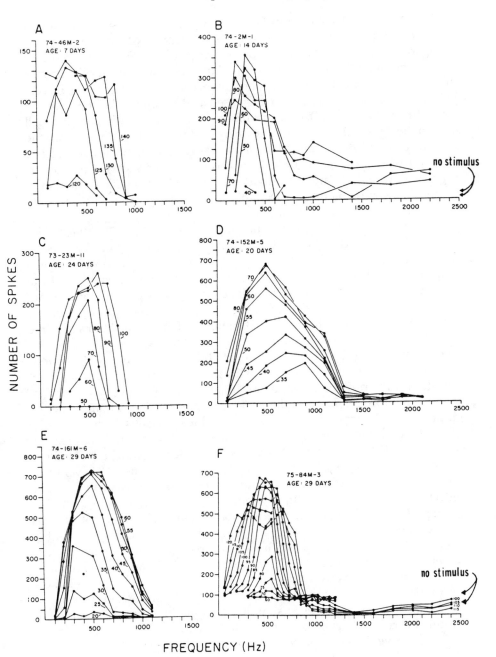

FREQUENCY (Hz)

FIGURE 9. Response areas of six neurons in AVCN from kittens of indicated ages. CFs are all below 1.0 kHz. Tone burst stimulation. (*A*) 100 ms, 50 trials; (*B*) 50 ms, 50 trials; (*C*) 100 ms, 10 trials; (*D,F*) 100 ms, 20 trials. Number beside each function indicates sound pressure level. (Modified from Brugge et al., 1978.)

The response area shown in Figure 9F is extremely systematic though somewhat atypical of response areas obtained from AVCN cells in the adult. Compared to the more usual response area shown in Figure 9E, this unit had a rather high threshold, and the discharge rate/stimulus level response functions were "nonmonotonic" for frequencies around CF. At the CF of 0.5 kHz, for example, discharge rate increased as the stimulus level was raised from threshold at 70 dB to a maximum at 100 or 105 dB and then fell systematically as stimulus level was increased further to 120 dB. Given the high discharge rate, extended dynamic range, and generally systematic behavior of this cell, it is difficult to know whether such nonmonotonic functions around CF are indicative of another characteristic of immature responsiveness or merely an example of a type of response area rarely observed in the AVCN of the adult.

Responses of auditory nerve fibers (Carlier et al., 1975; Walsh and McGee, 1986) and cells in the dorsal and posteroventral cochlear nucleus (Brugge and O'Connor, 1984) isolated in cats less than 10 days of age frequently display a rhythmicity that is unrelated to the frequency of the stimulus. In response to tonal stimuli several hundred milliseconds long, the discharge pattern consists of bursts of activity at 100–150-ms intervals that are time locked to the onset of the stimuli. That is, the bursts are time locked to the onset of the stimulus, but the intervals between the bursts, being of such long durations, are unrelated to the frequency of the sound. The intervals between the bursts diminish with increasing stimulus level but are always present, even at the highest stimulus levels. In contrast to this immature response to the prolonged portion of a stimulus, the beginning of such rhythmic responses of cochlear nucleus units often display rather adultlike patterns, such as the the so-called "chopper" pattern (Brugge and O'Conner, 1984). Since this rhythmicity occurs in the auditory nerve, it is likely that similar behavior is also present in the AVCN and that the rhythmicity observed throughout the cochlear nuclear complex is a reflection of the rhythmicity in its input.

Lippe (1986) has reported that the spontaneous discharges of nucleus magnocellularis and laminaris cells in day 14–18 embryonic chickens frequently occur in bursts. The rhythmic pattern of spontaneous activity was not observed in chickens older than embryonic day 19 and was eliminated in the younger chickens by destruction of the cochlea. It might be more appropriate, therefore, to view the rhythmicity in a prolonged response as the *entrainment* by an acoustic stimulus of some kind of periodic process within the cochlea. The mechanism that provides rhythmic bursting in auditory nerve fibers is presently unknown. It might be mechanical in origin, resulting from a structural immaturity within the organ of Corti, or neural in origin, resulting from immature interactions between the hair cell and its afferent processes, such as an underdeveloped pattern of transmitter release by the hair cells or some consequence of the late arrival of efferent synapses from the olivocochlear system. Whatever the mechanism turns out to be, since many fibers do not show such behavior, it is unlikely to result from a mechanism operating throughout the cochlea at any one time.

The response of auditory nerve fibers to tones below about 4 kHz is determined to a large extent by the periodic structure of the sound in that discharges tend to occur during a restricted portion of the stimulus waveform (e.g., Rose et al., 1967). Whereas the probability of a discharge during any given cycle of the stimulus is low, when a discharge does occur, it will tend to occur during a particular phase of the stimulus cycle. Consequently, the intervals between discharges tend to equal multiples of the stimulus period. Thus, it is very likely that the temporal cadence of the discharges comprising a response provides information about the frequency of stimuli below 4 kHz.

The best way to illustrate this ability of auditory nerve fibers to "phase lock" to the stimulus waveform is in a "period histogram," which represents the timing of the discharges relative to a single period of the stimulus, that is, as if the stimulus had consisted of a single cycle of the stimulus waveform. Period histograms of auditory nerve responses to a 0.5-, 1.0-, 2.0-, or 3.0-kHz stimulus obtained in an age-graded series of kittens and adult cats are shown in Figure 10. In each case stimulus level was sufficient to evoke a vigorous response. Vector strength (R), introduced by Goldberg and Brown (1969), is a measure of the degree of phase locking to a stimulus and varies between 0 and 1. Examination of the period histograms indicates that at each age, including the adults, the degree of phase locking diminishes as stimulus frequency is increased, and phase locking diminishes more quickly for younger animals. Viewed in another way, these histograms indicate that for each stimulus frequency the degree of phase locking increases with developmental age. By the end of the third week the degree of phase locking and the frequency range over which it occurs are indistinguishable from the values obtained in adult cats (Kettner et al, 1985).

The factors that limit phase locking in auditory nerve fibers of adult cat to about 4 kHz are not well understood, just as the factors that allow auditory nerve fibers in the barn owl to phase lock up to about 8 kHz are not well understood (Sullivan, 1985). The factors that limit the extent of phase locking in immature animals are, therefore, quite obscure. Nevertheless, three likely candidates can be identified. First, our discussion of the representation of stimulus frequency on the basilar membrane indicates that the micromechanics and, therefore, the resonance properties of the organ of Corti undergo progressive changes during development. It is reasonable to hypothesize, therefore, that the effective stimulus to the hair cells, that is, the deflection of the stereocilia, in the immature cochlea might be sufficient to evoke many discharges but not sufficiently synchronous with the waveform of the acoustic stimulus to produce a phase-locked response. This result could arise from perturbations in the pattern of stereocilia deflection or from the resonance properties of an immature basilar membrane that cause the deflection of the stereocilia. The shape of tuning curves obtained

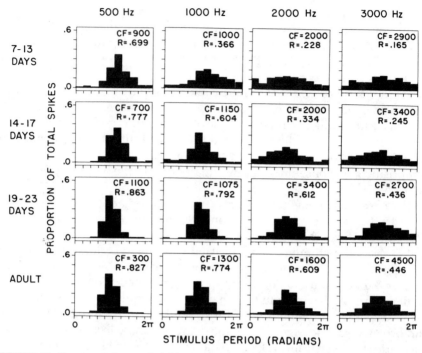

FIGURE 10. Representative period histograms for auditory nerve fibers from cats of the indicated ages stimulated at 0.5, 1.0, 2.0, and 3.0 kHz. The bin width for each histogram is 0.1 of the stimulus period. The CF of the fiber and the vector strength (*R*) of the response are illustrated above each histogram. Note the reduction of *R* with increasing stimulus frequency at each age and that adult levels of phase locking occur by the end of the third week. (From Kettner et al., 1985.)

in very young animals does suggest the resonance properties of the organ of Corti as the likely source of the poor phrase locking. Evaluation of these hypotheses must await measurements of the basilar membrane displacement pattern in an age-graded series of animals. Second, intracellular recordings from inner hair cells of guinea pig (Russell and Sellick, 1978) indicate that phase locking might be limited by the electrical time constant of the hair cell membrane. At low stimulus frequencies the release of transmitter by the hair cell is dominated by the AC component of the receptor potential, which is synchronous with the stimulus waveform. At high stimulus frequencies the AC component is reduced by the capacitance of the hair cell membrane and the release of transmitter is consequently dominated by a DC component, which, of course, does not reflect the periodicity in the stimulus waveform. The progressive increase in phase locking in young animals might thus reflect changes in the passive electrical properties of the hair cell membrane that occur during development. Third, temporal jitter in the excitation of the auditory nerve terminal or variability in the conduction velocity of the auditory nerve fiber would reduce the upper frequency limit of phase locking while leaving the synchrony of responses to low-frequency signals relatively unaffected. Examination of the period histograms in Figure 10 reveals that this is precisely the pattern that typifies phase locking in very immature kittens. Enhanced temporal jitter is more likely to be related to the immaturity of afferent and efferent synapses at the base of inner hair cells, as described in Chapter 5 by Coleman, than to the conduction of action potentials by an auditory nerve fiber. Myelination of these fibers in cat continues to increase for at least 6 months postpartum (Walsh et al., 1985; Walsh and McGee, 1986). While the number of myelin lamellae might determine conduction velocity and therefore influence the latency of a response, it is unclear how this parameter would determine the *variability* of conduction velocity and thereby influence response synchrony.

Information is conveyed from the auditory nerve to cells in AVCN through the endbulb of Held, a very large and secure terminal. The vector strength of responses recorded from an age-graded series of kittens is illustrated in Figure 11. Panel *A* illustrates these values for 59 auditory nerve fibers in adult monkey and panel *B* illustrates these values for 20 AVCN cells recorded in adult cat. Two of these cells exhibited phase locking to only about 1 kHz. Panels *C–F* indicate the progressive improvement of phase locking of kitten AVCN cells from the first to the seventh week of postnatal life. While some responses fall within the adult range of phase locking during the third week, the majority of responses fall below this range even at the end of the seventh week. The open circles in panel *F* indicate the vector strength of responses from 14 fibers studied in one 45-day-old kitten. Whereas some of them fall within the adult range, the great majority of responses recorded from this animal remain at low or intermediate levels of synchronization.

Phase locking is the last response property of these cells to achieve adult values. The observation that the synchronization of some of the responses of a 45-day-old cat persists at immature levels is perhaps surprising given the nature of the endbulb of Held and the fact that phase locking in the auditory nerve is mature by the end of the third week of postnatal life. However, the endbulb of Held and the principal cell of AVCN are still developing beyond postnatal day 45 in cat (Ryugo and Fekete, 1982). Furthermore, the late development of phase locking in AVCN of the cat might result from a neuron receiving supernumerary terminals from multiple auditory nerve fibers during development. Input from multiple terminals that is even slightly out of phase would, of course, diminish both the degree of phase locking and the upper frequency limit at which locking occurs. Jackson and Parks (1982) demonstrated that a single auditory nerve fiber contacts a larger number of nucleus magnocellularis cells in the very young chicken than it will in the adult. These data are illustrated in Figure 12. Intracellularly recorded postsynaptic responses reveal the influence of up to six terminals synapsing on a magnocellularis cell in an embryonic day 13

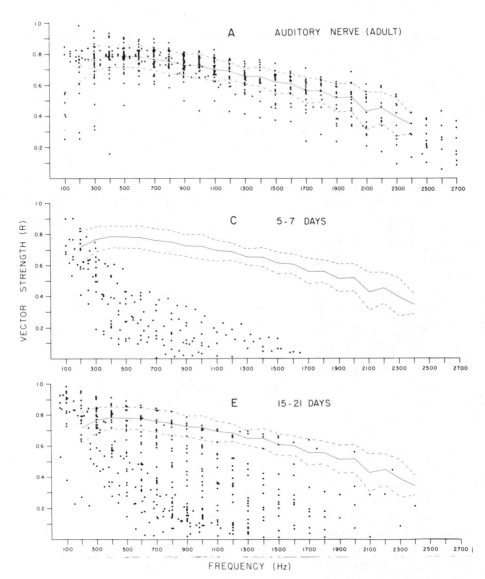

FIGURE 11. Scatter plots of vector strength as a function of frequency and age. (*A*) The *R* values for 59 auditory nerve fibers in adult squirrel monkey. Solid line connects mean *R* values; dashed lines are ±1 SD. These lines are repeated in each panel for comparative purposes. (*B*) The *R* values from 20 AVCN units in adult cat (unpublished observations of J.E. Rose, J. E. Hind, M. M. Gibson, and L. M. Kitzes). (*C-F*) The *R* values for 112 AVCN units isolated in cats of the indicated ages. The open circles in panel *F* derive from 14 units isolated in one 45-day-old cat; the filled circles derive from cats ranging from 22 to 30 days old. Note the progressive increase in R with age and that even at the end of the fourth week (*F*) these values typically remain below adult levels. (From Brugge et al., 1978.)

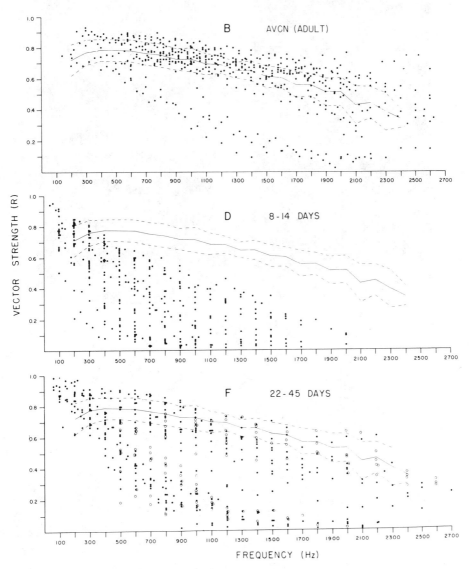

FIGURE 11. (*Continued*)

chicken (Figures 12 *A,B*). The mean number of terminals falls from 4.0 at embryonic day 13 to 2.2 terminals at embryonic days 17 and 18 and posthatching day 4 (Figures 12 *D,E*). Consistent with this physiological evidence for the developmental reduction in the number of synapses upon a cell, these authors described the diminution during this time period of the collateralization of auditory nerve fibers within nucleus magnocellularis (Figures 12 *C–F*). Unfortunately, the development of phase locking by cells

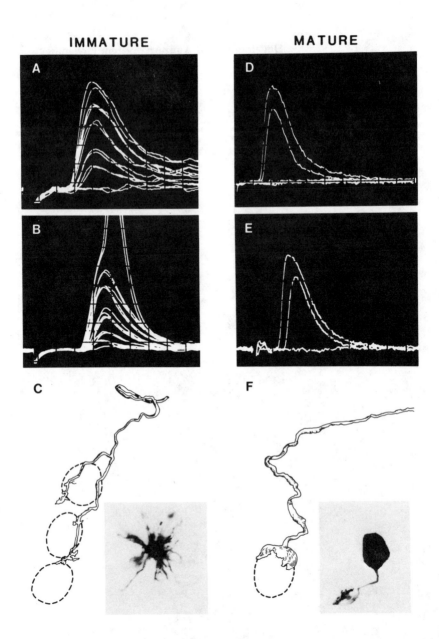

IMMATURE

A

B

C

MATURE

D

E

F

FIGURE 12. Developmental reduction in the number of cochlear nerve axons innervating nucleus magnocellularis neurons and the concomitant reduction in terminal branching of auditory nerve fibers. (*A,B*) Intracellular recording from nucleus magnocellularis neurons from embryonic day 13 chickens as electrical stimulus to auditory nerve was raised gradually. Note stepwise increase in response indicating influence of five or six terminals. (*C*) Camera lucida representation of HRP-filled auditory nerve fiber in embryonic day 14 chicken. Note branching of axon and innervation of multiple neurons. A Golgi-stained neuron with multiple somatic protuberances is also shown. (*D,E*) Intracellular recording from 4-day-old posthatching chicken (*D*) and embryonic day 18 chicken indicating influence of only two input terminals. (*F*) Camera lucida drawing of HRP-filled auditory nerve fiber from 4-day-old posthatchling chicken. No terminal branches were seen at this age; axons terminate in calycine ending on single neuron. Golgi-stained embryonic day 17 cell shows lack of somatic processes. Electrophysiology calibration: 2 ms; 2 mV (*A*) and 5 mV (*B,D,E*). (From Jackson and Parks, 1982.)

in nucleus magnocellularis has not been described. However, it is clear that the delayed ontogeny of phase locking in AVCN of cat would be explicable if the innervation of the principal cells in AVCN undergoes developmental changes similar to those that occur in nucleus magnocellularis of chicken.

VI BINAURAL INTERACTIONS

The foregoing discussion has been concerned with the coding of stimuli delivered to one ear. The term "binaural interactions" refers to the coding of stimuli that impinge upon both ears, more specifically, to the interactions between responses evoked by concurrent stimulation of the two ears. It has proven convenient, if not entirely accurate, to classify neurons as being "monaural," that is, responsive to stimulation of only one ear; "EE," excited by stimulation of either ear; or "EI," excited by stimulation of one ear and inhibited by stimulation of the other ear. The inhibitory effect of stimulating the nonexcitatory ear for EI cells may be evident in the suppression of spontaneous activity or in the reduction of responses to binaural stimuli relative to responses evoked by stimulation of the excitatory ear alone. Since sufficient spontaneous activity is usually lacking in anesthetized animals, particularly in very young animals, the inhibitory influence is assessed almost invariably in extracellularly recorded activity by comparing the magnitude of responses evoked by stimulation of the excitatory ear alone with the magnitude of responses evoked by stimulation of both ears.

Traditionally, EE cells are viewed as being sensitive to the average binaural stimulus level impinging on the two ears and relatively insensitive to the location of a stimulus source around the head (Goldberg and Brown, 1969). As a stimulus source is displaced in an arc around the head, the reduced stimulus level at one ear is compensated for by the increased stimulus level at the other ear, resulting theoretically in an unchanged amount of excitation impinging on the EE cell. On the other hand, EI cells are viewed as being more sensitive to the difference between the stimulus levels impinging on the two ears. An increase or decrease of stimulus level arising from a source located at a particular location would, theoretically, leave the response of an EI cell unchanged because the relative strengths of the evoked excitation and inhibition would remain unchanged. However, displacement of the source in an arc around the head, that is, the azimuthal location of the source, would alter the evoked response because the relative levels of the stimulus impinging on the two ears, and consequently the relative strengths of the excitatory and inhibitory influences, depend upon the azimuth of the source. Thus, EE cells would be most responsive to changes in stimulus level while EI cells would be most responsive to changes in stimulus azimuth. Recently published data obtained in ICC of the adult gerbil demonstrates, however, that this conceptually convenient scheme is somewhat oversimplified (Semple and Kitzes, 1987a).

Sanes and Rubel (1988) conducted an impressive study in which they assessed for the first time the development of both excitatory and inhibitory events in the lateral superior olive (LSO) in an age-graded series of gerbils. The LSO receives excitatory input from the ipsilateral ventral cochlear nucleus and inhibitory input from the ipsilateral medial nucleus of the trapezoid body. The medial nucleus of the trapezoid body is innervated by the contralateral ventral cochlear nucleus. These anatomical relationships permit the selective activation of excitatory events by stimulation of the ipsilateral ear and the selective activation of inhibitory events by stimulation of the contralateral ear. Cells in the LSO receiving this sort of input would be designated EI neurons according to the scheme described above.

Sanes and Rubel compared monaural and binaural responses of 13–14- and 15–16-day-old gerbil pups with adult gerbils. At 12 days postpartum only 15% of ventral cochlear nucleus cells in gerbil respond to sound; at 14 days postpartum the great majority of these cells can be activated by acoustic stimuli (Woolf and Ryan, 1985). As has been reported in the auditory nerve and ventral cochlear nucleus, excitatory response thresholds and minimal latency diminish while maximal discharge rate and dynamic range increase during development. By comparing responses evoked by stimulation of the excitatory, ipsilateral ear alone with responses evoked by binaural stimulation, these authors demonstrated that the inhibitory influence evoked by contralateral stimulation developed during the same period in parallel with the excitatory influence.

The influence of inhibition evoked by contralateral stimulation is illustrated in Figure 13. For each response function the level of the ipsilateral stimulus was held constant at 15–25 dB above threshold while the contralateral stimulus was raised at the indicated increments from levels less than (minus values) to levels greater than (positive values) the ipsilateral stimulus level. In each case, discharge rate fell as the relative level of the contralateral stimulus increased. The functions illustrated in Figure 13C demonstrate that inhibition is at least as developed at 13–15 days of age as is excitation. The fact that most of these functions appear to terminate when the ipsilateral stimulus level is still greater than the contralateral stimulus level suggests that in animals of this age the disynapic inhibitory pathway is actually more effective than the monosynaptic excitatory pathway.

In order for the binaural interactions apparent in Figure 13 to occur, the relevant excitatory and inhibitory pathways must be responsive to the same range of stimulus frequencies. The CFs of the excitatory and inhibitory influences were found by these authors to be highly correlated. In animals 13–14 days of age the correlation was 0.69 for all units with a CF below 4 kHz, the great majority of their sample for this age group. This correlation rose to 0.87 for animals 15–16 days of age and to 0.97 for adults. The lower correlation for the two younger groups might be related to the difficulty faced by the experimenter in assigning the proper CF to a tuning curve that is rather broad and perhaps noisy, as is often the case in such young animals.

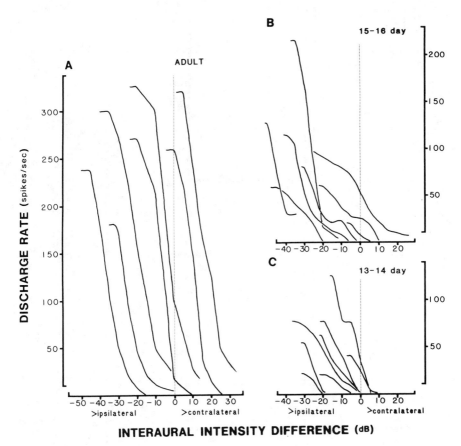

FIGURE 13. Representative interaural intensity difference functions for units in the lateral superior olive of adult (*A*), 15–16-day-old (*B*), and 13–14-day-old (*C*) gerbils. The ipsilateral, excitatory stimulus was held constant at 15–25 dB above threshold and the level of the contralateral, inhibitory stimulus was increased from levels less than (minus values) to greater than (positive values) the ipsilateral stimulus. Stimulus was set at CF for each unit. (From Sanes and Rubel, 1988.)

The correspondence of excitatory and inhibitory response areas is illustrated in Figure 14. A high- and a low-CF response area for each age group of gerbils is shown in the upper panels and the inhibitory response area for each of these units is shown in the lower panels. The inhibitory response areas were constructed by presenting a CF stimulus delivered at 15–25 dB above threshold to the excitatory, ipsilateral ear concurrently with tones delivered to the contralateral ear at the indicated frequencies and levels. The alignment of the inhibitory and excitatory response areas extends the data generated at CF (Figure 13) by demonstrating the congruity of the range of frequencies to which the excitatory and inhibitory circuits are responsive. It is of interest that for each unit the inhibitory response area tends to be

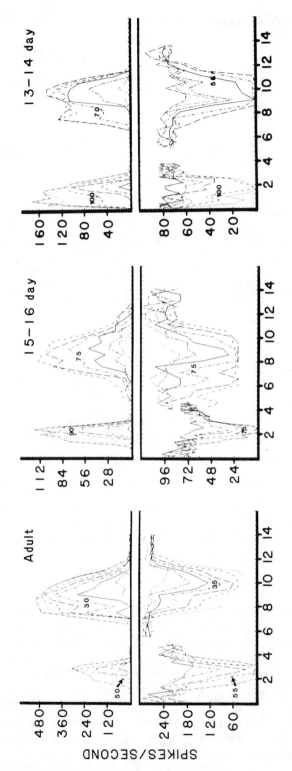

FIGURE 14. Corresponding excitatory and inhibitory response areas of pairs of lateral superior olive units isolated in three age groups of gerbils. Below each excitatory response area is the inhibitory response area for the same unit generated by holding the excitatory, ipsilateral stimulus constant at 15–25 dB above threshold at CF and varying the inhibitory, contralateral stimulus over the indicated frequencies and levels. For each response area the level of the intensity function 15 dB above threshold at CF is indicated. Stimulus level varies in 10-dB steps for the adult response areas and in 5-dB steps for the juvenile response areas. (From Sanes and Rubel, 1988.)

broader than the corresponding excitatory area. While the acoustic shadow produced in the environment by the gerbil head is unlikely ever to provide the interaural intensity differences employed in the experiment to generate the inhibitory response areas for the low-CF cells, it is clear that the structural and functional mechanisms that subserve the low-frequency inhibition in the adult are already present in the very young gerbil.

The neuronal circuitry that must underlie these physiological data exemplify the great precision that is characteristic of the auditory system. At the same time, minimal consideration of this circuitry reveals our great ignorance of the mechanisms that determine its development. For example, how is the output of neurons with the same CF in each ventral cochlear nucleus guided to the same neuron in LSO? The precision of these developmental mechanisms is best appreciated by considering the fact that each circuit actually begins with the auditory nerve fibers that determine the CF of the relevant neurons in each ventral cochlear nucleus. Moreover, the ipsilateral pathway is monosynaptic while the contralateral pathway includes a second, very large and specialized synapse in MNTB, the calyx of Held.

The functional development of the inferior colliculus has been the subject of several studies. Interest in the inferior colliculus is based primarily on the fact that this nucleus is a critical integrative focus in the ascending auditory neuroaxis. Since all pathways ascending from lower auditory brainstem nuclei synapse there, it is very likely that both monaural and binaural information arising from these nuclei are integrated within the inferior colliculus before being passed on to the medial geniculate body. Thus, analyses of the inferior colliculus provide insights into the development of stimulus coding within the entire auditory brainstem. Intracellular studies within the inferior colliculus or comparative analyses of its afferent systems would be required to separate developmental changes occurring within these lower nuclei from developmental changes occurring within the inferior colliculus itself. As there is some evidence that information is processed in a hierarchical manner (Semple and Kitzes, 1987b) rather than totally along parallel channels, such comparative analyses will have to be undertaken, challenging as they might be.

Analyses of ICCs in 5- and 6-day-old kittens reveal that the nucleus is organized tonotopically even at this very young age, with, as in the adult, lowest stimulus frequencies represented dorsally and higher frequencies represented ventrally (Aitkin and Reynolds, 1975). As response thresholds at this age normally exceed 110 dB, it is clear that the connectivity that must underlie this organization develops independent of any acoustically driven function. The progression of CFs for sequences of single units recorded during single dorsal-to-ventral penetrations of ICCs from an age-graded series of kittens is shown in Figure 15 (Aitkin and Moore, 1975). In each case lowest CFs occurred dorsally and CF increased as more ventrally located cells were isolated. The increase in the upper limit of the represented stimulus frequencies during development is evident in these data. The

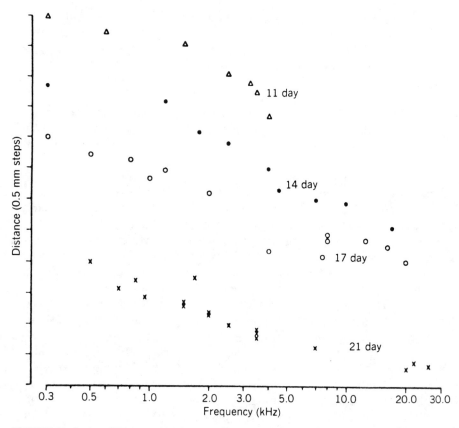

FIGURE 15. Series of CFs recorded during individual dorsoventral penetrations of the inferior colliculus in cats of the indicated ages. Each series begins at the point where a tonotopic sequence of CFs began, probably at the dorsal limit of the central nucleus of the inferior colliculus. Each series is offset on the ordinate for purposes of presentation. Note the increasing upper limit of CF as a function of age. (From Aitkin and Moore, 1975.)

highest CF recorded in the 11-day-old kitten was about 4.2 kHz, while the highest CF recorded in the 21-day-old kitten was about 26 kHz. Since these penetrations traversed the entire dorsal-to-ventral extent of the ICC, such data indicate that the CF of the most ventrally located neurons increases by about 2.5 octaves during this 10-day period of development, undoubtedly reflecting the progressive changes in the representation of stimulus frequency in the cochlea discussed earlier. Shnerson and Willott (1979) described very similar events occurring in the ICC of the mouse. Between 12 and 13 days postpartum CFs were always below 20 kHz. The upper limit of CF extended to approximately 30 kHz in animals between 13 and 14 days postpartum and to more than 40 kHz for animals between 15 and 17 days of age.

The proportions of EE and EI cells present in ICC of the adult are present in the ICC of perinatal kittens as soon as the neurons become responsive to acoustic stimulation (Aitkin and Reynolds, 1975; Moore and Irvine, 1980). Thus, at 5–7 days of age 47% of the recorded units were classified as being EE and 40% were classified as being EI (Aitkin and Reynolds, 1975). The respective values from adult cat were 41 and 39%. Furthermore, these authors presented data suggesting that for each cell, the CFs defined by stimulation of the contralateral and the ipsilateral ears were highly correlated. The distribution of values relating ipsilaterally and contralaterally defined CFs fall well within the range of similar data obtained in the ICC of the adult gerbil (Semple and Kitzes, 1985).

The prior discussion of binaural interactions has been concerned with the level of the stimulus impinging on the two ears. This cue is pertinent only for high-frequency stimuli, for the head and pinnae are insignificant obstructions when the wavelength of the sound is very long, that is, when the frequency of the sound is low. The relevant cue for the localization of low-frequency sounds is the difference in the time of arrival of the stimulus at the two ears. Thus, a sound will arrive at the two ears at the same time when the source is located at the midline; when the source is located away from the midline, a sound will arrive at the proximal ear earlier than at the distal ear, and the difference in arrival time provides the perception of the azimuthal location of the source.

The sensitivity of the inferior colliculus to temporal disparities was first analyzed in a seminal paper by Rose and his colleagues (Rose et al., 1966) and later extended in several publications by Yin and Kuwada and by others (Kuwada and Yin, 1983; Yin and Kuwada, 1983a,b). These workers demonstrated that in response to low-frequency tonal stimuli, discharge rate is a periodic function of interaural delay and the period of the rate function is equal to the period of the stimulating sinusoid. Aitkin and Reynolds (Aitkin, 1986) demonstrated such behavior in the activity of ICC cells isolated in 2-week-old kittens (Figure 16). Notice that the interval between the peaks or the troughs of the rate function in the left panel is approximately 2 ms of delay, the period of the 500-Hz stimulus. While the sinusoidal modulation of the rate function is clear, the depth of the modulation is perhaps less than that shown in the typical functions demonstrated in adult cats. That the rate function is the result of interactions between information conveyed from each ear is evident in the observation that neither contralateral nor ipsilateral stimulation presented alone evoked responses that exceeded the spontaneous discharge rate. Thus, the mechanisms that support such binaural interactions must be available already by the end of the second week of postnatal life in the kitten.

A coincidence detection model is commonly suggested to explain periodic interaural delay functions such as the ones shown in Figure 16. Stated simply, the probability of a discharge is greatest when input to a binaural cell is coincident and least when the input is temporally most disparate.

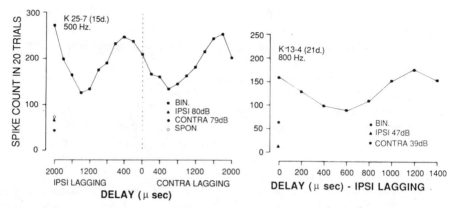

FIGURE 16. Interaural delay functions of two cells in the ICC of young kittens. Tones at the indicated frequencies and levels were presented simultaneously to the two ears. The stimulus to one ear was delayed relative to the stimulus to the other ear at the indicated steps. Age of kitten indicated at top line of each panel. Squares: binaural stimulation; triangles: ipsilateral stimulation; filled circles: contralateral stimulation; open circles: spontaneous discharge rate. Tone duration was 300 ms and the number of discharges accumulated over 20 presentations indicated. (Modified from Aitkin, 1986.)

This model requires that the monaural inputs to the binaural cell are phase locked to the stimulus. In the context of response functions in developing animals, the model would predict that the modulation of the interaural rate function is proportional to the degree of phase locking available in the monaural inputs to the binaural cell. The data presented in Figure 10 indicate that nearly adult levels of phase-locked input to the binaural cell should be available after the first week of postnatal life in the kitten. This is true, however, only at very low stimulus frequencies for phase locking diminishes rapidly as a function of frequency in very young animals. The data presented in Figure 10 would lead, therefore, to the prediction that the modulation of interaural delay functions would diminish rapidly as a function of increasing stimulus frequency in the very young kitten. This prediction remains to be tested. It is also of great interest to determine, as a separate but related issue, whether the binaural mechanisms that support the facilitative interactions that provide augmented responses to binaural stimuli are available at stimulus frequencies that are too high in very young animals to result in periodic interaural delay functions.

VII   SUMMARY AND CONCLUSIONS

These data from neonatal kittens and gerbils demonstrate two important points. First, in the youngest animals in which acoustically driven responses can be evoked, both excitatory and inhibitory influences are present in the brainstem. Second, the high correlation of contralaterally and ipsilaterally defined CFs and response areas at this age demonstrates that projections from a given locus on each cochlear partition have found their way to common neurons in the superior olivary complex and the ICC. In addition to the development of the tonotopic organization of these structures, these aspects of connectivity also must arise independently of acoustically driven function within the midbrain auditory system. It should be remembered, however, that the extracellular recording of excitatory and inhibitory events within ICC does not in itself prove that these events occurred within ICC, for such responses might be faithful reflections of binaural interactions occurring within lower order nuclei (like the superior olivary complex) that project to the ICC. Nevertheless, such projections from its afferent sources must be orderly by this early age in order for the organization within the ICC described in the preceding to occur.

It is clear from the behavioral research of Kelly and his colleagues presented earlier that very immature animals are able to localize a sound in space. Similarly, the electrophysiological data of Sanes and Rubel (1988), Aitkin and Reynolds (1975), Aitkin and Moore (1975), Moore and Irvine (1981), and others demonstrate that the physiological mechanisms that support this behavior are available at a very early age. The question that remains is whether the stimuli available to the adult to perform the task of localization are also available to the very young animal. The answer to this question is either no or that they are present but very attenuated.

In the previous discussion of the presumed utility of EI cells, it was stated that the relative magnitude of the stimulus impinging upon the two ears from a distant source was determined by the azimuth of the source, that is, the location of the source relative to the two ears. The difference between the levels at the two ears (IID) is due to the acoustic shadow of the head and pinna shielding the distal ear and the gain due to the "acoustic funnel" effect of the pinna at the proximal ear. The IID generally increases with stimulus frequency, and the magnitude of this effect of frequency depends upon the size of the head and the size of the pinnae. It should be intuitively clear that a larger head and larger pinnae will provide a greater IID than will a smaller head and pinnae.

These considerations have been confirmed experimentally by Moore and Irvine (1981). Depending upon stimulus frequency and azimuth, the largest IIDs measured for adult cats were 10–15 dB greater than those measured for 35-day-old kittens. However, there are technical reasons to believe that the IIDs reported in this study for the adults were underestimated by 5–15 dB (cf. Irvine, 1987) and, therefore, that the differences between the IIDs available to adults and to young kittens are much larger than have been described. This implies that a sound source located at a particular azimuth will provide a very different IID for the very young animal than it will for the fully grown animal. These data also imply that large IIDs available to the adult animal as cues for the localization of higher frequency stimulus sources are unavailable to the very young animal. These conclusions also apply to the interaural delay cue (ITD), which is critical for the localization of low-frequency stimuli. Obviously, the smaller distance between the ears of the very young animal restricts the magnitude of this cue relative to that available to the fully grown animal. Thus, as in the case of IID, a particular difference in the time of arrival of a sound at the proximal and distal ears will arise from a source located at one azimuth for very young animals and at quite a different azimuth for fully grown animals.

These considerations raise interesting questions about the interpretation of auditory physiology in the adult and in the developing animal. For example, since IIDs and ITDs arise from sources located at different azimuths as the animal grows, are physiological responses to these cues "interpreted" by the nervous system in a manner that takes into account the size of the head and pinnae? Clearly, the excitatory and inhibitory responses evoked by a particular IID or ITD do not arise from the same azimuth throughout the life of the animal and, presumably, cannot therefore be interpreted as being unequivocal neural information about source location. Do physiological and anatomical systems develop independently of the environmental cues available to the animal or is their development driven by environmental events, as suggested by Aitkin (1986). Evidence that cochlear function and, therefore, responsiveness to the environment is unnecessary for the development of certain functions of the auditory system has been presented previously in this chapter. Do binaural functions in the very young animal differ from those observed in the adult? If the answer to this empirical question is positive, then the question arises whether responses in the young animal are appropriate to the physical dimensions of the young animal or are merely immature, that is, less pronounced responses appropriate to the adult? Finally, and to come full circle in this chapter, what is the relationship between the ability of developing animals to localize a sound in space and the physiology of their binaural systems? Can we say that the physiology of binaural interactions is understood without being able to specify the relationship between our measures of auditory system physiology and the behavior of the animal?

We have seen that the physiology of the developing auditory system involves progressive changes in the available physical cues and dynamic interactions between structural and functional systems in the periphery and central nervous system. Understanding these developmental interactions is the goal of this unfolding field of research.

ACKNOWLEDGMENTS

The author wishes to thank Malcolm Semple and Ann Markham for their helpful discussions. Preparation of this chapter was supported by National Institutes of Health grant NS-17596.

REFERENCES

Aitkin, L. M. (1986) The Auditory Midbrain: Structure and Function in the Central Auditory Pathway. Clifton, NJ: Humana Press.

Aitkin, L. M., and D. R. Moore (1975) Inferior colliculus. II. Development of tuning characteristics and tonotopic organization in central nucleus of the neonatal cat. J. Neurophysiol. 38:1208–1216.

Aitkin, L. M., and A. Reynolds (1975) Development of binaural responses in the kitten inferior colliculus. Neurosci. Lett. 1:315–319.

Blatchley, B. J., W. A. Cooper, and J. R. Coleman (1987) Development of auditory brainstem response to tone pip stimuli in the rat. Dev. Brain Res. 32:75–84.

Bosher, S. K., and R. L. Warren (1971) A study of the electrochemistry and osmotic relationships of the cochlear fluids in the neonatal rat at the time of the development of the endocochlear potential. J. Physiol. (Lond.) 212:739–761.

Brugge, J. F., and T. A. O'Conner (1984) Postnatal functional development of the dorsal and posteroventral cochlear nuclei of the cat. J. Acoustic. Soc. Amer. 75:1548–1562.

Brugge, J. F., E. Javel, and L. M. Kitzes (1978) Signs of functional maturation of peripheral auditory system in discharge patterns of neurons in anteroventral cochlear nucleus of kitten. J. Neurophysiol. 41:1557–1579.

Brugge, J. F., L. M. Kitzes, and E. Javel (1981) Postnatal development of frequency and intensity sensitivity of neurons in the anteroventral cochlear nucleus of kittens. Hear. Res. 5:217–229.

Carlier, E., M. Abonnenc, and R. Pujol (1975) Maturation des responses unitaires a la stimulation tonale dans le nerf cochleaire du chaton. J. Physiol. (Paris). 70:129–138.

Clements, M., and J. B. Kelly (1978) Auditory spatial responses of young guinea pigs (Cavia porcellus) during and after ear blocking. J. Comp. Physiol. Psych. 92:34–44.

Dallos, P., and D. Harris (1978) Properties of auditory nerve responses in absence of outer hair cells. J. Neurophysiol. 41:365–383.

Davis, H. (1959) Excitation of auditory receptors. In J. Field, H. W. Magoun, and V. E. Hall (eds.): Handbook of Physiology, Sect. 1, Vol. 1, Neurophysiology. Baltimore, MD: Waverly Press, pp. 565–584

Davis, H. (1968) Mechanisms of the inner ear. Annals Otol., Rhinol., Laryngol. 77:644–655.

Dolan, D. F., D. C. Teas, and J. P. Walton (1985) Postnatal development of physiological responses in auditory nerve fibers. J. Acoustic. Soc. Amer. 78:544–554.

Echteler, S. M., E. Arjmand, and P. Dallos (1989) Developmental alterations in the frequency map of the mammalian cochlea. Nature 341:147–149.

Ehret, G., and R. Romand (1981) Postnatal development of absolute auditory thresholds in kittens. J. Comp. Physiol. Psych. 95:304–311.

Fernandez, C., and R. Hinojosa (1974) Postnatal development of endocochlear potential and stria vascularis in the cat. Acta Otolaryngol. 78:173–186.

Finck, A., C. D. Schneck, and A. F. Hartman (1972) Development of cochlear function in the neonate Mongolian gerbil (*Meriones unguiculatus*). J. Comp. Physiol. Psych. *78*:375–380.

Goldberg, J. M., and P. B. Brown (1969) Responses of binaural neurons of dog superior olivary complex to dichotic tonal stimuli: Some physiologic mechanisms of sound localization. J. Neurophysiol. *32*:613–636.

Harris, D. M., and P. Dallos (1984) Ontogenetic changes in frequency mapping of a mammalian ear. Science *225*:741–742.

Irvine, D. R. F. (1987) Interaural intensity differences in the cat: Changes in sound level at the two ears associated with azimuthal displacements in the frontal horizontal plane. Hear. Res. *26*:267–286.

Jackson, H., and T. N. Parks (1982) Functional synapse elimination in the developing avian cochlear nucleus with simultaneous reduction in cochlear nerve axon branching. J. Neurosci. *2*:1736–1743.

Kelly, J. B., and M. Potash (1986) Directional responses to sounds in young gerbils (*Meriones unguiculatus*). J. Comp. Physiol. Psych. *100*:37–45.

Kettner, R. E., J.-Z. Feng, and J. F. Brugge (1985) Postnatal development of the phase locked response to low frequency tones of auditory nerve fibers in the cat. J. Neurosci. *5*:275–283.

Kuwada, S., and T. C. T. Yin (1983) Binaural interaction in low frequency neurons in the inferior colliculus of the cat. I. Effects of long interaural delays, intensity, and repetition rate on the interaural delay function. J. Neurophysiol. *50*:981–999.

Liberman, M. C., and Dodds, L. W. (1984) Single-neuron labeling and chronic cochlear pathology. II. Stereocilia damage and alterations of spontaneous discharge rates. Hear. Res. *16*:43–53.

Liberman, M. C., and N. Y.-S. Kiang (1984) Single-neuron labeling and chronic cochlear pathology. IV. Stereocilia damage and alterations in rate- and phase-level functions. Hear. Res. *16*:75–90.

Lippe, W. R. (1986) Development changes in the pattern of spontaneous activity in the avian auditory system. Assoc. Res. Otolaryngol. Ninth Midwinter Research Meeting, p. 176.

Lippe, W. R. (1987) Shift of tonotopic organization in brain stem auditory nuclei of the chicken during late embryonic development. Hear. Res. *25*:205–208.

Lippe, W. R., and E. W. Rubel (1985) Ontogeny of tonotopic organization of brainstem auditory nuclei in the chicken: Implications for development of the place principle. J. Comp. Neurol. *237*:273–289.

Moore, D. R., and D. R. F. Irvine (1980) Development of binaural input, response patterns, and discharge rate in single units of the cat inferior colliculus. Exp. Brain Res. *38*:103–108.

Moore, D. R., and D. R. F. Irvine (1981) Development of responses to acoustic interaural intensity differences in the cat inferior colliculus. Exp. Brain Res. *41*:301–309.

Pickles, J. O. (1985) Recent Advances in Cochlear Physiology. In G. A. Kerkut and J. W. Phillis (eds.): Progress in Neurobiology, Vol. 24. Oxford: Pergamon Press, pp. 1–42.

Pujol, R. (1972) Development of tone-burst responses along the auditory pathway in the cat. Acta Otolaryngol. *74*:383–391.

Relkin, E. M., and J. C. Saunders (1980) Displacement of the malleus in neonatal golden hamsters. Acta Otolaryngol 90:6–15.

Rhode, W. S. (1971). Observations of the vibration of the basilar membrane in squirrel monkeys using the Mossbauer technique. J. Acoust. Soc. Amer. 49:1218–1231.

Rhode, W. S. (1973) An investigation of post-mortem cochlear mechanisms using the Mossbauer effect. In A. Møller (ed.): Basic Mechanisms in Hearing. New York: Academic Press, pp. 49–68.

Robles, L., M. A. Ruggero, and N. C. Rich (1986) Basilar membrane mechanics at the base of the chinchilla cochlea. I. Input-output functions, tuning curves, and response phases. J. Acoust. Soc. Amer. 80:1364–1374.

Romand, R. (1983) Development of the cochlea. In R. Romand (ed.): Development of Auditory and Vestibular Systems. New York: Academic Press, pp. 47–88.

Romand, R. (1984) Functional properties of auditory-nerve fibers duing postnatal development in the kitten. Exp. Brain Res. 56:395–402.

Rose, J. E., N. B. Gross, C. D. Geisler, and J. E. Hind (1966) Some neural mechanisms in the inferior colliculus of the cat which may be relevant to localization of a sound source. J. Neurophysiol. 29:288–314.

Rose, J. E., J. F. Brugge, D. J. Anderson, and J. E. Hind (1967) Phase-locked responses to low-frequency tones in single auditory nerve fibers of the squirrel monkey. J. Neurophysiol. 30:769–793.

Rubel, E. W. (1978) Ontogeny of structure and function in the vertebrate auditory system In M. Jacobson (ed.): Handbook of Sensory Physiology Vol. IX, Development of Sensory Systems. New York: Springer-Verlag.

Rubel, E. W., and B. M. Ryals (1983) Development of the place principle: Acoustic trauma. Science 219:512–514.

Rubel, E. W., W. R. Lippe, and B. M. Ryals (1984) Development of the place principle. Annals Otol., Rhinol., Laryngol. 93:609–615.

Russell, I. J., and P. M. Sellick (1978) Intracellular studies of hair cells in the mammalian cochlea. J. Physiol. (Lond) 284:261–290.

Ryugo, D. K., and K. M. Fekete (1982) Morphology of primary axosomatic endings in the anteroventral cochlear nucleus of the cat: A study of the endbulbs of Held. J. Comp. Neurol. 210:239–257.

Sanes, D. H., and E. W. Rubel (1988) The ontogeny of inhibition and excitation in the gerbil lateral superior olive. J. Neurosci. 8:682–700.

Sanes, D. H., M. Merickel, and E. W. Rubel (1989) Evidence for an alteration of the tonotopic map in the gerbil cochlea during development. J. Comp. Neurol. 279:436–444.

Schmiedt, R. A., J. J. Zwislocki, and R. P. Hamernik (1980) Effects of hair cell lesions on responses of cochlear nerve fibers. I. Lesions, tuning curves, two-tone inhibition, and responses to trapezoidal-wave patterns. J. Neurophysiol. 43:1367–1389.

Semple, M. N., and L. M. Kitzes (1985) Single-unit responses in the inferior colliculus: Different consequences of contralateral and ipsilateral auditory stimulation. J. Neurophysiol. 53:1467–1482.

Semple, M. N., and L. M. Kitzes (1987a) Binaural processing of sound pressure level in the inferior colliculus. J. Neurophysiol. 57:1130–1147.

Semple, M. N., and L. M. Kitzes (1987b) Hierarchical processing of binaural level cues in the ascending auditory system. Soc. Neurosci. Abstr. *13*:467.

Sewell, W. F. (1984a) The effects of furosemide on the endocochlear potential and auditory-nerve fibers tuning curves in cats. Hear. Res. *14*:305–314.

Sewell, W. F. (1984b) The relation between the endocochlear potential and spontaneous activity in auditory nerve fibers of the cat. J. Physiol. (Lond). *347*:685–696.

Shnerson, A., and J. F. Willott (1979) Development of inferior colliculus response properties in C57BL/6J mouse pups. Exp. Brain Res. *37*:373–385.

Sullivan, W. E. (1985) Classification of response patterns in cochlear nucleus of barn owl: Correlation with functional response properties. J. Neurophysiol. *53*:201–216.

Walsh, E., and J. McGee (1986) The development of function in the auditory periphery. In R. A. Altschuler, D. W. Hoffman and R. P. Bobbin (eds.): Neurobiology of Hearing: The Cochlea. New York: Raven Press.

Walsh, E. J., and J. McGee (1987) Postnatal development of auditory nerve and cochlear nucleus neuronal responses in kittens. Hear. Res. *28*:97–116.

Walsh, E. J., J. McGee, D. Wagahoff, and V. Scott (1985) Myelination of auditory nerve, trapezoidal, and brachium of the inferior colliculus axons in the cat. Assoc. Res. Otolaryngol. Eighth Midwinter Meeting, p. 33.

Woolf, N. K., and A. F. Ryan (1984) The development of auditory function in the cochlea of the mongolian gerbil. Hearing Res. *13*:277–283.

Woolf, N. K., and A. F. Ryan (1985) Ontogeny of neural discharge patterns in the ventral cochlear nucleus of the Mongolian gerbil. Dev. Brain Res. *17*:131–147.

Yancey, C., and P. Dallos (1985) Ontogenic changes in cochlear characteristic frequency at a basal turn location as reflected in the summating potential. Hear. Res. *18*:189–195.

Yin, T. C. T., and S. Kuwada (1983a) Binaural interaction in low frequency neurons in the inferior colliculus of the cat. II. Effects of changing rate and direction of interaural phase. J. Neurophysiol. *50*:1000–1019.

Yin, T. C. T., and S. Kuwada (1983b) Binaural interaction in low frequency neurons in the inferior colliculus of the cat. III. Effects of changing frequency. J. Neurophysiol. *50*:1020–1042.

Chapter Seven

DEVELOPMENT OF BEHAVIORAL RESPONSES TO SOUND

GÜNTER EHRET*

Zoologisches Institut, Universität Konstanz,
Universitat Bonn
Bonn, Federal Republic of Germany

Present address: Abteilung Vergleichende Neurobiologie, Universität Ulm, Ulm, Federal Republic of Germany

I   INTRODUCTION

The onset and further development of behavioral responses to sounds can be expected only on the basis of a functioning auditory system that gives rise to at least some sound perception. Thus perception of sound is a necessary condition for responding to it. The ability to hear, however, is not sufficient to initiate a behavioral response; and this is true for young developing animals in particular. In young animals two categories of factors can intervene, modify, and obstruct a simple stimulus–response relationship. These are arousal, attention, motivation, and other state-dependent factors on the one hand and restrictions due to immaturity of the developing motor system on the other. In any behavioral test of auditory development, therefore, state- and motor-system-dependent factors are potential variables in addition to those resulting from the maturation in the auditory system. As a result, full stimulus control of the behavior of a young animal in a test of auditory capability is often impossible to reach.

These difficulties with state- and motor-system-dependent factors in psychophysical tests of auditory maturation become relevant mainly if absolute capacities of the auditory system are measured, such as absolute thresholds of sensitivity, differential sensitivity, or spectral and temporal resolution. State- and motor-system-dependent factors can be used, however, as indicators of developmental changes if questions are raised concerning the extent to which an intact animal can make use of and adjust its behavior in response to received acoustic information. The adaptiveness of auditory response behavior in the ontogeny of an animal can be evaluated only in view of the animal's social behavior and ecology to which state- and motor-system-dependent factors are major determinants. Thus measurements of the development of behavioral responses to sound not only provide evidence for processes of maturation in the auditory system but also demonstrate improvement of auditory competence and the ability to participate, for example, as a receiver of intraspecific communication. One might suggest, therefore, that the development of response behavior to sound may have a time course different from that of auditory system maturation.

This chapter is especially designed for review of the following in mammals and humans: (a) behavioral methods used to measure auditory development and the types of results each produces; (b) the relationship between behavioral response development and the physiological maturation of the auditory system, which may help to separate factors that depend on development of the auditory system from those of nonauditory sources; and (c) possible interrelationships between the development of hearing and that of sound production.

II METHODOLOGICAL APPROACHES

In this section, a review of methods for testing hearing abilities in young developing mammals and humans will be presented. These methods must be designed to optimize both the behavioral control of the animal by the stimulus and the adaptiveness of the experimental task to the behavioral repertoire of the subject [see Ehret (1983a) for a review on mammals and Ehret (1988) for one on humans].

These methods imply that interference between the internal state of the subject and the experimental paradigm as well as between the behavior to be performed and the subject's innate behavioral tendencies should be reduced to a minimum. Since behavioral repertoires and abilities change permanently during ontogeny, methods and testing strategies have to be continuously adapted to the time course of these developments. Thus a good knowledge of the developmental biology of the animal being tested is very helpful for the planning of a meaningful experiment.

Both unconditioned and conditioned responses have been used to test hearing abilities in young mammals.

A Unconditioned Responses

This category comprises naturally occurring responses to sounds.

1 Startle Responses, Preyer Reflexes

Most often used in auditory research are so-called startle responses and Preyer reflexes. A startle response can be any behavioral change frequently observed as a sudden motor response of any part of the body to a loud sound. It is important that the actual response observed or measured by some criteria be specified in studies using startle responses. The Preyer reflex comprises movements of the pinnae and/or facial muscles and thus is part of a startle response pattern. The term "Preyer reflex" should be used if observations of motor responses to sounds are restricted to movements of these areas (Ehret, 1983a).

Startle response thresholds of hearing have been obtained in the opossum (Larsell and McCrady, 1935; Larsell et al., 1935; McCrady et al., 1937); in various strains of house mice (Powers et al., 1966; Hack, 1968; Shnerson and Willott, 1980); in the rat (Wada, 1923; Parisi and Ison, 1979); in the rabbit, dog, and mink (Foss and Flottorp, 1974); and in the cat (Foss and Flottorp, 1974; Olmstead and Villablanca, 1980). Preyer reflexes were observed in house mice (Alford and Ruben, 1963; Mikaelian and Ruben, 1965) and in cats (Ehret and Romand, 1981).

The advantages of startle response and Preyer reflex measurements are their simplicity and high speed of data acquisition. The data produced, however, are very much dependent on (a) the kind of stimuli used (e.g., familiar or unfamiliar to the subject; pure tones or broadband spectra);

(b) the internal state of the animal, especially on its vigilance; (c) the manipulation of the animal in the test (e.g., free moving, hand held, fixed in an apparatus); and (d) how the responses are observed (e.g., by unaided eye, through a microscope, by electronic movement detectors). Thus these two types of responses neither are particularly suitable for quantitative measurements nor do they provide accurate absolute auditory sensitivity if the data points are compared with those generated using more sensitive methodology (Knecht, 1958; Denes and Kocher, 1961; Anderson and Wedenberg, 1965; Markl and Ehret, 1973; Francis, 1975, 1979; Ehret 1983b). A further complication is that young developing individuals appear to be even more variable than adults in showing a response of defined appearance and magnitude. Unless special care is taken in experimental control procedures to facilitate reliability and validity, startle responses and Preyer reflexes should be taken only as indicators of some hearing ability (if they can repeatedly be elicited) but not as measures of absolute sensitivity. Furthermore, Preyer reflex audiograms seem to be more closely related to equal loudness contours than to absolute thresholds (Francis, 1979).

Startle responses in the form of movements of limbs and body (e.g., Fleischer, 1955; Tanaka and Arayama, 1969) and of eyelids (Birnholz and Benacerraf, 1983) have also been observed in studies of human prenatal hearing. Hearing tests *in utero* are inherently complicated by the presence of intrauterine noise (e.g., Querleu et al., 1981), which makes it impossible to exactly define the stimulus at the ear of the fetus.

2 Heart Rate Responses

Heart rate responses to sounds as rate accelerations or decelerations from a baseline have been used as indicators for hearing in young rats (Haroutunian and Campbell, 1981) and in human fetal (e.g., Tanaka and Arayama, 1969; Grimwade et al., 1971) and postnatal (Steinschneider et al., 1966; Turkewitz et al., 1972) testing. Since heart rate can be measured objectively over long periods from very young animals to adults, a continuous record of developmental changes of responsiveness can be obtained by this method. The measured changes, however, may not necessarily reflect processes in the auditory system but could also be due to cognitive processing and interpretation of sound stimuli.

3 Orientation Responses

Movements of the pinnae in response to soft sounds, head and body turns in response to sound, and movements toward or away from a sound source all are orientation responses that indicate auditory sensitivity and sound localization ability. Such responses were used to measure thresholds of hearing in young mouse pups (Ehret, 1976, 1977) and directional hearing in infant guinea pigs (Clements and Kelly, 1978a), rats, (Potash and Kelly,

1980; Kelly et al., 1987), and cats (Clements and Kelly, 1978b; Olmstead and Villablanca, 1980).

4 Behavioral Observation Audiometry

"Behavioral observation audiometry" is a term used for a variety of methods applied to human babies, infants, and children to study some aspect of unconditioned movement of eyes, eyelids, mouth, head, limbs, and body in response to presentation of sound (e.g., Suzuki and Sato, 1961; Thompson and Weber, 1974; Bench et al., 1976a,b; Kaga and Tanaka, 1980). In animal studies, responses in this category would often be called startle or orientation responses.

B Conditioned Responses

In all procedures under this heading, either a response to a certain sound is habituated (with dishabituation occuring when the sound is changed) or subjects are trained to respond to an acoustic stimulus that did not elicit a consistent response before. Meaningful data can be obtained only if false alarm rates are low and responses are stable with time. Conditioned responses are unsuitable for the measurement of hearing onset or for development in the first days thereafter because conditioning can start only after the subject can hear, and this often takes a few days to reach a stable response criterion.

1 Habituation–Dishabituation

Methods of this kind have proven to be very successful in chicks (Rubel and Rosenthal, 1975; Kerr et al., 1979; Gray and Rubel, 1981). Application of these methods to mammals, however, has thus far failed, obviously because a reliable and regularly occurring behavior to be habituated (except heart rate; Haroutunian and Campbell, 1981) could not be found. Cardiac and nonnutritive sucking-response habituation and dishabituation are promising methods for measuring differential auditory sensitivity in human babies (e.g., Eimas et al., 1971; Eisele et al., 1975; Bundy et al., 1982).

2 Conditioned Reflexes

A conditioned eyeblink reflex has successfully been used for auditory threshold measurements in young house mice (Ehret, 1976, 1977) and kittens (Ehret and Romand, 1981). Eyeblinks are released by mild electric shocks (unconditioned stimulus). Conditioning with sound–shock pairs may begin after eye opening, and it takes about 3–4 days until animals show a consistent reflex to the sound without shock presentation. Animals usually require frequent reconditioning in order to stabilize the response, especially if sounds close to threshold of perception are presented. In all three studies, unconditioned responses to sounds were also observed at the same times as the conditioned reflexes, thus permitting a comparison of threshold sensitivities of the two types of responses. After eyeblink conditioning, threshold responses were always lower (sensitivities higher) than those from unconditioned responses; that is, conditioning techniques appear to be better suited for identification of capabilities of the auditory system.

A conditioned suppression of movements (freezing) has been applied in tests of tone frequency generalization in rat pups (Hyson and Rudy, 1987). The rats (15-day-old animals) were trained with a tone of a certain frequency as the conditioned stimulus, which was then paired with a footshock (unconditioned stimulus). Later the strength of the conditioned freezing response was tested with tones of other frequencies. This method also seems promising for the testing of absolute and differential auditory thresholds in other mammals as well.

Conditioned orientation reflexes of several kinds have been used in human infant audiometry (e.g., Suzuki and Ogiba, 1961; Suzuki and Origuchi, 1969; Schneider et al., 1980; Trehub et al., 1980; Kaga and Tanaka, 1980). As with studies on mammals, conditioning was begun well after the onset and first developmental period of hearing.

3   Operant Conditioning

To date, operant conditioning techniques have been applied only in studies on human infants and older children and not in those on young mammals. Since these methods require stable behavioral patterns to build upon and a higher degree of cooperation by the subject than the other conditioning procedures, it is conceivable that operant conditioning might not reliably work in developing mammals or in human babies soon after birth. The most frequently used method involves an operant head turn response (e.g., Berg and Smith, 1983; Sinnott et al., 1983) and forced-choice paradigms (Roche et al., 1978; Elliott and Katz, 1980).

III   ACQUISITION OF RESPONSES TO ACOUSTIC STIMULI IN MAMMALS

In the previous section we have seen that behavioral responses can be used as *tools* for measuring auditory development. Now, discussion turns to the behaviors themselves as they occur in response to sound stimulation during the ontogeny of mammals.

The acquisition of behavioral responses to acoustic stimuli is often studied as a part of the natural behavioral development of an individual and becomes most obvious when a young animal takes active part as a sender and receiver in sound communication. There is an extensive literature (which will not be reviewed here) on how early experience with specific sounds can alter the further development of sound production, as, for example, with songs by birds and speech by humans (e.g., Marler, 1977, 1983; Petersen and Jusczyk, 1984; Bischof, 1985). Methods used in studies on acoustically controlled sound production include deprivation, substitution, and modification of normal sound input (experiments with dummies) and variations of the period of sound presentation (tests of sensitive or critical periods). The plasticity of acoustic behavior and the learning of new patterns in response to certain sounds reported for many birds and for humans seem to be exceptions where mammals are concerned. Plasticity of sound production has been described only for humpback whales, which change their song patterns over the years (Payne, 1979), and for Japanese macaques, which learn local call dialects associated with provisioning (Green, 1975). In other studies on monkeys (Winter et al., 1973), cats (Romand and Ehret, 1984), and house mice (Rottberger, 1980), an influence of specific sound experience, even of hearing ability, on the production of basic species-specific vocal patterns was not found. Nevertheless, changes in vocalizations of young mammals can be related to the perception of species-specific calls. Examples are young bats (*Antrozous, Eptesicus, Myotis*), which change their isolation calls in a predictable way when they can hear the calls of their mothers (Gould, 1971; Brown, 1976); wolf pups, which respond with an increased calling rate to the howls of their own species (Shalter et al., 1977); and kittens, which vocalize in response to calls and other behaviors of their mother (Haskins, 1979). Thus the calling of adults can elicit vocalization responses in the young that may contribute through an acoustic communication loop to secure maternal behavior.

Well-coordinated behavioral adjustments, which are obvious in sound communication, indicate an already advanced level of call recognition and response acquisition. Behavioral responsiveness to sounds usually starts with rather undirected reflexes such as the acoustic startle response and Preyer reflex described in the previous section. The time of appearance of startle and Preyer reflexes depends, in addition to sufficient hearing, very much upon the developmental state of neural substrates for sensorimotor interfacing and motor coordination (e.g., Fox, 1966; Burghardt and Bekoff, 1978) as well as and on the intensity of the sound. Reflex ontogeny and central motor development as described, for example, for the mouse (Fox, 1965), rat (Altman and Sudarshan, 1975), dog (Fox, 1964), and man (e.g., Fitzgerald et al., 1977; Wilson, 1978) have to precede the coupling of auditory input to motor responses. Such a coupling may not become apparent unless sophisticated methods of observation are used. Condon and Sander (1974) found that 1-day-old human babies respond to human speech by coordinating their movements with the rhythm of the speech irrespective of the language used. Such a coordination can be observed only by microanalysis and frame-by-frame scanning of sound films. To my knowledge, procedures of this kind have not been applied in studies of sound-elicited behavior in mammals. They are necessary, however, to achieve major progress in the field of the development of acoustically controlled behavior in mammals.

During ontogeny, the rather simple reflexes and responses to sounds generally become more refined and directed, and thus soon after the onset of hearing, orientation responses and directional movements to well-specified sounds can be released (see Section II) or even conditioned (Fox, 1966). Neither the types of behavioral patterns that can be associated with the perception of certain sounds nor the time course of possible developmental changes between perceived sounds and released behaviors are, to my knowledge, reported for mammals. A broad and interesting field awaits scientific efforts.

IV   ABSOLUTE THRESHOLDS TO TONE STIMULI

Inherent in behavioral audiometry is the problem that different methods of measurement often yield different thresholds of sensitivity (e.g., Ehret, 1983b). Measured thresholds are a product of sensory and motor response thresholds of the subject and of observational and criterion-dependent thresholds of the measuring system. As already mentioned in Section II, startle responses and Preyer reflexes are less sensitive indicators of hearing than orientation responses and conditioned reflexes. If behavioral data are taken to indicate auditory capabilities, the lowest thresholds from any experiment can be regarded as the closest approximations to the true sensitivity of the auditory system. Since hearing tests of most young mammals were performed by means of startle and Preyer reflexes (see Section II), other related data will not presented here. A complete record can be found in Ehret (1983a). In this section, results from kittens and mouse pups will be presented because they are the most complete sets of data obtained utilizing sensitive methods. These data will be used later as a meaningful basis for comparisons with structural and physiological development in the auditory system.

Behavioral responses to tone bursts over a limited frequency range (0.5–2 kHz) could be obtained in 4 of 11 kittens tested on the first postnatal day (Ehret and Romand, 1981). Most kittens of the sample responded on the second day although with very high (above 100 dB sound pressure level, SPL) thresholds (Figure 1). Subsequent development is characterized by three phases (Figure 1):

1. Up to day 6, behavioral threshold levels for all frequencies to which a response could be obtained remain consistently high while the frequency range of hearing is rather restricted. This range has widened only from 0.5–3 to 0.2–6 kHz on postnatal day 6; this is the only development observed during this phase.

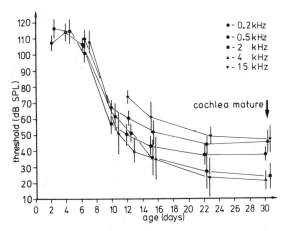

FIGURE 1. Cat: postnatal development of absolute auditory thresholds (dB SPL re 20 μPa) versus age for five representative frequencies. Standard deviations of the means are also shown. (Data from Ehret and Romand, 1981; modified from Ehret, 1985.)

2. Between days 6 and 12, thresholds decrease rapidly by more than 50 dB, and the range of hearing widens toward higher frequencies. Also within this period the maximum sensitivity of hearing (threshold minimum) appears at 4 kHz.

3. After day 12, thresholds decrease more slowly toward constant levels that are reached between days 22 and 30 depending on the frequency. During this period the hearing range widens again, now including ultrasonic frequencies up to 50 kHz (Ehret and Romand, 1981).

With the methods applied (conditioned eyeblink and pinna reflexes), threshold development does not continue beyond 30 days after birth as adult levels seem to be reached. A comparison of these thresholds (Figure 1) with others obtained by different behavioral methods from adult cats (Neff and Hind, 1955; Miller et al., 1963) shows, however, that the adult sensitivity is about 30–50 dB higher over the whole frequency range than the 30-day thresholds in Figure 1 indicate (Ehret and Romand, 1981). Unless further measurements clarify this subject, we can assume that this threshold difference is related to different sensitivities of behavioral methodology and not to a different gradient of maturation that could have been detected by a more sensitive method. If Figure 1 reproduces the development of the auditory system of cats correctly, one would expect that the curves shift along the abscissa while keeping their shapes constant when different methods of measurement are applied.

The threshold development for the house mouse is shown in Figure 2 (Ehret, 1976, 1977). Unlike the kitten, in the mouse the first phase of consistently high thresholds over several days was not observed. Phase 2 of

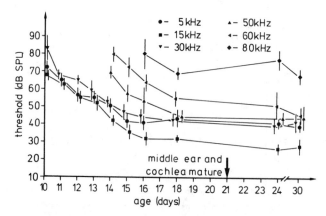

FIGURE 2. House mouse: postnatal development of absolute auditory thresholds versus age for six representative frequencies. Standard deviations of the means are also shown. (Data from Ehret, 1976, 1977; modified from Ehret, 1985.)

rapidly decreasing thresholds extends from the onset of hearing at day 10 to about day 15; phase 3 ends at about day 18 when adult levels (measured by unconditioned orientation responses) are reached. While the threshold levels decrease, the frequency response range widens from 5–40 kHz at day 11 to 1–80 kHz at day 16. The sensitivity maximum near 15 kHz in adult mice occurs within phase 2 at day 14 after birth (Ehret, 1976). Again, as in the cat, adult thresholds measured with more sensitive methods (Ehret, 1974) are about 10–30 dB lower than those shown in Figure 2. The tentative interpretation for this difference is the same as given for the cat (see the preceding).

As with many developmental processes that asymtotically approach adult states, the threshold decreases shown in Figure 1 and 2 can be approximated by a power function of the form (Eggermont, 1985a,b)

$$L_t = L_a + Ae^{-t/B} \tag{1}$$

in which L_t is the auditory threshold at a certain age (t), L_a is the adult threshold (measured by the same method as in the young), A is a scaling factor, and B is a time constant. The values for the cat are $A = 200$, $B = 4.55$ and for the mouse $A = 1.36 \times 10^3$, $B = 2.8$. The time constants of cat and mouse differ by a factor of 1.63, which indicates that development of auditory sensitivity proceeds about 1.6 times faster in the mouse as compared with the cat. In both mammals the length of the period from the beginning of phase 2 (rapid threshold decrease) to the adult thresholds is equal to 3–4 times the time constants.

V   SOUND LOCALIZATION

The development of orientation and directional responses to sounds has been studied to some extent in cats. In Figure 3 data from two studies on turning responses and directional movements of kittens are combined.

Olmstead and Villablanca (1980) showed that unconditioned turning toward attractive stimuli (mother and kitten calls) occurred earlier at about postnatal day 13 than turning away from unattractive sounds (threat, growl, air blast) at about day 18. Only by day 25 did the ability to discriminate and localize different sounds become stable. Since unconditioned responses were used, habituation to the stimuli, especially in older animals, was a problem and resulted in low scores of responding animals after day 20 (Figure 3) due to a loss of interest in the stimuli and not to principal inabilities to respond differently and to localize sounds.

Clements and Kelly (1978b) studied directional movements of kittens by an operant–reward paradigm. In a two-choice situation, the approach of a sound source playing kitten calls was rewarded with milk. The percentage of approach response above chance increased with increasing age of the animals and became statistically significant in 18–24-day-old kittens. At the age of 30 days, the performance reached about 60%, and one would suggest a further improvement in older animals. Thus, in this study, the maturation seems not to be reached at day 30 after birth.

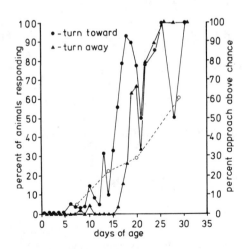

FIGURE 3. Cat: development of unconditioned orientation responses "turn toward" or "turn away" from a sound source (left ordinate, closed symbols; adapted from Olmstead and Villablanca, 1980) and development of conditioned orientation toward a loudspeaker (right ordinate, open circles; adapted from Clements and Kelly, 1978b). The increase of percentage of responding animals can be described by Equation 2.

The curves in Figure 3, which depict development of turn-toward and turn-away responses by kittens, can be approximated by an equation similar to Equation 1:

$$L_t = L_a - Ae^{-t/B} \qquad (2)$$

in which the inversed course (increase of values with increased age) is considered; L_t is the percentage of animals responded at a certain age (t), L_a is the adult value (100%), A is a scaling factor, and B a time constant. For turning toward an attractive sound source we obtain $A = 1187$, $B = 3.85$ and for turning away from unattractive sounds $A = 8 \times 10^5$, $B = 1.8$ (Ehret, 1985). Interestingly, attraction starts earlier than aversion, which leads to the conclusion that maturation processes beyond those in the auditory system may play a role in the establishment of differential responses to sounds.

A comparison of the development of sound quality discrimination and localization (Figure 3) with the development of absolute thresholds of hearing (Figure 1) reveals further interesting aspects. Discrimination of sounds and orientation toward or away from an identified sound starts rather late, at postnatal days 13–18, after the auditory sensitivity has markedly increased (thresholds decreased). The time constants from the orientation behaviors are, however, smaller than the one from auditory threshold development. This indicates that the identification of the quality of a perceived sound and the release of directional movements need a predeveloped auditory system with an effective transmission of potential information into higher brain centers. Further, the difference in the time constants suggests that two independent processes of maturation take place, one at lower levels of the auditory system characterized by the larger time constant for threshold development, the other at higher levels of the brain (auditory and more complex centers) characterized by the shorter time constant for the development of specific orientation abilities. We shall go deeper into this subject in Section VI, in which behavioral response development will be compared with structural and functional maturation in the auditory system.

VI STRUCTURAL AND PHYSIOLOGICAL MATURATION AND HEARING

With the onset of hearing, a process becomes manifested that started much earlier and continues further, namely, the structural and physiological maturation in the auditory pathway. Hearing in cat and mouse starts before the external ear canal is fully open (Mikaelian and Ruben, 1965; Olmstead and Villablanca, 1980), when properties of the middle ear are not yet adultlike (Saunders et al., 1983), when the inner ear structures are only partly (near the base of the cochlea) developed (Romand, 1983; Kraus and Aulbach-

Kraus, 1981), and while development in higher auditory centers is well in progress (Brugge, 1983; Moore, 1983; Mysliveček, 1983; Coleman, Chapter 5, this volume; Kitzes, Chapter 6, this volume). Thus behavioral data on the inception of hearing requires only a minimum of function at several levels: outer ear, middle ear, cochlea, VIIIth nerve, auditory brain centers, sensori-motor connections, and motor centers of the brain. If the development of only one necessary level of these is delayed, behavioral responses to sounds might not be releasable even though electrical response activity could be present somewhere in the pathway. If different time courses of maturation occur at different levels, superposition of the time constants should become obvious in behavioral response development. Behavior, therefore, is the most comprehensive measuring tool for auditory development, but the results are probably the most difficult to interpret. A development of behavioral thresholds of sensitivity could in principle be due to maturation at any level of the pathway. In order to compare and correlate the steps of structural and physiological maturation with the biological functions that become obvious in behavior, we have to look for parallels in the time courses of development features.

These parallels can be easily recognized from Figures 4 and 5, in which the development of response thresholds of neurons in several centers of the auditory pathway is shown together with behavioral threshold development for cat and mouse. The time courses and the threshold levels of the maturation in the cochlear nerve, cochlear nucleus, and inferior colliculus are very similar and comparable with those of the behavioral development.

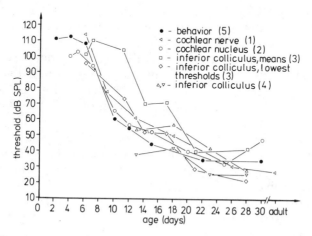

FIGURE 4. Cat: comparison of the development of behavioral absolute auditory thresholds (curve shows averages at frequencies of 0.2–15 kHz) with average single-neuron thresholds obtained from centers in the auditory pathway. The threshold decreases can be described by Equation 1. Numbers in parentheses refer to the references given in Table 1. (Modified from Ehret, 1985.)

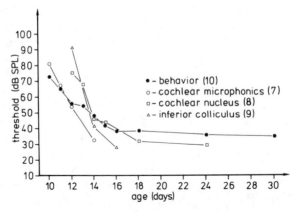

FIGURE 5. House mouse: comparison of the development of behavioral absolute auditory thresholds (curve shows average at frequencies of 5–30 kHz) with average response thresholds from centers in the auditory pathway. The threshold decreases can be described by Equation 1. Numbers in parentheses refer to the references given in Table 1. (Modified from Ehret, 1985.)

The correspondence between the curves shown in Figures 4 and 5 is the more striking as it emerges from different studies in which different methods and threshold criteria were used. It is interesting to note that behavioral thresholds in cats (Figure 4) agree better with the lowest thresholds from inferior colliculus neurons up to about day 18, and afterward with the mean thresholds of neurons (data from the study of Aitkin and Moore, 1975). Similarly, average single-neuron thresholds from the inferior colliculus of the mouse (Figure 5) are first higher (days 12–13) and then lower than the behavioral thresholds. This means that shortly after the onset of hearing the highest available sensitivity in the auditory system is used to elicit behavior, whereas later behavioral thresholds do not necessarily reflect the lowest neuronal thresholds in the auditory system. A divergence of adult threshold values is very obvious when one compares behavioral thresholds obtained by different methods from one animal species (e.g., Ehret, 1983b).

The close relationship between the maturation of response thresholds in the auditory brainstem and midbrain and the development of behavioral sensitivity can be expressed quantitatively by calculating and comparing time constants. Table 1 shows such data (partly taken from Ehret, 1985) for the curves illustrated in Figures 4 and 5. The similar time constants and maturation points in development, especially for thresholds of the inferior colliculus and behavior, suggests that auditory threshold development as determined by unconditioned and conditioned reflexes is related to threshold maturation at or below the midbrain level. Consistent with this suggestion are findings that movements of pinnae, facial muscles, and head, which were observed as behavioral responses, are controlled at or below the

TABLE 1. Development of Auditory Pathway Electrophysiology and Auditory Response Behavior in Cat and Mouse.[a]

Electrophysiological and Behavioral Measures[b]	A	B	Onset	Maturation
Cat				
Cochlear nerve, single-unit threshold (1)	307	5.55	5	26
Anteroventral cochlear nucleus, single-unit threshold (2)	300	4.46	5	22
Inferior colliculus, single-unit mean threshold (3)	446	4.35	?	21
Inferior colliculus, single-unit lowest threshold (3)	339	5.0	?	26
Inferior colliculus, single-unit mean threshold (4)	1166	4.62	?	33
Behavior, absolute threshold (5)	200	4.55	6	24
Behavior, orientation toward probability (6)	1187	3.85	13	18
Behavior, orientation away from probability (6)	8×10^5	1.8	18	23
Mouse				
Cochlear microphonic, threshold (7)	1.56×10^4	1.8	8	14
Cochlear nucleus, evoked potential threshold (8)	3.1×10^4	1.9	?	19
Inferior colliculus, single-unit threshold estimated (9)	8600	2.4	?	24
Behavior, absolute threshold (10)	1360	2.8	?	16–18

[a] The scaling factors (A) and time constants (B) are from equations 1 and 2; the onset and maturation of behavioral and electrophysiological events in postnatal days are presented in last two columns.

[b] References are indicated in parentheses: (1) Dolan et al., 1985; (2) Brugge et al., 1978; (3) Aitkin and Moore, 1975; (4) Moore and Irvine, 1979; (5) Ehret and Romand, 1981; (6) Olmstead and Villablanca, 1980; (7) Mikaelian and Ruben, 1965; (8) Saunders et al., 1980; (9) Shnerson and Willott, 1979; (10) Ehret, 1976, 1977.

midbrain level (Henkel and Edwards, 1978; Thompson and Masterton, 1978; Stein and Claman, 1981).

A comparison of the development of orientation behavior (time constants, onset and maturation of response to sound) with auditory threshold maturation in the brainstem and midbrain of the cat (Table 1) reveals clear differences, especially for the time constants and the beginning of functional development. This strengthens the preceding argument that identification and differential responding (toward or away) to sound quality requires advanced sensitivity in the auditory system up to the midbrain and that the development of these more complex abilities is not related to threshold maturation up to this level in the brain. Either maturation in higher centers and the influence of experience with sounds of different qualities or the development of some aspects other than sensitivity (e.g., tuning, temporal coding) in the brainstem and midbrain are responsible for the occurrence of differential sensitivity and orientation to sounds. The fact that auditory thresholds reach adult levels before the cochlea appears completely mature (Figures 1, 2, 4, and 5) points to the same idea, namely, that different developmental processes take place at different levels of the auditory pathway of which only some may influence auditory thresholds.

This statement is confirmed by several studies on the cat in which different time constants and maturation points of development for different measures in the auditory pathway have been found (compare Ehret, 1985; see also Blatchley et al., 1987 in the rat). Structural maturation of the auditory nerve (Romand et al., 1976) and cochlear nucleus (Larsen, 1985), spontaneous rate in the auditory nerve (Romand, 1984), tuning and discharge rate in the inferior colliculus (Moore and Irvine, 1979, 1980), evoked potential amplitudes (Mair et al., 1978; Walsh et al., 1986a), and latencies (Pujol, 1972; Mair et al., 1978; Shipley et al., 1980; Walsh et al., 1986b) in brain centers at or above the inferior colliculus all take substantially longer (longer time constants, later points of maturity) than the development of behavioral response thresholds. Another example for the divergence between physiological and behavioral results is binaural processing in the cat. The development of binaural neural responses, which are important for sound localization and orientation, are already beginning in the first postnatal week (Aitkin and Reynolds, 1975; Moore and Irvine, 1980) and continue after day 30 (Moore and Irvine, 1981) in the inferior colliculus. This is a time course very different from that of the development of behavioral orientation to sounds (Figure 3). Thus, many developmental processes in the auditory system have not, thus far, been shown to be highly correlated with behavioral measures. The major reason is that adequate behavioral tests have not been designed, and it will be very difficult to do so in the future. The best existing correlation between physiological and behavioral measurements of auditory development is that of thresholds as shown in Figures 4 and 5 and in Table 1.

One factor of auditory threshold determination has still to be considered. It is the external ear canal, which is closed by several membranes at birth and opens progressively until at about postnatal day 12 in the cat sound can pass unattenuated to the tympanum (Olmstead and Villablanca, 1980). Thus the high behavioral thresholds up to day 6 (Figures 1 and 4) can be attributed primarily to the attenuation of sound transfer to the middle ear by membranes in the ear canal (see also Chapter 5 by Coleman, this volume).

VII INFLUENCE OF HEARING DEVELOPMENT ON SPEECH ACQUISITION IN HUMANS

As stated earlier, feedback through the auditory system is not necessary for the production of rather normal species-specific sounds in mammals. This seems to be true for nonspeech sounds in humans (e.g., crying, laughing) although little is known (at least to the author) about possible development of such sounds. It is common knowledge, however, that speech acquisition is impossible without hearing. In this last section, therefore, we shall investigate possible influences of hearing development on speech acquisition in humans.

Hearing starts in the uterus as early as the 25th week of gestation when eyeblink responses can be recorded (Birnholz and Benacerraf, 1983). Consistent eyeblink, heart rate, and motor responses to tones and noises occur from the seventh month of pregnancy onward (e.g., Fleischer, 1955; Tanaka and Arayama, 1969; Grimwade et al., 1971; Birnholz and Benacerraf, 1983). Threshold sound pressure levels of perception *in utero* are 80–100 dB (Querleu et al., 1981). This is about 20–25 dB above the intrauterine noise level of 55–60 dB measured in octave bands (Querleu et al., 1981). Compared with the sound pressure levels at the onset of hearing in cat and mouse (Figures 1 and 2), the late human fetus is already very sensitive to sounds. Shortly after birth, in the absence of intrauterine noise, thresholds in the range of 30–60 dB are achieved (Figure 6). At the same time, newborn babies can orient toward a sound source (Wertheimer, 1961), synchronize movements to the rhythm of adult speech (Condon and Sander, 1974), discriminate their mother's voice from that of other persons (DeCasper and Fifer, 1980: DeCasper and Prescott, 1984), and be conditioned to prefer human voices to other sounds (Noirot and Alegria, 1983). All these abilities imply that in humans the major development of the auditory system with regard to absolute sensitivity, sound localization, complex pattern perception, and discrimination takes place *before birth*. A comparable state of auditory function in the cat is reached about 15 days after the onset of hearing (Figures 1 and 3).

The postnatal development of auditory threshold sensitivity in response to tones, complex sounds, and speech is shown for humans in Figures 6 and

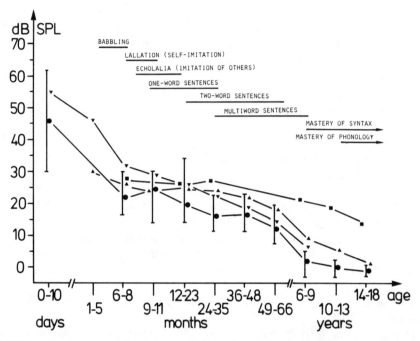

FIGURE 6. Man: postnatal development of absolute auditory thresholds versus age for three representative frequencies (▲, 0.5 kHz; ●, 2 kHz with range of data; ■, 10 kHz) and for noise and complex sounds not including speech (▼). Values are calculated from references given in the text. (Modified from Ehret, 1988.) Also shown is the development of speech acquisition. (Modified from Ehret, 1980.)

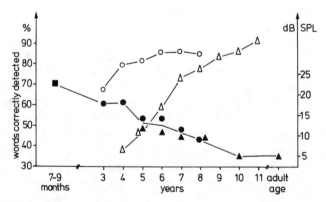

FIGURE 7. Man: development of absolute thresholds for speech perception versus age. Right ordinate, closed symbols: ■, Elliott et al. (1979); ●, Siegenthaler (1969); ▲, Samples and Franklin (1978). Development of intelligibility for normal (○) and fragmented (△) speech. Left ordinate, adapted from Siegenthaler (1969).

7. Threshold curves in Figure 6 are composed of measurements by several authors in which many kinds of methods (see Section II) were applied: tone thresholds (Kennedy, 1957; Suzuki and Ogiba, 1961; Suzuki and Sato, 1961; Eisele et al., 1975; Bench et al., 1976a,b; Schneider et al., 1980; Kankkunen, 1982; Berg and Smith, 1983; Sinnott et al., 1983) and noise and complex sound thresholds without speech (Steinschneider et al., 1966; Suzuki and Origuchi, 1969; Siegenthaler, 1969; Tybergheim and Forrez, 1971; Thompson and Weber, 1974; Samples and Franklin, 1978; Wilson, 1978, Kaga and Tanaka, 1980). Speech response thresholds from data of Siegenthaler (1969), Samples and Franklin (1978), and Elliott et al. (1979) are combined in Figure 7. Thresholds decrease from birth until, by about 10 years of age, adult values are reached. The curves in Figure 6 indicate three major phases of threshold development: a rapid decrease between 10 days and 6 months, a shallow decrease between 6 and 48 months, and a further final decrease between 48 months and 10 years. This pattern, however, seems to be influenced very much by the methods of measurement. Threshold estimations for children under 2 months of age are generally based on unconditioned responses, whereas conditionings of various kinds were used for children up to 6 years old and then regular audiometric procedures thereafter. Thus, the marked threshold decreases between 10 days and 6 months and between 66 months and 6 years could, at least partly, be due to improvement of the testing procedures.

The extraordinarily long developmental period for hearing abilities in man (Figures 6 and 7; see also Ehret, 1988) as compared with mammals (Figures 1–3) certainly does not include maturation processes in the auditory system alone. In Figure 7, time courses for the intelligibility of normal and fragmented speech at 10 dB above hearing threshold are presented (Siegenthaler, 1969). Adult scores for normal speech are reached by about 6 years and for fragmented speech not before 11 years of age. Hence, considerable experience with speech sounds is necessary for full mastery of message identification. A major aspect of the improvement of speech perception and discrimination as shown in Figure 7 is the development of interpretative strategies for treating sounds as a linguistic message (Peterson and Jusczyk, 1984) that have to build upon but certainly go beyond processing in the auditory pathway. Thus, the postnatal improvement of such abilities in man, which are coupled to sound perception, suggests that developmental strategies are used to take *full advantage* of the already present capacity of the auditory system.

In view of these facts, it can be stated that sufficient hearing, which is achieved by 6 months at the latest, is necessary for speech acquisition, but speech development, as shown in Figure 6, has little if anything to do with the further development of absolute auditory sensitivity (Figures 6 and 7). Speech acquisition may be guided by the development of abilities such as concept formation, which becomes apparent in precedence effect sensitivity (Clifton et al., 1984) and pitch perception (Bundy et al., 1982; Clarkson and

Clifton, 1985) in 5–7-month-old babies. This is about the time when babies start imitating vocalizations of their own and of others (lallation and echolalia; Figure 6), which indicates that they can process, recognize, and reproduce well-defined sound units such as syllables. Besides concept formation, a necessary condition for speech acquisition is categorical perception of voice onset time by which syllables, for example, "pa" and "ba," can be discriminated. Categorical perception of voice onset time (Eimas et al., 1971) and discrimination of vowel dimensions (Trehub, 1973; Kuhl and Miller, 1982) have already been identified in 1-month-old children. It seems that analytical capacities of the auditory system necessary as prerequisites for speech recognition, and thus for speech production, are present well before a baby can voluntarily utter his or her first word. Hence, we may end with the simple conclusion that hearing development precedes speech acquisition but does not directly influence it. It is remarkable, however, that both speech development and hearing development reach adult levels by the same age of about 10 years. This coincidence points to influences of developmental brain processes in the prepubescent phase that control the time courses of development of coordinative, motivational, and intellectual function on a general level.

VIII SUMMARY

Inherent in the title of this chapter are approaches to two different fields of research. The first comprises the development of various behaviors in young mammals that can be released by species-specific or other kinds of sounds. Research in the second field could not exist without knowledge collected by studies in the first because it deals with behavioral response audiometry, that is, behavioral responses used as tools for investigating properties of the auditory system. Except with regard to sound communication, there has been little interest in the ontogeny of behavior that may occur in response to sound, or that is coupled with the perception of or release by only acoustic stimuli. Thus the methodological basis for behavioral auditory testing in mammals is still small and comprises mainly unconditioned startle, Preyer, and orientation responses. New sound-dependent behaviors and more sophisticated methods of behavioral observation such as those applied for human babies are necessary for the achievement of significant process in behavioral response audiometry of mammals.

Nevertheless, behavioral studies have contributed valuable insights into the maturation of hearing and have documented, in combination with structural and physiological data, time courses of differential functioning in the auditory pathway and their effects on sound perception. Developmental progress can be described by an exponential function that presents a basis for quantitative comparisons of developmental speed and magnitude. Such comparisons reveal that the development of auditory sensitivity, as measured by unconditioned and conditioned reflexes to sounds, is clearly related to sensitivity increases (threshold decreases) of sound processing up to the auditory midbrain. Differential behavior response to sound stimulation such as directional responses and sound quality discrimination is possible only after a marked sensitivity increase and improvement of frequency selectively in the auditory system. Thus, the time course for development of rather basic properties (e.g., sensitivity) differs from that of more advanced hearing abilities. This also becomes obvious for development of human sound and speech perception in that early processing of the auditory system is supplanted by later development of cognitive function that gives rise to the acquisition of speech.

Behavioral studies can demonstrate nicely the time periods in which major developments of hearing take place. Likewise they do allow comprehensive statements about whether or not an animal can hear and recognize sounds of different qualities and can use these to adjust its behavior in a meaningful way. This can hardly be achieved by anatomical and physiological methods and thus provides impetus for further behavioral investigations of the development of hearing in mammals and other animals.

ACKNOWLEDGMENTS

M. Plummer's helpful comments are gratefully appreciated.

REFERENCES

Aitkin, L. M., and D. R. Moore (1975) Inferior colliculus. II. Development of tuning characteristics and tonotopic oranization in central nucleus of the neonatal cat. J. Neurophysiol. 38:1208–1216.

Aitkin, L. M., and A. Reynolds (1975) Development of binaural responses in the kitten inferior colliculus. Neurosci. Lett. 1:315–319.

Alford, B. R., and R. J. Ruben (1963) Physiological, behavioral and anatomical correlates of the development of hearing in the mouse. Ann. Otol. Rhinol. Laryngol. 72:237–247.

Altman, J., and K. Sudarshan (1975) Postnatal development of locomotion in the laboratory rat. Anim. Behav. 23:896–920.

Anderson, H., and E. A. Wedenberg (1965) A new method for hearing tests in the guinea pig. Acta Otolaryngol. 60:375–393.

Bench, J., Y. Collyer, L. Mentz, and I. Wilson (1976a) Studies in infant behavioural audiometry I. Neonates. Audiology 15:85–105.

Bench, J., Y. Collyer, L. Mentz, and I. Wilson (1976b) Studies in infant behavioural audiometry III. Six-month-old infants. Audiology 15:384–394.

Berg, K. M., and M. Smith (1983) Behavioral thresholds for tones during infancy. J. Exp. Child Psychol. 35:409–425.

Birnholz, J. C., and B. R. Benacerraf (1983) The development of human fetal hearing. Science 222:516–518.

Bischof, H. J. (1985) Environmental influences on early development: A comparison of imprinting and cortical plasticity. In P. P. G. Bateson, and H. Klopfer (eds.): Perspectives in Ethology. New York: Plenum Press, pp. 169–217.

Blatchley, B. J., W. A. Cooper, and J. R. Coleman (1987) Development of auditory brainstem response to tone pip stimuli in the rat. Dev. Brain Res. 32:75–84.

Brown, P. E. (1976) Vocal communication in the pallid bat, Antrozous pallidus. Z. Tierpsychol. 41:34–54.

Brugge, J. F. (1983) Development of the lower brainstem auditory nuclei. In R. Romand (ed): Development of Auditory and Vestibular Systems. New York: Academic Press, pp. 89–120.

Brugge, J. F., E. Javel, and L. M. Kitzes (1978) Signs of functional maturation of peripheral auditory system in discharge patterns of neurons in anteroventral cochlear nucleus of kitten. J. Neurophysiol. 41:1557–1579.

Bundy, R. S., J. Colombo, and J. Singer (1982) Pitch perception in young infants. Dev. Psychol. 18:10–14.

Burghardt, G. M., and M. Bekoff (1978) The Development of Behavior: Comparative and Evolutionary Aspects. New York: Garland Press.

Clarkson, M. G., and R. K. Clifton (1985) Infant pitch perception: Evidence for responding to pitch categories and the missing fundamental. J. Acoust. Soc. Amer. 77:1521–1528.

Clements, M., and J. B. Kelly (1978a) Auditory spatial responses of young guinea pig (Cavia porcellus) during and after ear blocking. J. Comp. Physiol. Psychol. 92:34–44.

Clements, M., and J. B. Kelly (1978b) Directional responses by kittens to an auditory stimulus. Dev. Psychobiol. 11:505–511.

Clifton, R. K., B. A. Morongiello, and J. M. Dowd (1984) A developmental look at an auditory illusion: the precedence effect. Dev. Psychobiol. 17:519–536.

Condon, W. S., and L. W. Sander (1974) Neonate movement is synchronized with adult speech: interactional participation and language acquisition. Science 183:99–101.

DeCasper, A. J., and W. P. Fifer (1980) Of human bonding: newborns prefer their mothers' voices. Science 208:1174–1176.

DeCasper, A. J., and P. A. Prescott (1984) Human newborns' perception of male voices: Preference, discrimination and reinforcing value. Dev. Psychobiol. 17:481–491.

Denes, P., and W. Kocher (1961) The reliability of the Preyer's ear reflex in the mouse (Mus musculus). Naturwissenschaften 48:82–83.

Dolan, D. F., D. C. Teas, and J. P. Walton (1985) Postnatal development of physiological responses in auditory nerve fibers. J. Acoust. Soc. Amer. 78:544–554.

Eggermont, J. J. (1985a) Physiology of the developing auditory system. In S. E. Trehub, and B. Schneider (eds): Auditory Development in Infancy. New York: Plenum Press, pp. 21–45.

Eggermont, J. J. (1985b) Mathematical models for developmental changes. Acta Otolaryngol. (Suppl.) 421:102–107.

Ehret, G. (1974) Age-dependent hearing loss in normal hearing mice. Naturwissenschaften *61*:506.

Ehret, G. (1976) Development of absolute auditory thresholds in the house mouse (*Mus musculus*). J. Amer. Audiol. Soc. *1*:179–184.

Ehret, G. (1977) Postnatal development in the acoustic system of the house mouse in the light of developing masked thresholds. J. Acoust. Soc. Amer. *62*:143–148.

Ehret. G. (1980) Development of sound communication in mammals. Adv. Study Behav. *11*:179–225.

Ehret, G. (1983a) Development of hearing and response behavior to sound stimuli: behavioral studies. In R. Romand (ed.): Development of Auditory and Vestibular Systems. New York: Academic Press, pp. 211–237.

Ehret, G. (1983b) Psychoacoustics. In J. F. Willott (ed.): The Auditory Psychobiology of the Mouse. Springfield: Thomas, pp. 13–56.

Ehret, G. (1985) Behavioral studies on auditory development in mammals in relation to higher nervous system functioning. Acta Otolaryngol. (Suppl.) *421*:31–40.

Ehret, G. (1988) Auditory development: psychophysical and behavioral aspects. In E. Meisami and P. S. Timiras (eds.): Handbook of Human Growth and Developmental Biology. Vol. 1, Part B Boca Raton: CRC Press, pp. 141–154.

Ehret, G., and R. Romand (1981) Postnatal development of absolute auditory thresholds in kittens. J. Comp. Physiol. Psychol. *95*:304–311.

Eimas, P. D., E. R. Siqueland, P. Jusczyk, and J. Vigorito (1971) Speech perception in infants. Science *171*:303–306.

Eisele, W. A., R. C. Berry, and T. H. Shriner (1975) Infant sucking response patterns as a conjugate function of changes in the sound pressure level of auditory stimuli. J. Speech Hear. Res. *18*:296–307.

Elliott, L. L., and D. R. Katz (1980) Children's pure-tone detection. J. Acoust. Soc. Amer. *67*:343–344.

Elliott, L. L., S. Connors, E. Kille, S. Levin, K. Ball, and D. Katz (1979) Children's understanding of monosyllabic nouns in quiet and in noise. J. Acoust. Soc. Amer. *66*:12–21.

Fitzgerald, H. E., E. A. Strommen, and J. P. McKinney (1977) Developmental Psychology: The Infant and Young Child. Homewood: Dorsey Press.

Fleischer, K. (1955) Untersuchungen zur Entwicklung der Innenohrfunktion. Z. Laryngol. Rhinol. Otol. *34*:733–740.

Foss, I., and G. Flottorp (1974) A comparative study of the development of hearing and vision in various species commonly used in experiments. Acta Otolaryngol. *77*:202–214.

Fox, M. W. (1964) The ontogeny of behaviour and neurologic responses in the dog. Anim. Behav. *12*:301–310.

Fox, M. W. (1965) Reflex-ontogeny, and behavioural development of the mouse. Anim. Behav. *13*:234–241.

Fox, M. W. (1966) Neuro-behavioral ontogeny. A synthesis of ethological and neurophysiological concepts. Brain Res. *2*:3–20.

Francis, R. L. (1975) Behavioural audiometry in mammals: review and evaluation of techniques. Symp. Zool. Soc. London *37*:237–289.

Francis, R. L. (1979) The Preyer reflex audiogram of several rodents, and its relation to the "absolute" audiogram in the rat. J. Aud. Res. 19:217–233.

Gould, E. (1971) Studies of the maternal-infant communication and development of vocalizations in the bats Myotis and Eptesicus. Commun. Behav. Biol. 5:263–313.

Gray, L., and E. W. Rubel (1981) Development of responsiveness to supra-threshold acoustic stimulation in chickens. J. Comp. Physiol. Psychol. 95:188–198.

Green, S. (1975) Dialects in Japanese monkeys: vocal learning and cultural transmission of local-specific vocal behavior? Z. Tierpsychol. 38:304–314.

Grimwade, J. C., D. W. Walker, M. Bartlett, S. Gordon, and C. Wood (1971) Human fetal heart rate change and movement in response to sound and vibration. Amer. J. Obstet. Gynecol. 109:86–90.

Hack, M. H. (1963) The developmental Preyer reflex in the sh-1 mouse. J. Aud. Res. 8:449–457.

Haroutunian, V., and B. A. Campbell (1981) Development and habituation of the heart rate orienting response to auditory and visual stimuli in the rat. J. Comp. Physiol. Psychol. 95:166–174.

Haskins, R. (1979) A causal analysis of kitten vocalization: an observational and experimental study. Anim. Behav. 27:726–736.

Henkel, C., and S. B. Edwards (1978) The superior colliculus control of pinna movements in the cat: possible anatomical connections. J. Comp. Neurol. 182:763–776.

Hyson, R. L., and J. W. Rudy (1987) Ontogenetic change in the analysis of sound frequency in the infant rat. Dev. Psychobiol. 20:189–207.

Kaga, K., and Y. Tanaka (1980) Auditory brainstem response and behavioral audiometry. Arch. Otolaryngol. 106:564–566.

Kankkunen, A. (1982) Pre-school children with impaired hearing. Acta Otolaryngol. (Suppl.) 391:1–124.

Kelly, J. B., P. W. Judge, and I. H. Fraser (1987) Development of the auditory orientation response in the albino rat (Rattus norvegicus). J. Comp. Psychol. 101:60–66.

Kennedy, H. (1957) Maturation of hearing acuity. Laryngoscope 67:756–762.

Kerr, L. M., E. M. Ostapoff, and E. W. Rubel (1979) Influence of acoustic experience on the ontogeny of frequency generalization gradients in the chicken. J. Exp. Psychol. 5:97–115.

Knecht, S. (1958) Ist der Preyersche Ohrmuschelreflex als Hörtest verwendbar? Z. Vgl. Physiol. 41:331–341.

Kraus, H.-J., and K. Aulbach-Kraus (1981) Morphological changes in the cochlea of the mouse after onset of hearing. Hear. Res. 4:89–102.

Kuhl, P. K., and J. D. Miller (1982) Discrimination of auditory target dimensions in the presence or absence of variation in a second dimension by infants. Percept. Psychophys. 31:279–292.

Larsell, O., and E. McCrady (1935) Acoustic function in pouch young of the opossum. Proc. Soc. Exp. Biol. Med. 32:774–776.

Larsell, O., E. McCrady, and A. A. Zimmerman (1935) Morphological and functional development of the membraneous labyrinth in the opossum. J. Comp. Neurol. 63:95–118.

Larsen, S. A. (1985) Postnatal maturation of the cat cochlear nuclear complex. Acta Otolaryngol. (Suppl.) 417:1–43.

Mair, I. W. S., H. H. Elverland, and E. Laukli (1978) Development of early auditory-evoked responses in the cat. Audiology 17:469–488.

Markl, H., and G. Ehret (1973) Die Hörschwelle der Maus (Mus musculus). Eine kritische Wertung der Methoden zur Bestimmung der Hörschwelle eines Säugetiers. Z. Tierpsychol. 33:274–286.

Marler, P. (1977) The structure of animal communication sounds. In T. H. Bullock (ed.): Recognition of Complex Acoustic Signals. Berlin: Abakon Verlagsgesellschaft, pp. 17–35.

Marler, P. (1983) Some ethological implications for neuroethology: the ontogeny of bird song. In J.-P. Ewert, R. R. Capranica, and D. J. Ingle (eds.): Advances in Vertebrate Neuroethology. New York: Plenum Press, pp. 21–52.

McCrady, E., E. G. Wever, and C. W. Bray (1937) The development of hearing in the opossum. J. Exp. Zool. 75:503–317.

Mikaelian, D., and R. J. Ruben (1965) Development of hearing in the normal CBA-J mouse. Acta Otolaryngol. 59:451–461.

Miller, J. D., C. S. Watson, and W. P. Covell (1963) Deafening effects of noise on the cat. Acta Otolaryngol. (Suppl.) 176:1–91.

Moore, D. R. (1983) Development of inferior colliculus and binaural audition. In R. Romand (ed.): Development of Auditory and Vestibular Systems. New York: Academic Press, pp. 121–166.

Moore, D. R., and D. R. F. Irvine (1979) The development of some peripheral and central auditory responses in the neonatal cat. Brain Res. 163:49–59.

Moore, D. R., and D. R. F. Irvine (1980) Development of binaural input, response patterns and discharge rate in single units of the cat inferior colliculus. Exp. Brain Res. 38:103–108.

Moore, D. R., and D. R. F. Irvine (1981) Development of responses to acoustic interaural intensity differences in the cat inferior colliculus. Exp. Brain Res. 41:301–309.

Mysliveček, J. (1983) Development of the auditory evoked responses in the auditory cortex in mammals. In R. Romand (ed.): Development of Auditory and Vestibular Systems. New York: Academic Press, pp. 167–209.

Neff, W. D., and J. E. Hind (1955) Auditory thresholds of the cat. J. Acoust. Soc. Amer. 27:480–483.

Noirot, E., and J. Alegria (1983) Neonate orientation towards human voice differs with type of feeding. Behav. Proc. 8:65–71.

Olmstead, C. E., and J. R. Villablanca (1980) Development of behavioral audition in the kitten. Physiol. Behav. 24:705–712.

Payne, R. (1979) Humpbacks: their mysterious songs. Nat. Geograph. 155:18–25.

Parisi, T., and J. R. Ison (1979) Development of the acoustic startle response in the rat: ontogenic changes in the magnitude of inhibition by prepulse stimulation. Dev. Psychobiol. 12:219–230.

Petersen, M. R., and P. W. Jusczyk (1984) On perceptual predispositions for human speech and monkey vocalizations. In P. Marler, and H. S. Terrace (eds.): The Biology of Learning. Berlin: Springer, pp. 585–616.

Potash, M., and J. B. Kelly (1980) Development of directional responses to sounds in the rat (*Rattus norvegicus*). J. Comp. Physiol. Psychol. *94*:864–877.

Powers, B. M., D. Warfield, and R. J. Ruben (1966) Development of the Preyer response to different frequencies in normal CBA-J mice. J. Aud. Res. *6*:425–435.

Pujol, R. (1972) Development of tone-burst responses along the auditory pathway in the cat. Acta Otolaryngol. *74*:383–391.

Querleu, D., X. Renard, and G. Crépin (1981) Perception auditive et réactivité foetal aux stimulations sonores. J. Gyn. Obst. Biol. Repr. *10*:307–314.

Roche, A. F., R. M. Siervogel, J. H. Himes, and D. L. Johnson (1978) Longitudinal study of hearing in children: baseline data concerning auditory thresholds, noise exposure, and biological factors. J. Acoust. Soc. Amer. *64*:1593–1601.

Romand, R. (1983) Development of the cochlea. In R. Romand (ed.): Development of Auditory and Vestibular Systems. New York: Academic Press, pp. 47–88.

Romand, R. (1984) Functional properties of auditory-nerve fibers during postnatal development in the kitten. Exp. Brain Res. *56*:395–402.

Romand, R., and G. Ehret (1984) Development of sound production in normal, isolated, and deafened kittens during the first postnatal months. Dev. Psychobiol. *17*:629–649.

Romand, R., A. Sans, M. R. Romand, and R. Marty (1976) The structural maturation of the stato-acoustic nerve in the cat. J. Comp. Neurol. *170*:1–16.

Rottberger, P. (1980) Die Rolle von akustischer Erfahrung bei der Entwicklung des Lautrepertoires der Hausmaus (*Mus musculus*). Master's thesis, University of Konstanz, Konstanz.

Rubel, E. W., and M. Rosenthal (1975) The ontogeny of auditory frequency generalization in the chicken. J. Exp. Psychol.: Anim. Behav. Proc. *1*:287–297.

Samples, J. M., and B. Franklin (1978) Behavioral responses in 7 to 9 month old infants to speech and non-speech stimuli. J. Aud. Res. *18*:115–123.

Saunders, J. C., K. G. Dolgin, and L. D. Lowry (1980) The maturation of frequency selectivity in C57BL/6J mice studied with auditory evoked response tuning curves. Brain Res. *187*:69–79.

Saunders, J. G., J. A. Kaltenbach, and E. M. Relkin (1983) The structural and functional development of the outer and middle ear. In R. Romand (ed.): Development of Auditory and Vestibular Systems. New York: Academic Press, pp. 3–25.

Schneider, B., S. E. Trehub, and D. Bull (1980) High-frequency sensitivity in infants. Science *207*:1003–1004.

Shalter, M. D., J. C. Fentress, and G. W. Young (1977) Determinants of response of wolf pups to auditory signals. Behaviour *60*:98–114.

Shipley, C., J. S. Buchwald, R. Norman, and D. Guthrie (1980) Brainstem auditory evoked response development in the kitten. Brain Res. *182*:313–326.

Shnerson, A., and J. F. Willott (1979) Development of behavioral response properties in C57BL/6J mouse pups. Exp. Brain Res. *37*:373–385.

Shnerson, A., and J. F. Willott (1980) Ontogeny of the acoustic startle response in C57BL/6J mouse pups. J. Comp. Physiol. Psychol. *94*:36–40.

Siegenthaler, B. M. (1969) Maturation of auditory abilities in children. Int. Audiol. *8*:59–71.

Sinnott, J. M., D. B. Pisoni, and R. N. Aslin (1983) A comparison of pure tone auditory thresholds in human infants and adults. Inf. Behav. Dev. 6:3–17.

Stein, B. E., and H. P. Clamann (1981) Control of pinna movements and sensorimotor register in cat superior colliculus. Brain Behav. Evol. 19:180–192.

Steinschneider, A., E. L. Lipton, and J. B. Richmont (1966) Auditory sensitivity in the infant. Effect of intensity on cardiac and motor responsitivity. Child Dev. 37:233–252.

Suzuki, T., and Y. Ogiba (1961) Conditioned orientation reflex audiometry. Arch. Otolaryngol. 74:192–198.

Suzuki, T., K. Origuchi (1969) Averaged evoked response audiometry (ERA) in young children during sleep. Acta Otolaryngol. (Suppl.) 252:19–28.

Suzuki, T., and I. Sato (1961) Free field startle response audiometry. Ann. Otol. Rhinol. Laryngol. 70:997–1007.

Tanaka, Y., and T. Arayama (1969) Fetal responses to acoustic stimuli. Pract. Oto-Rhino-Laryng. 31:269–273.

Thompson, G. C., and R. B. Masterton (1978) Brain stem auditory pathways involved in reflexive head orientation to sound. J. Neurophysiol. 41:1183–1202.

Thompson, G., and B. A. Weber (1974) Responses of infants and young children to behavior observation audiometry (BOA). J. Speech. Hear. Dis. 39:140–147.

Trehub, S. E. (1973) Infants' sensitivity to vowel and tonal contrasts. Dev. Psychol. 9:91–96.

Trehub, S. E., B. A. Schneider, and M. Endman (1980) Developmental changes in infants' sensitivity to octave-band noises. J. Exp. Child Psychol. 29:282–293.

Turkewitz, G., H. G. Birch, and K. K. Cooper (1972) Responsiveness to simple and complex auditory stimuli in the human newborn. Dev. Psychobiol. 5:7–19.

Tyberghein, J., and G. Forrez (1971) Objective (ERA) and subjective (COR) audiometry in the infant. Acta Otolaryngol. 71:249–252.

Wada, T. (1923) Anatomical and physiological studies on the growth of the inner ear of the albino rat. Mem. Wistar Inst. Anat. Biol. 10:1–74.

Walsh, E. J., J. A. McGee, and E. Javel (1986a) Development of auditory-evoked potentials in the cat. III. Wave amplitudes. J. Acoust. Soc. Amer. 79:745–754.

Walsh, E. J., J. A. McGee, and E. Javel (1986b) Development of auditory-evoked potentials in the cat. II. Wave latencies. J. Acoust. Soc. Amer. 79:725–743.

Wertheimer, M. (1961) Psychomotor coordination of auditory and visual space at birth. Science 134:1692.

Wilson, W. R. (1978) Behavioral assessment of auditory function in infants. In F. D. Minifie and L. L. Lloyd (eds.): Communicative and Cognitive Abilities—Early Behavioral Assessement. Baltimore: University Park Press, pp. 37–59.

Winter, P., R. Handley, D. Ploog, and D. Schott (1973) Ontogeny of squirrel monkey calls under normal conditions and under acoustic isolation. Behaviour 47:230–239.

Chapter Eight

EXPERIENTIAL FACTORS IN AUDITORY DEVELOPMENT

BEN M. CLOPTON AND COLLEEN R. SNEAD

University of Michigan
Ann Arbor, Michigan

I   INTRODUCTION

Over the past decade increasing evidence has indicated that early auditory experience, or the lack of it, affects auditory development. Most of the experimental and clinically related research that bears on this question concerns auditory deprivation in early life, although a few studies have attempted to use special auditory environments to influence the functional development of the auditory system. Observations on changes in peripheral and brainstem anatomy and physiology due to the early auditory environment are examined in this chapter.

The necessity of early sound stimulation for the normal development of peripheral and central auditory pathways is the most prevalent concern. Beyond that, lesser interest has focused on the effectiveness of selective exposure to unique or especially rich auditory environments on this development. Ancillary topics concern periods during development when deprivation or special experience might be most effective, and these bring into question the possibility of recovery from deprivational effects or loss of enhanced function.

The motivation behind these inquiries is an interest in how much of the function of adult human hearing is determined by early experience. As will be seen, it is unlikely that early exposure to simple sounds has much potential for shaping adult auditory processing. No support exists for an early impact from such stimuli as tones, which carry little information but serve as benchmarks against which to measure basic auditory function. On the other hand, we know little about how processes underlying the perceptions of complex sounds are established. Clearly some of them are learned and, in the case of speech, can have distinctive cultural components. In overview, we can entertain the concept that higher organisms undergo a period of environmental tuning that optimizes their response to their surrounds, tailoring their neural processes to complexities they would normally encounter and with which they would have to deal.

The published work on the functional development of the auditory system is limited, and observations on its plasticity under conditions of varying acoustic environments are very limited. If one further attempts to derive implications for information processing in auditory pathways so that mechanisms of plasticity might be designated for study, the evidence is very incomplete on almost every question that might be raised. What follows is a consideration of the strategies for probing and gaining information about early experiential influences on anatomical and physiological measures of cochlear and brainstem structure and function.

II STRATEGIES FOR DETERMINING EXPERIENTIAL FACTORS

The strategy one takes in approaching the effect of experiential factors on development depends on the process or structure under scrutiny. Anatomical structures illustrate one extreme of focus for developmental study. Closely associated with them are physiological measures of basic function such as cochlear microphonics and whole-nerve responses to clicks. A finer level of physiological observation is reached with such techniques as tone-on-tone masked tuning curves and single-fiber or neuron spike activity. Measures of tuning and phase locking to sinusoids and combinations of sinusoids are generally thought to relate to the capacity of the system to carry information about biologically important sounds such as speech and species-specific sounds, but more direct indicators of these higher levels of processing are needed.

Two major classes of experimental intervention into early auditory development have been used. They differ in the degree of intervention. One involves biochemical, metabolic, and surgical manipulation of the cochlea to influence normal development. These include such procedures as the administration of ototoxic drugs, alteration of normal biochemistry, and destruction of structures of the inner ear. Most of these provide a basis for restricting or eliminating sound experience. The second class involves manipulations that would be more easily termed "experiential." These are acoustic manipulations of the environment or of the mechanisms that underlie normal auditory experience. This class includes relative auditory deprivation over restricted periods of development, enrichment of early auditory experience, and subtotal acoustic trauma. The goal of these manipulations is to modify but not totally eliminate input to the system.

If sounds of the early environment are varied experimentally, three largely independent dimensions can be identified. The first is related to the intensity of sound, ranging from total quiet through reduced sound, normal intensities, more intense sounds, and finally, traumatic levels of sound exposure. The second pertains to the informational content of the sound, ranging from random background sounds that are poor or lacking in information through normal to information-rich sounds such as intraspecies communication sounds. The range of sounds along this dimension is effectively infinite. A third possible dimension is that of salience, that is, linkage to an animal's behavior. This involves changes in the relative locus of a sound source with movement, acoustic feedback from other animals, and similar aspects of sounds that depend on what the developing animal does. It might be expected that an extensive array of brain mechanisms would be tapped by control of environmental feedback to an animal.

Only the first dimension has been manipulated in most development studies, primarily as a way to deprive the auditory system of input. It is probably the least likely to induce adaptive tuning due to experience because it is not inherently a strong dimension for informational content in sounds. There is no apparent need to optimize relative intensity cues except for certain operations affecting signal-to-noise ratios for the detection of weak or noisy signals. On the other hand, a few physiological and behavioral measures have been used to examine early sound experience that are especially indicative of the auditory system's detection, discrimination, or localization capabilities for sounds. These include neural frequency tuning, synchrony to the temporal structure of sounds, and differential responses to binaural cues as well as behavioral paradigms to evaluate localization.

However, no attention has been paid to systematic variation of feedback cues in the early acoustic environment. The paucity of work in the auditory system stands in contrast to the numerous detailed investigations in the visual system (see Chapter 4).

III STRUCTURAL CHANGES

A Cochlea and Auditory Nerve

Along with limited information about inner ear histopathology from auditory deprivation, there is evidence from drug, hormone, and noise studies supporting the concepts of plasticity and sensitive periods for cochlear structures. Uziel (1986) has demonstrated periods of maximal sensitivity to thyroid hormone deficiency for several organ of Corti structures. These periods coincide with the individual structure's period of maximal morphological development in rat pups (6–13 days postnatal for inner sulcus epithelium, 6–10 days for pillar cells, and the second and third weeks for outer hair cells and their efferent innervation).

Several investigators have shown an increased sensitivity to noise damage in developing cochleae. Falk et al. (1974), Douek et al. (1976), and Dodson et al. (1978) demonstrated significantly more outer hair cell damage from noise exposure in guinea pigs under 8 weeks old. Bock and Saunders (1977) reported a similar sensitivity in young hamsters. Rat pups 16–40 days old exposed to white noise showed greatest noise damage to the organ of Corti if exposed at 22 days after birth (DAB), and the damage from a single exposure (30 minutes at 120 dB) exhibited continued degeneration for more than 2 months postexposure (Lenoir et al., 1979).

There also appears to be a period during development when the cochlea is especially susceptible to ototoxic antibiotics (Pujol, 1986). This maximally sensitive period corresponds with the period of rapid cochlear development, beginning with the onset of function and ending when adult morphology is achieved (Akiyoshi et al., 1974; Uziel et al., 1977, 1979).

Although early qualitative investigations suggested that mouse and rat cochlear structures were unaffected by auditory deprivation (Webster and Webster, 1977; Coleman and O'Connor, 1979), a more recent quantitative study has found a 17% decrease in mouse spiral ganglion cell size at 45 DAB following ligation of the external auditory meatus at 4 DAB (Webster, 1983a). However, Moore and colleagues (1989) found no significant change in spiral ganglion cell number, area, or nucleolar eccentricity in the ferret following 3–15 months of ear plug-induced conductive hearing loss.

Although no gross anatomical changes have been seen in cochlear hair cells or supporting cells at the light microscopic level, the first-order neurons as well as those in the auditory brainstem are impacted by changes in activity of a deprived cochlea. Electron microscopic evaluation of cochlear structures may demonstrate subtle intracellular changes in hair cells, supporting cells, or stria vascularis that would provide information about their relationship to auditory nerve function. It is clear that further investigation of deprivation effects on the developing cochlea and its afferent and efferent innervation is needed to better evaluate experimentally induced changes in neurons of the auditory pathways.

B   Cochlear Nuclei

Several groups have studied the effects of monaural and/or binaural auditory deprivation on cells in the cochlear nuclei of mammals and their homologues in birds. Deprivation procedures have included the use of earplugs, surgical ligation of the external auditory meatus, and ossicular removal to produce broadband conductive deficits of 40–55 dB (Killackey and Ryugo, 1977; Webster and Webster, 1977, 1979; Coleman and O'Connor, 1979; Feng and Rogowski, 1980; Conlee and Parks, 1981, 1983; Coleman et al., 1982; Blatchley et al., 1983; Smith et al., 1983; Webster, 1983a,b; Brugge et al., 1985; Schweitzer and Cant, 1985; Tucci and Rubel, 1985; Tucci, et al., 1987; Trune and Morgan, 1988a,b; Moore et al., 1989). Another means of producing a conductive reduction of auditory input has been the rearing of mice in sound-attenuating chambers with mothers rendered avocal (Webster and Webster, 1977, 1979; Evans, et al, 1983). Complete deafferentation has been accomplished by removal of the embryonic otocyst or destruction of the cochlea (Levi-Montalcini, 1949; Parks, 1979, 1981; Trune, 1982a,b, 1983; Jackson and Parks, 1983; Parks and Jackson, 1984; Schweitzer and Cant, 1985; Parks et al., 1987; Moore and Kowalchuk, 1988; Hashisaki and Rubel, 1989).

Most studies of the effects of conductive deprivation on the anteroventral cochlear nucleus (AVCN) or its avian homologue the nucleus magnocellularis (NM) have found a substantial decrease in the overall volume of the ipsilateral nuclei (Coleman et al., 1982), and at least a 12% decrease in the cross-sectional area of spherical cell somata (Webster and Webster, 1977, 1979; Coleman and O'Connor, 1979; Conlee and Parks, 1981; Blatchley et al., 1983; Webster, 1983a,b). However, Moore et al. (1989) reported no change in AVCN volume in the ferret following conductive deprivation. Position-dependent effects on spherical cell size in both birds and mammals have suggested a deprivation gradient roughly corresponding to the tonotopic arrangement, with the greatest reductions in the somata of cells located in the highest frequency areas of the chick (Conlee and Parks, 1981) and the rat (Blatchley et al., 1983). Trune and Morgan (1988b) reported significant reductions in cytoplasm, but not nuclei, of spherical and globular cells in deprived mice. Although there was a trend toward greater reduction in the high frequency regions, the differences were not statistically significant.

Conlee and Parks (1981) also demonstrated a significant (32–38%) decrease in the dendritic length of NM neurons. Other investigators (Tucci and Rubel, 1985; Tucci et al., 1987) found no changes in cell size in the NM following purely conductive deprivation but did see an 18–20% decrease in cell size when the oval window was punctured in addition to columellar removal. These findings raise the question of methodology. The apparent discrepancies among experimental results may be related to the difficulty in producing a pure conductive hearing loss without affecting the cochlea. In a study of ultrastructural effects of conductive hearing loss, Trune and Morgan (1988a) reported a significant reduction in auditory nerve terminals in the deprived mouse AVCN and an increased number of non-primary terminals, suggesting stimulus regulation of auditory nerve arborization and competition for synaptic space. They also found the mitochondria within the deprived neurons to be smaller, darker and apparently less active metabolically (Trune and Morgan, 1988a).

In addition, a few studies have examined the effects of deprivation on cells of the contralateral CN. These neurons show either no change (Conlee and Parks, 1981; Trune and Morgan, 1988b) or slight increase in size (Coleman and O'Connor, 1979) as a result of deprivation procedures of the opposite ear. Using a retrograde tracer injected into IC to label projection neurons, Moore et al. (1989) found an increased number labeled in the CN contralateral to the conductive hearing loss.

Deafferentation causes about a 40% reduction in the volume of the ipsilateral NM, a 30% loss of second-order neurons, and a 20% decrease in neuron soma size in chickens (Levi-Montalcini, 1949; Parks, 1979). Trune (1982a) found a decrease in number of cells in the mouse AVCN but no change in cell size. More recently, Hashisaki and Rubel (1989) found a 58% reduction in neuron number and a 38% decrease in size of remaining neurons in the AVCN of gerbils with cochleas unilaterally ablated in the first postnatal week and sacrificed 2 weeks later. Despite the obvious effects of auditory deprivation on development in the NM, Parks and Jackson (1984) found that otocyst ablation had no effect on the transformation of cells from multipolar (10 dendrites per cell) at E3 to unipolar by day E18. Noncochlear afferents do not arrive at the NM until P16 (Jhaveri and Morest, 1982). Therefore, they cannot contribute to this transformation or to the maintenance of the approximately 70% of the cells that remain. However, Jackson and Parks (1983) discovered a new projection to deafferented NM neurons from the contralateral (nondeprived) NM between E11 and P10 as well as similar sprouting on both sides after bilateral ablation. This suggests that synaptic specificity may not be important for cell maintenance but that any functional synaptic input may be sufficient. However, the viability of the new projection is yet to be determined physiologically.

The effects of deprivation on cells of the posteroventral cochlear nucleus (PVCN), the dorsal cochlear nucleus (DCN) in mammals, and the corresponding nucleus angularis (NA) in birds have not been studied as thoroughly as on AVCN cells. Coleman et al. (1982) found significant decreases in total volume of both the ventral and dorsal cochlear nuclei in rat ipsilateral to a conductive blockage when the deprivation was initiated at 10 (DAB), just prior to normal opening of the external meatus and onset of function. Webster and his co-workers compared the effects of ligation of the external auditory meatus with that of rearing mice in a sound-attenuated chamber with avocal mothers. They reported similar findings with both methods of deprivation, including decreases in some size of octopus cells, globular cells, multipolar cells, fusiform cells, and granule cells (Webster and Webster, 1977, 1979; Webster 1983a,b). When the deprivation was reversed at 45 DAB, the octopus cells increased to their normal size but the other cell types remained significantly smaller than their normal control counterparts (Webster and Webster, 1979). They also found that mice subjected to the same deprivation at 45 days exhibited no changes in somal size in the ventral cochlear nuclei, the medial nucleus of the trapezoid body, or the inferior colliculus (Webster, 1983c), indicating that deprivation effects are limited to a sensitive period during development. Further evidence for this sensitive period is provided by Blatchley et al. (1983), who unilaterally deprived rats of different ages beginning at postnatal day 10. If rats are deprived from postnatal day 10, spherical cell size of the AVCN is greatly reduced compared to cells of animals deprived from day 16, just a few days following the opening of the external acoustic neatus. Therefore, the first few days of hearing may be especially important for morphological development of these, and likely, other cells of the auditory system.

Deafferentation via cochlear ablation has been shown to cause a 46% decrease in volume of the ventral and dorsal cochlear nuclei, and a 34% decrease in number of cells without significant changes in cell soma size (Trune, 1982a; see also Moore and Kowalchuk, 1989). Dendritic field cross-sectional area was decreased in the deprived globular cell area, and multipolar cell dendrites were significantly shorter than nondeprived and normal controls throughout the cochlear nuclei (Trune, 1982b). Schweitzer and Cant (1985) demonstrated a disruption of the normal spatial orientation of dendrites in hamsters following early deprivation via ossicular removal and/or cochlear ablation. Although the absolute numbers of neurons projecting to the IC were reduced by deprivation, the proportion of neurons projecting to the IC from the cochlear nuclei was equal to that of control animals (Trune, 1983). Furthermore, there is an increase in the number and terminal distribution of ipsilaterally projecting CN neurons to the IC opposite the side of cochlear lesion (Trune, 1983; Moore and Kitzes, 1985; Moore and Kowalchuk, 1988).

In the chicken, otocyst ablation has been associated with a significant reduction (70%) in the size of NA (Levi-Montalcini, 1949; Parks, 1979), the avian homologue to the mammalian PVCN and DCN. Both studies found significant decreases in the number of neurons in NA, but Levi-Montalcini found an 83% decrease while Parks found only a 40% decrease. Both groups reported drastic changes in the shape of the nucleus, and Parks found a group of cells that were separated by several hundred micrometers ventro-medial and rostral from the normal location of the main nucleus. The difference in neuron counts between the two investigations is most likely because Parks included this ectopic group of cells in his count.

A recent study of jerker mutant mice, which never develop hearing, by Anniko and colleagues (1989) demonstrated incomplete maturation of the VCN. The volume of VCN was reduced as was the cross-sectional area of globular cell somata. Although the VCN in the heterozygote, which has normal hearing, was significantly larger than that of the deaf homozygote, it was smaller than that of a normal mouse. This suggests that there may be a genetic link to the smaller VCN size in the jerker mouse which is further reduced by auditory deprivation. There were no reported differences in DCN volume between the deaf homozygote, the normal hearing hetero-zygote, and the normal mouse (Anniko, et al., 1989). Webster et al. (1986) reported normal VCN and DCN maturation up to 14 postnatal days in the Shaker-2 mouse, with no further growth after that. The cessa-tion of CN growth coincides with the onset of cochlear degeneration. Because non-auditory areas of the brainstem continue to grow in volume, it is suggested that the failure of the CN to fully mature is due to the absence of stimulation. However, programmed genetic effects cannot be ruled out.

C Superior Olive and Inferior Colliculus

The effects of monaural deprivation on the structure of the olivary complex and IC have been studied to a very limited extent. Webster's group has reported reductions in cell size in the medial nucleus of the trapezoid body and the lateral superior olive contralateral to the monaurally deprived ear (Webster, 1983a,b).

Feng and Rogowski (1980) classified neurons of the rat medial superior olive (MSO) into three categories based on the relative amount of dendritic material on each side of the neuron. In control animals there were a small number of neurons with equally balanced dendritic trees and larger but equal numbers of right and left dominant neurons in each MSO. Monaural occlusion of the right ear produced an increased number of neurons with larger left-sided dendritic fields and equally balanced dendrites in the MSO both ipsi- and contralateral to the deprived ear, indicating a bias toward input from the normal ear. Interestingly, when both ears were occluded, the MSO on each side was no different than in the control animals. Similarly, in the chicken, the nucleus laminaris (NL) dendrites receiving input from the deprived ear were significantly shorter than normal controls, although the diameter of the dendrites was unchanged (Parks, 1981; Smith et al., 1983). Smith et al. (1983) also reported a tonotopic gradient in their study, with dendrites shortened in the high-frequency areas and lengthened in the low-frequency areas receiving input from the deprived side. This frequency-specific effect is probably related both to the different rates of maturation of high- and low-frequency areas and to the earplug itself reducing high-frequency stimulation to a greater degree. The reduction in dendritic length is much less dramatic if both otocysts are removed (Parks, et al., 1987) indicating that it is the symmetry of input, rather than absolute level of input, which apparently regulates dendritic length.

Surprisingly few anatomical studies have investigated the IC despite the emphasis of physiological studies on this structure. Monaural conductive hearing loss has been reported to cause a decrease in soma size in the contralateral CNIC (central nucleus of the IC) in mice deprived during the period between 12 and 24 days after birth (Webster, 1983a,b). In rats monaurally deprived at birth, both sides of the IC are reportedly reduced in size and lose their characteristic lamination (Killackey and Ryugo, 1977). In contrast, the IC on each side is essentially normal and there is no significant reduction in cell size following binaural deprivation (Killackey and Ryugo, 1977; Webster and Webster, 1977, 1979). These findings, like the evidence from the superior olive complex, suggest the probability of competitive interactions between ears as an important factor in development in the brainstem nuclei receiving binaural afferent innervation.

D Sensitive Periods

The anatomical data available relating auditory deprivation to development clearly suggests a period during development when the cochlea and auditory brainstem neurons are particularly susceptible to the effects of auditory deprivation. Prior to this period, experiential influences appear to be negligible. The cell types migrate appropriately and differentiate, with no impact from experimental manipulation of sound stimulation. And after auditory function has fully matured, stimulus deprivation has little or no effect on structure. The cochlear structures are most sensitive to noise and ototoxic damage during the period when they are undergoing their most rapid development (Pujol, 1986). Similarly, the periods of increased morphological sensitivity to deprivation in the auditory brainstem neurons coincide with the onset and rapid development of function as well as synapse formation.

Anatomical investigations of experiential influences on auditory structural development have been limited to the assessment of the impact of auditory deprivation. Several manipulations have been employed to this end. It is important to evaluate these methods of deprivation in order to distinguish between true experiential effects and alterations that may be attributed to the experimental manipulation itself as well as to an understanding of the relative degree of sound attenuation provided by the manipulation and its relation to frequency. Systematic studies of the intermediate stages of development in normal animals as well as experimentally manipulated animals need to be accomplished in order to more fully determine the role of auditory experience in development and plasticity of anatomical development.

IV   PHYSIOLOGICAL CHANGES

It is necessary to distinguish among physiological measures with regard to their implication for the representation and processing of information in the auditory system. Some measures, such as latency of response, characterize a feature of field potentials or spike activity that is referenced to a stimulus parameter—timing in the case of latency. Latency does, in fact, change in some cases due to a specific early sound environment. It is not, however, apparent how the population of neurons in the auditory system change in their relative latencies of responses, and it is this population function of latency that is most informative about the representation and processing of biologically important sounds. In contrast, the relational measures between neural responses to two or more stimuli such as tuning convey an index of resolution that has a more obvious implication for those sounds. Paradigms estimating binaural interaction are another example of relational measures of neural responses. As increasing attention is focused on the impact of normal or abnormal acoustic experience during development for information processing, the requirements of the neuronal response measure will be critical.

The influence of early conditions of acoustic stimulation on the physiology of the auditory system has been investigated primarily for the effects of deprivation. Measures of these effects have concentrated on the classical indices of neural responses: latency, threshold, tuning, and relationships to stimulus intensity. The major exceptions to this involve estimates of binaural interaction or related behavioral measures of localization. While the primary measures suggest deprivational effects that are interesting, their importance for auditory processing for normal development is unclear in most cases.

A   Cochlea and Auditory Nerve

The cochlea undergoes significant changes with maturation, but there is minimal evidence for experiential effects on its physiology other than damaging ones (Bock and Saunders, 1977; Bock and Seifter, 1978; Lenoir et al., 1979). Some observations indirectly suggest that cochlear function may be influenced by early deprivation. The latency of the N_1 potential decreases with age (Uziel et al., 1981) to the short latencies of the adult. Decreased latencies to clicks have been repeatedly observed in rodents deprived of early sound stimulation through meatal blockade (Clopton and Silverman, 1977) or rearing in a quiet environment (Evans et al., 1983). This decrease is associated with field potentials of the auditory nerve indicating more rapid spike generation in neurons of the spiral ganglion. In mice, the size of the spiral ganglion neurons is smaller than normal after conductive acoustic blocks (Webster, 1983a). This and more central observations raise implications of smaller cell sizes for transmission velocity through the auditory system, which will be discussed later.

Concepts of cochlear processing are changing rapidly, and dynamic elements and efferent control are implicated (Winslow and Sachs, 1987). For example, micromechanical tuning in hair cell systems is well established, and its existence in mammalian cochleas is likely (Clopton, 1986). Efferent influences appear to affect the processing of signals in noisy environments (Dewson, 1968; Winslow and Sachs, 1987). Tuning curves derived from tone-on-tone masking indicate that the sharpness of tuning increases in kittens over the first week through the third after birth (Carlier and Pujol, 1978; Carlier et al., 1979). Should early sound deprivation influence dynamic filter characteristics of the cochlea either directly or through effects on efferent control, both frequency resolution and temporal measures such as latency might be affected. Filter bandwidth, for example, is inversely related to the latency of response to a transient and might underlie the deprivational latency decrease observed.

B Cochlear Nuclei and Superior Olivary Complex

The primary indices of physiological function show that threshold, tuning, and synchrony undergo maturational approximations to adult values (Brugge et al., 1978; Carlier and Pujol, 1978). The anatomical changes in the cochlear nuclei resulting from developmental deprivation would suggest that physiological sequelae would be evident. Direct observations are largely lacking, however. Functional implications have, nevertheless, been inferred from a number of observations on anatomical changes in the cochlear nuclei, physiological changes in the inferior colliculus, and behavioral changes that are all induced by deprivation. Spherical cells in the anteroventral cochlear nucleus projecting to the MSO, as noted previously, depend on balanced binaural input during development to maintain their size (Coleman and O'Connor, 1979). In conjunction with the other evidence to be described, a competitive process between spherical cells in the left and right cochlear nuclei appears to occur during development, resulting in different balances of facilitatory input to higher centers. This conclusion, to be elaborated, implies plasticity that is predicated on contralateral input that does not directly activate the nucleus undergoing change.

Current functional views of the cochlear nuclei are largely derived from a combination of three anatomical features—locus in the cochlear nuclei, soma-dendritic shape, and connectivity—and two functional measures—a frequency–intensity response area and the spike–time response pattern (peristimulus–time histogram) to tone bursts. The globular and spherical bushy cells have been identified as being reduced in size due to deprivation (Webster and Webster, 1977; Coleman and O'Connor, 1979; Blatchley et al., 1983; Webster, 1983a,b,c). It is interesting to note that both project to portions of the superior olivary complex that are identified with binaural processing; the medial superior olive and the medial nucleus of the trapezoid body, which projects to the lateral superior olive.

C Inferior Colliculus

More observations have been made in the IC of single-unit activity after manipulations of the early acoustic environment than for any other site. Deprivation causes distinctive changes in IC responses (Clopton and Silverman, 1978; Kitzes and Semple, 1985). Units in the IC of rodents are normally activated primarily by contralateral stimulation, but after cochlear ablation in gerbils at 2 DAB ipsilateral stimulation at 6 months evokes responses that are comparable to contralaterally evoked ones on the basis of threshold, latency, peak rate, and pattern of response (Kitzes and Semple, 1985). Deprivation by meatal ligation in rats from 10 DAB produced changes in responses evoked later from the deprived ear, the major effects being an increase in the latency of responses to clicks for high-frequency units and a decrease in the duration of the response (Clopton and Silverman, 1978). This should be contrasted to smaller interpeak latencies seen in mice after deprivation for the auditory-evoked far-field potentials (Evans et al., 1983). Reconciliation of these two measures is uncertain but, as discussed earlier, may have involved cochlear as well as central effects of deprivation.

A more complete view of the impact of deprivational effects on IC responses is seen when binaural processing is evaluated. In rats (Silverman and Clopton, 1977), as illustrated in Figures 1 and 2, monaural deprivation through reversible meatal blockade has its major effect on unit responses of the IC on the side ipsilateral to the deprivation. Whereas clicks to an ear would normally suppress spike activity evoked by simultaneous clicks to the opposite ear for normal adults, the very young and for an ear opposite a deprived ear (Figure 1), this influence is reduced or lost with deprivation from 10 DAB (Silverman and Clopton, 1977). Binaural deprivation does not have this effect. If deprivation is begun much after day 30, the loss of ipsilateral suppression of IC responses from the deprived ear is much less, and after day 60 the effects of deprivation are minimal (Figure 2). These results indicate that reduced sound input to one ear during a sensitive period (10–30 DAB for the rat) disrupts binaural interaction for clicks, specifically causing an imbalance in ipsilateral suppression, which normally signals the relative intensity of sounds at the two ears. The lack of effect with binaural deprivation, in conjunction with the structural changes at cochlear nuclei noted earlier, points to a competitive process during development that normally ends in a precise signaling of sound locus cues, especially near midline positions.

This effect may depend partially on the nature of the click stimuli. Brugge et al. (1985) used more prolonged meatal atresias to examine monaural deprivation effects in the cat. Tone-evoked responses in area AI of the auditory cortex showed reduced binaural interaction after removal of the atresia, but the effect of deprivation was less. Threshold elevation for the deprived ear also was greater than in the rat. These results point to stimulus and perhaps species differences that affect the evaluation of deprivation

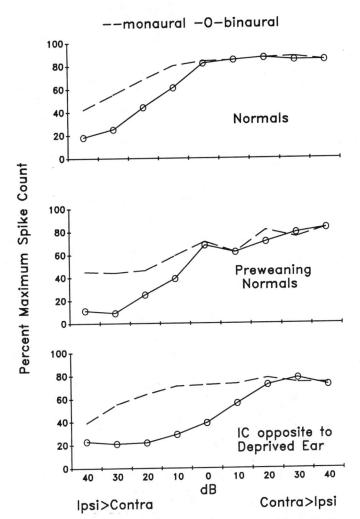

FIGURE 1. Binaural interaction at one inferior colliculus for clicks delivered to the opposite ear or to both ears in rat. Stimuli of increasing intensity (left to right in 5-dB steps) delivered only to the opposite ear caused an increasing spike rate that saturates. The addition of clicks to the ipsilateral ear in a balanced manner to mimic normally occurring binaural intensity differences reduces the monaural response when more intense than the contralateral click. This effect, shown as an average of many units, occurs for normal adults, pups immediately after the onset of hearing, and at the colliculus opposite a deprived ear.

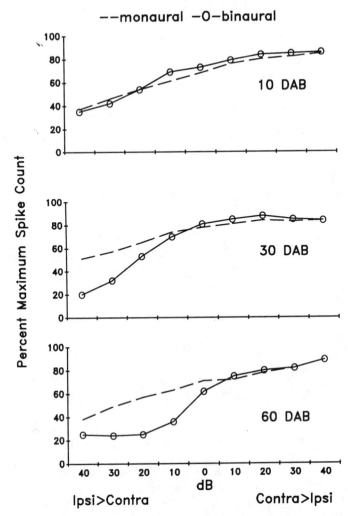

FIGURE 2. Binaural interaction after meatal atresia at 10, 30, and 60 days after birth (DAB). Recording was ipsilateral to unilateral atresia after its removal. Early monaural deprivation reduces ipsilateral suppression of contralaterally evoked responses.

effects. They also emphasize the value of a careful characterization of monaural changes due to deprivation.

Behavioral observations support the existence of binaural mechanisms tuned during development in both mammals (Clements and Kelly, 1978) and avians (Knudsen et al., 1982, 1984a,b). The behavioral observations support the existence of a sensitive period during which monaural occlusion can strongly influence binaural processing but after which little if any comparable plasticity exists.

Attempts to bias neural responses of the IC through early exposure to sounds having specific spectral or temporal features have been minimal (Moore and Aitkin, 1975; Clopton and Winfield, 1976; Sanes and Constantine-Paton, 1985). Simple exposure to selected frequencies does not appear to influence tonotopic organization (Moore and Aitkin, 1975). Biasing was reported for exposure to a repeating sequence of tone sweeps of increasing or decreasing frequency alternating with noise bursts (Clopton and Winfield, 1976). Rats were exposed during the first months of life to the upward or downward sweeping pattern, and relative responses to the patterns were measured for spike activity in the IC of adults. A biasing of responses toward the pattern of exposure was found superimposed on a decrement in overall responsiveness. Unexpectedly, the effect was most apparent in responses to the noise segment of the pattern.

D Postnatal Influences on Functional Development

Experimental evidence supports as well-established only two developmentally sensitive effects of the acoustic environment on auditory development in the periphery and brainstem: cochlear trauma caused by excessive sound intensities and tuning of the binaural system. Only the second is of interest if we restrict our attention to effects that arise from plasticity of central processing. The support for the binaural effects are, however, extensive, including anatomical, physiological, and behavioral observations, many in both mammals and avians.

Binaural paradigms lend themselves to testing the integration of stimuli because of the control available due to ear separation. In addition, binaural interaction is perhaps the closest analogy to the concept of the visual receptive field, which has guided much of the work in that modality. The bulk of acoustic processing, however, is readily accomplished with monaural input pointing to the lack of knowledge about experiential effects on the utilization of complex sounds such as speech. The heuristic value of looking for the interaction of binaural stimuli or of monaural stimulus components defined temporally and spectrally would suggest that the sweep–tone pattern is a reasonable first attempt at detecting biasing to a spectrotemporal feature. The space from which such patterns might be drawn is, unfortunately, multidimensional and very large.

The obviously devastating effects of congenital deafness on language acquisition have long been recognized by educators and clinicians. Observations of an apparent relationship of the age at onset and severity of hearing loss with the degree of impact on language acquisition initiated the concept of a "sensitive period" for language learning in the first 3 years of life. Studies of children with normal hearing and language development revealed the preschool years as a period of extremely rapid growth in form and use of language (deVilliers and deVilliers, 1978). These investigations have also determined that language is acquired almost exclusively via auditory input.

Since middle ear effusion and its resultant fluctuating conductive hearing loss are quite prevalent in the preschool years (Paradise, 1980; Teele et al. 1980), there is considerable interest in learning their effects on speech and language acquisition. Early retrospective studies utilizing school records, physician's files, and parental reports indicated a relationship between auditory processing deficits and a high incidence of chronic otitis media (Holm and Kunze, 1969; Lewis, 1976; Zinkus et al., 1978; Gottlieb et al., 1979; Freeman and Parkins, 1969; Bennett et al., 1980; Zinkus and Gottlieb, 1980). More recent investigations using subjects matched for intelligence, age, sex, and socioeconomic status have revealed language delays as well as deficits in overall verbal ability and in specific tasks requiring complex auditory memory or selective auditory attention in children with histories of recurrent middle ear effusion (Brandes and Ehinger, 1981; Sak and Ruben, 1981; Friel-Patti et al., 1982). Hoffman-Lawless et al. (1981) found that children whose early recurrent middle ear disease was treated surgically performed as well as matched controls on a number of auditory processing tests at ages 7 and 9 years, supporting the premise that elimination of the auditory deprivation associated with otitis media allows processing to develop normally. Schery (1985) surveyed over 700 children, highlighting the relationship between hearing status and both receptive and expressive language development. The magnitude of the language deficits correlated well with degree of hearing loss, and even mild losses (15–25 dB), if persistent in early childhood, affected language acquisition. This study, and one by Hall and Hill in 1986, demonstrated significant effects of early chronic otitis media on language development, but the effects varied considerably among individual children.

Clearly the relationship between middle ear disease and language learning is a complicated one, and it is dependent upon several factors including age of onset, duration of episodes, severity of hearing loss, intrinsic qualities of the child, and the linguistic environment (Hall and Hill, 1986). For more thorough discussion of this topic, excellent review articles are available (Ventry, 1980; Eimas and Kavanagh, 1986; Ruben, 1986).

Unilateral hearing loss, and its resultant one-sided auditory deprivation, has long been considered inconsequential. However, unilaterally hearing-impaired adults consistently report difficulty understanding speech in noise, and several recent studies have shown that children with unilateral hearing loss exhibit significant delays in educational achievement, communication disorders, and behavior problems (Bess et al., 1986; Culbertson and Gilbert, 1986; Klee and Davis-Dansky, 1986).

A relationship between early auditory deprivation and language/cognitive function has been established. However, it is complicated by many other factors in the child's life. If the human auditory brainstem is altered by deprivation as has been described in birds and lower mammals, there are strong implications for early intervention and further investigation of this phenomenon.

V SUMMARY

Anatomical, physiological, and behavioral observations validate plasticity in cochlear and brainstem pathways. While some is best described as a heightened susceptibility to damage during a certain period of development, much of the evidence directly or indirectly implicates mechanisms that underlie the integration of and selective responses to stimulus components. By far the strongest case is made from observations of monaural deprivation and its effect on neuronal anatomy in the cochlear nuclei and superior olivary complex, binaural interaction in the inferior colliculus, and behavioral deficits of localization. Some results support the possibility that early exposure to specific sound patterns can bias central responsiveness toward those patterns. Observations on humans, while often difficult to evaluate due to their correlative nature, point to important periods during language acquisition when a degradation of the auditory environment can have detrimental effects.

REFERENCES

Akiyoshi, M., K. Sato, K. Sugahirok, and T. Tajima (1974) Ototoxic effects of 3', 4'-dideoxykanamycin B on the inner ear in the intrauterune guinea pig embryo. Jap. J. Antibiot. 27: 745.

Anniko, M., B. Sjöström, and D. B. Webster (1989) The effects of auditory deprivation on morphological maturation of the ventral cochlear nucleus. Arch. Otorhinolaryngol. 246:43–47.

Bennett, F. C., S. H. Ruuska, and R. Sherman (1980) Middle ear function in learning-disabled children. Pediatrics 6:254–260

Bess, F. H., A. M. Tharpe, and A. M. Gibler (1986) Auditory performance of children with unilateral sensorineural hearing loss. Ear & Hearing. 7:20–26.

Blatchley, B. F., J. E. Williams, and J. R. Coleman (1983) Age-dependent effects of acoustic deprivation on spherical cells of the rat anteroventral cochlear nucleus. Exp. Neurol. 80:81–93.

Bock, G. R., and J. C. Saunders (1977) A critical period for acoustic trauma in the hamster and its relation to cochlear development. Science 197:396–398.

Bock, G. R., and E. J. Seifter (1978) Developmental changes of susceptibility to auditory fatigue in young hamsters. Audiology 17:193–203.

Brandes, P. J., and D. M. Ehinger (1981) The effects of early middle ear pathology on auditory perception and academic achievement. J. Sp. Hear. Dis. 46:301–307.

Brugge, J. F., E. Javel, and L. M. Kitzes (1978) Signs of functional maturation of peripheral auditory system in discharge patterns of neurons in anteroventral cochlear nucleus of kitten. J. Neurophysiol. 41:1557–1579.

Brugge, J. F., S. S. Orman, J. R. Coleman, J. C. K. Chan, and D. P. Phillips (1985) Binaural interactions in cortical area AI of cats reared with unilateral atresia of the external ear canal. Hear. Res. 20:275–287.

Carlier, E., and R. Pujol (1978) Role of inner and outer hair cells in coding sound intensity: An ontogenetic approach. Brain Res. *147*:174–176.

Carlier, E., M. Lenoir, and R. Pujol (1979) Development of cochlear frequency selectivity tested by compound action potential tuning curves. Hear. Res. *1*:197–201.

Clements, M., and J. B. Kelly (1978) Auditory spatial responses of young guinea pigs (*Cavia porcellus*) during and after ear blocking. J. Comp. Physiol. Psychol. *92*:34–44.

Clopton, B. M. (1986) Micromechanics of the cochlea. Sem. Hearing. *7*:15–25.

Clopton, B. M., and M. S. Silverman (1977) Plasticity of binaural interaction. II. Critical period and changes in midline response. J. Neuropysiol. *40*:1081–1089.

Clopton, B. M., and M. S. Silverman (1978) Changes in latency and duration of neural responding following developmental auditory deprivation. Exp. Brain Res. *32*:39–47.

Clopton, B. M., and J. A. Winfield (1976) Effect of early exposure to patterned sound on unit activity in rat inferior colliculus. J. Neurophysiol. *39*:1081–1089.

Coleman, J. R., and P. O'Connor (1979) Effects of monaural and binaural sound deprivation on cell development in the anteroventral cochlear nucleus of rats. Exp. Neurol. *64*:553–566.

Coleman, J., B. J. Blatchley, and J. E. Williams (1982) Development of the dorsal and ventral cochlear nuclei in rat and effects of acoustic deprivation. Dev. Brain Res. *4*:119–123.

Conlee, J. W., and T. N. Parks (1981) Age and position-dependent effects of monaural acoustic deprivation in nucleus magnocellularis of the chicken. J. Comp. Neurol. *202*:373–384.

Conlee, J. W., and T. N. Parks (1983) Late appearance and deprivation sensitive growth of permanent dendrites in the avian cochlear nucleus (nuc. magnocellularis). J. Comp. Neurol. *217*:216–226.

Culbertson, J. L., and L. E. Gilbert (1986) Children with unilateral sensorineural hearing loss: Cognitive academic and social development. Ear & Hearing *7*:38–42.

deVilliers, J. C., and P. A. deVilliers (1978) Language Acquisition. Cambridge: Harvard University Press.

Dewson, J. H. (1968) Efferent olivocochlear bundle: Some relationships to stimulus discrimination in noise. J. Neurophysiol. *31*:122–130.

Dodson, H. C., L. H. Bannister, and E. E. Douek (1978) Further studies of the effects of continuous white noise of moderate intensity (70–80 dB SPL) on the cochlea in young guinea pigs. Acta Otolaryngol. *86*:195–200.

Douek, E., L. H. Bonnister, H. C. Dodson, P. Ashcroft, and K. N. Humphries (1976) The effects of incubator noise on the cochlea of the newborn. Lancet. *ii*:1110–1113.

Eimas, P. D., and J. F. Kavanagh (1986) Otitis media, hearing loss, and child development: A NICHD conference summary. Pub. Health Rep. *101*:289–293.

Evans, W. J., D. B. Webster, and J. K. Cullen, Jr. (1983) Auditory brainstem responses in neonatally sound deprived CBA/J mice. Hear. Res. *10*:269–277.

Falk, S. A., R. O. Cook, J. K. Hoseman, and G. M. Sanders (1974) Noise-induced inner ear damage in newborn and adult guinea pigs. Laryngoscope 84:444–453.

Feng, A. S., and B. A. Rogowski (1980) Effects of monaural and binaural occlusion on the morphology of neurons on the medial superior olivary nucleus of the rat. Brain Res. 189:530–534.

Freeman, B. A., and C. Parkins (1979) The prevalence of middle ear disease amoung learning impaired children. Clin. Ped. 18:205–212.

Friel-Patti, S., T. Finitzo-Hieber, G. Canti, and K. C. Brown (1982) Language delay in infants associated with middle ear disease and mild, fluctuating hearing impairment. Ped. Inf. Dis. 1:104–109.

Gottlieb, M. I., P. W. Zinkus, and A. Thompson (1979) Chronic middle ear disease and auditory perceptual deficits. Clin. Ped. 18:725–732.

Hall, D. M. B., and P. Hill (1986) When does secretory otitis media affect language development? Arch. Dis. Child. 61:42–47.

Hashisaki, G. T., and E. W. Rubel (1989) Effects of unilateral cochlea removal on anteroventral cochlear nucleus neurons in developing gerbils. J. Comp. Neurol. 283:465–473.

Hoffman-Lawless, L., R. W. Keith, and R. T. Cotton (1981) Auditory processing abilities in children with previous middle ear effusion. Ann. Otol. 90:543–545.

Holm, V. A., and L. H. Kunze (1969) Effects of chronic otitis media on language and speech development. Pediatrics 43:833–839.

Jackson, H., and T. N. Parks (1983) Functional synapse elimination in the developing avian cochlear nucleus with simultaneous reduction in cochlear nerve axon branching. J. Neurosci. 2:1736–1793.

Jhaveri, S., and D. K. Morest (1982) Neuronal architecture in nucleus magnocellularis of the chicken auditory system with observations on nucleus laminaris: A light and electron microscope study. Neuroscience 7:809–836.

Killackey, H. O., and D. K. Ryugo (1977) Effects of neonatal peripheral auditory system damage on the structure of inferior colliculus of the rat. Anat. Rec. 187:624.

Kitzes, L. M., and M. N. Semple (1985) Effects of neonatal unilateral cochlear ablation: Single unit responses in the inferior colliculus. J. Neurophysiol. 53:1483–1500.

Klee, T. M., and E. Davis-Dansky (1986) A comparison of unilaterally hearing impaired children and normal hearing children on a battery of standardized language tests. Ear & Hearing 7:38–42.

Knudsen, E. I., P. F. Knudsen, and S. D. Esterly (1982) Early auditory experience modifies sound localization in barn owls. Nature 295:238–240.

Knudsen, E. I, S. D. Esterly, and P. F. Knudsen (1984a) Monaural occlusion alters sound localization during a sensitive period in the barn owl. J. Neurosci. 4:1001–1011.

Knudsen, E. I., P. F. Knudsen, and S. D. Esterly (1984b) A critical period for the recovery of sound localization accuracy following monaural occlusion in the barn owl. J. Neurosci. 4:1012–1020.

Lenoir, M., G. Bock, and R. Pujol (1979) Supranormal susceptibility to acoustic trauma of the rat pup cochlea. J. Physiol. 75:521–524.

Levi-Montalcini, R. (1949) Development of the acoustico-vestibular centers in the chick embryo in the absence of the afferent root fibers and of descending fiber tracts. J. Comp. Neurol. 91:209–242.

Lewis, N. (1976) Media and linguistic incompetence. Arch. Otolaryngol. 102:387–390.

Moore, D. M., and L. M. Aitkin (1975) Rearing in an acoustically unusual environment—Effects on neural auditory responses. Neurosci. Lett. 1:29–34.

Moore, D. R., and L. M. Kitzes (1985) Projections from the cochlear nucleus to the inferior colliculus in normal and neonatally cochlea-ablated gerbils. J. Comp. Neurol. 240:180–195.

Moore, D. R., and N. E. Kowalchuk (1988) Auditory brainstem of the ferret: Effects of unilateral cochlear lesions on cochlear nucleus volume and projections to the inferior colliculus. J. Comp. Neurol. 272:503–515.

Moore, D. R., M. E. Hutchings, A. J. King, and N. E. Kowalchuk (1989) Auditory brain stem of the ferret: Some effects of rearing with a unilateral ear plug on the cochlea, cochlear nucleus, and projections to the inferior colliculus. J. Neurosci. 9:1213–22.

Paradise, J. L. (1980) Otitis media in infants and children. Pediatrics 65:917–943.

Parks, T. N. (1979) Brainstem auditory nuclei of the chicken. J. Comp. Neurol. 183:665–667.

Parks, T. N. (1981) Changes in the length and organization of nucleus laminaris dendrites after unilateral otocyst ablation in chick embryos. J. Comp. Neurol. 202:47–57.

Parks, T. N., and H. Jackson (1984) A developmental gradient of dendritic loss in the avian cochlear nucleus occurring independently of primary afferents. J. Comp Neurol. 227:459–466.

Parks, T. N., S. S. Gill, and H. Jackson (1987) Experience-independent development of dendritic organization in the avian nucleus laminaris. J. Comp. Neurol. 260:312–319.

Pujol, R. (1986) Periods of sensitivity to antibiotic treatment. Acta Otolaryngol. (Suppl.) 429:29–33.

Ruben, R. J. (1986) Unsolved issues around critical periods with emphasis on clinical application. Acta Otolaryngol. (Suppl.) 429:61–64.

Sak, R. J., and R. J. Ruben (1981) Recurrent middle ear effusion in childhood: Implications of temporary auditory deprivation for language and learning. Ann. Otol. Rhinol. 90:546–551.

Sanes, D. H., and M. Constantine-Paton (1985) The sharpening of frequency tuning curves requires patterned activity during development in the mouse, Mus Musculus. J. Neurosci. 5:1152–1166.

Schery, T. K. (1985) Correlates of language development in language disordered children. J. Sp. Hear. Dis. 50:73–83.

Schweitzer, L., and N. B. Cant (1985) Development of oriented dendritic fields in the dorsal cochlear nucleus of the hamster. Neuroscience 16:969–978.

Silverman, M. S., and B. M. Clopton (1977) Plasticity of binaural interaction: I. Effect of early auditory deprivation. J. Neurophysiol. 40:1266–1274.

Smith, Z. D. J., L. Gray, and E. W. Rubel (1983) Afferent influences on brainstem auditory nuclei of the chicken: n. laminaris dendritic length following monaural conductive hearing loss. J. Comp. Neurol. *220*:199–205.

Teele, D. W., J. O. Klein, and B. A. Rosenes (1980) Epidemiology of otitis media in children. Ann. Otol. Rhinol. Laryngol. *89* (Supp.68):5–6.

Trune, D. R. (1982a) Influence of neonatal cochlear removal on the development of mouse cochlear nucleus: I. Number, size and density of its neurons. J. Comp. Neurol. *209*:409–424.

Trune, D. R. (1982b) Influence of neonatal cochlear removal on the development of mouse cochlear nucleus: II: Dendritic morphometry of its neurons. J. Comp. Neurol. *209*:425–434.

Trune, D. R. (1983) Influence of neonatal cochlear removal on the development of mouse CN. III: Its efferent projections to inferior colliculus. Dev. Brain Res. *9*:1–12.

Trune, D. R., and C. R. Morgan (1988a) Influence of developmental auditory deprivation on neuronal ultrastructure in the mouse anteroventral cochlear nucleus. Brain Res. *470*:304–308.

Trune, D. R., and C. R. Morgan (1988b) Stimulation-dependent development of neuronal cytoplasm in mouse cochlear nucleus. Hear. Res. *33*:141–150.

Tucci, D. L., and E. W. Rubel (1985) Afferent influences on brain stem auditory nuclei of the chicken: Effects of conductive and sensorineural hearing loss on n. magnocellularis. J. Comp. Neurol. *238*:341–381.

Tucci, D. L., D. E. Born, and E. W. Rubel (1987) Changes in spontaneous activity and CNS morphology associated with conductive and sensorineural hearing loss in chickens. Ann. Otol. Rhinol. Laryngol. *96*:343–350.

Uziel, A. (1986) Periods of sensitivity to thyroid hormone during the development of the organ of Corti. Acta Otolaryngol. (Suppl.) *429*:23–27.

Uziel, A., R. Romand, and J. Gabrion (1977) Intrauterine ototoxicity of kanamycin in the guinea pig. In: Portmann, M. and J. M. Aran (eds.): Inner Ear Biology. Les Colloques de l'I.N.S.E.R.M.: INSERM *68*:347–358.

Uziel, A., J. Gabrion, and R. Romand (1979) Hair cell degeneration in guinea pigs intoxicated with kanamycin during intrauterine life. Arch. Otorhinolaryngol. *224*:187–191.

Uziel, A., R. Romand, and M. Marot (1981) Development of cochlear potentials in rats. Audiology *20*:89–100.

Ventry, I. M. (1980) Effects of conductive hearing loss: Fact or fiction. J. Sp. Hear. Dis. *45*:143–156.

Webster, D. B. (1983a) Auditory neuronal sizes after a unilateral conductive hearing loss. Exp. Neurol. *79*:130–140.

Webster, D. B. (1983b) A critical period during postnatal auditory development of mice. Int. J. Ped. Otorhinolaryngol. *6*:107–118.

Webster, D. B. (1983c) Late onset of auditory deprivation does not affect brainstem auditory neuron soma size. Hear. Res. *12*:145–147.

Webster, D. B., and M. Webster (1977) Sound deprivation affects brain stem auditory nuclei. Arch. Otolaryngol. *103*:392–396.

Webster, D. B., and M. Webster (1979) Effects of neonatal conductive hearing loss on brain stem auditory nuclei. Ann. Otol. Rhinol. Laryngol. *88*:684–688.

Webster, D. B., A. Sabin, and M. Anniko (1986) Incomplete maturation of brainstem auditory nuclei in genetically induced early postnatal cochlear degeneration. Acta Otolaryngol. *101*:429–438.

Winslow, R. L., and M. B. Sachs (1987) Effect of electrical stimulation of the crossed olivocochlear bundle on auditory nerve response to tones in noise. J. Neurophysiol. *57*:1002–1021.

Zinkus, P. W., and M. I. Gottlieb (1980) Patterns of perceptual and academic deficits related to early chronic otitis media. Pediatrics *66*:246–253.

Zinkus, P. W., M. I. Gottieb, and M. Schapiro. (1978) Development and psycho-educational sequelae of chronic otitis media. Am. J. Dis. Child. *132*:1100–1104.

Part Three

THE VESTIBULAR SYSTEM

Chapter Nine

DEVELOPMENT OF THE VESTIBULAR SYSTEM

MATTI ANNIKO

University of Umeå
Umeå, Sweden

I   INTRODUCTION

The only function attributed to the ear, from ancient times to the early nineteenth century, was that of processing of acoustic energy. The anatomy of the inner ear was described in part during the sixteenth and seventeenth centuries (Fallopius, 1561; Caserio, 1600; Riolanus, 1649; all cited in DuVerney, 1683). DuVerney (1683) was the first to publish drawings of the cochlea with the lamina spiralis ossea and the semicircular canals and their ampullae. It was not, however, until the beginning of the nineteenth century that the vestibular organs of the ear became recognized as the organs of equilibrium (Flourens, 1824; cited in Bast and Anson, 1949). In 1870 Goltz too concluded that the semicircular canals were concerned with equilibrium. He supported his view largely on the finding that extirpation of the labyrinth in the frog is followed by disturbance of equilibrium, though without the disordered movement of the head observed in his previous experiments on pigeons. He proposed the theory of hydrostatic equilibrium which is associated with his name. According to this theory the canals are stimulated by the weight of the contained fluid. The weight is greatest when the canal is in the vertical position and zero when horizontal, while intermediate canal positions give intermediate weight values.

Thus, Goltz's theory suggests that the canals are specific organs whose task is to sense the position of the head. Later, Ewald (1892, 1899, 1903) suggested a directional sensitivity by vestibular receptor organs in the semicircular canals. However, it was not until the mid-1950s with the introduction of electron microscopy into inner ear research that the morphologic basis was laid for detailed correlations between structure and function of individual vestibular organs (Engström and Wersäll, 1952; Wersäll, 1956).

One of the most thoroughly studied features of mammalian organogenesis is the early development of the otic labyrinth. In 1885 Sharp pointed out that invagination seems to be one of the simplest as well as one of the most common methods by which sensory organs are formed in animals. The formation of the eye (both lens and optic vesicle) and ear are no exception to this rule. A developmental analysis of the early relation between the otic vesicle and the ectoderm in human embryos was described by Anson in 1934.

During inner ear organogenesis, three infoldings of the wall of the otic vesicle subdivide it into the main parts of the ultimate otic labyrinth: the endolymphatic duct and sac, the utriculus with its semicircular ducts and the sacculus with its outgrowth of the ductus reuniens, and the cochlear duct. For general reviews, see Bast and Anson (1949) and Anniko (1983).

II   ANATOMICAL OVERVIEW OF THE VESTIBULAR SYSTEM

The osseous labyrinth encompasses the sense organs for hearing and balance. The inner ear consists of the saccule and utricle, the three vestibular canals with their ampullae, the vestibular and cochlear aqueducts, and the cochlea with its organ of Corti. The membranous labyrinth is an epithelial system with similarly formed spaces and tubes containing endolymph. It is surrounded by perilymphatic fluid labyrinth that is enclosed in the bony labyrinth of the otic capsule. The membranous labyrinth is interconnected by small canals: the utricular duct, the saccular duct, and the ductus reuniens (Figure 1).

The expanded (ampullary) end of each semicircular duct contains a crista ampullaris. In the utricle and the saccule there are also areas of specialized epithelia, the maculae. The utricular macula lies in the horizontal plane, whereas that of the saccule is in the vertical plane. The sensory epithelia of all vestibular organs contain two types of sensory cells together with nerves, blood supply, and supporting cells. The two types of hair cells were originally characterized in detail at the ultrastructural level by Wersäll (1956), who classified them as type I and type II sensory cells (Figure 2). For detailed ultrastructural descriptions, see Wersäll and Bagger-Sjöbäck (1974) and Hunter-Duvar and Hinojosa (1984).

The type I hair cell is flask shaped and is surrounded up to the surface by a nerve chalyx formed from the terminal end of an afferent nerve fiber. In general, only one nerve chalyx surrounds each hair cell. The upper surface

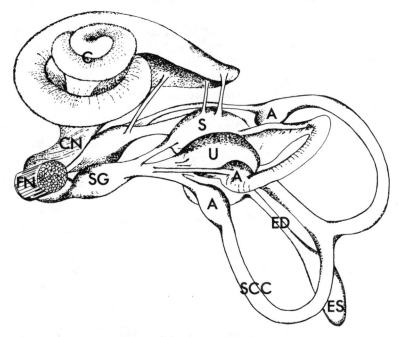

FIGURE 1. Schematic drawing illustrating the principal structures of the membranous labyrinth. C, cochlea; CN, cochlear nerve; SG, Scarpa's ganglion; U, utricle; S, saccule; A, crista ampullaris; FN, facial nerve; ES, endolymphatic sac; ED, endolymphatic duct; SCC, semicircular canal.

of the hair cell contains between 20 and 100 stereocilia and one kinocilium. The stereocilia are contiguous with the surface membrane of the hair cell and can be morphologically considered as enlarged and specialized microvillae. They are arranged in an organ pipe fashion according to length, that is, the longest being positioned adjacent to the kinocilium. The stereocilia contain actin filaments. Each kinocilium is narrower at the base and ends in rootlets that extend into the cuticular plate. The infracuticular region is often rich in mitochondria and multivesicular bodies. The cytoplasm surrounding the nucleus contains mitochondria, endoplasmic reticulum, and Golgi complexes and numerous polysomes. The infranuclear region close to the base of the cell also contains a great number of mitochondria. Synaptic bodies occur at the cell membrane, usually in the vicinity of an invagination in the cell membrane. The nerve chalyx that surrounds all type I hair cells is rich in mitochondria. Efferent nerve endings terminate on the afferent nerve chalyx.

Type II hair cells, which are genetically older than type I cells, have a cylindrical shape and can vary considerably in length. The arrangement of stereocilia and the kinocilium is identical with that found in type I cells. The nucleus is located in the middle third of the cell. The cytoplasmic components are similar to those described for type I sensory cells. Both afferent and efferent nerve endings synapse with type II cells, mainly in the lower and middle third of the hair cell. Only occasionally do nerve endings occur at higher levels.

The receptors in the vestibular organs are secondary sensory cells. The associated afferent nerve fibers originate in the vestibular ganglion (ganglion of Scarpa), which is situated in the temporal bone close to the vestibular organs. The fibers project into the region of the vestibular nuclei in the medulla oblongata (Figure 3). There are four different nuclei on each side. Since the vestibular organs participate in maintaining the balance of the body, essential connections occur between the vestibular nuclei and appropriate motor centers. The major outputs from the vestibular nuclei are the vestibular spinal tract (influencing the motor neurons to the extensor muscles), motor neurons of the cervical cord, eye muscle nuclei, cerebellum, vestibular nuclei on the opposite side (thus, the inputs of the two sides can be processed together), reticular formation, thalamus (mediating connections to the posterior central gyrus of the cortex), and hypothalamus.

Balance is maintained by reflexes without conscious intervention. The reflexes elicited by the vestibular organs are the static and statokinetic reflexes. The macular organs are responsible for static reflexes that maintain an equilibrium in a great variety of extending and reclining positions of the body. Compensatory rolling of the eyes is a static reflex. It ensures that the horizontal and vertical lines are imaged on the retina in the same way. Of course, the neck receptors (muscle spindles, Golgi receptors) are also involved in this reflex. Statokinetic reflexes occur during movements. These reflexes can be elicited both by the macular organs and by the semicircular

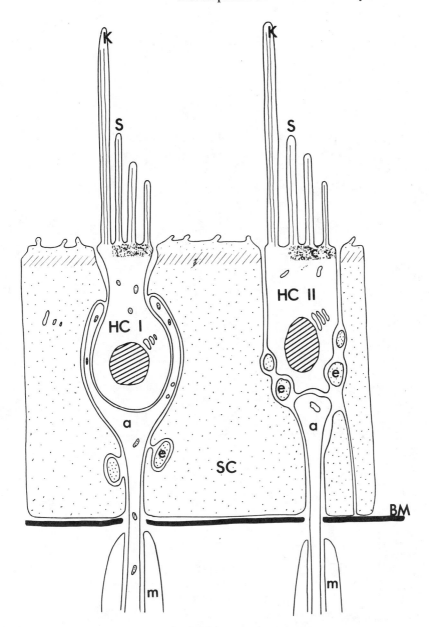

FIGURE 2. Schematic drawing showing the type I (HC I) and type II (HC II) hair cells. a, afferent nerve; e, efferent nerve ending; m, myelin sheet; c, cuticle; K, kinocilium; S, stereocilia; BM, basal membrane; SC, supporting cell.

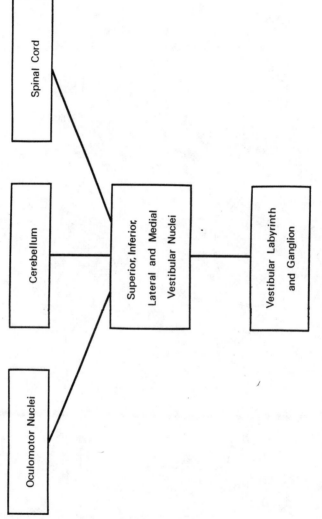

FIGURE 3. Schematic diagram showing basic projections in the vestibular system.

canals. A clinically applied statokinetic reflex is vestibular nystagmus. This is a consequence of eye movements elicited by vestibular input, which causes the eyes to move counter to the direction of body rotation so that the direction of gains is preserved.

The vestibular nuclear complex is comprised of the superior nucleus (nucleus of Bechterew), the lateral nucleus (nucleus of Ditus), the medial nucleus, and the inferior nucleus (descending or spinal nucleus). The central branches of the bipolar vestibular ganglion cells in Scarpa's ganglion project to the vestibular nuclear complex (Figure 3). The branching of these projections has been described by Lorente de Nó (1933), Hauglie-Hansen (1968), and others. The anatomy of the vestibular nuclei and their connections has been reviewed by Brodal (1974) and the physiology of the vestibular nuclei by Precht (1974).

III GENESIS OF VESTIBULAR STRUCTURES

The early morphogenesis of the central nervous system (CNS) involves the distortion of a sheet of cells, the neuroepithelium. A neural plate forms from the embryonic ectoderm, rolls into a tube, and then expands at the brain end, forming bulges and furrows. In embryos of mammals, birds, and many amphibians, the neuroepithelium remains one cell layer thick throughout these transformations (Connelly et al., 1981). The early stages of CNS formation in mammals, including the human embryo, have been described but not measured (O'Rahilly and Gardner, 1971). Studies on the early development of the inner ear anlage have been performed mainly by classic anatomists, but only a few have used modern morphologic techniques (for review, see Anniko, 1983). Comparative summaries of formation of inner ear structures are presented in Tables 1 and 2.

The earliest sensory anlage in humans is the otic plate, which can be recognized in an embryo of two or three somites as a diffuse thickening of ectoderm in the hindbrain region (Bartelmez, 1922). Recently, Anniko and Wikström (1984) described the pattern formation of the otic placode and morphogenesis of the otocyst. The first indication of the otic anlage is the very shallow depression lateral to the everted edge of the neural fold, which is still widely separated from the contralateral fold. The cells of the otic anlage are considerably smaller than adjacent cells of the surface ectoderm including the cells delineating the otic placode. At this gestational stage, prior to morphogenesis of the otocyst, pattern formation is likely to occur. In genetically induced abnormalities of inner ear development, distortion of the overall configuration of the otic anlage has been reported (Wilson, 1983).

Studies on tissue interactions during inner ear development have focused on the relation and inductive influence between the otocyst and adjacent mesenchyme and/or rhombencephalon. With the in vitro techniques presently available, morphogenetic differentiation of different organ

TABLE 1. Early Development of the Inner Ear in Some Common Species Used in Inner Ear Research and for Which Data Are Available with Regard to Early Identification of Anatomical Structures[a]

Species	Gestational Length (days)	Otic Placode	Otic Invagination	Otocyst	Endolymphatic Duct	Semicircular Canals	Statoacoustic Ganglion	Cochlear Duct	Reference
Opossum	13, stage 35	8–10 somites, stage 24, 9 days[b]	14–16 somites, stage 25, 9½ days	16–18 somites, stage 28, 10 days	16–18 somites, stage 28, 10 days	16–18 somites, stage 28, 10 days	—	—	Larsell et al., 1935
Chick	20–21, stage 46	1 somite, stage 11	16 somites, 45–49 h	22 somites, 50–53 h	—	—	—	—	Hamberger and Hamilton, 1951
Chick	20–21, stage 46	—	Stage 13, 45–52 h	stage 15–17, 50–64 h	—	stage 21, 3½ days	stage 21, 3½ days	—	Knowlton, 1967
Chick	20–21, stage 46	6–7 somites, 28–30 h	33 h	40–45 h	—	—	—	—	Meier, 1978
Golden hamster	16	—	8 DBB	7 DBB	5 DBB	5 DBB	—	5 DBB	Stephens, 1972
Mouse	(20)–21	—	—	—	12 days	13 days	—	—	Sher, 1971
Mouse	(20)–21	—	8½ days	9 days	10½ days	12½–13 days	—	—	Anniko, unpublished

[a] Table does not apply to the maturation process. Abbreviation: DBB, days before birth.
[b] Days of gestation.

TABLE 2. Morphogenesis of Vestibular Organs[a]

Species	Gestational Age	Crista Ampullaris		Macula Utriculi		Macula Sacculi		Reference
		First Detectable	Mature	First Detectable	Mature	First Detectable	Mature	
Human	270 days	—	—	18–20-mm embryo	—	18–20-mm embryo	—	Streeter, 1906
Human	270 days	Streeter's horizon, XIV-5 mm	—	—	—	—	—	Yokoh, 1974
Opossum	13 days	Birth	16 DAB	Birth	16 DAB	Birth	16 DAB	Larsell et al., 1935
Chick	20–21 days	Stages 24–28	—	Stages 24–28	—	Stage 22	—	Knowlton, 1967
Golden hamster	16 days	5 DBB	12 DAB	5 DBB	1 DBB	5 DBB	1 DBB	Stephens, 1972
Mouse	21 days	14 days	1 DAB	(13?) 14th	—	Late 13th	—	Sher, 1971
Mouse	21 days	Late 13th day, early 14th day	20–21 days[b]	Late 13th day, early 14th day	18 days	Late 13th day, early 14th day	—	Anniko, unpublished

[a] Abbreviations: DAB, days after birth; DBB, days before birth.
[b] Gross structure.

systems—including the inner ear—can be studied in organ culture. Knowledge of *in vitro* culture of the embryonic inner ear dates back to the 1920s (Fell, 1928). During the following decades it was mainly the avian embryonic labyrinth that was used for organ culture. Emphasis was placed on histological differentiation of individual cells and tissues, but the techniques yielded poor morphogenesis–organogenesis. In the 1950s a very important field of research emerged that concerned the morphogenetic relationship between cells and different types of tissues (Yntema, 1950; Lawrence and Merchant, 1953). Great progress in the basic understanding of *in vitro* conditions for normal and tumor tissues from mammalian species, including man, was made during the 1960s. The first application of organ culture techniques to the analysis of factors influencing mammalian inner ear ontogeny was reported by Van De Water and Ruben (1973). Sobkowicz et al. (1975) reported on the organotypic development in postnatal segments of mammalian cochlear ducts. Organ culture combined with the anatomical techniques of light and electron microscopy constitute important and fundamental scientific tools with which to investigate the embryogenesis of the mammalian inner ear and those factors that may act as causative agents in the production of the congenitally malformed inner ear, which results in deafness.

Organ culture techniques have been applied to the study of embryonic development of the mouse inner ear anlage and, to a lesser extent, early postnatal development (Anniko, 1984). *In vitro* studies on other species are few. This method has been applied to inner ear studies involving observations on morphology and to some extent on chemical parameters such as phospholipid composition, transport enzyme adenylate cyclase, and so on. With the introduction of organ culture techniques for the inner ear of the mouse and guinea pig (higher vertebrates) many of the experiments earlier restricted to lower vertebrates and performed *in vivo* as recombination homologous transplants could now be performed with great accuracy *in vitro* using material from higher vertebrates under considerably better controlled and well-defined conditions: neural induction, epitheliomesenchymal interactions, neurotrophic interaction, fate mapping, tissue interactions for normal morphogesis, studies on especially vulnerable stages of inner ear development, and applied research such as ototoxicity. It must be emphasized that applications of the organ culture technique cannot provide information on the systemic effect of an agent but only about its direct effect on a given tissue.

Principles for morphogenesis of the various vestibular organs are similar in different mammalian species (Figure 4). In comparison with the human, embryonic development in many other animal species is rapid. However, during the period of development immediately following fertilization, this is often less evident (Tables 1 and 2). For recent reviews, see Anniko (1983) and Lim and Anniko (1985).

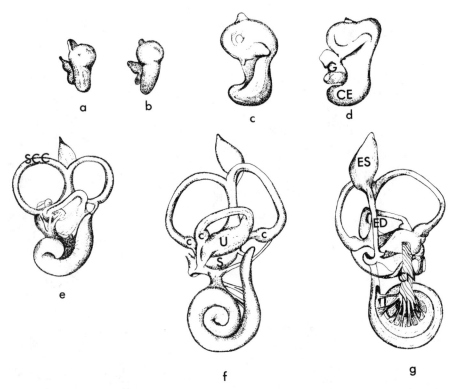

FIGURE 4. Schematic drawing showing the embryonic development of the inner ear from the otocyst stage (*a, b*) to the mature inner ear; (*f*) lateral view; (*g*) medial view. CE, cochlear end; SCC, semicircular canal; ED, endolymphatic duct; ES, endolymphatic sac; S, saccule; U, utricle; C, cristae ampullares; CN, cochlear nerve; G, statoacoustic ganglion.

IV   DEVELOPMENT AND DIFFERENTIATION OF PERIPHERAL AND CENTRAL STRUCTURES

A   Hair Cells

The morphologic differentiation of vestibular hair cells can be subdivided into five not always sequential developmental events depending on the structures involved: terminal mitoses, characterization of the hair cell itself, and specific structures (surface morphology, junctional complexes, and innervation) involved in the transductional process. These principles are rather similar across a number of species (Table 3).

1   Terminal Mitoses

Ruben (1967) reported in mouse (which has a gestational period of 20–21 days) that the labeling activity of hair cells and supporting cells of the three

TABLE 3. Comparative Timing of Vestibular Receptor Development[a]

Structural Feature	Guinea Pig	Cat	Dog	Mouse	Rabbit
Recognizable HC	—	—	—	7 DBB	9 DBB
Beginning of afferent nerve calyx	30 DBB	—	—	3–4 DAB	4 DBB
Afferent NE recognizable	—	—	—	—	8–9 DBB
Efferent NE recognizable	—	—	—	3 DBB	Birth
Synapse formation	12–15 DBB	2–3 DBB	4 DAB	3–5 DBB	—
Mature stage					
HC I	3–5 DBB	10–12 DAB	20 DAB	3–5 DAB	Birth?
HC II	3–5 DBB	10–12 DAB	—	—	—
Differentiation into HC type I and type II	—	27 DBB	—	3–4 DBB	—

[a] Abbreviations: DBB, days before birth; DAB, days after birth; NE, nerve ending; HC, hair cell.

cristae followed a similar pattern. There was very little labeling in the inner ear between gestational days 12 and 13. The labeling index increased on gestational day 14, reached a maximum on day 16, and continued slightly into the early postnatal period. Thus, most hair cells passed their terminal mitoses within a period of a few days, although a few hair cells continued to develop even postnatally. Cells differentiating into future hair cells pass their terminal mitoses close to the otocyst lumen (Figure 5) (Van De Water et al., 1978; Anniko et al., 1979). Except for position within the epithelium, it is not possible morphologically to distinguish future hair cells from adjacent supporting structures at this very early stage of embryonic development.

2   Characterization of the Hair Cell

At the otocyst stage the epithelium facing the otocyst lumen comprises cuboidal or slightly pillar-shaped cells. Except for their surfaces being covered with an irregular arrangement of microvillae, these cells have the same shape as in the layers below the surface layers of cells. The cell organelles are homogeneously distributed and a large number of polyribosomes are found, indicating a high rate of metabolic activity. The morphologic pattern of the otocyst (as observed in sectional material) is related directly to the developmental potential of these regions, that is, the site of origin of the embryonic inner ear concerning sensory and nonsensory structures (Li, 1978). According to scanning electron microscopic studies, such

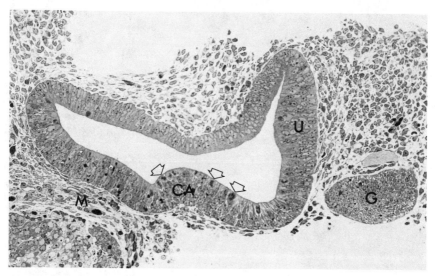

FIGURE 5. Light micrograph of late-13-gestational-day mouse showing the otocyst stage of the embryonic inner ear. Formation into a crista ampullaris (CA) and utricle (U) is indicated. Hair cells pass their terminal mitoses (arrows) close to the otocyst lumen. M, mesenchyme; G, statoacoustic ganglion.

differences in developmental potential between different regions of the otocyst may also be identified by differences in surface morphology (Figures 6 and 7) (Anniko and Wikström, 1984).

In many species the earliest morphologic sign of differentiation into future hair cells is the arrangement of microvillae in a regular fashion which covers the cell surface. Generally speaking, hair cell cytodifferentiation takes place along a gradient from the hair cell surface to the base. Concomitant with the maturation of sensory hairs a rebuilding of the intracellular matrix occurs: the number of polyribosomes and the amount of rough endoplasmic reticulum both decrease, the nucleus moves basally, and mitochondria accumulate in the supranuclear region (Nakai, 1970; Heywood et al., 1976; Favre and Sans, 1978, 1979a,b; Anniko et al., 1979; Nordemar, 1983). Further morphologic rebuilding of the hair cell itself does not occur. Differentiation into the two types of hair cells is indicated by their innervation patterns.

Sans and Dechesne (1985) studied development of vestibular receptors in 7–9-week-old human embryos by light microscopy and scanning and transmission electron microscopy. The greater part of the vestibular epithelium is still undifferentiated in the 7-week-old embryo and is composed of polystratified epithelial cells. A small number of afferent nerve endings are found between epithelial cells, but no synaptic specializations are detected. Only a few of these afferent nerve endings reach the upper part of the epithelium.

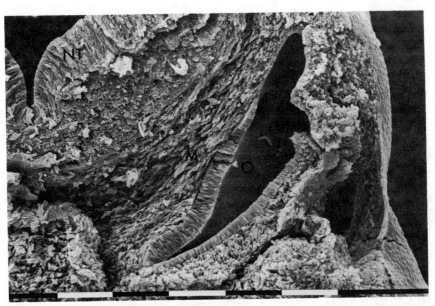

FIGURE 6. Scanning electron micrograph (SEM) of the otocyst (O) on the 11th gestational day of mouse. Considerable variations occur in the thickness of the otocyst epithelial layer. NT, neural tube; M, mesenchyme. Bar = 0.1 mm.

Thus, at this stage the nerve fibers are present within the vestibular epithelium prior to differentiation of the sensory cells. The apical pole of the epithelial cells presents basal bodies linked with striated rootlets and other typical vestibular epithelium cell structures. Short hair bundles are found in a very small part of the vestibular epithelium, likewise indicating the formation of future hair cells. At 8–9 weeks of gestation, numerous nerve endings surround the base of developing sensory cells. Densifications of the pre- and postsynaptic membranes and synaptic bodies are seen. The newly afferented hair cells display polarized hair bundles. It was assumed that the hair cells are important for guidance of afferent terminals, perhaps even before morphologic differentiation of hair cells.

The cytoskeletal protein composition of a cell can reflect both its embryonic origin and, if present, a specialized cell function. The cytoskeleton in all eukaryotic cells is comprised of microfilaments (actin filaments; 4–6 nm in diameter), intermediate filaments (8–10 nm), microtubules (22–25 nm), and a very large number of various interconnecting proteins. Actin filaments constitute the structural basis of eukaryotic cellular and subcellular motility, such as locomotion, contraction, membrane mobility, and organelle transport. The specificity required to induce and control these different movements most likely depends not only on the molecular properties of actin but also on its interaction with other structural proteins such as actin-binding proteins. So far, approximately 30 actin-associated proteins have been de-

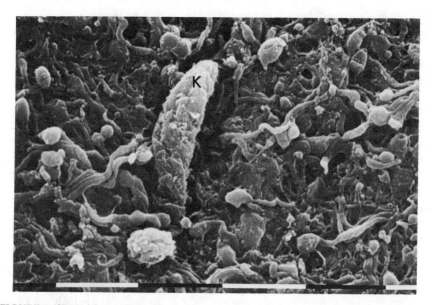

FIGURE 7. SEM of the medial surface of the 13-gestational-day otocyst of mouse. Morphologically, considerable secretory activity is identified: large amounts of organic material are present close to numerous microvilli. A giant kinocilium (K) protrudes above the otocyst surface. Bar = 10 μm.

scribed. Several of these (e.g., vinculin, alpha-actinin, and alpha-spectrin) regulate the spatial arrangement and packing of microfilaments and their association with the cell membrane, while others connect to the two remaining major cytoskeletal components.

Immunohistochemical techniques have been applied in inner ear research mainly for the identification of contractile proteins at the mature hair cell surface (Zenner et al., 1985; Flock et al., 1986) and for immunoreactivity of hair cell innervation and its central projection (Fex and Altschuler, 1981; Altschuler et al., 1984, 1986). The distribution of actin filaments and actin-associated proteins and their role in hearing has been extensively studied (Drenckhahn et al., 1982; Tilney et al., 1983; Slepecky and Chamberlain, 1985). Considerably less is known about the two other components of the cytoskeleton—microtubules and intermediate filaments.

In the inner ear of several rodents including the guinea pig, actin, vinculin, fimbrin, tropomyosin, myosin, and alpha-actinin are present in the cuticular plate region in cochlear hair cells (Drenckhahn et al., 1982, 1985; Flock et al., 1982; Flock and Orman, 1983). In contrast, vestibular hair cells lack fimbrin in the cuticular plate, which may indicate different physiological mechanoreceptor properties of cochlear and vestibular hair cells (Sobin and Flock, 1984). Flock and Strelioff (1984) showed physiologically that cochlear hair cell stereocilia are 20 times as stiff as stereocilia on vestibular hair cells.

Anniko and Thornell (1987) analyzed the presence of alpha-actinin, vinculin, alpha-spectrin, beta-spectrin, and fibronectin in 14–21-week-old fetal human inner ears, using fluorescence with rhodamine–phalloidin-bound antibodies. Alpha-actinin was identified fairly evenly distributed at the surface of all five vestibular organs but mainly at the surface of the receding greater epithelial ridge in the cochlea and in some foci apically at the lesser epithelial ridge. Thus, alpha-actinin seemed to be distributed in the human inner ear in a way similar to that earlier described for rodents (Drenckhahn et al., 1985; Slepecky and Chamberlain, 1985). Fluorescence for vinculin occurred mainly at the surfaces of vestibular organs but was lacking in the lesser epithelial ridge (containing at least outer hair cells) of the cochlea, as is also found in other mammalian species. Intense fluorescence for alpha-spectrin was observed at the apical surfaces of individual cells of the cristae and maculae (Figure 8). It can be speculated that alpha-spectrin may be present in the cuticular plate of vestibular hair cells and that it connects actin filaments of the cuticle and sensory hairs with the internal organization of the vimentin-containing hair cells or cytokeratins in the hair cells; alpha-spectrin may also be involved in the attachment of microfilaments to the plasma membrane. Beta-spectrin stained only the endothelial cells of blood vessels. Thus, the fluorescence patterns for actin-associated proteins indicate differences in structure—at least between cochlear and vestibular hair cells of the human fetus. Fibronectin was identified only between mesenchymal cells and its functional importance still remains to be clarified.

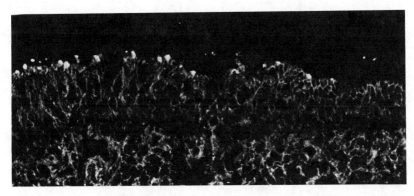

FIGURE 8. Macula utriculi from a 14-week-old human fetus using fluorescence staining for alpha-spectrin. The resulting fluorescent activity is found at the cell borders of many cell types but is particularly intense at the apical surfaces of individual cells (identified as hair cells) in the macula.

Actin filaments and microtubules both consist of globular protein subunits that can assemble and disassemble rapidly in the cell. Delicate control mechanisms exist for the assembly from pools of unpolymerized subunits in the cytoplasm. In contrast, intermediate filaments consist of fibrous protein subunits and are much more stable than most actin filaments and microtubules. The mature type of intermediate filament composition of the various structures of both the cochlear and vestibular parts of the inner ear is found very early during embryonic development (Wikström et al., 1988), usually very soon after cytodifferentiation commences. Principally the same type of intermediate filaments and actin are found in the human inner ear and in a number of other animal species (Figures 9–12) (Anniko et al., 1986, 1987a,b, 1988; Thornell et al., 1987). Recent studies have shown that even in the 14th gestational week, human fetal vestibular hair cells contain cytokeratins (a subclass of intermediate filaments) as a major component of the hair cell cytoskeleton (Figure 13), although in this respect differing from cochlear hair cells by less vigorous immunoreactivity for cytokeratins (Anniko et al., 1987a).

3 Specific Structures Involved in Sensory Transduction

a Surface Morphology. The early development of human vestibular receptors is only partially documented (Bast and Anson, 1949; Altmann, 1950; Anson et al., 1966). Vestibular receptor differentiation has been postulated to begin at 7.5 weeks and to end at 12–14 weeks. Recent studies by Dechesne and Sans (1985) on the development of the vestibular receptor surfaces in human fetuses have shown that maturation of vestibular receptors is delayed, as compared with older studies. The vestibular epithelium appears at about 7 weeks, and maturation is still not complete at 14 weeks,

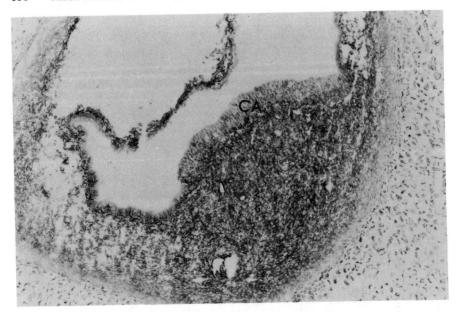

FIGURE 9. Crista ampullaris (CA) from a 14-week-old human fetus. Immunostaining for vimentin using monoclonal antibodies of clone FV24BAG. Mesenchymal cells show an intense staining whereas epithelial cells have a weaker staining.

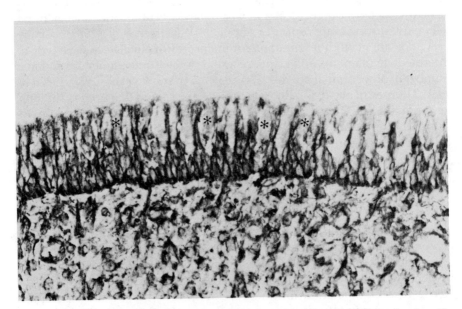

FIGURE 10. Macula utriculi from a 14-week-old human fetus. Immunostaining for vimentin using monoclonal antibodies of clone V24BAG. The supporting cells of the epithelial layer stain more intensely than the hair cells (asterisks), which show only weak immunoreactivity.

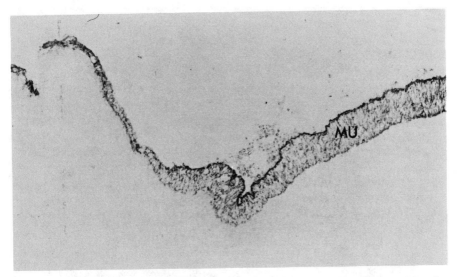

FIGURE 11. Macula utriculi (MU) from a 16-week-old human fetus. Immunostaining for cytokeratins (monoclonal antibodies from clone PKK-2 identifying cytokeratins nos. 7, 17, and 19). An intense immunoreactivity is found at the apical surface of the macula.

at which time the cristae have only reached 55% of their adult size and the hair cell ciliary apparatus is far from being mature. Growing hair bundles can be seen on the cristae and hair cells, but have not reached adult length. The persistence of numerous and tall microvilli of the sensory surface even at 14 weeks is a sign of immaturity of the crista itself, although many individual hair cells show a mature morphology. Maturation of hair bundles appears sequentially in a gradient from the more mature ones at the top to the base of the cristae where a more immature stereociliary pattern is found. A similar pattern of hair cell development and maturation has also been described in the rat (Sans and Chat, 1982) and the mouse (Li, 1978; Mbiene et al., 1984; Lim and Anniko, 1985).

Hair cell stereociliary development appears orderly, with well-defined polarization of the kinocilia and graded arrangement of the stereocilia. The whole hair cell surface is initially covered with microvilli, which gradually either recede or develop into stereocilia. In some cases the kinocilium is initially found in the center of the stereocilia. Thus, a physical reorganization of the stereocilia and the kinocilium on individual hair cells occurs during maturation, either by regression of some immature stereocilia or by rearrangement.

Vestibular maturation in humans involves the same principal sequences and comparable maturational stages as in other mammals. For example, parallels in the receptor differentiation sequence can be observed in mice and humans. An important observation on vestibular receptor surface maturation was reported by Dechesne and Sans (1985), namely, that there are

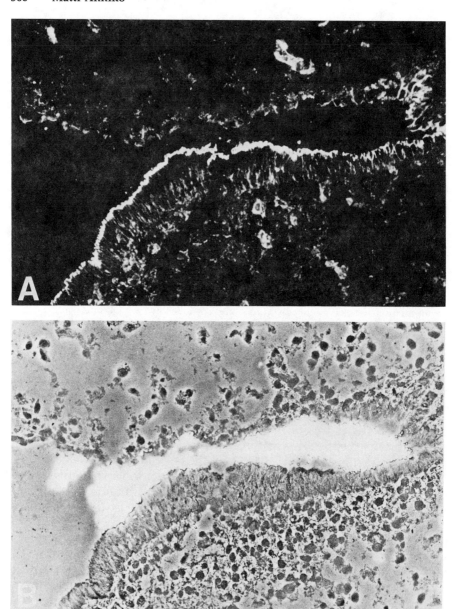

FIGURE 12. Crista ampullaris of a 14-week-old human fetus. (*A*) Intense fluorescence for F-actin at the surface of the crista but not in the dark cell region or in the epithelial lining of the ampulla. (*B*) Phase contrast microscopy of the specimen in (*A*).

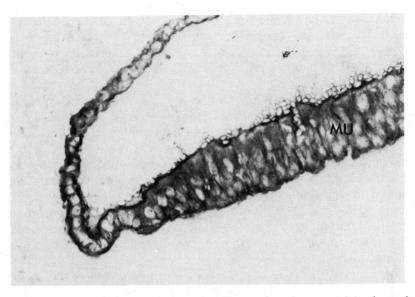

FIGURE 13. Macula utriculi (MU) of a 14-week-old human fetus. Immunostaining for cytokeratin no. 8 using monoclonal antibodies from clone T-1 (chain specific). Both supporting cells and hair cells show immunoreactivity as well as do cells in the epithelial lining of the endolymphatic space.

both rapid and slow periods of cell surface maturation in humans; there is a pause in growth of the crista between 9 and 12 weeks and in the utricle between 8 and 11 weeks.

During the pause in growth in the vestibular organs of the mouse, the utricular epithelium thins out, retarding overall surface growth of the vestibular structures (Mbiene et al., 1984). Utricular maturation occurs prior to the pause phenomenon in the three cristae. During the pause, overall receptor sizes do not increase much, but their shape changes strikingly, from an immature to an adult configuration. This pause probably corresponds to a critical period of development. The pause period in the utricle occurs in the mouse between gestational days 17 and 18. On gestational day 18 in mouse, the utricle and cristae are at the same stage of development as corresponding receptors in the human during weeks 11–12.

In the adult vestibular epithelium there are two hair cell types present. However, it is difficult to detect any differential maturation of the surfaces of these two cell populations. Adult type I and type II sensory cells in mammalian vestibular sensory organs are distinguishable by surface morphology of the sensory cilia (Lindeman et al., 1973; Lim, 1976, 1977; Hunter-Duvar and Hinojosa, 1984). Although there are differences between the central and peripheral zones regarding the height of type I cell stereocilia, these stereocilia are generally thicker and taller than those of the neighboring type II hair cells. Individual stereocilia of type I cells resemble an inverted baseball bat, with a thicker top and tapered, thinner shaft. Judging from these characteristics, the short (type II) and tall (type I) hair cells can be recognized in the vestibular organs as early as gestational day 16 in mouse. The postnatal development of vestibular receptor surfaces is gradual in a number of species (Lim and Anniko, 1985). Sans and Chat (1982), using autoradiography to follow the chronology of normal development of rat vestibular receptors, demonstrated temporal and spatial gradients of hair cell differentiation from the top to the bottom of the cristae and from the center to the periphery of the utricular maculae. The sensory cells at the top of the cristae and the center of the maculae are the first to be contacted by nerve fibers and also the first to differentiate, whereas the cells at the bottom of the cristae and sides of the utricular maculae are the youngest and the last to be contacted and to differentiate. Dechesne et al. (1986) showed in rat (in which labyrinthine receptor development is similar to that of mouse) that hair bundles are still developing in the cristae, mainly at the bottom, during the first few postnatal days.

Hypothyroidism leads to disturbances in maturation of the vestibular receptors by influencing differentiation of the hair cells into two types, and innervation and growth of stereociliary bundles (Dechesne et al., 1984). Dememes et al. (1986) showed that congenital hypothyroidism resulted in immaturity of vestibular ganglion cells characterized by an absence of myelin sheath around the perikarya. Type I hair cells have delayed development of innervation. The last cells to differentiate and the last synaptic contacts to develop are the most affected. The most remarkable result of hypothyroidism is the persistent immaturity of synaptic contacts.

Mbiene et al. (1984) performed a qualitative and quantitative scanning electron microscopic study on the pattern of ciliary development in fetal mouse vestibular receptors. The number of differentiated tufts in the macula utriculi increased significantly between gestational days 13 and 16. However, the number of ciliary tufts remained stable between gestational days 16 and 17. This pause was later compensated by an accelerated increase in the number of ciliary tufts between gestational days 17 and 18. The increase in the entire sensory surface exhibited a progression similar to that of the number of differentiated ciliary tufts, but the pause for this surface increase occurred 1 day later, between gestational days 17 and 18. The increase in cellular density during macular development, with the exception of gestational day 17, indicates that the rate at which individual sensory cells appeared was higher than that for macular surface growth. Hair cell density was also always greater in the center than at the periphery. A pause in growth of the cristae ampullares in the mouse during the fetal period made it difficult to count the total number of hair cells, and it was not possible to demonstrate a pause in the differentiation of hair cells. At the end of the gestation period, which in the mouse is 21 days, a new wave of sensory cells developed over the whole surface of the epithelium (Mbiene et al., 1984). Similar observations were reported by Lim and Anniko (1985).

b Hair Cell Junctions. By using the freeze-fracture technique, intercellular junctions can be visualized with regard to tight junctions and gap
junctions. At the otocyst stage, junctional elements are present but appear
immature (Ginsburg and Gilula, 1979; Khan and Marowitz, 1979; Bagger-
Sjöbäck and Anniko, 1984). Tight junctions in the vestibular portion of the
inner ear gradually attain mature appearance (Figures 14 and 15). In the
mouse, tight junctions of the supporting cells develop slightly faster than
those of hair cells. Remodeling and differentiation of both tight and gap
junctions precedes formation of contacts between nerve fibers and hair cells
(Bagger-Sjöbäck and Anniko, 1984). In contrast, Ginsburg and Gilula (1979,
1980) found that differentiation of epithelial cells into hair cells and supporting cells in the domestic fowl was initiated as nerve fibers enter the epithelium and that hair cell cytodifferentiation continued with neuronal expansion and synaptogenesis. Species-dependent variations may account for
differences between these two studies. The disappearance of gap junctions
was suggested as a mechanism for uncoupling epithelial cells as they differentiate into innervated hair cells. An uncoupling phenomenon is also observed in the mouse. The maturation of tight junctions on hair cells and
supporting cells is completed before the ionic composition of endolymph
becomes mature (Anniko and Wróblewski, 1981).

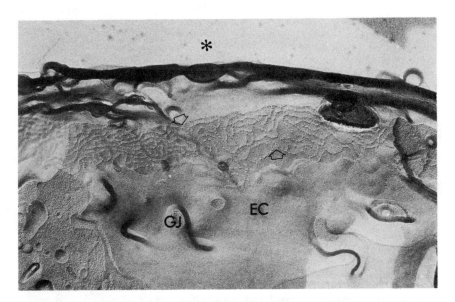

FIGURE 14. Transmission electron micrograph (TEM) showing freeze fracture replica of 14-
gestational-day mouse inner ear. Tight junctions consist of several layers of immature strands
that allow ionic flow between the interrupting strands (arrows). GJ, gap junctions; EC, epithelial cell. The otocyst lumen is indicated with an asterisk.

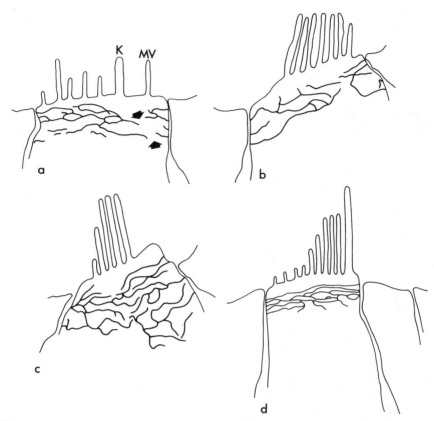

FIGURE 15. Schematic drawing illustrating the maturation of tight junctions during embryonic development of the inner ear. (*a*) Otocyst stage. MV, microvillae; the kinocilium (*K*) at this developmental stage is still in an immature position without polarization of stereocilia as in the adult stage in (*d*). Tight junctions at the otocyst stage are immature and allow ionic flux (arrows) between the individual sealing strands. (*b*) The first morphological sign of future hair cells is the regularization of the stereocilia on the cell surface. The tight junction, although consisting of several sealing strands, is still immature, permitting ionic flux between individual strands. (*c*) While the surface morphology of the hair cell matures (showing a stepwise increase in height of stereocilia), the tight junction itself is still immature, although the number of sealing strands has increased. However, the individual strands are not yet parallel and still allow passage of ions, but not as extensively as before. (*d*) Adult configuration of the tight junction complex at the upper surface of a hair cell. The sealing strands are parallel and do not allow ionic flow. Mature features of the surface morphology of stereocilia and the kinocilium are also shown.

c Innervation Pattern. In several species the first morphologic contact between the vestibular hair cell and ingrowing nerve fibers occurs when the hair cell has reached a considerable degree of cytologic maturation. The hair cell innervation is often the last morphologic structure to become mature in the sensory transduction chain. A gradual maturation of innervation is evident in mouse (Sher, 1971; Anniko et al., 1979). Similar features have been described in cat (Favre and Sans, 1978, 1979), guinea pig (Heywood et al., 1976; Sobin and Anniko, 1979; Shnerson and Pujol, 1983), rabbit (Nakai, 1970), and other species. In the cat the afferent and efferent innervations develop in parallel (Favre and Sans, 1977, 1979a,b). In the mouse and rabbit, development of efferent nerve endings occurs after the appearance of afferent innervation. These differences in sequence of afferent and efferent innervation apparently represent species variation.

The initial appearance of several nerve terminals on type I hair cells and later detachment of some of these reflects a polyneural type of primary innervation (Figures 16A–C, 17, and 18). The adult hair cell has, in principle, a mononeural innervation. The polyneural type of innervation apparently includes competition between ingrowing afferent nerve fibers. When the first nerve endings appear on hair cells, there is no competition between afferent fibers. Thus, competition is a phenomenon of the later stages of hair cell maturation. Formation of an initial "primitive" innervation of type I hair cells similar to that of type II hair cells supports the hypothesis that during ontogenesis, innervation of type I hair cells passes through a stage corresponding to that of type II hair cells. By comparison, the establishment of temporary synapses has also been described in other organ systems (e.g., cerebellum, skeletal muscle, and cochlea), as well for detachment phenomenon of synaptic contacts (Ronnevi, 1977, 1979). The maturation of innervation involves a dual mechanism (Figure 19). The independent formation of synaptic bodies in the basal parts of the sensory cell can occur before nerve endings reach the sensory cell itself. Clusters of synaptic bodies can often be identified even in the embryonic hair cell.

It is now well established that, at least in some species, sensory cell differentiation is not under neural influence (Van De Water, 1976; Anniko et al., 1979; Raymond, 1987). However, further development of neurons may be dependent upon interactions with synaptic targets. While in some systems the interdependence of neurons and their targets has yet to be established, in other cases isolation of molecules responsible for trophic effects is under investigation (Barde et al., 1983). The first such molecule discovered, nerve growth factor (Levi-Montalcini and Angeletti, 1963), has been purified and its amino acids sequenced (Angeletti and Bradshaw, 1971). Nevertheless, it is not clear in all cases whether trophic agents are diffusible molecules or whether direct contact between hair cells and ingrowing nerve fibers is necessary. In a recent study, Ard et al. (1985) showed that in the chick inner ear the peripheral targets of the neurons in the sensory epithelium exert a trophic effect on the ganglion cells. Direct contact between ganglion cells and hair cells was a factor in neuronal survival and differentiation. Although there is no evidence to suggest a trophic requirement for the presence of the ganglion cells in the differentiation of the sensory epithelium, Van De Water and Ruben (1984) proposed that, prior to overt cytodifferentiation, the developing sensory receptors undergo a biochemi-

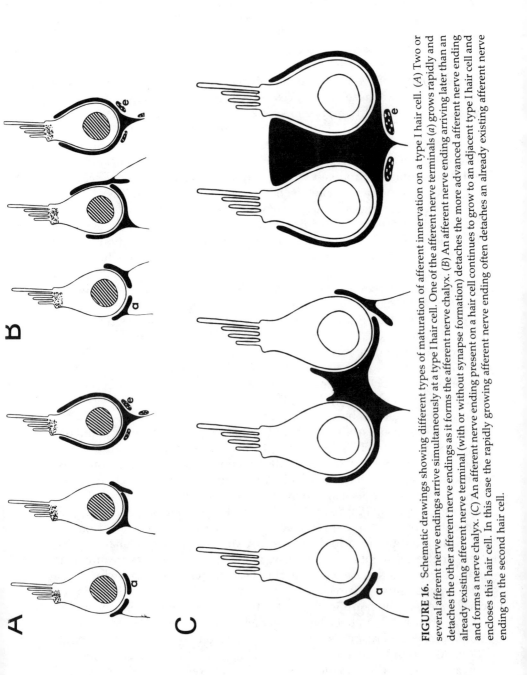

FIGURE 16. Schematic drawings showing different types of maturation of afferent innervation on a type I hair cell. (*A*) Two or several afferent nerve endings arrive simultaneously at a type I hair cell. One of the afferent nerve terminals (*a*) grows rapidly and detaches the other afferent nerve endings as it forms the afferent nerve chalyx. (*B*) An afferent nerve ending arriving later than an already existing afferent nerve terminal (with or without synapse formation) detaches the more advanced afferent nerve ending and forms a nerve chalyx. (*C*) An afferent nerve ending present on a hair cell continues to grow to an adjacent type I hair cell and encloses this hair cell. In this case the rapidly growing afferent nerve ending often detaches an already existing afferent nerve ending on the second hair cell.

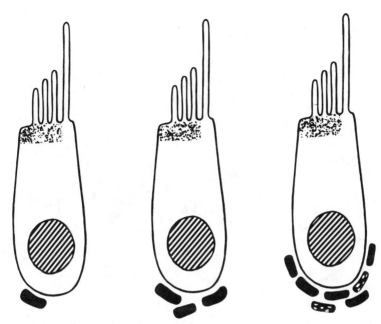

FIGURE 17. Schematic drawings illustrating how afferent nerve endings reach a type II hair cell. All the nerve terminals make synaptic contacts with the hair cell. The detachment phenomenon does not occur. Dotted nerve endings indicate efferent nerve endings.

cal differentiation and thus establish a chemoattractant field to direct ingrowth of neuronal elements from a nearby source to the target site. Later, Anniko and Van De Water (1987) showed not only that nerve outgrowth occurred at the sites of differentiating vestibular sensory epithelium but also that synaptic contacts were established between vestibular sensory hair cells and ingrowing statoacoustic ganglion neurites, even in cases where the original statoacoustic ganglion had been removed and replaced by the statoacoustic ganglion from the contralateral ear. The plasticity of the central nervous system is considerable, and whether such nerve fiber and hair cell connections can still be preserved at later stages remains speculative. However, there is little evidence of absolute specificity in the formation of synaptic connections between different receptor cell types since a wide variety of heterologous connections can occur (Berry et al., 1981).

Both afferent and efferent synaptic transmission in the vertebrate vestibular system is chemical in nature. However, the corresponding neurotransmitters are not yet fully characterized. In the adult, gamma-butyric acid (GABA) is one of the afferent neurotransmitters and acetylcholine is a possible efferent neuromediator. The cellular localization of neuromediators or their precursors cannot be inferred from experiments performed on a homogenate of a vestibular organ. A technique for separation of the

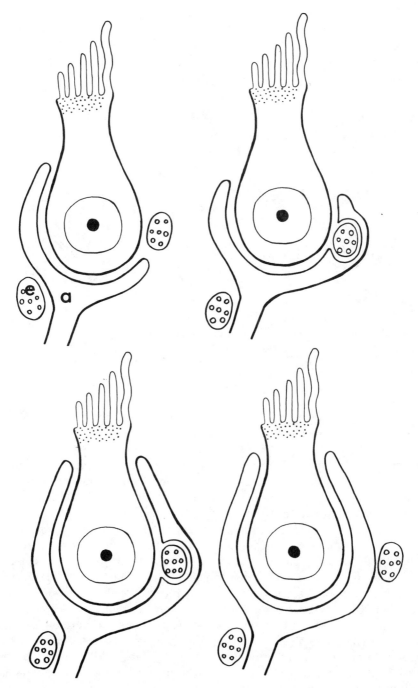

FIGURE 18. Schematic drawings showing how the growth cone of an afferent nerve ending detaches an efferent nerve ending (already having a synaptic contact) during the formation of the afferent nerve chalyx for a type I hair cell.

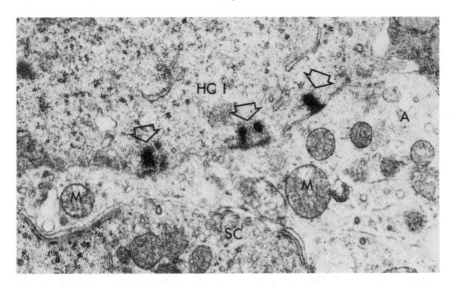

FIGURE 19. TEM. During initial formation of synaptic contacts between ingrowing afferent nerve endings (A) and a type I hair cell (HC I), a great number of synaptic bodies (arrows) appear. Later, as the nerve chalyx matures, the number of synpatic bodies decreases. M, mitochondria; SC, supporting cells.

various types of cells comprising the sensory epithelium in the chick vestibule was recently described (Ohmori, 1984). However, this technique cannot be used in biochemical experiments because of the low cell yield. An alternative approach is an ontogenic one recently described by Meza and Hinojosa (1987). The content of GABA-synthesizing enzyme and of choline acetyltransferase, the enzyme for synthesis of acetylcholine, was analyzed in the ampullary cristae of embryonic chicks at different stages of development. These measurements were made in parallel with electron microscopic studies on the development and maturation of sensory cells and their adjacent afferent and efferent nerve connections. This ontogenic approach to cellular localization of neurotransmitters in the chick vestibule confirmed that GABA and acetylcholine are the neuromediators for the afferent and efferent systems, respectively.

The appearance of neuron-specific enolase is concomitant with the differentiation of the first synaptic formations (Whitehead et al., 1982). The role of calbindin in vestibular receptors can be associated with either the particular functioning of the sensory cells or their synaptic activity (Rabié et al., 1983; Sans et al., 1986). At 10 weeks of gestation weak neuron-specific enolase reactivity is observed in human vestibular hair cells, whereas these cells express strong immunoreactivity for calbindin (Dechesne et al., 1987b). It can be concluded that by 10 weeks of gestation many human vestibular receptors show biochemical signs of maturation, which implies the possibility of synaptic activity.

A trophic influence by neuronal elements on inner ear sensory receptor development is not required. In contrast, comparisons of the rates of survival and cytodifferentiation of isolated statoacoustic ganglia with that of the ganglia with peripheral and/or central targets show a trophic effect of target tissue on the survival and differentiation of the neurons (Zhou and Van De Water, 1987). It seems that the presence of brainstem target tissue has no significant effect on the survival of ganglion neurons when the peripheral target tissue is present. Isolated statoacoustic ganglion cells from the 12-gestational-day mouse do not continue their morphologic differentiation into vestibular and cochlear ganglion cells, although they survive for 8–10 days *in vitro* and show an outgrowth of nerve fibers (Berggren and Anniko, 1989). The same features have been observed for the isolated 13th gestation day statoacoustic ganglion explant (Raymond, 1987). When the statoacoustic ganglion has developed into a cochlear and vestibular part and has reached a certain degree of maturity (in principle without establishing synpatic contacts with its targets), explantation to organ culture (e.g., close to birth in the mouse) becomes possible with even a gradual development of electrophysiological potentials (Desmadryl et al., 1986). In the vestibular ganglion, onset of electrophysiological activity was thus recorded even prior to myelination of ganglion cells and their neurons (Anniko, 1985a; Dechesne et al., 1987).

B   Cupula and Otoconia

Sensory cells of the inner ear, whether they are involved in hearing or in vestibular function, are all mechanoreceptors provided with geometrically organized and directionally sensitive sensory ciliary bundles. Their ciliary organization has a direct functional implication in the process of sensory transduction (Wersäll et al., 1965; Flock, 1971; Hudspeth and Corey, 1977). Recent evidence indicates that the stereocilia from different hair cells in the auditory organ of the alligator lizard are mechanically tuned to the frequencies to which they respond (Frischkopf and De Rosier, 1983; Holton and Hudspeth, 1983). During development there is considerable morphogenetic change in the formation of ciliary organization, which is under direct cell control. The stereociliary bundles of all sensory cells of the inner ear are closely associated with an overlying membrane, such as the tectorial membrane, the otoconial membrane, and the cupula. This coupling between the stereocilia and an overlying membrane influences the micromechanical properties of the mechanoreceptor organs. Although these membranes are considered to consist of an amorphous gel, recent studies indicate that they are organized by different substructures (Lim, 1984; Lim and Anniko, 1985, 1986). During embryonic development, all overlying membranes undergo remarkable morphogenetic changes and establish predetermined relationships with the underlying stereociliary bundles.

1 Cupula

Formation of the cupular substance has been attributed to hair cells (Vilstrup, 1950), supporting cells of the crista ampullaris (Kolmer, 1926), combinations of hair cells, supporting cells, and intercellular substance (Werner, 1940), cells of the planum semilunatum (Farkas, 1936), or to an extracellular part of the hair cell itself (Wittmaack, 1937). In adults the stereociliary bundle of each hair cell is inserted into the tubules within the cupula (Wersäll, 1956; Dohlman, 1971).

The chemical composition of the cupula is only partially known. For example, histochemical studies indicate the presence of acid mucopolysaccharides. X-ray diffraction of cupular material revealed two bands, between 4.57 and 4.81 Å and between 10 and 14 Å. This pattern is superimposable on that given by the tectorial membrane, that is, double lines at 4.6–4.8 Å and 10–14 Å (Iurato, 1960). However, elemental analysis of the tectorial membrane and the cupula reveals at least qualitative differences (Anniko and Wróblewski, 1980). Distinct elemental histogram peaks are identified for sodium, phosphorus, sulfur, chlorine, potassium, and calcium in the tectorial membrane, whereas only minor peaks for chlorine and potassium are obtained for the cupula. However, this technique does not allow analysis of elements with an atomic weight below that of sodium, which must influence the interpretation of the results obtained from a structure composed mainly of organic material.

Serial studies on the formation of the cupula crista ampullaris have been performed in the mouse (Anniko and Nordemar, 1982). The development of the cupula starts on gestational day 14 and proceeds mainly during gestational days 15 and 16. The cupula is formed from the underlying epithelium when there are only a small number of differentiated hair cells present. The secretion of organic material occurs from supporting cells (Figures 20 and 21). The surface of the epithelium, which corresponds in location to the planum semilunatum in the adult organ, has a thick layer of microvilli and shows particularly high secretory activity on gestational day 15. After gestational day 16 there are few morphologic signs of secretion. The cupula also develops in inner ear explants cultured *in vitro* (Figure 22). A subcupular space is identified early during development as well as a fibrillar substructure in the cupular substance (Figures 23 and 24).

The cupula is highly susceptible to tissue shrinkage during tissue preparation, which makes it difficult to assess accurately the stereocilia–cupula relationships. Embedding this material in epoxy followed by the freeze-fracture technique (Tanaka, 1972) allows this relationship to be examined by scanning electron microscopy, even under *in situ* conditions, as demonstrated in adult guinea pig, human fetuses, and developing mice (Tanaka et al., 1975; Lim and Anniko, 1985).

Using scanning electron microscopy it was reconfirmed that in the mouse, the cupula starts to develop at 14 days of gestation as an amorphous

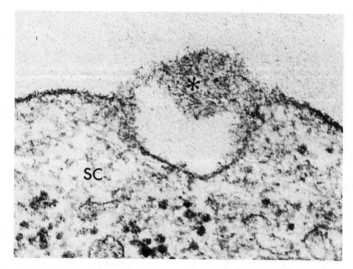

FIGURE 20. TEM. Organic intracellular material (asterisk) secreted from a supporting cell (SC) during the formation of the cupula at the 14th gestational day in mouse.

granular substance covering the sensory cell area, and by gestation day 16 the cupula forms a thin membrane. The amorphous substance covering the sensory cilia forms a small clearing surrounding the sensory cell, and the amorphous substance becomes fibrillar. In 16-day embryos the developing cupula is already attached to the transitional cells. At birth the cupula has almost reached its adult form. Up to 1 day after birth the base of the cupula is in close contact with the stereociliary bundles. The supporting cells with tall microvillae are secreting a gelatinous meshwork and cupular substance. However, at around 6 days after birth the secretory activity is reduced and a distinct subcupular space becomes evident (Figure 25). In mice, the tall ciliary bundles are inserted into cupular canals as in guinea pig and human fetus, but the short ones are in general free-standing. In mouse as in other species, the canals are larger in the central part and smaller at the periphery of the cupula. The diameter of each individual canal is larger at the base and smaller toward the apex.

In the 26-week human fetal inner ear, each sensory hair bundle appears in the canaliculus. During embryonic development the tall stereociliary bundles in the periphery of the crista ampullaris become inserted into the tubules, while the shorter ciliary bundles in the central zone of the crista remain free-standing. This anatomic arrangement suggests that the cells with short hair bundles are best stimulated by endolymph drag (dynamic receptors), whereas the cells with long hair bundles are inserted into the cupular tubules, which makes the stereocilia best stimulated by the displacement of the cupula (static receptors). In general, maturation of the cupula appears parallel to that of the sensory cilia.

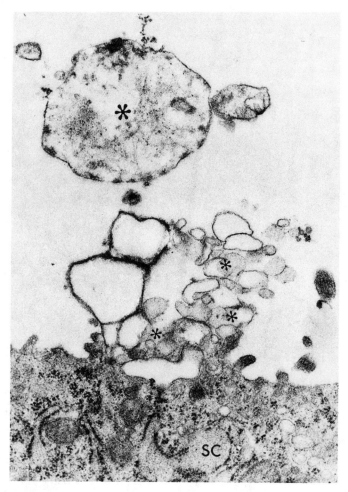

FIGURE 21. TEM. Crista ampullaris of the 15-gestational-day mouse inner ear. Secretion of intracellular material (asterisks) from supporting cell (SC) surfaces into the endolymphatic space.

2   Otoconia

The otolith layer is a distinct feature of the utricle and saccule. The morphology and elemental composition of mature otoconia are well documented in the literature (Carlström et al., 1953; Carlström and Engström, 1955; Igarashi and Kanda, 1969; Lim, 1974). Otoconia are found in the gravity receptor organs of a number of invertebrates and all vertebrates. However, there are considerable species differences in the shape, size, chemical composition, and mode of otoconial formation. Otoconia consists of calcium carbonate crystallized in the form of calcite in mammals, birds, and sharks,

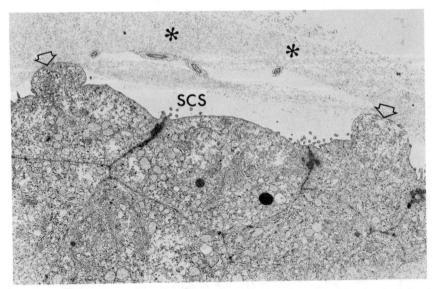

FIGURE 22. TEM. Cupular material (asterisks) above the surface of a crista ampularis developed *in vitro*. Mouse otocyst at the 12th gestational day cultured *in vitro* for 9 days. Prominent protrusions from supporting cells (arrows) are in contact with the cupula. A subcupular space (SCS) is evident. The cells are filled with polyribosomes, Golgi material, and extended endoplasmic reticulum.

calcium carbonate in the form of aragonite in amphibia, and calcium phosphate in the lamprey. The statoconial membrane is composed of the otoconial layer, the gelatinous layer, and a subcupular meshwork. Some otoconia are partly embedded in the gelatinous substance, whereas the rest of the otoconia are simply held together by gelatinous material. Histochemical studies have revealed that the gelatinous layer and subcupular meshwork are composed of acid mucopolysaccharides and glycoproteins (Veenhof, 1969). Recent immunomorphologic investigations have shown that at least some gelatinous substances react with monoclonal antibodies directed against cytokeratins (Thornell et al., 1987; Anniko et al., 1988).

Statoconia provide indispensable cues for sensory perception of the environment. Although abnormalities of the vestibular nerve and nuclei contribute to postnatal imbalance and ataxia, the vestibular end organs and statoconia provide the primary input for detecting gravity. Without the utricular and saccular maculae and/or statoconia in these structures, vertebrates have great difficulty maintaining body balance. Several species with genetically defective otoliths show erratic behavior and are sometimes unable to walk upright (Lyon, 1955; Erway et al., 1970; Purichia and Erway, 1972; Rouse et al., 1984).

During embryonic development, secretion of organic material occurs from the epithelial cell layer of the macula utriculi and macula sacculi and is

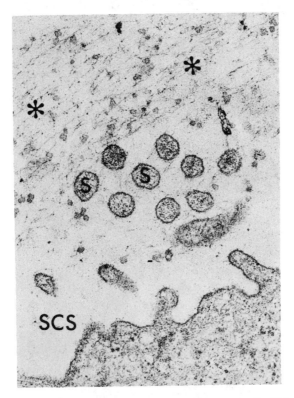

FIGURE 23. TEM. Cupular material (asterisks) surrounding stereocilia (S) in 15-gestational-day inner ear of the mouse. A subcupular space (SCS) is also apparent.

regarded as an organic matrix for otoconial formation (Lim, 1973; Ross and Peacor, 1975; Nakahara and Bevelander, 1979). Anniko (1980b) showed in undecalcified mouse specimens that although large accumulations of secreted cytoplasmic material occurred above the surface of the developing macula, a rebuilding of the organic material must take place in this region (Figures 26 and 27). The otoconial matrix frequently revealed an extensive fibrillar substructure that was not present either in hair cells or in supporting cells. The critical nucleation concept for the initiation of crystal formation has been supported by several investigators (Veenhof, 1969; Lim, 1973; Anniko, 1980b). According to this theory, preexisting heterogeneous nucleation initiates the growth of crystals. In contrast, Nakahara and Bevelander (1979) proposed that primitive otoconia form a nonmineralized organic mass that serves as a template on which calcium carbonate is deposited. In a study on the formation of otoconia in rats, Salamat et al. (1980) demonstrated multinucleation sites of crystal seeding during early development of the calcified crystal. The morphology of primitive otoconia is closely related to that of the organic nuclei of the crystals.

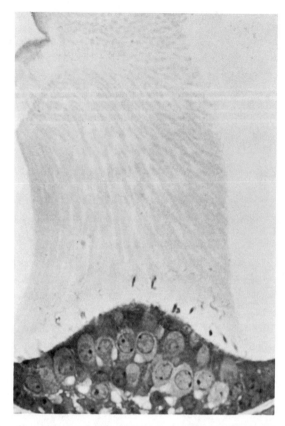

FIGURE 24. Cupular canals are identified by light microscopy in the 18-gestational-day mouse crista ampullaris.

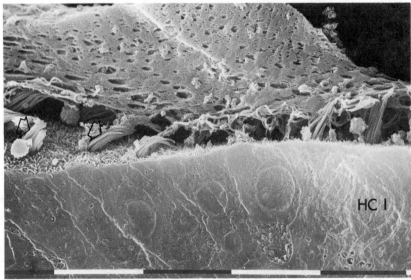

FIGURE 25. SEM. Mouse crista ampullaris photographed on PND 6. Tall stereociliary bundles in the periphery of the crista are inserted into cupular canals, whereas shorter stereocilia (arrows) at the middle of the crista are often free-standing. HC I, type I hair cells. Bar = 10 μm.

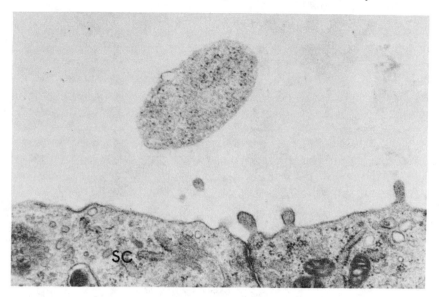

FIGURE 26. TEM. Macula utriculi of mouse on 16th gestational day. An otoconia-like structure consisting of organic material appears above the surface of the macula. SC, supporting cells.

The question of which is formed first, the gelatinous layer or otoconia, still remains unsolved. Lim and Anniko (1985) used the epoxy fracturing technique to show that otoconia were found prior to the identification of the gelatinous layer (Figure 28). However, use of this special morphologic technique does not preclude early appearance of the gelatinous layer as well.

A directed secretion of calcium is likely to occur from epithelial cells into developing otoconia (Anniko, 1980b; Anniko et al., 1987b). Harada (1979) showed that large quantities of calcium were present in protoplasmic protrusions of supporting cells in the maculae during otoconial development. However, this material was processed for ordinary scanning electron microscopy prior to X-ray microanalysis. Such a procedure is likely to distort the elemental composition of cells *in situ*. Recent X-ray microanalytic studies on developing otoconia from material only cryofixed and cryosectioned shows that morphologically distinct cell protrusions are not fixation artefacts but indicate high secretory activity (Anniko et al., 1987). Cell protrusions in the maculae are evident for only a short period during the most active phase of otoconial development. Elemental analyses of the epithelial cell blebbings revealed an extremely high calcium content in many, but not all, cell blebbings analyzed. This indicates that the incorporation of calcium into otoconia occurs as a directed flow from the epithelial cells of the macula (either together with secreted organic material or as a flow of calcium ions) and is not due to a general oversaturation with calcium in the endolymphatic fluid.

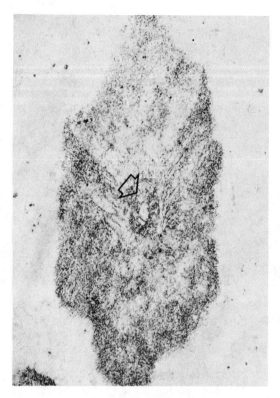

FIGURE 27. TEM. Immature otoconium with a (probably organic) nucleus (arrow) in 17-gestational-day macula utriculi of mouse.

In the developing chick labyrinth, a primitive organic matrix of future otoconia was identified in the supporting cells of the saccule and utricle (Fermin and Igarashi, 1986; Fermin et al., 1987). Statoconial units emerged from the upper surface of supporting cells but without a central core. Statoconia thickened at the periphery, and a central core formed. Calcium was deposited between the fibrils of older statoconia. Exposure to carbonic anhydrase inhibitors prevented statoconia formation and/or prevented calcium and the matrix from associating. The fact that both components of statoconia (organic matrix and calcium) could be separated and not associated with each other might indicate that a limiting factor is the culprit. Thus, it can be hypothesized that during otoconial formation, organic calcium in granular form may be attracted to the organic matrix and subsequently incorporated (Anniko, 1980b; Fermin and Igarashi, 1985).

C Biochemistry of the Inner Ear

Biochemical studies on the vestibular part of the developing inner ear are still rather sparse. Since the membranous labyrinth in mammals, including

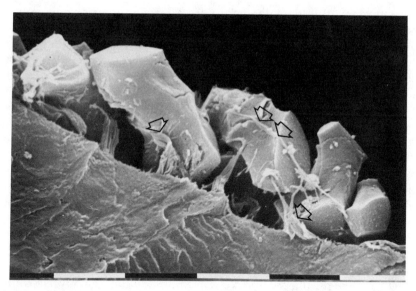

FIGURE 28. SEM. Late-17-gestational-day macula utriculi of mouse. Immature otoconia immediately above the macular surface in close contact with sensory hair bundles (arrows). A fibrillar network (double arrows) extends between adjacent otoconia, which probably keeps otoconia together. Bar = 10 μm.

man, is enclosed within the temporal bone at the skull base, access to the inner ear is technically difficult. Because of the complexity of various cells and tissues in the inner ear, isolation of pure cell populations for traditional biochemical analysis has been unsuccessful. Quantitative histochemistry and cytochemistry of the adult inner ear has largely been performed by Thalmann and coworkers (1976) and Schacht (1986).

Anniko et al. (1981b) analyzed transport enzyme adenylate cyclase activity in fetal and early postnatal inner ears of mice in which vestibular and cochlear parts were studied separately. Two periods of increased activity were documented: from gestational days 16–19 in both the cochlear and vestibular parts of the labyrinth and from birth to postnatal day (PND) 6 in the lateral wall tissues of the scala media. During the first period the anatomical boundaries of the secretory epithelia are developing. The dark cell epithelium around the vestibular organs reaches an electron optically mature configuration except for an incompletely developed number of cell projections toward the basal membrane (Anniko, 1980a). The stria vascularis starts to differentiate on day of gestation 17, that is, the anatomical location can be distinguished from surrounding structures. The epithelium consists of cuboid cells that stain histologically more intensely than cells in adjacent parts of the lateral wall of the scala media that do not develop into stria vascularis (Sher, 1971). It is therefore possible that changes in the concentrations of adenylate cyclase are related to morphologic and biochemical differentiation of the secretory epithelia. The postnatal increase in adenylate cyclase activity in the lateral wall tissues correlates in time with the morphologic maturation of the stria vascularis at the cellular and subcellular levels. Elemental analysis of endolymph at birth and 2 days after birth shows a slightly more mature composition in the vestibular part than in the cochlear part (Anniko and Wróblewski, 1981). This may indicate some physiological function in the dark cell epithelium at this stage of maturation. The increase in enzyme activity in the cochlea during maturation of endolymph supports a link between adenylate cyclase and control of inner ear fluids. In general, however, it is difficult to establish any absolute correlations between specific structures and function. During embryonic development, maturation of the inner ear proceeds in parallel to maturation of a variety of cell and tissue types. The onset of function (often registered electrophysiologically as changes in different electrical potentials) begins gradually.

Inner ears developed *in vitro* show very little growth with regard to total protein content during the first week in culture. In contrast, protein content in the labyrinth increases threefold during the corresponding period *in vivo*. The activity of adenylate cyclase develops synchronously *in vivo* and *in vitro* until gestational day 19, after which the specific activity of the enzyme *in vitro* exceeds that of the enzyme *in vivo* some three- to fivefold, suggesting a lack of control mechanisms in organ culture (Anniko et al., 1981a).

Phospholipid labeling revealed less dramatic differences between the two systems: the same lipids are labeled in an essentially similar quantitative manner. The presence of polyphosphoinositide metabolism and ototoxicity has been demonstrated for the adult guinea pig (Schacht et al., 1977, Schacht, 1979; Lodhi et al., 1980). The organ culture system may thus serve as a suitable model for morphologic and biochemical studies on aminoglycoside ototoxicity. However, the fact that some quantitative differences exist between the labeling of cultured inner ears and labyrinths developed *in vivo* again demonstrates that the two systems are not fully comparable.

Study of the phosphoinositide content in the developing inner ear shows that phosphatidylinositol phosphate and phosphatidylinositol biphosphate are rapidly labeled by ^{32}P orthophosphate in the developing inner ear of the mouse (Anniko and Schacht, 1981). In chase experiments the label is lost from polyphosphoinositides but not from other lipids. The lipids are already present in the 13-gestational-day otocyst and behave similarly in the cochlear and vestibular part of the labyrinth. A rapid turnover of these lipids, as previously determined in adult nerves and secretory tissues, is thus already present in functionally immature tissues.

Several enzymes, such as Na^+, K^+–APTase, carbonic anhydrase (Watanabe and Ogawa, 1984), and adenylate cyclase systems (Paloheimo and Thalmann, 1977; Anniko et al., 1981b) are located in the inner ear organelles. The Na^+, K^+–ATPase has been demonstrated cytochemically in the strial marginal cell (Mees, 1983; Yoshihara et al., 1987b) and the vestibular dark cell (Yoshihara and Igarashi, 1987; Yoshihara et al., 1987b). Several of these systems are influenced by calcium ions; for example, Ca^{2+}–ATPase activity occurs on the plasma membranes of vestibular cells and is closely related to Ca^{2+} transport across the plasma membrane (Yoshihara et al., 1987a). However, studies have so far been focused on the mature inner ear and, there is a great need for analysis of embryonic material.

The ideal procedure for biochemical analysis is one in which both tissue morphology and the *in vivo* distribution of ions and elements in specimens are preserved. The method of choice is to quickly freeze and thereafter handle the tissue in the frozen state. These general principles have been applied in analytical electron microscopy. The use of X-ray microanalysis technique (XRMA) in studies on the developing inner ear has recently been reviewed (Anniko and Wróblewski, 1983). Cryosectioning allows one to study a large number of different structures of the membranous labyrinth and to analyze these structures with good topographical precision. XRMA is particularly suitable for embryonic material and for temporal bones from small laboratory animals such as mice and guinea pigs. Special emphasis has been placed on documentation of inner ear fluid maturation and on the formation of otoconia. We have recently reported (Anniko et al., 1988) advances in inner ear cytochemistry with regard to microanalytical and immunomorphological investigations.

D Central Pathways

Kölliker (1891) and later Ramón y Cajal (1909) described how the vestibular nerve enters the brainstem and bifurcates into ascending and descending branches. The first attempt to investigate how the different parts of the vestibular organ project on the vestibular ganglion and further into the brainstem was made by Lorente de Nó (1933) in Golgi material in the mouse. His findings, however, are rather difficult to interpret as he used a terminology for brainstem structures different from that commonly used today. Nevertheless it was obvious that fibers from the various labyrinthine receptor organs have, in part, a different central representation. In a more recent study, Siegborn and Grant (1983) described brainstem projections of different branches of the vestibular nerve in the adult cat. The present understanding is that the fibers innervating the cristae of the semicircular canals terminate mainly in the interstitial nucleus and the superior and oral parts of the medial and descending vestibular nuclei, whereas fibers deriving from otolithic organs end mainly in the descending nucleus, medial vestibular nucleus, ventral parts of the lateral vestibular nucleus, and group "Y" (Stein and Carpenter, 1967; Gacek, 1969).

The vestibular nuclei are among the first to become differentiated in the brainstem. At birth many mammals show the different morphologic types of neurons that have been described for the four vestibular nuclei.

However, in species with relatively short gestational periods, such as the rat and cat, these neurons are not mature and undergo distinct postnatal changes, both qualitatively and quantitatively (Karhunen, 1973; Sans and Chat, 1976). This process is associated with increasing dendritic length, a general increase in the density of dendritic spines, and a reorganization of synaptic contacts. In the adult, most of the spines are not concentrated on the proximal parts of the dendrites but are located 200–300 μm from the soma. At present it is not known if the differentiation of neurons of the vestibular nucleus in higher vertebrates depends on the trophic influence of primary vestibular efferents as has been demonstrated by Peusner and Morest (1977) in the chick.

Most studies on the development of the central vestibular system have focused on parameters of functional development in humans and in a few other species (Lannou et al., 1983; Ornitz, 1983). Although relatively little is known about structural features of developing central pathways of the vestibular system, some fundamental properties of functional development in this system have been examined.

V   FUNCTIONAL ORGANIZATION OF THE SEMICIRCULAR CANAL

All mechanoreceptor epithelia in a labyrinth and in the lateral line system basically exhibit the same architecture, being composed of sensory cells embraced by supporting cells that rest upon a basement membrane. The receptor cells contain sensory hairs coupled to auxiliary structures that transmit vibratory or gravitational stimuli to the sensory cells. The responses of the receptor cell regulate flow of impulses to the innervating nerve fibers. Each hair cell possesses a morphologic polarization determined by the relative positions of the kinocilium and stereocilia (Wersäll et al., 1965). Even in hair cells of the adult mammalian cochlea, where the kinocilium is lacking, polarization is observed as defined by position of the basal body.

The adult kinocilium is always located in the periphery of the sensory hair bundle. In the crista ampullaris of the horizontal ampulla, the kinocilium is found on the side of the bundle facing the utricle, whereas it is found on the canal side of the cristae in the outer two semicircular canals. The location of the kinocilium thus coincides with the direction of excitation of the hair cell. As a consequence the morphologic polarization of the hair cell reflects its functional polarization (Loewenstein and Wersäll, 1959). The macula utriculi exhibits a more complicated pattern of orientation. Beginning at the medial macula, the kinocilia point in gradually altering directions from anterior to lateral to posterior in a nearly semiannular pattern (Flock, 1965). In a zone along the anterior, lateral, and posterior margins of the macula, the hair cells are oriented with the kinocilia pointing in opposite directions.

The basic electrophysiological principle of hair cell organs is the bidirectional response to stimuli approaching from opposite directions. Displacement of the sensory hairs toward the kinocilium is accompanied by depolarization of the cell and increased discharge rate by innervating nerve fibers, whereas displacement in the opposite direction is accompanied by hyperpolarization and decreased discharge frequency (Figure 29). This theory is consistent with the orientation of the cristae.

The functional polarization and directional selectivity of individual hair cells as originally described by Loewenstein and Wersäll (1959) in the ray (*Raja clavata*) has now been extended to the canals of a wide variety of species ranging from cyclostomes (Loewenstein, 1970) to mammals (Goldberg and Fernandez, 1971). The theory is also applicable to otolith (Fernandez et al., 1972; Loe et al., 1973) and lateral line organs (Flock, 1965). Peripheral canal neurons in warm-blooded animals have a remarkably high resting discharge rate, averaging 65 spikes per second in gerbils (Schneider and Andersson, 1976) and 90 spikes per second in pigeons (Correia and Landolt, 1973) and squirrel monkeys (Goldberg and Fernandez, 1971). Lower resting discharges are found in cold-blooded animals. The afferent innervation exhibits a bidirectional response. The directions of excitatory and inhibitory accelerations are identical for all afferents innervating a single semicircular canal ampulla and are consistent with Ewald's first law.

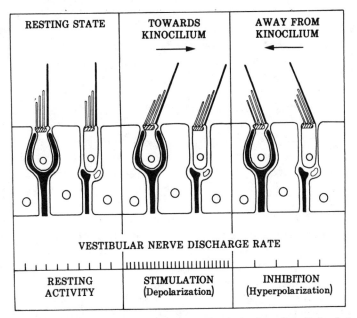

FIGURE 29. Schematic drawing showing anatomical polarization of vestibular hair cells and vestibular nerve discharge rate due to displacement of sensory hairs. Modified from Wersäll et al. (1967).

Traditionally, the response dynamics of peripheral neurons were thought to reflect dynamics of the cupula–endolymph system. However, it has now been established that additional mechanisms influence responses in both peripheral and central vestibular neurons.

Head movements in the horizontal plane around the vertical axis cause angular accelerations that displace endolymph in the membranous horizontal semicircular duct of the inner ear. The magnitude of fluid displacement is greatest when the plane of the head movement coincides with the plane of the semicircular duct and decreases in a cosine function as the angle between these planes increases (Curthoys et al., 1977). The cupula has an elastic restorative force so that at the end of angular acceleration it returns to its normal resting position. The sequences of the cupular bending and return have been described as a mechanical operation of the semicircular canal. For a given head movement of angular acceleration a number of anatomical and mechanical factors influence the extent to which the cupula will be bent and the time course of this bending: the radius of the duct, the viscosity and density of endolymph, and the stiffness of the cupula (Steinhausen, 1933; Oman, 1981). In response to head rotation, horizontal canal neurons increase their firing rate during angular acceleration to the ipsilateral side and decrease firing during angular acceleration to the contralateral side.

According to Goldberg and Fernandez (1972), a steady potential exists across the luminal surface of the hair cell. The potential may have two sources: an intrinsic polarization of the membrane of the hair cell and an extrinsic (or endolymphatic) potential. The two potentials taken together result in a current flow directed through the hair cell from its luminal to its basal surface. An adequate stimulus results in a shearing displacement of the sensory hairs. The displacement is envisioned as modulating the resistance of the luminal surfaces and hence the current flow.

The interactions of acoustic stimuli with the vestibular system are only partially known. Recently Wit et al. (1986) showed that acoustic stimuli caused electrical responses in the vestibular system of the pigeon. The vestibular response was described as a "vestibular microphonics" generated by the vestibular hair cells. Which groups of hair cells (cristae, maculae utriculi, or sacculi) actually contribute to this response was not clarified. The fact that the ratio of the first and second harmonic response component depends strongly on the recording site suggests that more than one sensory area is involved within the membranous labyrinth.

In a series of studies Suzuki and co-workers (1984) and Suzuki and Harada (1985a,b) analyzed the physiological significance of the mode of cupular movement. It was suggested that the swing door deflection is physiologically most relevant in giving the optimum increase in response rate as well as in maintaining the time course of the tonic response. Perception of rotatory movement can thus be achieved primarily by swing door deflection, which elicits both phasic and tonic responses that can eventually signal both the change and magnitude of angular velocity.

VI   RECORDINGS OF PRIMARY AFFERENT AND BRAINSTEM ACTIVITY: DEVELOPMENTAL PERSPECTIVE

Studies in this field are relatively few and have been performed mainly in rat (review: Curthoys, 1983), cat (Romand and Dauzat, 1982), and squirrel monkey (Goldberg and Fernandez, 1971).

A   Resting Activity

Responses of rat horizontal semicircular canal primary afferents during postnatal development have been described by Curthoys in a series of papers (Curthoys, 1978, 1979, 1981a,b). At birth, primary horizontal canal afferent neurons in the rat show slow, irregular, spontaneous activity as well as insensitive, sluggish, and variable responses to angular acceleration stimuli. During the first 4–5 days after birth, rapid changes occur in the gross morphology of the rat semicircular canal. During this time there is a rapid increase in neural sensitivity to both constant and sinusoidal acceleration. However, after gross morphologic changes are complete and duct dimensions have reached adult size, there are still further changes in neural response properties. Neurons with regular spontaneous activity begin to appear after PND 4 in rat. During subsequent days there is a steady increase in the proportion of neurons classified as regular. At about PND 20 some 25% of primary afferents show regular activity as compared with adult animals having 31% regularly firing neurons. A study on newborn and postnatal cats has confirmed this maturation pattern (Romand and Dauzat, 1982). The bases for these developmental changes in neurophysiological activity are not clearly understood. Developmental alterations in physiologically defined regular cells probably reflect changes in the receptor–neural fiber complex. For example, Nordemar (1983) showed that a complete and mature type of vestibular hair cell innervation is not present until the beginning of the second postnatal month in mouse (which has a similar time sequence for morphologic maturation of vestibular organs as the rat).

B   Response to Angular Acceleration

Theoretically, long-duration acceleration behaves essentially as a square-wave stimulus to the cupula. During such stimulation the cupula would be displaced from its resting position to a new position depending on the magnitude of the acceleration. Thereafter, the cupula should maintain that displaced position during the remainder of the acceleration.

In the adult rat the average incremental sensitivity of irregular neurons is significantly higher than that of regular neurons, a phenomenon consistent throughout postnatal development. For regular neurons, no consistent trend of incremental sensitivity appears during postnatal life. Regular neurons are first encountered at about 4 days of age and the incremental sensitivity of these early cells is about the same as that of adults. For further discussion of asymmetry of sensitivity and time constants in regular and irregular neurons during growth, see Curthoys (1983).

C   Optokinetic Response

In principle, three major sensory inputs converge on central vestibular neurons: those from peripheral labyrinthine receptors, inputs elicited by optokinetic stimulation, and proprioceptive inputs originating mainly from joint and muscle afferents in the neck. All three systems are used to trigger and control ocular and postural reflexes. The functional development of neurons of the vestibular nucleus following vestibular and optokinetic stimulation has been mainly studied in the rat, an altricial species which manifests about the same sequence of postnatal morphologic and functional maturation as the mouse.

In contrast to the vestibular system that is already functioning to some extent at birth, the optokinetic input to the vestibular nuclei is not functional until after eye opening in the rat. So far it has not been established whether this absence of optokinetic responses of vestibular neurons during the first week following eye opening, and the slow development thereafter, is only a true developmental process of the optokinetic system or whether this phenomenon reflects the vigilance level of young animals. For detailed studies, see Precht and Cazin (1979), Cazin et al. (1980), and Lannou et al. (1983).

VII   DEVELOPMENT OF VESTIBULAR REFLEXES

Principles of functional development of vestibular reflexes have recently been described by Lannou et al. (1983) in the rat, cat, and rabbit. It is concluded that vision is not essential for the development of the vestibulo-ocular reflex (VOR). Visual deprivation has no effect on the development of vestibular receptors and primary vestibular afferents. The vestibular inputs fed into the VOR system are normal during visual deprivation. The VOR matures as the peripheral and central vestibular systems develop in the complete absence of any visual input. The gain of the VOR takes on an arbitrary value according to the bias of the system (Collewijn, 1977). Vision is necessary, however, to achieve perfect compensatory eye movements over a wide frequency range. Early visual deprivation impairs the influence of vision on VOR gain. It seems likely that there is a critical period for both the achievement of a normal bias of the VOR proper and the ability of optokinetic feedback to adjust VOR gain and phase during head movements. Thus, the final shaping of vestibular reflex behavior requires optokinetic inputs during early life.

Maturation of vestibular spinal reflexes has been studied by Sans et al. (1968), Hård and Larsson (1975), Parrad and Cottereau (1977), and others. In principle, vestibular spinal reflexes in rat undergo postnatal changes similar to those observed for the VOR system. Gradual maturation takes place, although these changes have not yet been correlated to any specific event of the maturing CNS.

In man, the vestibular system is both anatomically complete and functionally responsive at or before birth. However, vestibular responses to an equivalent stimulus (caloric or rotational) are markedly different between preadolescent children and adults (Conraux and Collard, 1970; Jongkees and Gasthuis, 1973). The most marked maturation changes occur in preschool children (Ornitz et al., 1979). Newborn infants show distinct nystagmus characterized by alternating slow and fast components that can be elicited by acceleration, optokinetic stimuli, or caloric stimuli provided that arousal is maintained. An interesting phenomenon is that after the first few months of life the vestibular system is functioning at its highest level of reactivity, a level that will wane with subsequent maturation. Important modifications of central vestibular mechanisms occur during the first few years of life and continue more gradually throughout childhood. For further details concerning the normal and pathologic maturation of vestibular function in humans see Ornitz (1983).

VIII   DEVELOPMENT OF VESTIBULAR APPARATUS UNDER WEIGHTLESS CONDITIONS

Development of the structure and function of the vestibular apparatus in vertebrates precedes the formation of other sense organs. The morphologic development of the inner ear is genetically preprogrammed; after induction of the rhombencephalic area the isolated inner ear organ can reach close-to-full maturation in organ culture (Van De Water, 1976; Anniko and Schacht, 1984; Anniko, 1985b).

Development of the vestibular apparatus and cochlea is not dependent on the influence of earth's gravitational field (Vinnikov et al., 1983). Using light microscopy and transmission electron microscopy, it has been documented in a number of species that both organogenesis and cytodifferentiation occur normally under weightless conditions; these features include polarization of sensory cells with regard to the peripheral location of the kinocilium in vestibular hair cells or of the basal body in cochlear hair cells. The statoacoustic ganglion develops and differentiates under weightless conditions, and nerve fibers also grow to their predetermined regions as under normal gravity conditions. In addition, utricular and saccular otoconia develop without morphologic deviation under these nongravitational conditions. Using the electron microprobe technique, Vinnikov et al. (1979) showed that with regard to the distribution of elements in otoconia, no qualitative differences were observed between otoconia formed on earth and under weightless conditions. A specific stimulus, namely, gravity, is not needed for initial formation or structural maturation of the vestibular apparatus.

While morphologic development of the vestibular apparatus under weightless conditions has been analyzed in a number of studies, considerably less is known about corresponding behavioral development. When the fish *Fundulus heteroclitus* is allowed to develop in space, it later undergoes unusual loop-shaped motion in space flight. However, structural development of the vestibular apparatus was completely normal in these animals. Deviations in the geotactic reaction were also observed after 6 months of adaption on earth in fish fertilized up to 32 h after launch (von Baumgarten et al., 1975; Sheld et al., 1979). Fish in orbit were also more sensitive to habituation than were control animals.

The studies cited in this section have to be classified as short-term sets of observations using species that develop rapidly within a few days. Effects of prolonged weightlessness are not known, particularly if several generations develop under these conditions.

IX SUMMARY

The developmental sequence of inner ear organs is similar among mammals as well as in vertebrates generally. The order of formation is first anterior, then posterior, and lateral semicircular canals. Next the anterior crista and macula sacculi become separate units, followed by the posterior crista, lateral crista, and macula utriculi. The cytodifferentiation of vestibular organs also follows general principles of maturation in mammals. These principles are particularly well understood for structural development of peripheral vestibular organs in a number of rodent species and in the cat. Considerably less is known about primates, which suggests that future areas of research on embryonic development of the inner ear should especially focus on primate species, including man. Present knowledge based upon recent studies of the human embryonic inner ear (Hoshino, 1982; Dechesne and Sans, 1985; Sans and Dechesne, 1985; Thornell et al., 1987; Anniko et al., 1988) does, however, generally confirm that developmental sequences in man are comparable to other mammals. Analyses of physiological maturation in the vestibular part of the inner ear are particularly sparse and have focused mainly on functional maturation of the lateral (horizontal) semicircular canal and its crista ampullaris (Curthoys, 1983).

There is a paucity of studies on structural and physiological maturation of central vestibular pathways that to date have concentrated on few species. Further studies especially need to focus on pathways beyond the receptor level in mammals, including primate species.

Maturation of vestibular reflexes reflects an integrated function of peripheral and central pathways. In man the developmental sequences of these behaviors are well documented from birth on (Ornitz, 1983). However, it is difficult to separate the importance of individual cell and tissue development from total integrated maturation of vestibular reflexes.

Thus far, studies on maturation of vestibular reflexes have been mainly descriptive, without direct comparisons with individual morphologic and physiological events during maturation. It is clear that extraordinary plasticity of vestibular function occurs during postnatal development in humans. Vestibular mechanisms may play a pervasive role in general maturation, a role that transcends various functions including preservation of gaze and maintenance of equilibrium. Fruitful areas for future research would focus on maturation of vestibular–proprioceptive and vestibular–visual interactions. More data are clearly needed on the relationship between spontaneous vestibular behavior and motor development in infancy.

The extent to which morphologic and electrophysiological development can be correlated to onset of integrated function of the inner ear is at present only speculative. Behavioral development is also dependent on the maturation of central vestibular pathways as well as on the developmental stage of other organ systems, such as proprioception and other sensory organs. Therefore studies of behavioral development alone cannot provide many answers to mechanisms of development of vestibular function. It can be assumed that the onset of behavioral function comes gradually, in a way that can be described by various morphologic and electrophysiological components.

ACKNOWLEDGMENTS

Supported by grants from the Swedish Medical Research Council (12X-7305), the Foundation Tysta Skolan, the Ragnar and Torsten Söderberg Foundation, and the University of Umeå.

REFERENCES

Altmann, F. (1950) Normal development of the ear and its mechanics. Arch. Otolaryngol. (Chic.) 52:725–766.

Altschuler, R. A., M. H. Parakkal, J. A. Rubio, D. W. Hoffman, and J. Fex (1984) Enkephalin-like immunoreactivity in the guinea pig organ of Corti: Ultrastructural and lesion studies. Hear. Res. 16:17–31.

Altschuler, R. A., D. W. Hoffman, and R. J. Wenthold (1986) Neurotransmitters of the cochlea and cochlear nucleus. Immunocytochemical evidence. Amer. J. Otolaryngol. 7:100–106.

Angeletti, R. H., and R. A. Bradshaw (1971) Nerve growth factor from mouse submaxillary gland: Amino acid sequence. Proc. Natl. Acad. Sci. USA. 68:2417–2420.

Anniko, M. (1980a) Embryonic development in vivo and in vitro of the dark cell region of the mammalian crista ampullaris. Acta Otolaryngol. (Stockh.) 90:106–114.

Anniko, M. (1980b) Development of otoconia. Amer. J. Otolaryngol. *1*:400–410.

Anniko, M. (1983) Embryonic development of vestibular sense organs and their innervation. In R. Romand (ed.): Development of Auditory and Vestibular systems. New York: Academic Press, pp. 375–423.

Anniko, M. (1984) Das "In-vitro-System" in der Innenohrforschung. Laryng. Rhinol. Otol. *63*:413–423.

Anniko, M. (1985a) Formation and maturation of the vestibular ganglion. Adv. Oto-Rhino-Laryngol. *47*:57–65.

Anniko, M. (1985b) Hair cell differentiation following tissue interactions for induction of otocyst morphogenesis. Arch. Oto-Rhino-Laryngol. *242*:287–294.

Anniko, M., and H. Nordemar (1982) Formation of the cupula cristae ampullaris: Development *in vivo* and *in vitro*. Amer. J. Otolaryngol. *3*:31–40.

Anniko, M., and J. Schacht (1981) Phosphoinositides in the developing inner ear with references to brain, kidney and liver of the mouse. Int. J. Biochem. *13*:951–953.

Anniko, M., and J. Schacht (1984) Inductive tissue interactions of mammalian inner ear development. Arch. Oto-Rhino-Laryngol. *240*:27–33.

Anniko, M., and L.-E. Thornell (1987) Cytoskeletal organization of the human inner ear. IV. Expression of actin in vestibular organs. Acta Otolaryngol. (Stockh.) Suppl. *437*:65–76.

Anniko, M., and L.-E. Thornell (1989) Actin-associated proteins and fibronectin in the fetal human inner ear. Amer. J. Otolaryngol. *10*:99–109.

Anniko, M., and T. R. Van De Water (1986) Synaptogenesis in cocultured inner ear explants which share a single statoacoustic ganglion. Acta Otolaryngol. (Stockh.) *102*:415–422.

Anniko, M., and S.-O. Wikström (1984) Pattern formation of the otic placode and morphogenesis of the otocyst. Amer. J. Otolaryngol. *5*:373–381.

Anniko, M., and R. Wróblewski (1980) Elemental composition of the mature inner ear. Acta Otolaryngol. (Stockh.) *90*:25–32.

Anniko, M., and R. Wróblewski (1981) Elemental composition of the developing inner ear. Ann. Otol. Rhinol. Laryngol. *90*:25–32.

Anniko, M., and R. Wróblewski (1983) X-ray microanalysis of developing and mature inner ear. Scan. Electr. Microsc. *2*:757–768.

Anniko, M., H. Nordemar, and T. R. Van De Water (1979) Embryogenesis of the inner ear. I. Development and differentiation of the mammalian crista ampullaris *in vivo* and *in vitro*. Arch. Oto-Rhino-Laryngol. *224*:285–299.

Anniko, M., H. Nordemar, M.-L. Spangberg, and J. Schacht (1981a) Biochemical studies on the embryonic development of the mammalian inner ear in organ culture. Arch. Oto-Rhino-Laryngol. *230*:237–243.

Anniko, M., M.-L. Spangberg, and J. Schacht (1981b) Adenylate cyclase activity in the fetal and the early postnatal inner ear of the mouse. Hear. Res. *4*:11–22.

Anniko, M., L.-E. Thornell, H. Gustafsson, and I. Virtanen (1986) Intermediate filaments in the newborn inner ear of the mouse. O.R.L *48*:98–106.

Anniko, M., L.-E. Thornell, and I. Virtanen (1987a) Cytoskeletal organization of the human inner ear. II. Characterization of intermediate filaments in the cochlea. Acta Otolaryngol. (Stockh.) Suppl. *437*:29–54.

Anniko, M., S.-O. Wikström, and R. Wróblewski (1987b) X-ray miroanalytic studies on developing otoconia. Acta Otolaryngol. (Stockh.) *104*:285–289.

Anniko, M., L.-E. Thornell, and R. Wróblewski (1988) Recent advances in inner ear cytochemistry. Microanalytical and immunomorphological investigatins. Progr. Neurobiol. *30*:209–269.

Anniko, M., L.-E. Thornell, T. Stigbrand, and F. C. S. Ramaelars (in press) Cytokeratin diversity in epithelia of the human inner ear. Acta Otolaryngol. (Stockh.).

Anson, B. J. (1934) The early development of the membranous labyrinth in mammalian embryos, with special reference to the endolymphatic duct and the utriculo-endolymphatic duct. Anat. Rec. (Suppl.) *59*:15–25.

Anson, B. J., D. G. Harper, and T. R. Winch (1966) Developmental and adult anatomy of the membranous labyrinth in man. In R. J. Wolfson (ed.): The Vestibular System and Its Diseases. Philadelphia: University of Pennsylvania Press, pp. 19–38.

Ard, M. D., D. K. Morest, and S. H. Hauger (1985) Trophic interactions between the cochleo-vestibular ganglion of the chick embryo and its synaptic targets in culture. Neuroscience *16*:151–170.

Bagger-Sjöbäck, D., and M. Anniko (1984) Development of intercellular junctions in the vestibular end-organ. A freeze-fracture study in the mouse. Ann. Otol. Rhinol. Laryngol. *93*:89–95.

Barde, Y.-A., D. Edgar, and H. Thoenen (1983) New neurotrophic factors. Ann. Rev. Physiol. *45*:601–612.

Bartelmez, G. W. (1922) The otic origin of the otic and optic primordia in man. J. Comp. Neurol. *34*:201–232.

Bast, T. M., and B. J. Anson (1949) The Temporal Bone and the Ear. Springfield, Illinois: Thomas.

Berggren, D., and M. Anniko, (1989) Lack of differentiation of the isolated murine statoacoustic ganglion during organ culture. O. R. L. *51*:124–129.

Berry, M., P. McConell, J. Sivers, S. Price, and A. Anwar (1981) Factors influencing the growth of cerebellar neural networks. Bibl. Anat. *19*:1–51.

Brodal, A. (1974) Anatomy of the vestibular nuclei and their connections. In H. H. Kornhuber (ed.): Handbook of Sensory Physiology, Vol. 6/1. Berlin: Springer-Verlag, pp. 239–352.

Carlström, B., H. Engström, and S. Hjorth (1953) Electron microscopic and X-ray diffraction studies of statoconia. Laryngoscope *63*:1052–1057.

Carlström, B., and H. Engström (1955) The ultrastructure of statoconia. Acta Otolaryngol. (Stockh.) *45*:14–18.

Cazin, L., W. Precht, and J. Lannou (1980) Optokinetic responses of vestibular nuclear neurons in the rat. Pflüg. Arch. *384*:31–38.

Collewijn, H. (1977) Optokinetic and vestibulo-ocular reflexes in dark-reared rabbits. Exp. Brain Res. *27*:287–300.

Connelly, T. G., L. L. Brinkley,, and W. M. Carlsson (1981) Morphogenesis and Pattern Formation. New York: Raven Press.

Conraux, C., and M. Collard (1970) L'éléctronystagmographie chez l'enfant. Acta Oto-Rhino-Laryngol. (Belg.) *24*:363–369.

Correia, M. J., and J. P. Landolt, (1973) Spontaneous and driven responses from primary neurons of the anterior semicircular canal of the pigeon. O. R. L. *19*:134–148.

Curthoys, I. S. (1978) Firing rate measurement. Electroenceph. Clin. Neurophysiol. *45*:793–794.

Curthoys, I. S. (1979) The development of function of horizontal semicircular canal primary neurons in the rat. Brain Res. *167*:41–52.

Curthoys, I. S. (1981a) The organization of the horizontal semicircular duct, ampulla and utricle in the rat and guinea pig. Acta Otolaryngol. (Stockh.) *92*:323–330.

Curthoys, I. S. (1981b) The response of primary semicircular canal neurons to angular accelerations of varying magnitudes. In T. Gualtierotti (ed): Vestibular Function and Morphology. New York: Springer, pp. 367–373.

Curthoys, I. S. (1983) The development of function of primary vestibular neurons. In: R. Romand (ed.): Development of Auditory and Vestibular Systems. New York: Academic Press, pp. 425–461.

Curthoys, I. S., R. H. I. Blanks, and C. H. Markham (1977) Semicircular canal functional anatomy in cat, guinea pig and man. Acta Otolaryngol. (Stockh.) *83*:258–265.

Dechesne, C. and A. Sans (1985) Development of vestibular receptor surfaces in human fetuses. Amer. J. Otolaryngol. *6*:378–387.

Dechesne, C., C. Legrand, and A. Sans (1984) Effects of experimental hypothyroidism on the surface structures of vestibular receptors in developing rats. Rev. Laryngol. *105*:237–241.

Dechesne, C., J.-P. Mbiene, and A. Sans (1986) Postnatal development of vestibular receptor surfaces in the rat. Acta Otolaryngol. (Stockh.) *101*:11–18.

Dechesne, J. C., G. Desmadryl, and D. Dememes (1987a) Myelination of the mouse vestibular ganglion. Acta Otolaryngol. (Stockh.) *103*:18–23.

Dechesne, C. J., P. Escudero, N. Lamande, M. Thomasset, and A. Sans (1987b) Immunohistochemical identification of neuron-specific enolase and calbindin in the vestibular receptors of human fetuses. Acta Otolaryngol. (Stockh.) Suppl. *436*:69–75.

Dememes, D., C. Dechesne, C. Legrand, and A. Sans (1986) Effects of hypothyroidism on postnatal development in the peripheral vestibular system. Dev. Brain Res.*25*:147–152.

Desmadryl, G., J. Raymond, and A. Sans (1986) *In vitro* electrophysiological study of spontaneous activity in neonatal mouse vestibular ganglion neurons during development. Dev. Brain Res. *25*:133–136.

Dohlman, B. F., (1971) The attachment of the cupulae otolith and tectorial membranes to the sensory cell areas. Acta Otolaryngol. (Stockh.) *71*:89–105.

Drenckhahn, D., J. Kellner, H. G. Mannerherz, U. Gröschel-Stewart, J. Kendrick-Jones, and J. Scholey (1982) Absence of myosin-like immunoreactivity in stereocilia of cochlear hair cells. Nature *300*:531–532.

Drenckhahn, D., T. Schäfer, and M. Prinz (1985) Actin, myosin, and associated proteins in the vertebrate auditory and vestibular organs: Immunocytochemical and biochemical studies. In D. G. Drescher (ed.): Auditory Biochemistry. Springfield, Illinois: Thomas, pp. 317–335.

DuVerney, M. (1683) Traite' de l'Organe de l'Ouie, Contenant la Structure le Ufages & les Maladies de toutes les Parties de l'Oreille. Paris: Chez Estienne Michalet.

Engström, H., and J. Wersäll (1952) The ultrastructural organization of the organ of Corti and of the vestibular sensory epithelia. Exp. Cell Res. 5:460–492.

Erway, L. C., L. S. Hurley, and A. S. Fraser (1970) Congenital ataxia and otolith defects due to manganese deficiency in mice. J. Nutr. 100:643–654.

Ewald, J. R. (1892) Physiologische Untersuchungen über das Endorgan des Nervus octavus. Wiesbaden: Bergmann Verlag.

Ewald, J. R. (1899) Zur Physiologie des Labyrinths, VI. Eine neue Hörtheorie. Pflüg. Arch. 76:147–188.

Ewald, J. R. (1903) Zur Physiologie des Labyrinths. VII. Die Ergenzung von Schallbilder in der Camera Acustica. Pflüg. Arch. 93:485–500.

Farkas, B. (1936) Das Gehör der Fische und die Cristae acusticae. Acta Otolaryngol. (Stockh.) 24:53–68.

Favre, D., and A. Sans (1977) Synaptogenesis of the efferent vestibular nerve endings of the cat: Ultrastructural study. Arch. Oto-Rhino-Laryngol. 215: 183–186.

Favre, D., and A. Sans (1978) The development of vestibular efferent nerve endings during cat maturation: Ultrastructural study. Brain Res. 142:333–337.

Favre. D., and A. Sans (1979a) Morphological changes in afferent vestibular hair cell synapses during the postnatal development of the cat. J. Neurocytol. 8:765–775.

Favre, D., and A. Sans (1979b) Embryonic and postnatal development of afferent innervation in cat vestibular receptors. Acta Otolaryngol. (Stockh.) 87:97–107.

Fell, H. B. (1928) Development "in vitro" of the isolated otocyst of the embryonic fowl. Arch. Exp. Zellforsch. 7:69–81.

Fermin, C. D., and M. Igarashi (1985) Development of otoconia in the embryonic chick (Gallus domesticus). Acta Anat. 123:148–152.

Fermin, C. D., and M. Igarashi (1986) Review of statoconia formation in birds and original research in chicks (Gallus domesticus). Scan. Electr. Microsc. 4:1649–1665.

Fermin, C. D., M. Igarashi, and T. Yoshihara (1987) Ultrastructural changes of statoconia after segmentation of the otolithic membrane. Hear. Res. 28:23–34.

Fernandez, C., J. M. Goldberg, and W. K. Abend (1972) Response to static tilts of peripheral neurons innervating otolith organs of the squirrel monkey. J. Neurophysiol. 35:978–997.

Fex, J., and R. A. Altschuler, (1981) Enkephalin-like immunoreactivity of olivocochlear nerve fibers in cochlea of guinea pig and cat. Proc. Natl. Acad. Sci. USA 78:1255–1259.

Flock, Å. (1965) Electron microscopic and eletrophysiological studies on the lateral line canal organ. Acta Otolaryngol. (Stockh.) Suppl. 199:1–90.

Flock, Å. (1971) Sensory transduction in hair cells. In W. R. Loewenstein (ed.): Handbook of Sensory Physiology, Vol. 1. Berlin: Springer-Verlag, pp. 384–442.

Flock, Å., and S. Orman (1983) Micromechanical properties of sensory hairs in receptor cells of the inner ear. Hear. Res. 11:249–261.

Flock, Å, and D. Strelioff (1984) Graded nonlinear mechanical properties of sensory hairs in the mammalian hearing organ. Nature 310:597–599.

Flock, Å, A. Bretscher, and K. Weber (1982) Immunohistochemical localization of several cytoskeletal proteins in inner ear sensory and supporting cells. Hear. Res. 7:75–89.

Flock, Å., B. Flock, and M. Ulfvendahl (1986) Mechanisms of movement in outer hair cells and a possible structural basis. Arch. Oto-Rhino-Laryngol. *243*:83–90.

Frischkopf, L. S., and D. J. DeRosier (1983) Mechanical tuning of free-standing stereociliary bundles and frequency analysis in the alligator lizard cochlea. Hear. Res. *12*:393–404.

Gacek, R. R. (1969) The course and central termination of first order neurons supplying vestibular end organs in the cat. Acta Otolaryngol. (Stockh.) Suppl. *254*:1–66.

Ginsburg, R. D., and N. B. Gilula (1979) Modulation of cell junctions during differentiation of the chicken otocyst sensory epithelium. Dev. Biol. *68*:110–129.

Ginsburg, R. D., and N. B. Gilula (1980) Synaptogenesis in the vestibular sensory epithelium of the chick embryo. J. Neurocytol. *9*:405–424.

Goldberg, J. M., and C. Fernandez (1971) Physiology of peripheral neurons innervating semicircular canals of the squirrel monkey. I. Resting discharge and response to constant angular accelerations. J. Neurophysiol. *34*:635–660.

Goldberg, J. M., and C. Fernandez (1972) Vestibular mechanisms. Ann. Rev. Physiol. *37*:129–162.

Goltz, F. (1870) Über die physiologishe Bedenhung der Bogengänge des Ohrlabyrinths. Pflüg. Arch. Ges. Physiol. *3*:172–192.

Hamburger, V., and H. L. Hamilton (1951) A series of normal stages in the development of the chick embryo. J. Morph. *88*:49–92.

Heywood, P., R. Pujol, and D. A. Hilding (1976) Development of the labyrinthine receptors in the guinea pig, cat and dog. Acta Otolaryngol. (Stockh.) *82*:359–367.

Holton, T., and A. J. Hudspeth (1983) A micromechanical contribution to cochlear tuning and tonotopic organization. Science *222*:508–510.

Hoshino, T. (1982) Scanning electron microscopic observation of the foetal labyrinthine vestibule. Acta Otolaryngol. (Stockh.) *93*:349–354.

Hudspeth, A. J., and D. P. Corey (1977) Sensitivity, polarity, and conductance changes in the response of vertebrate hair cells to controlled mechanical stimuli. Proc. Natl. Acad. Sci. USA *74*:2407–2411.

Hunter-Duvar, J. M., and R. Hinojosa (1984) Vestibule: Sensory epithelia. In I. Friedmann and J. Ballantyne (eds.): Ultrastructural Atlas of the Inner Ear. London: Butterworths, pp. 211–244.

Igarashi, M., and T. Kanda (1969) Fine structure of the otolithic membrane in the squirrel monkey. Acta Otolaryngol. (Stockh.) *68*:43–52.

Iurato, S. (1960) Submicroscopic structure of the membranous labyrinth. I. The tectorial membrane. Z. Zellforsch. *52*:105–128.

Jongkees, L. B. W., and W. Gasthuis (1973) La fonction de l'organe vestibulaire du nouveauné et de l'enfant. J. Fr. d'Oto-Rhino-Laryng. *22*:97–101.

Karhunen, E. (1973) Postnatal development of the lateral vestibular nucleus (Deiter's nucleus) of the rat. Acta Otolaryngol. (Stockh.) Suppl. *313*:1–87.

Khan, K. M., and W. F. Marowitz (1979) Intercellular junctions in the differentiating rat otocyst. Ann. Otol. Rhinol. Laryngol. *88*:540–544.

Knowlton, V. Y. (1967) Correlation of the development of membranous and bony labyrinthes, sensory ganglia, nerves, and brain centers of the chick embryo. J. Morph. *121*:179–208.

Kölliker, A. (1891) Der feinere Bau des verlängerten Markes. Anat. Anz. 6:427–431.

Kolmer, W. (1926) über das Verhalten der Dechmembranen zum Sinnesepithel. Arch. Ohrenheilk. 116:10–26.

Lannou, J., W. Precht, and C. Cazin (1983) Functional development of the central vestibular system. In R. Romand (ed.): Development of Auditory and Vestibular Systems. New York: Academic Press, pp. 463–478.

Larsell, O., E. McCrady, Jr., and A. A. Zimmerman (1935) Morphological and functional development of the membranous labyrinth in the opossum. J. Comp. Neurol. 62:95–118.

Lawrence, M., and D. J. Merchant (1953) Tissue culture techniques for the study of the isolated otic vesicle. Ann. Otol. Rhinol. Laryngol. 62:770–785.

Levi-Montalcini, R., and P. U. Angeletti (1963) Essential role of the nerve growth factor in the survival and maintenance of dissociated sensory and sympathetic embryonic nerve cells in vitro. Dev. Biol. 7:653–659.

Li, C. W. (1978) Hair cell development in the inner ear. Scan. Electr. Microsc. 2:967–974.

Lim, D. J. (1973) Formation and fate of the otoconia. Ann. Otol. Rhinol. Laryngol. 82:23–35.

Lim, D. J. (1974) The statoconia of the non-mammalian species. Brain Behav. Evol. 10:37–51.

Lim, D. J. (1976) Morphological and physiological correlates in cochlear and vestibular sensory epithelia. Scan. Electr. Microsc. 5:269–276.

Lim, D. J. (1977) Fine morphology of the tectorial membrane: Fresh and developmental. INSERM Symp. 68:47–60.

Lim, D. J. (1984) The development and structure of the otoconia. In I. Friedmann and J. Ballantyne (eds.): Ultrastructural Atlas of the Inner Ear. London: Butterworths, pp. 245–269.

Lim, D. J., and M. Anniko (1985) Developmental morphology of the mouse inner ear. A scanning electron microscopic observation. Acta Otolaryngol. (Stockh.) Suppl. 422:1–69.

Lim, D. J., and M. Anniko (1986) Correlative development of sensory cells and overlying membranes of the inner ear: Micromechanical aspects. In R. J. Ruben, T. R. Van De Water, E. W. Rubel (eds.): The Biology of Change in Otolaryngology. Amsterdam: Elsevier Science, pp. 55–69.

Lindeman, H. H., H. Ades, and R. W. West (1973) Scanning electron microscopy of the vestibular end organs. In: Proceedings 5th Symposium on the Vestibular Organs in Space Exploration. NASA, Washington, D.C., pp. 145–156.

Lodhi, S., N. D. Weiner, I. Mechigian, and J. Schacht (1980) Ototoxicity of aminoglycosides correlated with their action on monomolecular films of polyphosphinositides. Biochem. Pharmacol. 29:597–601.

Loe, P. K., D. L. Tomko, and G. Werner (1973) The neural signal of angular head position in primary afferent vestibular nerve axons. J. Physiol. (Lond.) 230:29–50.

Loewenstein, O. (1970) The electrophysiological study of the responses of the isolated labyrinth of the lamprey (Lampetra fluviatilis) to angular acceleration, tilting and mechanical vibration. Proc. Roy. Soc. (Lond.) B 174:419–434.

Loewenstein, O., and J. Wersäll (1959) A functional interpretation of the electron microscopic structure of the sensory hairs in the cristae of elasmobranch *Raja clarata* in terms of directional sensitivity. Nature *184*:1807–1808.

Lorente de Nó, R. (1933) Anatomy of the eight nerve. The central projection of the nerve endings of the internal ear. Laryngoscope *43*:1–38.

Lyon, M. F. (1955) The developmental origin of hereditary absence of otoliths in mice. J. Embryol. Exp. Morph. *3*:230–241.

Mbiene, J.-P., D. Favre, and A. Sans (1984) The pattern of ciliary development in fetal mouse vestibular receptors. A qualitative and quantitative SEM study. Anat. Embryol. *170*:229–238.

Mees, K. (1983) Ultrastructural localization of K$^+$-dependent, oubain-sensitive NPPase (Na-K-ATPase) in the guinea pig inner ear. Acta Otolaryngol. (Stockh.) *95*:277–289.

Meier, S. (1978) Development of the embryonic chick otic placode. I. Light microscopic analysis. I. Electron microscopic analysis. Anat. Rec. *191*:447–459.

Meza, G., and R. Hinojosa (1987) Ontogenic approach to cellular localization of neurotransmitters in the chick vestibule. Hear. Res. *28*:73–85.

Nakahara, H., and G. Bevelander (1979) An electron microscopy study of crystal calcium carbonate formation in the mouse otolith. Anat. Rec. *193*:233–242.

Nakai, Y. (1970) The development of the sensory epithelium of the cristae ampullares in the rabbit. Pract. Oto-Rhino-Laryngol. *32*:268–278.

Nordemar, H. (1983) Postnatal maturation of vestibular hair cells in mouse. Acta Otolaryngol. (Stockh.) *96*:1–8.

Ohmori, H. (1984) Studies of ionic currents in the isolated vestibular hair cell of the chick. J. Physiol. *350*:561–581.

Oman, C. M. (1981) The influence of duct and utricular morphology on semicircular canal response. In T. Gualitieroth (ed.): Vestibular Function and Morphology. Berlin: Springer-Verlag, pp. 251–274.

O'Rahilly, R., and E. Gardner (1971) The timing and sequence of events in the development of the human nervous system during the embryonic period proper. Z. Anat. Entwickl. Gesch. *134*:1–12.

Ornitz, E. M. (1983) Normal and pathological maturation of vestibular function in the human child. In R. Romand (ed.): Development of Auditory and Vestibular systems. New York: Academic Press, pp. 479–536.

Ornitz, E. M., C. W. Atwell, D. O. Walter, E. E. Hartmann, and A. R. Kaplan (1979) The maturation of vestibular nystagmus in infancy and childhood. Acta Otolaryngol. (Stockh.) *88*:244–256.

Paloheimo, S., and R. Thalmann (1977) Influence of "loop" diuretics upon Na$^+$ K$^+$-ATPase and adenylate cyclase of the stria vascularis. Arch. Oto-Rhino-Laryngol. *217*:347–359.

Parrad, J., and P. Cottereau (1977) Apparition des réactions rotatoires chez le rat nopuveauné. Physiol. Behav. *18*:1017–1020.

Peusner, K. D., and D. K. Morest (1977) Neurogenesis in the nucleus vestibularis tangentialis of the chick embryo in the absence of the primary afferent fibers. Neuroscience *2*:253–270.

Precht, W. (1974) The physiology of the vestibular nuclei. In H. H. Kornhuber (ed.): Handbook of Sensory Physiology, Vol. 6/1. Berlin: Springer-Verlag, pp. 353–416.

Precht, W., and C. Cazin (1979) Functional deficits in the optokinetic system of albino rats. Exp. Brain Res. *37*:183–186.

Purichia, N., and L. C. Erway (1972) Effects of dichlorophenamide, zinc, and manganese on otolith development in mice. Dev. Biol. *27*:395–405.

Rabié, A., M. Thomasset, and Ch. Legrand (1983) Immunocytochemical detection of 28 000-MW calcium-binding protein in the cochlear and vestibular hair cells of the rat. Cell Tiss. Res. *232*:891–896.

Ramón y Cajal, S. (1909) Histologie du Systeme Nerveaux de L'Homme et des Vertébrés. Paris: Maloine, pp. 754–773.

Raymond, J. (1987) *In vitro* differentiation of mouse embryo statoacoustic ganglion and sensory epithelium. Hear. Res. *28*:45–56.

Romand, R., and M. Dauzat (1982) Modification of spontaneous activity in primary vestibular neurons during development in the cat. Exp. Brain Res. *45*:265–268.

Ronnevi, L.-O. (1977) Spontaneous phagocytosis of boutons on spinal motoneurons during early postnatal development: An electron microscopic study in the cat. J. Neurocytol. *6*:487–504.

Ronnevi, L.-O. (1979) Spontaneous phagocytosis of C-type synaptic terminals by spinal alpha-motoneurons in newborn kittens: An electron microscopic study. Brain Res. *162*:189–199.

Ross, M. D., and D. R. Peacor (1975) The nature and crystal growth of otoconia in the rat. Ann. Otol. Rhinol. Laryngol. *84*:22–36.

Rouse, R. C., L.-G. Johnsson, C. G. Wright, and J. R. Hawkins (1984) Abnormal otoconia and calcification in the labyrinth of deaf Dalmatian dogs. Acta Otolaryngol. (Stockh.) *98*:53–60.

Ruben, R. J. (1967) Development of the inner ear of the mouse: A radioautographic study of terminal mitroses. Acta Otolaryngol. (Stockh.) Suppl. *220*:1–44.

Salamat, M. D., M. D. Ross, and D. R. Peacor (1980) Otoconial formation in the fetal rat. Ann. Otol. Rhinol. Laryngol. *89*:229–238.

Sans, A., and M. Chat (1976) Maturation postnatale des noyaux vestibularières chez le chat: Etude histologique par la méthode de Golgi-Cox. Brain Res. *111*:13–20.

Sans, A., and M. Chat (1982) Analysis of temporal and spatial patterns of rat vestibular hair cell differentiation by tritiated thymidine radioautography. J. Comp. Neurol. *206*:1–8.

Sans, A., and C. Dechesne (1985) Early development of vestibular receptors in human embryos. An electron microscopic study. Acta Otolaryngol. (Stockh.) Suppl. *423*:51–58.

Sans, A., R. Pujol, and R. Marty (1968) Etude du réflexe de redressement dans la période postnatale chez divers mammifières. Physiol. Fr. *13*:351–353.

Sans, A., B. Etchecopar, A. Brehier, and M. Thomasset (1986) Immunocytochemical detection of vitamin-D-dependent calcium-binding protein (Ca BP-28K) in vestibular sensory hair cells and vestibular ganglion neurons of the cat. Brain Res. *363*:190–194.

Schacht, J. (1979) Isolation of an aminoglycoside receptor from guinea pig inner ear tissues and kidney. Arch. Otol. Rhinol. Laryngol. *224*:129–134.

Schacht, J. (1986) Molecular mechanisms of drug-induced hearing loss. Hear. Res. *22*:297–304.

Schacht, J., S. Lodhi, and N. D. Weiner (1977) Effects of neomycin on polyphosphoi-nositides in inner ear tissues and monomolecular films. In M. W. Miller and A. E. Shamoo (eds.): Membrane Toxicity. New York: Plenum Press, pp. 191–198.

Schneider, L. W., and D. J. Anderson (1976) Transfer characteristics of first and second order lateral canal vestibular neurons in gerbil. Brain Res. 112:61–76.

Sharp, B. (1885) Homologies of the vertebrate crystalline lens. Proc. Nat. Acad. Sci. USA, pp. 300–310.

Sheld, H. W., J. F. Boyd, P. M. Fuller, R. B. Hoffman, J. R. Keefe, G. M. Oppen-heimer, and G. A. Salinas (1979) Development of fundulus heteroclitus in weightlessness. In Y. A. Illin and G. P. Parfenow (eds.): Biological Investigations on the Kosmos Biosputniks. Moscow: Nauka, pp. 54–62.

Sher, A. E. (1971) The embryonic and postnatal development of the inner ear of the mouse. Acta Otolaryngol. (Stockh.) Suppl. 285:1–77.

Shnerson, A., and R. Pujol (1983) Development: Anatomy, electrophysiology and behavior. In: Willott, J. F. (ed.): The Auditory Psychobiology of the Mouse. Springfield, Illinois: Thomas, pp. 395–425.

Siegborn, J., and G. Grant (1983) Brainstem projections of different branches of the vestibular nerve. An experimental study by transganglionic transport of horsera-dish peroxidase in the cat. I. The horizontal ampullar and utricular nerves. Arch. Ital. Biol. 121:237–248.

Slepecky, N., and S. C. Chamberlain (1985) Immunoelectron microscopic and im-munofluorescent localization of cytoskeletal and muscle-like contractile proteins in inner ear sensory hair cells. Hear. Res. 20:245–260.

Sobin, A., and M. Anniko (1979) Embryonic development of vestibular hair cells in the waltzing guinea pig. Proc. 16th Workshop on Inner Ear Biology. Bern: Switzerland.

Sobin, A., and Å. Flock (1984) Immunohistochemical identification and localization of actin and fimbrin in vestibular hair cells in the normal guinea pig and in a strain of the waltzing guinea pig. Acta Otolaryngol. (Stockh.) 96:407–412.

Sobkowicz, H. M., B. Bereman, and J. E. Rose, (1975) Organotypic development of the organ of Corti in culture. J. Neurocytol. 4:543–572.

Stein, B. M., and M. B. Carpenter (1967) Central projections of portions of the vestibular ganglia innervating specific parts of the labyrinth in the rhesus mon-key. Amer. J. Anat. 120:281–317.

Steinhausen, W. (1933) Über die Beobachtung der Cupula in den Borgengängsam-pullen des Labyrinths des leben Hechts. Pflüg. Arch. Gesamte Physiol. Menchen Tiere 232:500–512.

Stephens, C. B. (1972) Development of the middle and inner ear in the golden hamster. Acta Otolaryngol. (Stockh.) Suppl. 296:1–51.

Streeter, G. L. (1906) On the development of the membranous labyrinth and the acoustic and facial nerves in the human embryo. Amer. J. Anat. 6:139–165.

Suzuki, M., and Y. Harada (1985a) An experimental study on the physiological significance of the mode of cupular movement. Arch. Oto-Rhino-Laryngol. 242:57–62.

Suzuki, M., and Y. Harada, (1985b) An experimental study on cupular function: Mapping of the cupula by direct stimulation. Arch. Oto-Rhino-Laryngol. 241:237–242.

Suzuki, M., Y. Harada, and Y. Sugata (1984) An experimental study on a function of the cupula. Effect of cupula removal on the ampullary nerve action potential. Arch. Oto-Rhino-Laryngol. *241*:75–81.

Tanaka, T. (1972) Frozen resin cracking method for scanning electron microscopy of biological material. Nature *59*:77–78.

Tanaka, T., Y. Ozeki, T. Aoki, and Y. Ogura (1975) Morphological relation of the vestibular sensory hairs to the otolithic membrane and the cupula. A scanning electron microscopic study. Proc. 5th Extraordinary Meeting of the Bárány Society, pp. 406–409.

Thalmann, R. (1976) Quantitative histochemistry and cytochemistry of the ear. In C. A. Smith and J. A. Vernon (eds.): Handbook of Auditory and Vestibular Research Methods. Springfield, Illinois: Thomas, pp. 359–418.

Thornell, L.-E., and M. Anniko (1987) Cytoskeletal organization of the human inner ear. III. Expression of actin in the cochlea. Acta Otolaryngol. (Stockh.) Suppl. *437*:55–63.

Thornell, L.-E., M. Anniko, and I. Virtanen (1987) Cytoskeletal organization of the human inner ear. I. Expression of intermediate filaments in vestibular organs. Acta Otolaryngol. (Stockh.) Suppl. *437*:5–27.

Tilney, L. G., E. H. Egelman, D. J. DeRosier, and J. C. Saunders (1983) Actin filaments, stereocilia, and hair cells of the bird cochlea. II. Packing of actin filaments in the stereocilia and in the cuticular plate and what happens to the organization when stereocilia are bent. J. Cell Biol. *96*:822–834.

Van De Water, T. R. (1976) Effects of removal of the statoacoustic ganglion complex upon the growing otocyst. Ann. Otol. Rhinol. Laryngol Suppl. *33*:1–32.

Van De Water, T. R., and R. J. Ruben (1984) Neurotrophic interactions during *in vitro* development of the inner ear. Ann. Otol. Rhinol. Laryngol. *93*:558–564.

Van De Water, T. R., M. Anniko, H. Nordemar, and J. Wersäll (1978) Embryonic development of the sensory cells in maculae utriculae of mouse. INSERM Symp. *68*:25–36.

Veenhof, V. B. (1969) The development of statoconia in mice. Thesis, University of Amsterdam, pp. 1–49.

von Baumgarten, R. J., R. C. Simmonde, J. F Royd, and O. K. Garriott (1975) Effects of prolonged weightlessness on the swimming pattern of fish aboard Skylab 3. Aviat. Space Environ. Med. *46*:902–906.

Vilstrup, T. (1950) Studies on the histogenesis of the ampullary cupula. Ann. Otol. Rhinol. Laryngol. *59*:19–45.

Vinnikov, Ya. A., O. G. Gazenko, L. K. Titova, A. A. Bronstein, V. I. Govardovskii, F. G. Gribakin, R. A. Pevzner, M. Z. Aronova, T. A. Kharkeevich, T. P. Tsirulis, G. A. Pyakina, D. V. Lichakow, L. P. Palmbach, and V. F. Anichin (1979) The structural and functional organization of the vestibular apparatus of rats exposed to weightlessness for 20 days on board the sputnik "Kosmos-782." Acta Otolaryngol. (Stockh.) *87*:90–96.

Vinnikov Ya. A., O. G. Gazenko, D. N. Lychakow, and L. R. Palmbach (1983) Formation of the vestibular apparatus in weightlessness. In R. Romand (ed.): Development of Auditory and Vestibular Systems. New York: Academic Press, pp. 537–560.

Watanabe, K., and A. Ogawa (1984) Carbonic anhydrase activity in stria vascularis and dark cells in vestibular labyrinth. Ann. Otol. Rhinol. Laryngol. 93:262–266.

Werner, C. F. (1940) Das Labyrinth. Leipzig: Georg Thieme.

Wersäll, J. (1956) Studies on the structure and innervation of the sensory epithelium of the cristae ampullares in the guinea pig. Acta Otolaryngol (Stockh.) Suppl. 126:1–85.

Wersäll, J., and D. Bagger-Sjöbäck (1974) Morphology of the vestibular sense organ. In H. H. Kornhuber (ed.): Handbook of Sensory Physiology, Vol. 6/1. Berlin: Springer-Verlag, pp. 123–170.

Wersäll, J., Å. Flock, and P.-G. Lundquist (1965) Structural basis for directional sensitivity in cochlear and vestibular sensory receptors. Cold Spring Harb. Symp. Quant. Biol. 30:115–145.

Wersäll, J, L. Gleisner, and P.-G. Lundquist (1967) Myostatic, kinesthetic and vestibular mechanisms. Boston: Little, Brown.

Whitehead, M. C., P. J. Marangos, S. M. Connolly, and D. K. Morest (1982) Synapse formation is related to the onset of neron-specific enolase immunoreactivity in the avian auditory and vestibular systems. Dev. Neurosci. 5:298–305.

Wikström, S.-O., M. Anniko, L.-E. Thornell, and I. Virtanen (1988) Developmental stage-dependent pattern of inner ear expression of intermediate filaments. Acta Otolaryngol. (Stockh.) 106:71–80.

Wilson, D. B. (1983) Early development of the otocyst in an exencephalic mutant of the mouse. Acta Anat. 117:217–224.

Wit, H. P., H. F. Kahmann, and J. M. Segenhout (1986) Vestibular microphonic potentials in pigeons. Arch. Oto-Rhino-Laryngol. 243:146–150.

Wittmaack, K. (1937) Nachtrag zu meiner Arbeit über Aufbau und Funktion der Cupula. Acta Otolaryngol. (Stockh.) 24:424–447.

Yntema, C. L. (1950) An analysis of induction of the ear from foreign ectoderm in the salamanda embryo. J. Exp. Zool. 113:211–243.

Yokoh, Y. (1974) On sensory cells of the human otocyst. Acta Anat. 87:72–76.

Yoshihara, T., and M. Igarashi, (1987) Cytochemical study of K^+-NPPase in planum semilunatum and dark cells of the squirrel monkey. Acta Otolaryngol. (Stockh.) 104:22–28.

Yoshihara, T., M. Igarashi, S. Usami, and T. Kanda, (1987a) Cytochemical studies of Ca^{++}-ATPase activity in the vestibular epithelia of the guinea pig. Arch. Oto-Rhino-Laryngol. 243:417–423.

Yoshihara, T., S. Usami, M. Igarashi, and C. D. Fermin, (1987b) Ultracytochemical study of oubain-sensitive, potassium-dependent P-nitrophenylphosphatase activity in the inner ear of the squirrel monkey. Acta Otolaryngol. (Stockh.) 103:161–169.

Zenner, H. P., A. Giller, U. Zimmermann, U. Schmitt, and E. Frömter (1985) Die isolierte, lebende haarzelle—ein neues modell zur untersuchung der hör-funktion. Laryngol. Rhinol. Otol. 64:642–648.

Zhou, X.-N., and T. R. Van De Water (1987) The effect of target tissues in survival and differentiation of mammalian statoacoustic ganglion neurons in organ culture. Acta Otolaryngol. (Stockh.) 104:45–56.

Part Four

THE SOMATOSENSORY SYSTEM

Chapter Ten

DEVELOPMENT OF SOMATOSENSORY SYSTEM STRUCTURES

HERBERT P. KILLACKEY

University of California
Irvine, California

MARC F. JACQUIN

St. Louis University
St. Louis, Missouri

ROBERT W. RHOADES

Medical College of Ohio
Toledo, Ohio

I INTRODUCTION

At all levels of the mammalian central somatosensory system there is a characteristic topographic map that reflects the distribution and density of receptors on the body surface. While such somatotopic organization is usually inferred from neurophysiological recording procedures, it can be directly observed with routine anatomical techniques in the somatosensory system of a number of small rodents. This relationship between the periphery and central structure was first noted by Woolsey and Van der Loos (1970), who correlated the distribution of multicellular cytoarchitectonic units in layer IV of mouse somatosensory cortex, which they called "barrels," with the distribution of mystacial vibrissae on the snout. Since the initial description of this isomorphic relationship between the periphery and central structure, a number of investigators have studied the developmental events that underlie this relationship and how it can be modified during the course of development.

The focus of the present review is on morphological events that underlie the formation of somatotopic patterns within the central nervous system. An analysis of this problem, like most problems in developmental biology, involves two complementary approaches. The first is a description of the normal developmental events related to the system under investigation. The second is the experimental manipulation of some aspect of the system under investigation during the course of its development and assaying the outcome of the manipulation on the system under investigation. The premise underlying the second approach is that the aberrant organization resulting from the experimental manipulation will shed some light on normal developmental mechanisms. The present review will lean heavily toward the first approach, as the second is treated in detail in other chapters (see Chapters 11 and 12, this volume). However, some overlap is inevitable, as experimental manipulation provides necessary verification of hypotheses based on the description of normal developmental events.

The evidence reviewed in this chapter leads to several generalizations about the development of somatotopic patterns within the central nervous system. First, somatotopic patterns are formed in a sequential order beginning at the periphery and ending in the cerebral cortex. This sequence along with supporting experimental evidence has led to the view that a pattern at the periphery provides a primary template that is replicated in sequence at each level of the somatosensory system and that the process of pattern formation at a given level of the system is dependent on the previous level. Second, the formation of somatotopic patterns is a relatively late developmental event and is best regarded as an overlay on a preexisting topographic order. Together, these generalizations suggest that the periphery plays a limited but important instructive role in the organization of the central nervous system.

Finally, it should be pointed out that while the development of the three major sensory systems represented in the cerebral neocortex (audition, vision, and somatosensory) have much in common, there may be differences between these systems. For example, the distribution of peripheral somatosensory receptors is clearly punctuate, while the retina, on the other hand, although possessing some regional variations in receptor density, is more clearly a continuous receptor surface. Further, at the cortical level, the mammalian visual system has the added task of combining projections from both sides of the neural axis to form a coherent map of visual space, while in the somatosensory system the representation of each half of the body surface is confined to one-half of the neural axis. Such differences may well be reflected in the ontogeny of a given sensory system and exploited to provide a fuller picture of the development of the brain.

II OVERVIEW OF THE LEMNISCAL PATHWAYS

Somatosensory information is processed and represented both within the brain and the spinal cord. However, the development of patterns of somatotopic organization within the cerebral cortex appears to be most closely coupled with the development of the lemniscal pathways. The evidence for this statement is the major focus of this review, but before turning to this evidence, it is necessary to briefly outline the organization of the lemniscal pathways.

A Peripheral Organization

Tactile sensation is subserved by a diverse group of mechanoreceptors that are distributed throughout the body surface in a nonrandom fashion. In small rodents, a particularly important collection of receptors are located on the snout (Woolsey et al., 1975). These are associated with the mystacial vibrissae. In the mouse and rat, these large tactile hairs are organized into five rostral–caudally organized rows of four to seven large tactile hairs (designated rows A through E from dorsal to ventral). Other species possess a varying number of rows of vibrissae; for example, there are seven rows of vibrissae on the face of the gerbil. The mystacial vibrissae are not a passive organ of touch. Each mystacial vibrissa follicle is encased in a sling of muscle tissue that allows the vibrissae to be actively moved or whisked in concert at a species-specific rate (Dorfl, 1982). The ensemble of whiskers and the accompanying musculature form the vibrissal or whisker pad, a sensitive tactile organ for the exploration of the environment (Vincent, 1912; Welker, 1964). Each mystacial vibrissa follicle is complexly innervated at two levels of the hair shaft and contains a rich complement of mechanoreceptor types including Merkel discs, Golgi-Manzoni, lanceolate, and free nerve endings (Andres, 1966; Renehan and Munger, 1986). The vibrissa follicles are innervated by the infraorbital nerve, which is the largest peripheral nerve in the mouse and rat. In the rat, the infraorbital nerve contains approximately 33,000 nerve fibers (Jacquin et al., 1984). It is in turn a branch of the maxillary nerve, which becomes one of the three major subdivisions of the trigeminal nerve. Each vibrissa follicle is innervated by both myelinated and nonmyelinated fibers (Vincent, 1913). The number of myelinated nerve fibers innervating a given vibrissa follicle is related to the position of that follicle within a row. For example, the C-1 vibrissa, which is located in the rostral end of that row, is innervated by an average of 69 myelinated nerve fibers, while the more caudal C-6 vibrissa is innervated by 162 nerve fibers on average (Lee and Woolsey, 1975). Physiological studies indicate that each trigeminal ganglion cell is responsive to stimulation of a single vibrissa (Zucker and Welker, 1969).

Central patterns suggest that there are also discrete distributions of peripheral receptors on the glabrous surface of the forepaw and hindpaw as there are discrete representations of both the pads and digits of the distal extremities within the central nervous system (Welker, 1976; Belford and Killackey, 1978; Dawson and Killackey, 1987). The association between peripheral receptor distributions and central patterns has not been as clearly established for the limb representations as for the mystacial vibrissae. The dermal papilla of the glabrous skin of the mouse digital pads contain many digital or Meissner corpuscles (Ide, 1976). Most likely it is these receptor complexes that are associated with the primary afferents of the limbs and the corresponding central patterns. However, this needs to be more thoroughly investigated. The forepaw is innervated by the radial, ulnar, and medial nerve and the hindpaw by the sciatic and saphenous nerve. The cell bodies associated with these primary afferents are located in dorsal root ganglia found at cervical and lumbar portions of the spinal cord, respectively.

B   Subcortical Organization

The primary afferents conveying tactile information from the body surface terminate in the brainstem and spinal cord. In the brainstem, afferents associated with the face terminate in the brainstem trigeminal nuclei and those associated with the forelimb and hindlimb terminate in the dorsal column nuclei (see Figure 1). On entering the brainstem, trigeminal afferents bifurcate into ascending and descending branches (Cajal, 1911). The ascending branches terminate in the principal sensory nucleus and the descending branches in the spinal trigeminal nucleus, which can be further subdivided into the subnuclei oralis, interpolaris, and caudalis. A single trigeminal primary afferent innervates all of these subdivisions of the brainstem trigeminal complex (Hayashi, 1980). These afferents terminate in discrete clusters, which form bands running rostral to caudal in the horizontal plane and in the transverse plane replicate the pattern of mystacial vibrissae and sinus hairs on the face (Belford and Killackey, 1979a,b; Ar-

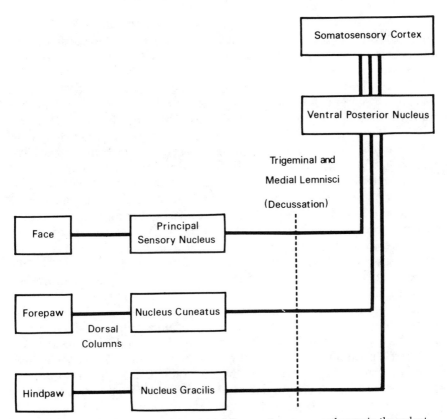

FIGURE 1. Diagrammatic representation of the somatosensory pathways in the rodent.

vidson, 1982; Bates and Killackey, 1985). This pattern is particularly obvious in the principal sensory nucleus and the subnuclei interpolaris and caudalis (Figure 2). This high degree of somatotopic organization is also demonstrable with physiological techniques (Nord, 1967).

Each of the subdivisions of the brainstem trigeminal complex projects in a unique fashion to other portions of the central nervous system. The major projections from the principal sensory nucleus are to the contralateral ventral posterior nucleus of the dorsal thalamus (Smith, 1973; Erzurumlu et al., 1980; Peschanski, 1984). The subnucleus interpolaris also projects to the contralateral ventral posterior nucleus as well as to the superior colliculus and the cerebellum (Smith, 1973; Fukushima and Kerr, 1979; Erzurumlu and Killackey, 1980; Killackey and Erzurumlu, 1981; Peschanski, 1984; Steindler, 1985; Bruce et al., 1987). The portion of subnucleus caudalis in which the vibrissae are represented projects to the lateral division of the facial nucleus, which in turn innervates the musculature of the vibrissae pad, suggesting that this is a pathway subserving reflex movements of the vibrissae (Erzurumlu and Killackey, 1979). The connections of the subnucleus oralis are largely confined to the brainstem trigeminal complex itself; in particular, the subnucleus oralis projects heavily to the subnucleus caudalis (Hockfield and Gobel, 1982).

Primary afferents associated with the limbs are organized in a similar fashion. On entering the spinal cord these fibers also bifurcate, and one branch terminates within the spinal cord. The other branch travels the length of the spinal cord in the dorsal fasciculus and terminates in the dorsal column nuclei in the caudal brainstem (Basbaum and Hand, 1973). The nucleus gracilis, located most medially, is related to the hindpaw and the more lateral nucleus cuneatus is related to the forepaw. Both of these nuclei contain a pattern that can be related to their respective peripheral input (Belford and Killackey, 1978) and in turn project to the contralateral ventral posterior nucleus (Lund and Webster, 1967; McAllister and Wells, 1981). Thus, stretching across the upper part of the lower brainstem is a complete map of the body surface with the head represented laterally in the brainstem trigeminal complex and the hindpaw most medially in the nucleus gracilis.

The trigeminal lemniscus and the medial lemniscus are the fiber pathways between the brainstem somatosensory nuclei and the dorsal thalamus. The trigeminal afferents terminate in the dorsal and medial portions of the ventral posterior nucleus (ventral posterior medial, VPM), while those of the medial lemniscus terminate in more lateral and ventral portions of this nucleus (ventral posterior lateral, VPL). The VPM is the largest portion of this nucleus, and it is separated from the VPL by a clear fiber plexus. The entire nucleus is characterized by a high degree of somatotopic order that can be demonstrated with both physiological (Emmers, 1965; Waite, 1973; Rhoades et al., 1987b) and anatomical (Van der Loos, 1976; Belford and Killackey, 1979a,b; Ivy and Killackey, 1982) techniques. In this nucleus, like in the brainstem, a peripheral structure such as a vibrissa is represented by a cylinder of neural tissue that runs roughly rostral to caudal through the nucleus. In the VPM, the receptive field of the vast majority of neurons is restricted to a single vibrissa, suggesting the system possesses a high degree of spatial resolution.

One feature of the rat ventral posterior nucleus worthy of note is its relatively simple organization. In contrast to some thalamic nuclei, the rat ventral posterior nucleus appears on morphological, immunohistochemical, and functional grounds to contain no interneurons (Spacek and Lieberman, 1974; McAllister and Wells, 1981; Barbaresi et al., 1986; Harris, 1986). It consists of a relatively pure population of projection neurons. Its synaptic organization is correspondingly simple, and the three types of synaptic profiles found in the nucleus can be correlated with inputs from the lemnisci, cortex, and thalamic reticular nucleus. The major target of the ventral posterior nucleus is the primary somatosensory cortex (Killackey, 1973; Donaldson et al., 1975).

C   Cortical Organization

The primary somatosensory cortex of all mammals is characterized by a map that reflects both the distribution and density of receptors on the body surface. Usually, such a somatotopic map results from determining the cortical loci of low-threshold tactile stimulation of the body surface. In small rodents, somatotopic organization is a directly observable feature of primary somatosensory cortex. This was first noted by Woolsey and Van der Loos (1970), who described the relationship between the distribution of large mystacial vibrissae on the face of the mouse and discrete groups of cells in the fourth layer of cortex, which they termed "barrels." A combined anatomical and physiological study of the rat somatosensory cortex by Welker (1976) suggested that there was a similar anatomically visible organization in other parts of somatosensory cortex as well. This has recently been confirmed by Dawson and Killackey (1987), who provided evidence that other portions of the body surface, particularly the distal extremities, are discretely represented in the cortex. Overall, this anatomical map is congruent with the physiological map obtained by other investigators (Welker, 1971, 1976; Chapin and Lin, 1984). It should also be pointed out that there are both species and strain differences in the organization of the peripheral pattern that is reflected in the cortical pattern and, presumably, the subcortical patterns as well. Different species of rodents possess varying numbers of rows of vibrissae. For example, the vibrissae of both the mouse (Figure 2) and rat are arranged in five rows, while in the gerbil they form seven rows, and this peripheral difference is reflected in the organization and number of cortical barrels (Woolsey et al., 1975). Similarly, some mice have extra vibrissae and corresponding extra cortical barrels (Yamakado and Yohro, 1979), and this trait can be selected for in a breeding program (Welker and Van der Loos, 1986).

Primary somatosensory cortex, like most other cortical areas, is composed of six layers. The anatomically discrete map of the body surface is characteristic of the fourth cortical layer. This cortical layer is composed of stellate cells, and it is the layer in which the majority of thalamic afferents from the ventral posterior nucleus terminate. Within this layer, thalamocortical afferents form synapses with the dendrites and somata of these stellate cells and, also, with the layer IV portions of dendrites of neurons whose somata are found in other layers (White, 1978). The somatotopic map is reflected in the discrete termination pattern of thalamocortical afferents (Killackey et al., 1976; Killackey and Belford, 1979; Dawson and Killackey, 1987). Indeed, individual thalamocortical afferent terminations are of the same size as the barrel in which they terminate (Jensen and Killackey, 1987a). Further, there is a variation in both the size of termination and of the corresponding barrel that is related to the position of the vibrissae on the face. Vibrissae that are caudal on the face are larger and are innervated by more myelinated fibers than more rostral ones. This relationship is reflected

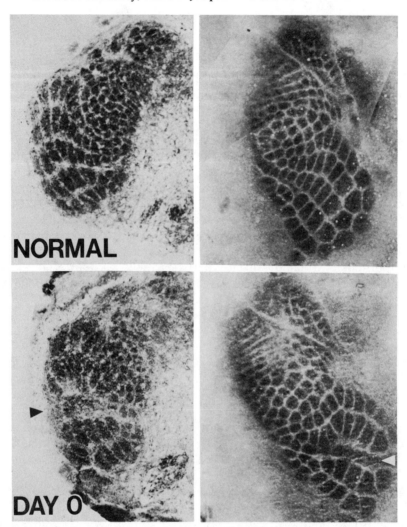

FIGURE 2. Each pair of photomicrographs shows the representations of the mystacial vibrissae at two levels of the somatosensory system of a single mouse. For each pair, the left micrograph shows the representation in the subnucleus interpolaris of the spinal trigeminal in coronal section and the right shows layer IV of the contralateral somatosensory cortex in flattened tangential section. Each animal was sacrified on postnatal day 9, and all sections were stained for succinic hydrogenase activity. *Normal:* This pair shows the normal pattern of vibrissae representation on postnatal day 9. *Day 0:* The pair in this figure and in the next two figures shows the vibrissae representation resulting from cautery of the vibrissae follicles in row C on the day shown in the label. The arrows point out the abnormal pattern related to the cauterized row of mystacial vibrissae. Note that (1) the extent of disruption of the row C representation decreases with cautery at progressively older ages and (2) for each day of cautery, the abnormal pattern in layer IV of somatosensory cortex mimics the abnormal pattern seen in the brainstem of the same mouse.

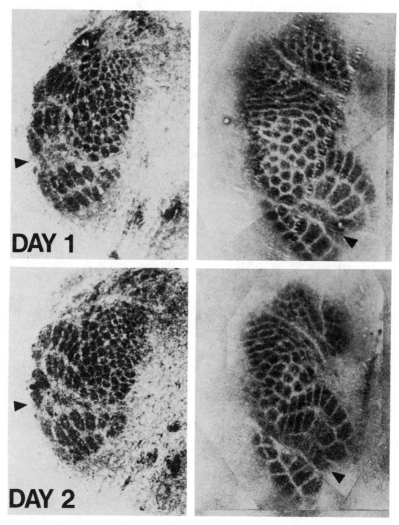

FIGURE 3. Effects of cautery of the vibrissae follicles in row C on postnatal days 1 and 2 (see Figure 2).

in the cortex by the number of cells that compose a given barrel, the volume of a barrel, and the size and branching density of the associated thalamocortical afferent (Lee and Woolsey, 1975; Welker and Van der Loos, 1986; Jensen and Killackey, 1987a). The dendrites of the barrel stellate cells are oriented toward the thalamocortical terminations. For example, the dendrites of a stellate cell on the side of a barrel are all oriented toward the center of that barrel and seldom cross the border between adjacent barrels (Lorente de Nó, 1922; Killackey and Leshin 1975; Steffen and Van der Loos,

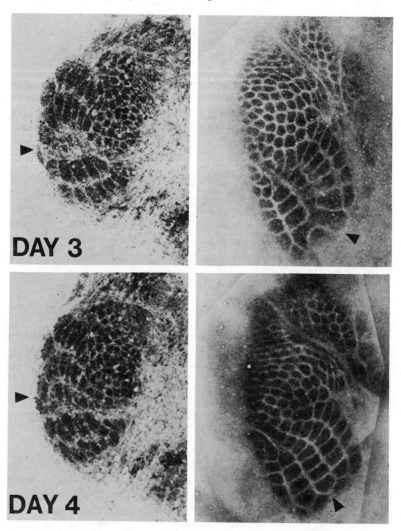

FIGURE 4. Effects of cautery of the vibrissae follicles in row C on postnatal day 3 and 4 (see Figure 3). Neural representation is less disrupted by surgical intervention on postnatal day 4 than on previous days.

1980; Harris and Woolsey, 1981). This highly specific morphological organization is also reflected in the functional properties of barrel neurons. The receptive field of individual barrel neurons is dominated by a single vibrissa (Simons, 1978). However, the tightness of this functional relationship has recently been questioned (Armstrong-James and Fox, 1987).

The discrete morphological organization of the fourth cortical layer is not obvious in the other layers of primary somatosensory cortex. The superficial cortical layers give rise to corticocortical projections as do portions of the deep cortical layers (Akers and Killackey, 1978). Subcortical projections arise from restricted portions of the deep cortical layers (Wise and Jones, 1977; Killackey and Erzurumlu, 1981; Killackey, 1983; Bates and Killackey, 1984; Killackey et al., 1989). The surrounding cortical areas are major targets of the primary somatosensory cortex. One area of particular interest is located lateral and caudal to primary somatosensory cortex. This is the second somatosensory area. This area is somatotopically organized and receives major projections from the ipsilateral primary somatosensory cortex and projections from the opposite hemisphere via the corpus callosum (Koralelek et al., 1990).

A final point with regard to the normal organization of the rat somatosensory cortex is the distribution of interhemispheric projections. These projections, which arise and terminate in both the supragranular and infragranular layers of the rat, surround and interdigitate the primary somatosensory cortex of the rat (Akers and Killackey, 1978). Overall, they form a pattern that is complementary to the pattern of thalamocortical afferents (Olavarria et al., 1984). This high degree of organization in these projections as well as in many other portions of the somatosensory system between the periphery and cortex raises a number of intriguing questions about the development of this system.

III DEVELOPMENT OF THE LEMNISCAL PATHWAYS

A The Periphery

The characteristic patterns of the rodent somatosensory system first develop in the periphery. The sequence in this process has been best detailed in the trigeminal system. The development of the vibrissa pad is a relatively early developmental event that begins about embryonic day 10 in the mouse and a day or two later in the rat. (In general, the developmental sequence in the rat lags behind that of the mouse by about 2 days; allowing for this time lag the developmental events in the two species appear to be quite similar.) On the muzzle, which at this time can be subdivided into a nasal and maxillary process, the pattern appears first as five longitudinal ridges of epithelium separated by grooves. Superimposed on the ridges a series of domes that are the precursors of the vibrissa follicles develop in a caudal-to-rostral sequence (Yamakado and Yohro, 1979; Van Exan and Hardy, 1980). The hair follicles are present by embryonic day 12 in the mouse, and the associated mechanoreceptors (the Merkel discs in particular) develop at a still later time (English et al., 1980). These events appear to be an extrinsic property of the epithelium. Andres and Van der Loos (1982) have presented evidence that facial epithelium that is isolated before trigeminal innervation and raised in tissue culture will express a pattern of vibrissa follicles. There is also recent evidence that the facial epithelium produces a growth factor capable of attracting the outgrowing trigeminal nerve fibers (Lumsden and Davies, 1986). This growth factor appears to be specific for trigeminal fibers and to be present for only a short time in the developmental process.

The neurons that compose the trigeminal ganglion are largely produced on embryonic days 12 and 13 in the rat (Forbes and Welt, 1981). In the mouse, peak production is on embryonic day 11 (Taber Pierce, 1970). As early as embryonic day 12 in the rat trigeminal primary neurons can be seen to be distributed in a polarized fashion with their peripheral and central processes arranged along the same axis (Erzurumlu and Killackey, 1983). This axis appears to radiate from the point at which the central processes contact the brainstem. The peripheral processes are pointed straight at their epithelial targets. During the next several days, the trigeminal ganglion differentiates into its three major components (the ophthalmic, maxillary, and mandibular subdivisions), and there is a straight outgrowth of the peripheral processes of ganglion cells to their epithelial targets. This occurs during the same time as epithelial differentiation is taking place. The epithelial events described in the preceding are first detectable in the rat on embryonic day 14. On this day, fine nerve fibers can be seen to contact mesenchymal condensations that are the first signs of follicle formation. It seems likely that the growth factor referred to in the preceding plays some role as a local signal in the final stages of the growth of the peripheral fiber toward its epithelial target. The general morphology and innervation of the vibrissa follicle at the light microscopic level resembles that of the adult around embryonic day 17.

A major unresolved question is how the epithelial-based pattern is coded in the trigeminal nerve and passed to the central nervous system. At present, it is only possible to speculate about the mechanisms involved. The pattern of fasciculation in the peripheral portion of the trigeminal ganglion fibers that is present at late prenatal stages may be a reflection of these mechanisms (Erzurumlu and Killackey, 1983). The spatial distribution of the peripheral targets of the trigeminal nerve is reflected in the fasciculation pattern, and this pattern develops after the epithelial pattern. In the mouse, approximately 50% of the original population of trigeminal ganglion neurons and fibers are eliminated during this period by naturally occurring neuronal death (Davies and Lumsden, 1984). There is also evidence that this occurs in the rat (Renehan and Rhoades, 1984). Lumsden and Davies (1986) have recently presented evidence that at early ages before an ordered pattern of fasciculation would presumably develop in the mouse some subpopulation of peripheral fibers shift fasciculi during their course. Perhaps it is this subpopulation of fibers that is eliminated. It should also be emphasized that the ordered pattern of fasciculation should be regarded as a relatively gross reflection of cellular adhesive interactions that may play a role in the transmittal of the pattern rather than as a causative agent. How the pattern in the peripheral portion of the trigeminal fibers comes to be expressed in their central processes has yet to be clearly elucidated. In this regard, it would be of extreme interest to determine the morphological organization of the central portions of primary trigeminal afferents during the course of development.

The central processes of trigeminal primary afferents reach the vicinity of their brainstem target quite early in development. In the rat they appear to have reached the brainstem by the embryonic day 12. The clustered pattern of terminations associated with these afferents develops much later, around the time of birth. This will be dealt with in the next section.

The development of primary afferents associated with the limbs have been studied in less detail. In the rat, genesis of dorsal root ganglion cells located at lower cervical and upper thoracic levels that later innervate the forelimb takes place between embryonic days 12 and 14 (Altman and Bayer, 1984). The time course of neurogenesis of dorsal root ganglion neurons located at lower lumbar levels and associated with the hindpaw is approximately 1 day later. Peripheral processes of dorsal root ganglion neurons reach the epithelium by embryonic day 16 or 17 but do not form functional connections with receptors until embryonic day 20 or later (English et al., 1980). The central processes of dorsal root ganglion neurons associated with the forepaw reach their target, the cuneate nucleus, on embryonic day 17. Hindlimb afferents reach the gracile nucleus on the following day (Altman and Bayer, 1984). Thus, by the time of birth primary somatosensory afferents have established contact with both their epithelial and brainstem targets. In addition primary afferents have also developed functional properties by this time. Fitzgerald (1987) has recently reported that primary afferents at the lumbar level are spontaneously active by embryonic day 16 and can be activated from small, well-defined peripheral receptive fields on the following day.

B The Brainstem

The neurons that compose the brainstem trigeminal nuclei are generated toward the end or after the time period during which the primary trigeminal afferent neurons are generated. In the rat, neurogenesis as determined by tritiated thymidine labeling takes place on embryonic days 13 and 14 (Altman and Bayer, 1982). The sequential order of generation of the primary and secondary neurons of the trigeminal system is continued in more central stations (see what follows), and overall, the trigeminal system is generated in a centripetal fashion.

The vibrissa-related pattern develops in the brainstem around the time of birth. On the day of birth (embryonic day 21) a pattern can only be detected in the lateral portions of the brainstem trigeminal nuclei where the most caudal vibrissae are represented. It should be noted that these are the vibrissae that develop first. Over the next day or two a pattern becomes visible in more medial portions of the trigeminal nuclei. Thus, in the brainstem the pattern develops along the same gradient as vibrissae develop on the face (Erzurumlu and Killackey, 1983). As near as can be determined, the vibrissa-related pattern develops concurrently in both the terminations of the primary afferents and in clusters of trigeminothalamic relays of the principal sensory nucleus. One would assume that the primary afferents play a causal role in the clustering of the relay neurons, but direct evidence for this is lacking, as is an understanding of the attractive interactions that would bring about the clustering of relay neurons. The indirect evidence that supports this notion is the fact that if a row of vibrissae are cauterized on the day of birth, the associated primary afferents degenerate (Bates and Killackey, 1985; Killackey, 1987) and the associated neurons in the principal sensory nucleus fail to cluster normally (Bates et al., 1982; see Figure 2 on the nucleus interpolaris).

The interaction between primary afferents and their target relay cells in the principal sensory nucleus have been hypothesized to be the primary event in pattern formation in central trigeminal structures (Belford and Killackey, 1980; Bates and Killackey, 1985). If vibrissae are damaged after the first few days of life when normal clustering has already occurred, more central patterns in the thalamus and cortex are unaffected (Figures 2–4). Thus, the system is characterized by a "sensitive" or "critical" period when peripheral damage can result in altered central organization. This period most likely coincides with the normal time course of primary afferent induction of clustering of principal sensory nucleus thalamic relay neurons. There are, however, alternate interpretations of sensitive and critical periods (see Woolsey, Chapter 12). It should also be mentioned that while vibrissa-related patterns are characteristic of three brainstem trigeminal nuclei (the principal sensory nucleus and subnuclei interpolaris and caudalis), only the principal sensory nucleus seems to play a role in pattern formation in more rostral structures. Neonatal lesions of the principal sensory nucleus result in a lack of pattern in the ventral posterior nucleus while similar lesions of the spinal trigeminal nuclei do not effect pattern formation in the ventral posterior nucleus (Killackey and Fleming, 1985).

The dorsal column nuclei are generated a day or two later than the brainstem trigeminal complex (Altman and Bayer, 1984). Forelimb primary afferents reach the cuneate nucleus on embryonic day 17; hindpaw afferents reach the gracilis nucleus on the following day. This difference in arrival time has been exploited to shed light on the role of primary afferents in specifying their targets. If a rat forelimb is amputated before primary afferent central processes have reached the cuneate nucleus, hindlimb afferents are capable of expanding their terminal territory to include portions of the cuneate as well as the gracile nucleus. Such an expansion of gracile afferents does not occur if the forelimb is removed after the forepaw afferents have reached the cuneate nucleus (Dawson and Killackey, 1986; Killackey and Dawson 1989). This suggests that once a target has been invaded by primary afferents, it is no longer capable of accepting afferents from a second source. This observation may also explain the difference between the response of the hamster and rat trigeminal system to section of the infraorbital nerve on the day of birth (Rhoades et al., 1983). Following infraorbital nerve section in the newborn hamster, the mandibular afferent terminations expand into the denervated maxillary territory. Such an expansion does not occur in the newborn rat. This difference is more likely due to the relative immaturity of the hamster at birth compared to the rat and, one would assume, the incomplete innervation of the hamster's brainstem trigeminal nuclei at birth. Together, these results underscore the similarity in developmental mechanisms throughout the entire somatosensory system.

C   The Thalamus

The neurons that compose the ventral posterior nucleus of the rat are generated rather abruptly on embryonic day 14 (McAllister and Das, 1977). As at other levels of the somatosensory system, this same event occurs a few days earlier in the mouse (Angevine, 1970). Brainstem lemniscal afferents grow into the ventral posterior nucleus during the late embryonic period. On embryonic day 20, lemniscal fibers can only be detected in the caudal and ventral portions of the ventral posterior nucleus. By the time of birth, they have reached the full extent of the nucleus although the density of fibers in portions of the nucleus continues to increase until postnatal day 4 (unpublished observations). During the first few postnatal days, these afferents first segregate into bands that can be related to the rat's five rows of vibrissae and then further segregate into individual discrete clusters within the bands. During this same period, the distribution of thalamocortical relay cells are undergoing a similar shift in their distribution from continuous to discrete (Ivy and Killackey, 1982a).

The other major afferent to the ventral posterior nucleus arises in the somatosensory cortex. Corticothalamic afferents invade the ventral posterior nucleus at a later time than the lemniscal afferents. One day after birth, these afferents surround rostral and lateral portions of the ventral posterior nucleus but have yet to invade it in a major way. This process occurs during the next several days. By postnatal day 4, these afferents are distributed throughout the nucleus in a latticelike pattern that is a mirror image of the vibrissa-related clusters of trigeminal afferents (Akers and Killackey, 1979). Over the next week, this latticelike pattern is obscured by the gradual encroachment of the corticothalamic afferents into the discrete clusters that are the domain of the trigeminal afferents and are not detectable in the adult (Hoogland et al., 1987). Other aspects of the vibrissa-related morphological pattern noted above also gradually become less distinct during this period. Evidence from Golgi studies (Scheibel et al., 1976) suggest that this gradual obscurement is correlated with the gradual increase in the complexity and overlap of afferent terminal arbors of these fiber systems as viewed at the light microscopic level during this period. It should also be emphasized that this relative obscurement of the very discrete patterns detectable during the early postnatal period is not in any sense a breakdown of the high degree of somatotopic organization that characterizes the ventral posterior nucleus.

Section of the infraorbital nerve on the day of birth results in the absence of a vibrissa-related pattern within the ventral posterior nucleus (Killackey and Shinder, 1981). The effects of more subtle peripheral manipulations such as the removal of a row of vibrissae are also clearly detectable in this nucleus. The effects of such a manipulation at birth can be detected within the ventral posterior nucleus with the succinic dehydrogenase (SDH) stain within 48 h of the time the peripheral damage is inflicted (Belford and Killackey, 1979b). Indeed, abnormal organization occurs with the same time course as normal discrete organization. This has been interpreted as evidence of the role of the periphery in guiding the formation of central somatotopic patterns. Given that the SDH stain is a reflection of the pattern of lemniscal terminations within the ventral posterior nucleus, it also suggests that it is the pattern of afferent terminations that is most closely controlled by the periphery. This point will be returned to in more detail later in the consideration of somatosensory cortex.

It is also important to emphasize the rather obvious point that the ventral posterior nucleus is further removed from the periphery than the brainstem somatosensory relay nuclei and that, consequently, the effects of a peripheral manipulation are somewhat different than at more peripheral levels. At the level of the primary afferent, peripheral manipulations such as follicle cautery (Savy et al., 1981; Bates and Killackey, 1985; Killackey, 1987) or nerve cut (Waite and Cragg, 1982) result in explicit degeneration or loss of fibers during the developmental period. The exact degree of loss, however, is difficult to determine, as primary afferents are capable of some degree of regeneration that complicates assessment (Rhoades et al., 1987b). It does seem reasonable to assume that the brainstem trigeminal targets of these afferents are relatively completely denervated for at least several days following peripheral manipulation (i.e., during the critical or sensitive period when the periphery plays its role in central pattern formation). This is supported by the finding that cortical-evoked potentials that can normally be elicited by vibrissa stimulation 2 or 3 days after birth are not elicited in nerve cut animals until at least 7 days after birth (Waite and Cragg, 1982).

At the level of the brainstem targets of the primary afferents there is some neuronal loss following complete vibrissa follicle destruction. Hamori et al. (1986) have reported an 18% cell loss and a 33% decrease in volume within the subnucleus interpolaris following such a manipulation in the mouse. This same study reported no loss of neurons within the ventral posterior nucleus in the same animals. On the contrary, they report an increased number and density of neurons in the ventral posterior nucleus in which the damaged periphery is represented, which they attribute to the failure of the normally occurring cell death process. In a previous study using a more restricted peripheral manipulation in the mouse, removal of a single row of vibrissae, Woolsey et al. (1979) report no changes in cell density between the affected region of the ventral posterior nucleus and the normal side. Whatever the basis of this discrepancy, these results do suggest that basic organizational features of the ventral posterior nucleus, such as the source and size of its afferent input and its basic cytological organization, are relatively normal in animals with neonatal peripheral trigeminal damage. The major change in the nucleus is in the pattern of afferent terminations formed in the nucleus, which in turn affects the distribution of the terminal arbors of its projection to the somatosensory cortex.

D   The Neocortex

The neurons that compose the neocortex of the rat are generated over a time period that extends from embryonic day 16 to 21 (Berry and Rogers, 1965; Hicks and D'Amato, 1968). Further, as first demonstrated in the mouse (Angevine and Sidman, 1961), time of origin of cortical cells is reflected in their laminar position. Cortical neurons in the deeper cortical layers are generated before neurons in the more superficial cortical layers, resulting in an "inside-out" sequence of cortical development. Given that laminar location of a cortical neuron is also correlated with its projection target (Wise and Jones, 1977), the time of origin of cortical neurons may also be correlated with its ultimate projection target. Jensen and Killackey (1984) have provided experimental evidence for this hypothesis.

The neurons of the fourth cortical layer that compose the barrels are generated on embryonic day 18 in the rat. The first signs of the barrels in layer IV are detectable on postnatal day 3 in Nissl-stained material (Rice et al., 1985). This coincides with the arrival of thalamocortical afferents in layer IV (Wise and Jones, 1978) and the first appearance of discrete clusters of SDH staining in this layer (Killackey and Belford, 1979). At the cortical level, there is no evidence of the pattern developing along a gradient as it does in the brainstem; rather, the whole pattern appears to develop at approximately the same time (see however, Rhoades et al., 1990). This is probably attributable to the concurrent ingrowth of thalamocortical afferents into the cortical layers as opposed to the staggered growth of primary afferents into the brainstem. The effects of a peripheral manipulation such as removal of a row of vibrissae can also be detected at the same time as the normal pattern. Once again, this suggests that it is normal developmental events that are perturbed by neonatal peripheral manipulations. Several experiments provide some insight into these events at the cortical level.

At the time of birth, thalamocortical projections have reached the cortex but are located in the white matter beneath the still-forming cortical layers (Wise and Jones, 1978). Recent preliminary evidence, however, suggests that thalamocortical fibers may penetrate the cortical plate as early as postnatal day 1 (Senft and Woolsey, 1987). At the time of birth, discrete topographic relations between the thalamus and cortex can be demonstrated by the retrograde transport of horseradish peroxidase from cortex to thalamus (Dawson and Killackey, 1985). Thus, topographic relations between the thalamus and cortex develop well before there are any hints of a vibrissa-related somatotopic pattern in either structure and even before the ventral posterior nucleus is fully innervated. This suggests that the overall topographic relations between these two structures are intrinsically determined before birth and that peripheral manipulations at birth affect events in this system that occur between birth and day 3. This is the time period during which thalamocortical afferents are growing into the fourth cortical layer and forming their terminal arbors.

It was previously noted that the afferent terminations of individual thalamocortical afferents completely fill the discrete cortical cluster with which they are associated and that cluster size can be correlated both with peripheral location and innervation density. This suggests that the major role of the periphery is in shaping the size of afferent terminations. Presumably, this process is in some way related to "activity" in the system and has occurred by between the third and fourth postnatal day when discrete clusters of SDH activity are apparent. Jensen and Killackey (1987b) have provided evidence favoring this hypothesis. Neonatal infraorbital nerve section that abolishes all evidence of a vibrissa-related pattern at the level of the brainstem and thalamus (Killackey and Shinder, 1981; Bates et al., 1982) also results in very anomalous cortical patterns that are not readily related to the periphery. Individual thalamocortical afferent terminations in adult rats subjected to neonatal nerve cut are also severely perturbed. Such terminations are much larger than normal and have a much reduced branching density. While this result directly supports the hypothesis that the role of the periphery in guiding somatotopic organization is exerted at the level of afferent terminations, two interpretations of the result are possible. First, the periphery plays a role in forming terminal arbors that are normally discrete at all stages including initial outgrowth. Second, the periphery functions in trimming back terminal arbors that are diffuse in their initial outgrowth. The short time period in which the terminal arbors are formed favors the first of these alternatives, but the question deserves further attention.

The periphery also appears to play some role in the sculpting of other aspects of cortical organization, namely, the distribution of cortical projection neurons. While this role has yet to be clearly defined, some hints of it are evident in the distribution of callosal projection neurons. As noted in the preceding, callosal projection neurons and terminations that in adult rat somatosensory cortex are located in the supra- and infragranular layers are distributed in a complementary fashion to the discrete thalamocortical afferents arising from the ventral posterior nucleus (Akers and Killackey, 1978; Olavarria et al., 1984). At birth the cells of origin of the immature callosal projection are continuously distributed in the deep layers below the cortical plate, and callosal afferents are evenly distributed in the underlying white matter (Ivy et al., 1979; Ivy and Killackey, 1982b). The discontinuous adult pattern is established during the next 10 days or so and is accompanied by the specific ingrowth of callosal afferents into appropriate regions. The mechanism underlying this change is the elimination of neuronal processes (O'Leary et al., 1981; Ivy and Killackey, 1982b). Double labeling has indicated that many neurons in the neonatal rat somatosensory cortex project both ipsilaterally to motor cortex, and presumably to other ipsilateral targets as well, and across the corpus callosum. During development neurons located within primary somatosensory cortex lose their callosal processes, resulting in the discontinuous distribution of callosal projections characteristic of the adult. This elimination process also seems to be influenced by the periphery. The complementary organization of thalamic and callosal projections in the normal adult may be taken as indirect evidence for this assertion. More direct evidence is provided by the distribution of callosal projection neurons after neonatal infraorbital nerve section, the same manipulation that profoundly disrupts the distribution of thalamocortical afferents. This same manipulation both reduces the density of callosal projection neurons and alters their distribution in a way that reflects the changed distribution of thalamocortical afferents (Koralek and Killackey, 1990). This manipulation also produces changes in the distribution of callosal projections outside of primary somatosensory cortex. The face region of the second somatosensory area which normally receives callosal projections is now devoid of callosal connections. This suggests that the train of organizational events that begins at the periphery and has been traced in some detail up to primary somatosensory cortex may continue in other cortical areas beyond primary somatosensory cortex.

The foregoing has focused on the trigeminal system as the unique distribution of peripheral receptors, and their central representations have generated considerable interest and can be experimentally manipulated with relative ease. However, the principles derived from the trigeminal system apply equally well to other portions of the somatosensory system. Dawson and Killackey (1987) have provided evidence that neonatal limb removal or section of the afferent innervation to the limbs at birth results in an anomalous organization of the associated cortical patterns. Amputation of a forelimb at or before embryonic day 17 results in an even more surprising cortical change (Dawson and Killackey, 1986; Killackey and Dawson, 1989). As noted in a previous section, this manipulation results in what has been interpreted as a partial invasion of the "virgin" cuneate nucleus by later arriving hindlimb primary afferents at the level of the brainstem. At the cortical level, the manipulation results in a doubling of the size of the cortical representation of the hindpaw. This expansion appears to be at the expense of cortical areas outside the primary somatosensory cortex. Such results further emphasize the point that no level of the central nervous system develops in isolation of other levels. The effects of a peripheral manipulation on a given level of the neural axis can only be interpreted within the larger framework of the entire system under study.

As a final point, it is obvious from the foregoing that the authors favor the hypothesis that the periphery plays a key instructive role in the formation of the central somatosensory system. This view has been challenged (Cooper and Steindler, 1986 and Cooper et al., 1989). These authors have postulated that glial associated adhesion molecules intrinsic to the developing neocortex play a primary role in forming borders between functional units such as "barrels". Further, they postulate that this glial event "results in the formation of 'premaps' which can be further sculped during early postnatal life by more precise map-conveying afferent systems, . . .". We regard this view as a very tenuous one for two reasons. First, the earliest detectable "barrel-like" patterns in the neocortex are clearly formed by extrinsic afferent systems and not intrinsic glial elements (Rhoades et al., 1990). Second, neonatal peripheral manipulations such as those reviewed above alter the patterns of glial boundaries just as patterns of neural elements are altered (Cooper and Steindler, 1989). Thus, at present the role of glial boundaries in pattern formation does not appear to be a primary one, rather their role is secondary to that of the extrinsic afferent input to a given level of the somatosensory neural axis.

IV SUMMARY

The studies reviewed in this chapter provide evidence that the overall development of the somatosensory system takes place in a sequential fashion beginning at the periphery and progressing centrally. These studies also demonstrate that the development of the system is accomplished by a number of diverse mechanisms, some of which are confined to particular levels of the system and others that operate at all levels. One of the most prominent features of the system at each level of the neural axis, somatotopic patterns, develops relatively late and seems to be most closely related to the formation of afferent terminations. Major unresolved questions involve the molecular mechanisms that play a role in sculpting of patterns of afferent terminals and their "transmittal" along the neural axis. Finally, the studies also point out that when focusing on a particular level of the system, it is important to do so within the larger context of the entire system, keeping in mind that what occurs at one level is the result of interactions intrinsic to that level as well as events that have occurred at previous levels.

REFERENCES

Akers, R. M., and H. P. Killackey (1978) Organization of corticocortical connections in the parietal cortex of the rat. J. Comp. Neurol. *181*:513–538.

Akers, R. M., and H. P. Killackey (1979) Segregation of cortical and trigeminal afferent to the ventrobasal complex of the neonatal rat. Brain Res. *161*:527–532.

Altman, J., and S. Bayer (1982) Development of the cranial nerve ganglia and related nuclei in the rat. Adv. Anat. Embryol. Cell Biol. *74*:1–90.

Altman, J., and S. A. Bayer (1984) The development of the rat spinal cord. Adv. Anat. Embryol. Cell Biol. *85*:1–166.

Andres, F. L., and H. Van der Loos (1982) Whisker patterns form in cultured non-innervated muzzle skin from mouse embryos. Neurosci. Lett. *30*:37–41.

Andres, K. H. (1966) Uber die feinstruktur der rezeptoren an sinus-haaren. Z. Zellforsch. *75*:339–365.

Angevine, J. B. (1970) Time of neuron origin in the diencephalon of the mouse: An autoradiographic study. J. Comp. Neurol. *139*:129–188.

Angevine, J. B., and R. L. Sidman (1961) Autoradiographic study of cell migration during histogenesis of cerebral cortex in the mouse. Nature *192*:766–768.

Armstrong-James, J. and K. Fox (1987) Spatiotemporal convergence and divergence in the rat S1 "barrel cortex." J. Comp. Neurol. *263*:265.

Arvidson, J. (1982) Somatotopic organization of vibrissae afferents in the trigeminal sensory nuclei of the rat studied by transganglionic transport of HRP. J. Comp. Neurol. *211*:84–92.

Barbaresi, P., R. Spreafico, C. Frassoni, and A. Rustioni (1986) GABAergic neurons are present in the dorsal column nuclei but not in the ventroposterior complex of rats. Brain Res. *382*:305–326.

Basbaum, A. I., and P. J. Hand (1973) Projections of cervicothoracic dorsal roots to the cuneate nucleus of the rat, with observations on cellular "bricks." J. Comp. Neurol. *148*:347–360.

Bates, C. A., and H. P. Killackey (1984) The emergence of a discretely distributed pattern of corticospinal projection neurons. Dev. Brain Res. *13*:265–273.

Bates, C. A., and H. P. Killackey (1985) The organization of the neonatal rat's brainstem trigeminal complex and its role in the formation of central trigeminal patterns. J. Comp. Neurol. *240*:265–287.

Bates, C. A., R. S. Erzurumlu, and H. P. Killackey (1982) Central correlates of peripheral pattern alterations in the trigeminal system of the rat. III. Neurons of the principal sensory nucleus. Dev. Brain Res. *5*:108–113.

Belford, G. R., and H. P. Killackey (1978) Anatomical correlates of the forelimb in the ventrobasal complex and the cuneate nucleus of the neonatal rat. Brain Res. *158*:450–455.

Belford, G. R., and H. P. Killackey (1979a) The development of vibrissae representation in subcortical trigeminal centers of the neonatal rat. J. Comp. Neurol. *188*:63–74.

Belford, G. R., and H. P. Killackey (1979b) Vibrissae representation in subcortical trigeminal centers of the neonatal rat. J. Comp. Neurol. *183*:305–322.

Belford, G. R., and H. P. Killackey (1980) The sensitive period in the development of the trigeminal system of the neonatal rat. J. Comp. Neurol. *193*:335–350.

Berry, M., and A. W. Rogers (1965) The migration of neuroblasts in the developing cerebral cortex. J. Anat. *99*:691–709.

Bruce, L. L., J. G. McHaffie, and B. E. Stein (1987) The organization of trigeminotectal and trigeminothalamic neurons in rodents: A double-labeling study with fluorescent dyes. J. Comp. Neurol. 262:315–330.

Cajal, S. Ramón y (1911) Histologie du Systeme Nerveux de l'Homme et des Vertebres, Vol. 2 (Maloine, Paris, 1911), reprinted by Consejo Superior de Investigaciones Cientificas. Madrid: 1972.

Chapin, J., and C.-S. Lin (1984) Mapping the body representation in the SI cortex of anesthetized and awake rats. J. Comp. Neurol. 229:199–213.

Cooper, N. G. F., and D. A. Steindler (1986) Lectins demarcate the barrel subfield in the somatosensory cortex of the early postnatal mouse J. Comp. Neurol. 249: 157–169.

Cooper, N. G. F., and D. A. Steindler (1989) Critical period-dependent alterations of the transient body image in the rodent cerebral cortex. Brain Res. 489: 167–176.

Davies, A., and A. Lumsden (1984) Relation of target encounter and neuronal death to nerve growth factor responsiveness in the developing mouse trigeminal ganglion. J. Comp. Neurol. 223:124–137.

Davies, A., and A. Lumsden (1986) Fasciculation in the early mouse trigeminal nerve is not ordered in relation to the emerging pattern of whisker follicles. J. Comp. Neurol. 253:13–24.

Dawson, D. R., and H. P. Killackey (1985) Distinguishing topography and somatotopy in the thalamocortical projections of the developing rat. Dev. Brain Res. 17:309–313.

Dawson, D. R., and H. P. Killackey (1986) Morphological changes in rat somatosensory cortex following prenatal limb removal. Soc. Neurosci. Abstr. 12:1436.

Dawson, D. R., and H. P. Killackey (1987) The organization and mutability of the forepaw and hindpaw representations in the somatosensory cortex of the neonatal rat. J. Comp. Neurol. 256:246–256.

Donaldson, L., P. J. Hand, and A. R. Morrison (1975) Corticothalamic relationships in the rat. Exp. Neurol. 47:448–458.

Dorfl, J. (1982) The musculature of the mystacial vibrissae of the white mouse. J. Anat. 135:147–154.

Emmers, R. (1965) Organization of the first and second somesthetic regions (SI and SII) in the rat thalamus. J. Comp. Neurol. 124:215–228.

English, K. B., P. R. Burgess, and D. Kavka-Van Norman (1980) Development of rat Merkel cells. J. Comp. Neurol. 194:475–496.

Erzurumlu, R. S., and H. P. Killackey (1979) Efferent connections of the brainstem trigeminal complex with the facial nucleus of the rat. J. Comp. Neurol. 188:75–86.

Erzurumlu, R. S., and H. P. Killackey (1980) Diencephalic projections of the subnucleus interpolaris of the brainstem trigeminal complex in the rat. Neuroscience 5:1891–1901.

Erzurumlu, R. S., and H. P. Killackey (1983) Development of order in the rat trigeminal system. J. Comp. Neurol. 213:365–380.

Erzurumlu, R. S., C. A. Bates, and H. Killackey (1980) Differential organization of thalamic projection cells in the brain stem trigeminal complex of the rat. Brain Res. 198:427–433.

Fitzgerald, M. (1987) Spontaneous and evoked activity of foetal primary afferents "in vivo." Nature 326:603–605.

Forbes, D. J., and C. Welt (1981) Neurogenesis in the trigeminal ganglion of the albino rat. A quantitative autoradiographic study. J. Comp. Neurol. 199:133–147.

Fukushima, T., and F. W. L. Kerr (1979) Organization of trigeminothalamic tracts and other thalamic afferent systems of the brainstem in the rat: Presence of gelatinosa neurons with thalamic connections. J. Comp. Neurol. 183:169–184.

Hamori, J., C. Savy, M. Madarasz, J. Somogyi, J. Takacs, R. Verley, and E. Farkas-Bargeton (1986) Morphological alterations in subcortical vibrissal relays following vibrissal follicle destruction at birth in the mouse. J. Comp. Neurol. 254:166–183.

Harris, R. M. (1986) Morphology of physiologically identified thalamocortical relay neurons in the rat ventrobasal thalamus. J. Comp. Neurol. 251:491–505.

Harris, R. M., and T. A. Woolsey (1981) Dendritic plasticity in mouse barrel cortex following postnatal vibrissa follicle damage. J. Comp. Neurol. 196:357–376.

Hayashi, H. (1980) Distributions of vibrissae afferent fiber collaterals in the trigeminal nuclei as revealed by intra-axonal injection of horseradish peroxidase. Brain Res. 183:442–446.

Hicks, S. P., and C. J. D'Amato (1968) Cell migrations to the isocortex in the rat. Anat. Rec. 160:619–634.

Hockfield, S., and S. Gobel (1982) An anatomical demonstration of projections to the medullary dorsal horn (trigeminal nucleus caudalis) from rostral trigeminal nuclei and the contralateral caudal medulla. Brain Res. 252:203–211.

Hoogland, P. V., E. Welker, and H. Van der Loos (1987) Organization of the projections from barrel cortex to thalamus in mice studied with phaseolus vulgaris-leucoagglutinin and HRP. Exp. Brain Res. 68:73–87.

Ide, C. (1976) The fine structure of the digital corpuscle of the mouse toe pad with special reference to nerve fibers. Amer. J. Anat. 147:329–356.

Ivy, G. O., and H. P. Killackey (1981) The ontogeny of the distribution of callosal projection neurons in the rat parietal cortex. J. Comp. Neurol. 195:327–389.

Ivy, G. O., and H. P. Killackey (1982a) Ephemeral cellular segmentation in the thalamus of the neonatal rat. Dev. Brain. Res. 2:1–17.

Ivy, G. O., and H. P. Killackey (1982b) Ontogenetic changes in the projections of neocortical neurons. J. Neurosci. 2:735–743.

Ivy. G. O., R. M. Akers, and H. P. Killackey (1979) Differential distribution of callosal projection neurons in the neonatal and adult rat. Brain Res. 173:532–537.

Jacquin, M. F., A. Hess, G. Yang, P. Adamo, M. F. Math, A. Brown, and R. W. Rhoades (1984) Organization of the infraorbital nerve in rat: A quantitative electron-microscopic study. Brain Res. 290:131–135.

Jensen, K. F., and H. P. Killackey (1984) Subcortical projections from ectopic neocortical neurons. Proc. Natl. Acad. Sci. USA 81:964–968.

Jensen, K. F., and H. P. Killackey (1987a) Terminal arbors of axons projecting to the somatosensory cortex of the adult rat. I. The normal morphology of specific thalamocortical afferents. J. Neurosci. 7:3529–3543.

Jensen, K. F., and H. P. Killackey (1987b) Terminal arbors of axons projecting to the somatosensory cortex of the adult rat. II. The altered morphology of thalamocortical afferents following neonatal infraorbital nerve cut. J. Neurosci. 7:3544–3553.

Killackey, H. P. (1973) Anatomical evidence for cortical subdivisions based on vertically discrete thalamic projections from the ventral posterior nucleus to cortical barrels in the rat. Brain Res. *51*:326–331.

Killackey, H. P. (1983) The somatosensory cortex of the rodent. Trends Neurosci. *6*:425–429.

Killackey, H. P. (1987) Three phases in the vulnerability of the somatosensory system to peripheral nerve damage. In L. Pubols and B. Sessle (eds.): Effects of Injury on Trigeminal and Spinal Somatosensory Systems. New York: Alan R. Liss, pp. 363–370.

Killackey, H. P., and G. R. Belford (1979) The formation of afferent patterns in the somatosensory complex of the neonatal rat. J. Comp. Neurol. *183*:285–304.

Killackey, H. P., and D. R. Dawson (1989) Expansion of the central hindpaw representation following fetal forelimb removal in the rat. European J. Neurosci *1*:210–221.

Killackey, H. P., and R. S. Erzurumlu (1981) Trigeminal projections to the superior colliculus of the rat. J. Comp. Neurol. *201*:221–242.

Killackey, H. P., and K. Fleming (1985) The role of the principal sensory nucleus in central trigeminal pattern formation. Dev. Brain Res. *22*:141–145.

Killackey, H. P., and S. Leshin (1975) The organization of specific thalamocortical projections to the posteromedial barrel subfield of the rat somatic sensory cortex. Brain Res. *86*:469–472.

Killackey, H. P., and A. Shinder (1981) Central correlates of peripheral pattern alterations in the trigeminal system of the rat. II. The effect of nerve section. Dev. Brain Res. *1*:121–126.

Killackey, H. P., G. R. Belford, and D. K. Ryugo (1976) Anomalous organization of the thalamocortical projections consequent to vibrissae removal in the newborn rat and mouse. Brain Res. *104*:309–315.

Killackey, H. P., K. A. Koralek, N. L. Chiaia, and R. W. Rhoades (1989) Laminar and areal differences in the origin of subcortical projection neurons in the rat somatosensory cortex. J. Comp. Neurol. *282*:428–445.

Koralek, K. A., and H. P. Killackey (1990) Callosal projections in rat somatosensory cortex are altered by early removal of afferent input. Proc. Nat. Acad. Sci. USA, in press.

Koralek, K. A., J. Olaveria, and H. P. Killackey (1990) Areal and laminar organization of corticocortical projections in rat somatosensory cortex. J. Comp. Neurol., in press.

Lee, K. J., and T. A. Woolsey (1975) A proportional relationship between peripheral innervation density and cortical neuron number in the somatosensory system of the mouse. Brain Res. *99*:349–353.

Lorente de Nó, R. (1922) La corteza cerebral del raton. Trab. Lab. Invest. Biol. Univ. Madrid *20*:1–38.

Lumsden, A. G. S., and A. M. Davies (1983) Earliest sensory nerve fibres are guided to peripheral targets by attractants other than nerve growth factor. Nature *306*:786–788.

Lumsden, A. G. S., and A. M. Davies (1986) Chemotropic effect of specific target epithelium in the developing mammalian nervous system. Nature *323*:538–539.

Lund, R. D., and K. E. Webster (1967) Thalamic afferents from the dorsal column nuclei. An experimental anatomical study in the rat. J. Comp. Neurol. *130*:301–312.

McAllister, J. P., and G. D. Das (1977) Neurogenesis in the epithalamus, dorsal thalamus, and ventral thalamus of the rat: An autoradiographic and cytological study. J. Comp. Neurol. *172*:647–686.

McAllister, J. P., and J. Wells (1981) The structural organization of the ventroposterolateral nucleus in the rat. J. Comp. Neurol. *197*:271–301.

Nord, S. G. (1967) Somatotopic organization in the spinal trigeminal nucleus, the dorsal column nuclei and related structures in the rat. J. Comp. Neurol. *130*:313–328.

Olavarria, J., R. C. Van Sluyters, and H. P. Killackey (1984) Evidence for the complementary organization of callosal and thalamic connections within rat somatosensory cortex. Brain Res. *291*:364–368.

O'Leary, D. D, B. B. Stanfield, and W. M. Cowan (1981) Evidence that the early postnatal restriction of origin of the callosal projection is due to the elimination of axonal collaterals rather than the death of neurons. Dev. Brain Res. *1*:607–617.

Peschanski, M. (1984) Trigeminal afferents to the diencephalon in the rat. Neuroscience *12*:465–487.

Renehan, W. E., and B. L. Munger (1986) Degeneration and regeneration of peripheral nerve in the rat trigeminal system. I. Identification and characterization of the multiple afferent innervation of the mystacial vibrissae. J. Comp. Neurol. *246*:129–145.

Renehan, W. E., and R. W. Rhoades (1984) A quantitative electron microscopic analysis of the infraorbital nerve in the newborn rat. Brain Res. *322*:369–373.

Rhoades, R. W., J. M. Fiore, M. F. Math, and M. F. Jacquin (1983) Reorganization of trigeminal primary afferents following neonatal infraorbital nerve section in hamsters. Dev. Brain Res. *7*:337–342.

Rhoades, R. W., G. R. Belford, and H. P. Killackey (1987a) Receptive field properties of VPM neurons before and after selective kainic acid lesions of the trigeminal brainstem complex. J. Neurophysiol. *57*:1577–1600.

Rhoades, R. W., N. L. Chiaia, R. D. Mooney, B. G. Klein, W. E. Renehan, and M. F. Jacquin (1987b) Reorganization of the peripheral projections of the trigeminal ganglion following neonatal transection of the infraorbital nerve. Somatosens. Res. *5*:35–62.

Rhoades, R. W., C. A. Bennet-Clarke, N. L. Chiaia, E. A. White, G. J. McDonald, J. H. Haring, and M. F. Jacquin (1990) Development and lesion induced reorganization of the cortical representation of the rat's body surface as revealed by imunocytochemistry for serotonin. J. Comp. Neurol., in press.

Rice, F. L., C. Gomez, C. Bartow, A. Burnet, and P. Sands (1985) A comparative analysis of the development of the primary somatosensory cortex: Interspecies similarities during barrel and laminar development. J. Comp Neurol. *236*:447–495.

Savy, C., S. Margules, E. Farkas-Bargeton, and R. Verley (1981) A morphometric study of mouse trigeminal ganglion after unilateral destruction of vibrissae follicles at birth. Brain Res. *217*:265–277.

Scheibel, M. E., T. L. Davies, and A. B. Scheibel (1976) Ontogenetic development of somatosensory thalamus. I. Morphogenesis. Exp. Neurol. 51:392–406.

Senft, S., and T. A. Woolsey (1987) Development of afferents to mouse somatosensory cortex. Soc. Neurosci. Abstr. 13:387.

Simons, D. J. (1978) Response properties of vibrissae units in rat SmI somatosensory neocortex. J. Neurophysiol. 41:798–820.

Smith, R. L. (1973) The ascending fiber projections from the principal sensory trigeminal nucleus in the rat. J. Comp. Neurol. 148:423–446.

Spacek, J., and A. R. Lieberman (1974) Ultrastructure and three-dimensional organization of synaptic glomeruli in rat somatosensory thalamus. J. Anat. 117:487–516.

Steffen, H., and H. Van der Loos (1980) Early lesions of mouse vibrissal follicles: their influence on dendrite orientation in the cortical barrelfield. J. Comp. Neurol. 196:357–376.

Steindler, D. A. (1985) Trigeminocerebellar, trigeminotectal, and trigeminothalamic projections: A double retrograde axonal tracing study in the mouse. J. Comp. Neurol. 237:155–175.

Steindler, D. A., N. G. F. Cooper, A. Faissner, and M. Schachner (1989) Boundaries defined by adhesion molecules during development of the cerebral cortex: The J1/tenascin glycoprotein in the mouse somatosensory cortical barrel field. Dev. Biol. 131:243–260.

Taber Pierce, E. (1970) Histogenesis of the sensory nucleus of the trigeminal nerve in the mouse: An autoradiographic study. Anat. Rec. 166:388.

Van der Loos, H. (1976) Barreloids in mouse somatosensory thalamus. Neurosci. Lett. 2:1–6.

Van Exan, R. J., and M. H. Hardy (1980) A spatial relationship between innervation and the early differentiation of vibrissae follicles in the embryonic mouse. J. Anat. 131:643–656.

Vincent, S. B. (1912) The function of the vibrissae in the behavior of the white rat. Behavior Monographs 1:1–81.

Vincent, S. B. (1913) The tactile hair of the white rat. J. Comp. Neurol. 23:1–36.

Waite, P. M. E. (1973) Somatotopic organization of vibrissal responses in the ventrobasal complex of the rat thalamus. J. Physiol. 228:527–540.

Waite, P. M. E., and B. G. Cragg (1982) The peripheral and central changes resulting from cutting or crushing the afferent nerve supply to the whiskers. Proc. Roy. Soc. Lond. B 214:191–211.

Welker, C. (1971) Microelectrode delineation of fine grain somatotopic organization of SMI cerebral neocortex in albino rat. Brain Res. 26:259–275.

Welker, C. (1976) Receptive field of barrels in the somatosensory neocortex of the rat. J. Comp. Neurol. 166:173–190.

Welker, E., and H. Van der Loos (1986) Quantitative correlation between barrel-field size and the sensory innervation of the whiskerpad: A comparative study in six strains of mice bred for different patterns of mystacial vibrissae. J. Neurosci. 6:3355–3373.

Welker, W. I. (1964) Analysis of sniffing in the albino rat. Behavior 22:223–244.

White, E. L. (1978) Identified neurons in mouse SmI cortex which are postsynaptic to thalamocortical axon terminals: a combined Golgi-electron microscopic and degeneration study. J. Comp. Neurol. *181*:627–662.

Wise, S. P., and E. G. Jones (1977) Cells of origin and terminal distribution of descending projections of the rat somatic sensory cortex. J. Comp. Neurol. *175*:129–158.

Wise, S. P., and E. G. Jones (1978) Developmental studies of thalamocortical and commissural connections in the rat somatic sensory cortex. J. Comp. Neurol. *178*:187–208.

Woolsey, C. N. (1956) Organization of somatic sensory and motor areas of the cerebral cortex. In H. Harlow and C. N. Woolsey (eds.): Biological and Biochemical Bases of Behavior. Madison: University of Wisconsin Press, pp. 63–82.

Woolsey, T. A., and H. Van der Loos (1970) The structural organization of layer IV in the somatosensory region (SI) of the mouse cerebral cortex. Brain Res. *17*:205–242.

Woolsey, T. A., C. Welker, and R. H. Schwartz (1975) Comparative anatomical studies of the SmI face cortex with special reference to the occurrence of "barrels"in layer IV. J. Comp. Neurol. *164*:79–94.

Woolsey, T. A., J. R. Anderson, J. R. Wann, and B. B. Stanfield (1979) Effects of early vibrissae damage on neurons in the ventrobasal (VB) thalamus of the mouse. J. Comp. Neurol. *184*:363–380.

Yamakado, M., and T. Yohro (1979) Subdivision of mouse vibrissae on an embryological basis, with descriptions of variations in the number and arrangement of sinus hairs and cortical barrels in BALB/c (nu/+ nude, nu/nu) and hairless (hr/hr) strains. Amer. J. Anat. *156*:153–174.

Zucker, E., and W. I. Welker (1969) Coding of somatic sensory input by vibrissae neurons in the rat's trigeminal ganglion. Brain Res. *12*:138–156.

Chapter Eleven

PHYSIOLOGICAL DEVELOPMENT AND PLASTICITY OF SOMATOSENSORY NEURONS

ROBERT W. RHOADES

Medical College of Ohio
Toledo, Ohio

HERBERT P. KILLACKEY

University of California
Irvine, California

NICOLAS L. CHIAIA

Medical College of Ohio
Toledo, Ohio

MARK F. JACQUIN

St. Louis University School of Medicine
St. Louis, Missouri

I   INTRODUCTION

The purpose of this chapter is to review the data that are currently available regarding the normal development and lesion-induced reorganization of somatosensory maps and the receptive field properties of single neurons in the mammalian somatosensory system. The studies discussed are limited to those that have examined lemniscal pathways and our review of "plasticity" experiments is restricted to those concerned with the physiological consequences of neonatal nervous system damage. Readers interested in experiments that have assessed the functional sequelae of somatosensory system lesions in adult animals are referred to the recent reviews of Kaas et al. (1983) and Wall and Cusick (1984).

Before initiating our review of this literature, it is important to consider, at least briefly, the method that has been employed to collect almost all of the data that will be discussed.

II   TECHNICAL PROBLEMS AND LIMITATIONS ASSOCIATED WITH EXTRACELLULAR SINGLE-UNIT RECORDING

Virtually all of the experiments reviewed in this chapter have employed some form of extracellular single-unit recording to assess the topographic organization of somatosensory nuclei and/or the receptive field properties of individual neurons. This method is by no means novel, and it has been used to generate most of the information that we have regarding the response characteristics of sensory neurons in all modalities. Nevertheless, there are several limitations to the technique that should be considered [see also Pubols (1984) and Rhoades et al. (1987a) for additional related discussion]. Most important among these limitations is electrode selectivity. A number of experiments carried out primarily in the visual system (e.g., Stone, 1973; Levick and Cleland, 1974; Shapley and So, 1980) have indicated that the resistance and tip size of the recording electrode can markedly alter the sample of neurons that is isolated in a nucleus containing cells of different sizes. This problem may be particularly acute in developmental studies where there is good reason to believe that neurons within a given structure mature, both physiologically and anatomically, at different times.

A second related problem is verification of the sites from which recordings were made. Small electrolytic lesions or dye marks are employed in most, but by no means all, experiments to denote the locations of electrode tracks or particular cells. While this would seem to be a straightforward process, it must be noted that a given neuron can be recorded over a substantial distance (often at more than 150 μm) even with relatively high-resistance electrodes. Electrode coordinates where neurons are killed (as indicated by a high-frequency "agonal" discharge) provide relatively unequivocal information regarding the locations of the somata of these cells. In other instances, exact assignment of recordings to specific loci is more difficult. This problem again becomes more acute in developing animals where the volumes of most nuclei are quite small.

A final problem that is particularly important in experiments designed to assess topography is the distinction between recordings from cell bodies and fibers of passage. While there are published criteria for distinguishing somal and axonal recordings (e.g., Hubel, 1960; Bishop et al., 1962), our own experience (Jacquin et al., 1986b) indicates that such distinctions are often extremely difficult.

III NORMAL DEVELOPMENT OF SOMATOSENSORY NEURON RECEPTIVE FIELDS

In view of the fact that ascending somatosensory and especially trigeminal pathways have become important models in which to address general questions about central nervous system development (see Chapter 10 by Killackey et al. and Chapter 12 by Woolsey in this volume), it is surprising that there have been only a relatively small number of experiments that have examined the responses of somatosensory neurons in developing animals.

One probable reason for this lack of studies is the difficulty involved in carrying out physiological recording experiments in newborns. Small body mass and immature metabolic processes often preclude the use of standard anesthetics and complicate precise thermoregulation. In addition, incomplete cranial development necessitates the use of novel procedures for stabilization of the head and subsequent stereotaxic localization of recording loci. Nevertheless, it must be noted that workers in other sensory systems have overcome these difficulties and provided data of the type that are sorely needed to understand development of response properties (e.g., Hubel and Wiesel, 1963; Stein et al., 1973).

A   Development of Responses of Primary Afferent Neurons

The receptive field properties of sensory ganglion cells in newborn animals have been assessed in only a handful of studies. While some immaturity has been noted for the response characteristics of these neurons (e.g., Kocsis et al., 1983), departures from adult organization are much less pronounced than those reported for central somatosensory neurons. Welker and his co-workers (Gibson et al., 1975; Beitel et al., 1977) recorded from primary afferents innervating the glabrous skin of the forepaw in kittens between the ages of 1 and 52 days and observed only relatively subtle changes in their responses as a function of maturation. They concluded that most of the physiological changes which occurred were a function of alterations in the mechanical properties of the skin rather than in the terminals of the nerve fibers themselves. One exception to this generalization is, of course, conduction velocity. Most peripheral nerve fibers are small and unmyelinated in newborn animals (Ekholm, 1967; Friede and Samorajski, 1968; Renehan and Rhoades, 1984) and thus conduct action potentials more slowly than their adult counterparts.

Ferrington and Rowe (1980), in experiments similar to those of Welker and his colleagues, observed somewhat more clear-cut differences between the responses of primary afferents in neonatal and mature cats. They found that the proportions of rapidly and slowly adapting fibers matched, quite closely, those obtained in adults but that the dynamic properties of rapidly adapting fibers in the neonates differed considerably from those observed in adult animals. They suggested that at least some of these differences might be due to morphological immaturity of the Pacinian corpuscles at the time of birth (Malinovsky and Sommerova, 1972).

Ekholm (1967) carried out the most extensive study to date of the response properties of primary afferents in newborn kittens, and like Ferrington and Rowe (1980), he observed a number of differences between the characteristics of these fibers in neonates and adult cats. As in their study, most of the differences he noted were for characteristics such as thresholds, frequency following, and peak firing rates.

While there are some discrepancies between the findings of Ekholm (1967) and Ferrington and Rowe (1980) on the one hand and Welker and co-workers (Gibson et al., 1975; Beitel et al., 1977) on the other, one important point of agreement is that receptive field sizes (relative to the area of the entire skin surface) were not radically different in newborn and adult animals and no qualitatively abnormal receptive fields were recorded. Fitzgerald (1987) has obtained similar results from her recordings of spinal primary afferents in fetal rats. These aspects of the physiological data are in good accord with anatomical findings that indicate that the *adult topography* of the primary afferent innervation of the skin is well established by birth (e.g., Van Exan and Hardy, 1980; Honig, 1982; Scott, 1982; Erzurumlu and Killackey, 1983; Klein et al., 1986).

B Development of Receptive Fields of Second-Order Neurons

A substantial number of investigators have examined the functional organization of the spinal cord in fetal and neonatal animals (e.g., Naka, 1964; Ekholm, 1967; Kellerth et al., 1971; Saito, 1979; Fulton et al., 1980; Otsuka and Konishi, 1980). Their studies have, however, concentrated primarily upon the development of motoneurons and spinal reflexes. The first investigation of the development of receptive field properties of dorsal horn neurons in mammals was carried out only recently by Fitzgerald (1985). Her results are typical of those that have been obtained for immature neurons in most sensory systems. She found that lumbar dorsal horn cells in the newborn rat gave only sluggish responses to either electrical or tactile stimulation and were typically unable to follow even moderate rates of stimulation. For the first 3 days of life, most of these neurons responded only to pinching of the skin and receptive field sizes were nearly four times as large as they would be when the animal reached 15 days of age (Figure 1). Ipsilateral, contralateral, and distant inhibitory afferents to dorsal horn neurons were observed from the day of birth, but the C fiber input to these cells did not develop fully until the second postnatal week.

The data that have been obtained from the cuneate nucleus of newborn kittens are considerably different (Ferrington and Rowe, 1981, 1982). Here, the functional cell classes observed in the adult animal could be readily distinguished in the newborn. There were some subtle differences between the receptive field properties of cuneate neurons of young kittens and mature cats, but Ferrington and Rowe (1981, 1982) concluded that the specificity of connections between primary afferents and cuneate cells observed in the adult animal was present by birth.

The substantial difference between the data that have been obtained in the rat spinal cord and the kitten cuneate nucleus is most probably a function of the difference in the gestational period for these two species. Rats are born 21 days after conception, and for cats this period is 65 days. The question that remains to be answered is whether the differences in the maturity of the receptive fields of second-order neurons observed in these two species is a function of differences in primary afferent input or central neuronal circuitry. The data presented in the preceding section indicate that sensory ganglion cells have relatively mature receptive field properties in newborn cats. This also appears to be the case in rodents (Fitzgerald, 1987). As noted above, the available anatomical information suggests that the topographic organization of the peripheral projections of sensory ganglion cells are very adultlike in newborn rodents. This also appears to be true of the central projections of these neurons, at least at the level of the light

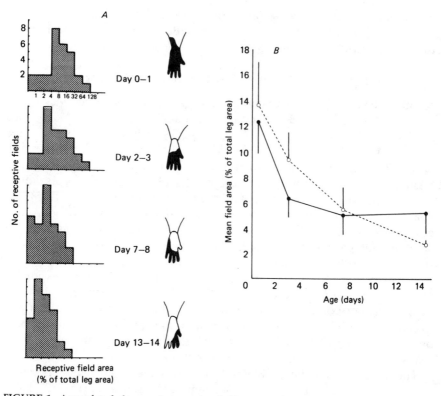

FIGURE 1. Age-related changes in receptive field size for dorsal horn neurons in the spinal cord of the perinatal rat. All measurements are relative to the area of the entire body surface. The histograms (A) summarize the data for different time points and the drawings show typical receptive fielded for each of these ages. The solid circles in (B) denote data for superficial layer neurons and the open circles data from deeper layer cells. (Reproduced from Fitzgerald, 1985.)

microscope (e.g., Fitzgerald and Swett, 1983; Smith, 1983; Jacquin and Rhoades, 1985).

Consideration of the anatomical and physiological data would thus prompt the conclusion that the relative lack of specificity of the receptive fields of spinal neurons in newborn rats may be primarily a function of immaturity of either descending systems or interneuronal connections. Fitzgerald (1985) has also suggested that the slower development of the C fiber input to the dorsal horn may be responsible, at least in part, for the relatively immature receptive fields observed in newborn rodents. In support of this argument, she notes that permanent destruction of C fibers by neonatal administration of capsaicin (Jansco et al., 1977) results in dorsal horn cells with permanently expanded receptive fields (Wall et al., 1982).

C   Development of Receptive Fields of Thalamic Neurons

To our knowledge, there have been no investigations of the development of somatosensory topography or neuronal response properties in the diencephalon.

D   Development of Receptive Fields of Neurons in Somatosensory Cortex

Somatosensory system development and damage-induced reorganization have been examined most extensively at the cortical level. As might be expected from the data that exist for the spinal cord and dorsal column nuclei in neonatal rats and kittens (see Section III,B), the functional status of the primary somatosensory cortex of newborns from these two species is quite different.

Rubel (1971) recorded from the primary somatosensory cortex of newborn kittens and reported that its organization is quite similar to that observed in mature cats. This was the case with respect to both topography and the response characteristics of individual neurons. The only appreciable differences between the neonate and adult that he observed were longer latencies to electrical stimulation of the skin and fewer discontinuities in receptive field maps in the former animals. The first difference is almost certainly a function of increases in the myelination of peripheral and central axons and reductions in the times of synaptic delays (Purpura et al., 1965; Ekholm, 1967). The latter difference may be a result of intracortical projections that are functional in the adult but not the newborn.

Both topography and the receptive field characteristics of the sensory responses of cortical neurons in rodents are quite immature at birth. Armstrong-James (1975) reported that reliable evoked responses could be obtained from primary somatosensory cortical cells only by the seventh postnatal day. At this time, the receptive fields of individual cells were extremely large relative to those observed in adult animals (Figure 2), and there was rapid habituation to repeated stimulation. While Armstrong-James (1975) suggested that the large receptive fields of the cells he recorded may have been due to a lack of surround inhibition at the cortical level, it is equally likely that they simply reflected the larger receptive fields of neurons interposed between primary afferents and the cortex (see the preceding). Recordings from brainstem and thalamic neurons in immature rodents would help to determine which of these two possibilities is correct.

There is another potential reason that the cells recorded by Armstrong-James (1975) in week-old rats all had such large receptive fields relative to those observed in mature animals. This possibility is related to the limitations of extracellular single-unit recording techniques already discussed. It is well known that lamina V neurons in the primary somatosensory cortex of adult rats have much larger receptive fields than those of cells in lamina

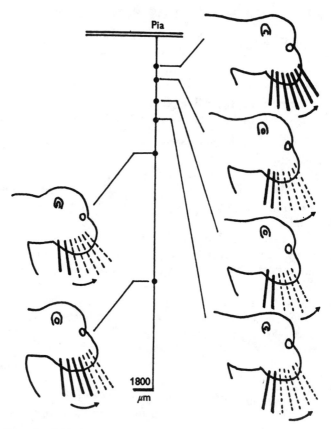

FIGURE 2. Receptive fields for vibrissa sensitive cells in the primary somatosensory cortex of a newborn rat. The solid vibrissae were those that activated the cell in question; those shown as dashed lines were not a part of the cell's receptive field. (Reproduced from Armstrong-James, 1975.)

IV or the supragranular layers (Simons, 1978; Ito, 1981). The apical dendrites of lamina V neurons pass through the superficial laminae, and it is relatively easy to record from these processes in adult animals (R. W. Rhoades, R. A. Mooney, and M. F. Jacquin, personal communication). The neurons that will occupy layer V in the adult are among the earlier generated cortical cells (Angevine and Sidman, 1961; Berry and Rogers, 1965), and it is not unreasonable to suggest that they may become responsive to peripheral stimuli before neurons in the superficial cortical layers. Given the small size of the cortex and the tight packing of its cells in perinatal rodents, it is possible that some of the findings reported by Armstrong-James (1975) may have been due to errors in the laminar assignment of the units that he recorded. The potential for such a problem was increased by the fact that he did not mark his electrode penetrations for histological verification of recording sites.

E Conclusions

The data reviewed in the preceding section, while somewhat limited, indicate that the maturity of the somatosensory system in newborns depends very much upon the the species that is being examined. In cats, departures from the functional organization observed in adult animals are relatively subtle while in more altricial rodents they are quite marked. These differences may be largely a function of the anatomical immaturity of central circuits in the latter species since the organization of the primary afferent projections to the periphery and brainstem appear, at the light microscopic level, to be relatively adultlike in these animals. It is also possible that species differences in the maturity of synaptic contacts between primary afferents and central neurons may contribute to the observed differences in functional organization [compare the data of Clark (1977) with those of Dunn and Westrum (1978)].

IV LESION-INDUCED CHANGES IN RESPONSE PROPERTIES OF SOMATOSENSORY NEURONS

The literature concerned with the effects of neonatal nerve damage upon somatosensory functional organization is considerably more extensive than that describing the normal development of somatotopy and the receptive fields of single somatosensory neurons. This is probably the case for two reasons. The first is the obvious clinical relevance of studies concerned with the effects of peripheral nerve damage, and the second is the simple fact that it is technically much easier to make a lesion in a neonatal animal and wait until it is an adult to carry out recordings than it is to accomplish similar physiological experiments in a neonate. One unfortunate aspect of the experiments that have been concerned with lesion-induced changes in the responses of somatosensory cells is that relatively little attention has been paid to primary afferents. The limited data that are available suggest that changes in the receptive fields of sensory ganglion cells may explain many of the functional alterations that have been observed in central structures.

A Lesion-Induced Changes in Response Properties of Primary Afferent Neurons

There is to our knowledge only a single study that has examined the effects of neonatal peripheral nerve damage upon the receptive field properties of sensory ganglion cells. Jacquin et al. (1986b) have recorded from trigeminal primary afferent neurons after transection of the infraorbital nerve in newborn rats. They identified neurons that, by maturity, had regenerated (or sprouted; see Rhoades et al., 1987b) axons into this trigeminal branch by electrical stimulation proximal to the point of the neonatal transection. They observed changes in both the topographic organization of the ganglion and the response characteristics of individual neurons. With respect to topography, mandibular and oral maxillary units exhibited an organization similar to that observed in normal adult rats, but ophthalmic primary afferents were recorded more ventrally and laterally in the ganglion than is normally the case. In addition, the dorsoventral topography observed for vibrissa-sensitive ganglion cells in normal adults was absent in the neonatally nerve-damaged rats.

Conclusions regarding ganglionic topography based upon data obtained in single-unit recording experiments must be tempered by the methodological limitations outlined at the beginning of this chapter. A particular problem in these experiments was distinguishing somal from axonal recordings. We have discussed in detail the manner in which we attempted to control for this problem and the way in which it may have influenced our data (Jacquin et al., 1986b), but it must still be noted that there are discrepancies between the ganglionic topography established by physiological and anatomical techniques (Klein et al., 1985; also see Killackey et al., Chapter 10, this volume).

Alterations in the response properties of individual ganglion cells are perhaps more interesting and certainly more readily interpreted than changes in ganglionic topography. Neonatal transection of the infraorbital nerve resulted in a marked decrease in the percentage of primary afferents that responded to vibrissa stimulation and an increase in the percentage that were excited by noxious stimulation of nonvibrissa infraorbital territory (Jacquin et al., 1986b). For those cells that remained responsive to vibrissa stimulation, there was a significant reduction in the percentages of slowly adapting and low-velocity-sensitive rapidly adapting units and a corresponding increase in the percentages of primary afferents that responded only to either high-velocity displacement of the vibrissa or the application of a noxious pinch or deep pressure to the vibrissa follicle.

It seems probable that these changes in the responses of primary afferent neurons reflected an inability of many regenerate (or late growing) axons to form (or reform) the peripheral receptor associations that they normally make. The vibrissa follicle is known to contain an elaborate array of cutaneous receptors (Andres, 1966; Patrizi and Munger, 1966; Renehan and Munger, 1986a), some of which are substantially reduced in number after transection of the infraorbial nerve in *adult* animals (Renehan and Munger, 1986b). It may be that a similar or even more extensive loss of receptors occurs after neonatal transection of this trigeminal branch.

An alternative hypothesis that should be considered is that the altered distribution of functional ganglion cell types reflects differential survival of the primary afferent neurons that would *normally* develop velocity or noxious biased receptive fields. While such a proposal is compatible with the findings described in the preceding paragraph, it cannot explain all of the changes observed after neonatal infraorbital nerve damage. Many infraorbital ganglion cells in neonatally nerve-damaged rats developed receptive field types that were never observed in normal adult animals. These included neurons that were responsive to deflection of multiple vibrissae (Figures 3A and B); ganglion cells that responded to both vibrissae and guard hairs (Figure 3C); neurons that were discharged by stimulation of guard hairs, skin, and vibrissae (Figure 3D); and primary afferents with split (Figure 3E) or abnormally large (Figure 3F) receptive fields. We also recorded a number of neurons that could only be excited by the application of pressure to the region of the infraorbital foramen (Figure 3G). These responses may have reflected regenerate axons that became trapped in neuromata.

B Lesion-Induced Changes in Receptive Field Properties of Second-Order Neurons

Neonatal damage to peripheral nerves has been shown to alter the receptive field properties of second-order neurons. The studies of Waite and Cragg (1982) and Waite (1984) and recent results from one of our laboratories (Jacquin, 1989) have demonstrated that this is clearly the case for cells in the rodent's trigeminal brainstem complex, and Kalaska and Pomeranz (1982) have shown that it is also true for neurons in the kitten's cuneate nucleus.

Waite and Cragg (1982) compared the effects of neonatal crushing and transection of the infraorbital nerve upon the somatotopic organization of the trigeminal brainstem complex of the adult animal. The only significant changes observed after nerve crush were an absence of cells responsive to some mystacial vibrissae at different levels and increases in the portion of principalis and each spinal subnucleus devoted to the representations of the supraorbital and auriculotemporal sinus hairs (Figure 4). Transection of the nerve, on the other hand, yielded profound changes in brainstem somatotopy. There were major increases in the areas in which the auriculotemporal and supraorbital sinus hairs were represented and a concomitant reduction in that area devoted to the mystacial vibrissae. One-third to one-half of these whiskers were not represented at all (Figure 5).

Waite (1984) and Kalaska and Pomeranaz (1982) carried out logically comparable experiments in rats and kittens and obtained quite similar results. Waite (1984) transected the infraorbital nerve in newborn rats and then recut it at weekly intervals to prevent reestablishment of connections with the periphery. Kalaska and Pomeranz (1982) denervated the forepaws of 2–3-week-old kittens by transecting and ligating the superficial radial, median, and ulnar nerves. Both manipulations produced subtantial changes in central somatotopy and in the receptive field characteristics of individual neurons. In the rats, neurons in the portion of the trigeminal brainstem complex in which the mystacial vibrissae were normally repre-

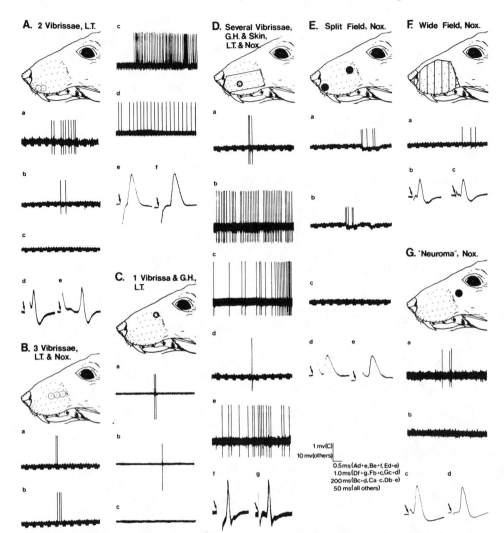

FIGURE 3. Abnormal receptive fields for infraorbital ganglion cells recorded from rats that sustained transection of this trigeminal branch on the day of birth. See text for description. (Reproduced from Jacquin et al., 1986b.)

sented became responsive to stimulation of the cheek, inside of the mouth, and lower jaw. Individual cells had abnormally large and often discontinuous receptive fields (Figure 6). There was also a greater convergence of submodalities onto individual neurons than normally observed. In the cats, many cells in the portion of the cuneate nucleus where the forepaw is normally represented responded to stimulation of the wrist, forearm, or trunk. Kalaska and Pomeranz (1982) also observed a small number of neurons with abnormally large or disjoint receptive fields.

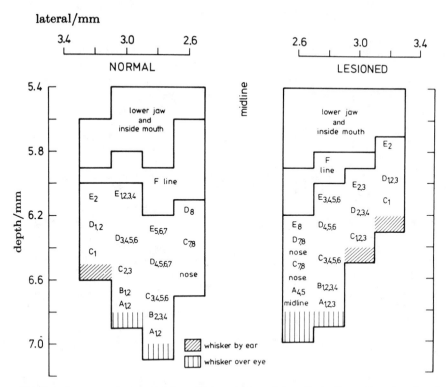

FIGURE 4. Somatotopic organization of trigeminal nucleus principalis on the normal and deafferented sides of the brainstem of a rat that sustained a crush lesion of the infraorbital nerve on the day of birth. (Reproduced from Waite and Cragg, 1982.)

An issue of considerable interest is the nature of the substrate for the physiological changes observed in experiments such as those of Waite (1984) and Kalaska and Pomeranz (1982). There are a number of nonmutually exclusive ways in which such reorganization might occur. Several of the more obvious of these are:

1. The changes observed in the receptive fields (and thus peripheral connectivity) of primary afferent neurons (see the preceding) might simply be passed on to brainstem circuitry that is not altered by perinatal nerve damage.

2. Alterations in the central arbors of damaged and/or undamaged primary afferents might change patterns of input onto second-order neurons (e.g., Rhoades et al., 1983).

3. There may be alterations in the growth of the dendritic arbors of second-order neurons that provides them with access to novel subsets of primary afferent input (e.g., Smith, 1974; Harris and Woolsey, 1981; Hoy et al., 1985).

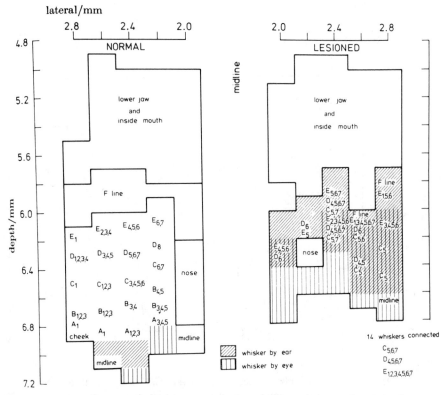

FIGURE 5. Somatotopic organization of subnucleus oralis on the normal and deafferented sides of the brainstem of a rat that sustained transection of the infraorbital nerve on the day of birth. (Reproduced from Waite and Cragg, 1982.)

4. Reorganization of interneuronal circuits may "unmask" normally subliminal inputs to brainstem cells (Wall, 1977; Merrill and Wall, 1978).

A variety of experimental paradigms have provided anatomical and physiological data that are consistent with all of the preceding hypotheses. It is instructive to see how these possibilities may apply to the lesion-induced physiological reorganization observed in the trigeminal brainstem complex by Waite (1984). Two additional facts regarding the changes that she observed are important with respect to this discussion. First, the somatotopic reorganization began 7 days after the initial nerve transection and was completed by day 21. Second, none of the effects observed after neonatal nerve lesions were seen after similar damage was induced in adult animals.

Several of the changes observed by Waite (1984) are very similar to the

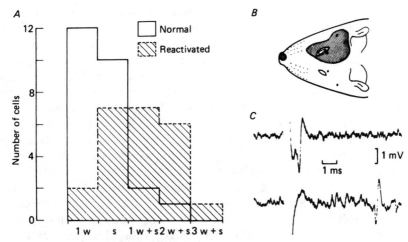

FIGURE 6. Changes in the organization of the receptive fields of nucleus principalis cells in rats that sustained neonatal transection and intermittent recutting of the infraorbital nerve. The histogram (*A*) shows the increases in receptive field size for the deafferented cells, and the data in (*B*) illustrate the location and responses of one principalis neuron with a split receptive field. (Reproduced from Waite, 1984.)

lesion-induced alterations in primary afferent receptive fields summarized in the preceding, and it is thus possible that a portion of the reorganization that she observed reflected these peripheral changes. It is probably not likely that the functional changes in the brainstem reflected *central* collateral sprouting by undamaged primary afferent axons. Jacquin and Rhoades (1985) examined this possibility using transganglionic transport techniques in similarly prepared rats and found no strong evidence to support the existence of such sprouting. The relatively long time course of the changes and the fact that they were observed after neonatal but not adult nerve damage both militate against the possibility that unmasking was responsible for the observed functional reorganization.

The suggestion that changes in the dendritic arbors of postsynaptic cells that provided them with access to novel inputs may be involved in reorganization of the type observed by Waite (1984) is attractive because there is strong precedent for it in simpler systems (Shankland et al., 1982; Hoy et al., 1985), and it can be readily tested in mammals by combining intracellular recording and horseradish peroxidase injection into single neurons. This approach has been employed to examine the effects of spinal cord deafferentations in adult animals (Brown et al., 1983; Sedivec et al., 1986), and we have begun to apply it to trigeminal brainstem neurons in rats that were subjected to neonatal transection of the infraorbital nerve. Our early results provide at least some support for the conclusion that alterations in receptive field properties of a given neuron *need not* be associated with dramatic changes in that cell's dendritic arbor.

Figure 7 illustrates the structural characteristics and receptive field properties of a trigeminocerebellar neuron from subnucleus interpolaris of an adult rat that sustained transection of the ipsilateral infraorbital nerve on the day of birth. The morphology of this neuron did not differ significantly from those of trigeminocerebellar neurons in normal animals (M. F. Jacquin, R. A. Mooney, and R. W. Rhoades, personal communication). Its receptive field, on the other hand, was considerably different from those of such cells in normal adult rats (e.g., Woolsten et al., 1982; M. F. Jacquin, R. A. Mooney, and R. W. Rhoades, personal communication). It was abnormally large and it responded to *both* guard hair and vibrissa deflection. Such convergence is not normally observed in these projection neurons.

Another interpolaris cell with a relatively restricted dendritic arbor is illustrated in Figure 8. The morphology of this trigeminothalamic neuron in a normal adult rat would predict a small receptive field. The cell shown was excited by stimulation of portions of the skin in all three trigeminal divisions. It thus represents another example of dramatic physiological reorganization without a concomitant change in dendritic morphology.

While the cells described in the immediately preceding paragraphs do not support the suggestion that changes in the dendritic arbors of postsynaptic cells provide the anatomical substrate for the functional reorganization observed in the neonatally deafferented brainstem, this was not invariably the case. The trigeminothalamic neuron illustrated in Figure 9 had a dendritic arbor that was very different from those observed for such cells in normal animals (Jacquin et al., 1986a). Instead of being radially symmetric about the cell body, the dendrites of this cell were oriented toward the lateral portion of subnucleus interpolaris, the region in which fibers from the auriculotemporal nerve terminate (Jacquin et al., 1983). The receptive field for this cell included the auriculotemporal sinus hair and extended onto the ear. The structural and functional characteristics of this neuron would thus *suggest* a reorientation of dendrites away from the deafferented (i.e., infraorbital) portion of the nucleus toward a source of residual input (see also Smith, 1974).

C   Lesion-Induced Changes in Receptive Field Properties of Thalamic Neurons

There are considerable data that indicate that neonatal nerve damage alters the anatomical organization of the ventrobasal thalamus (see Chapter 10 by Killackey et al. and Chapter 12 by Woolsey, this volume). Only one study to date has employed physiological techniques to address the issue of functional reorganization after such lesions. Verley and Onnen (1981) recorded from the ventrobasal thalamus (VB) of mice that sustained cauterization of the mystacial vibrissae on the day of birth. This lesion might be considered the equivalent of a partial and very distal transection of the infraorbital nerve. They observed a reduction in the representation of these whiskers

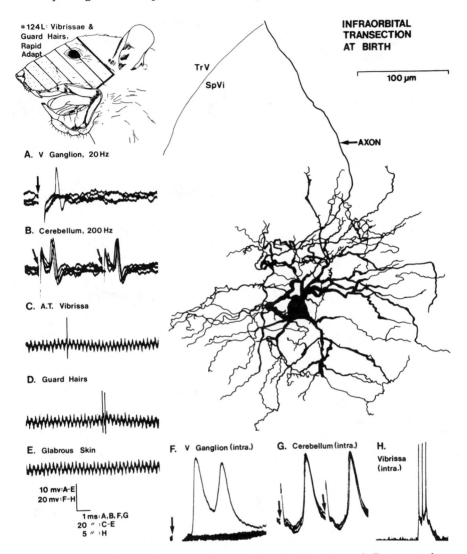

FIGURE 7. Morphology and response characteristics of a trigeminocerebellar neuron from subnucleus interpolaris of a rat that sustained transection of the ipsilateral infraorbital nerve on the day of birth. The morphology of the cell was normal, but its receptive field was abnormally large.

and an increase in the portion of VB that was devoted to the facial common fur.

It should be clear that all of the potential mechanisms suggested to explain lesion-induced alterations in the receptive fields of brainstem neurons could apply equally well to the thalamus. The paucity of information

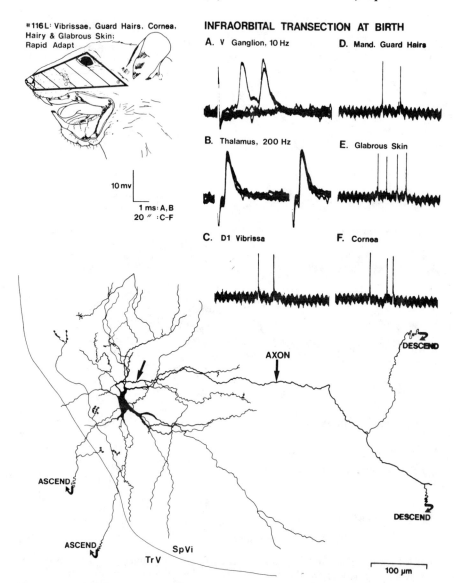

FIGURE 8. Morphology and response characteristics of a trigeminothalamic neuron from subnucleus interpolaris that was deafferented by neonatal transection of the infraorbital nerve. As for the cell shown in Figure 7, the somadendritic morphology is relatively normal, but the receptive field is abnormally large.

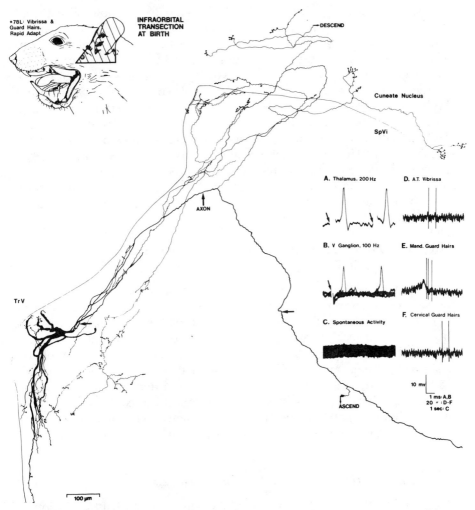

FIGURE 9. Morphology and response characteristics of a second trigeminothalamic cell from subnucleus interpolaris of a neonatally nerve-damaged rat. Here, both the morphology and receptive field characteristics of the cell are abnormal. See text for further details.

concerning the details of the functional changes that occur here would, however, make any proposals regarding mechanisms of reorganization extremely speculative at this point. It is, nevertheless, worth noting that the anatomical and functional organization of the VB, and in particular the ventral posteromedial nucleus (VPM), offers an excellent opportunity to assess potential substrates for the functional reorganization that follows nerve damage.

The anatomical organization of the VPM is relatively simple. Virtually all of the cells there are projection neurons (e.g., Saporta and Kruger, 1977), and their receptive field properties in the intact animal are quite uniform. The vast majority give rapidly adapting responses to deflection of a single mystacial vibrissa (Waite, 1973; Shosaku, 1985; Rhoades et al., 1987a). The ultrastructural organization of the nucleus is also uncomplicated (Tripp and Wells, 1978; McAllister and Wells, 1981; Wells and Tripp, 1987), and changes in synaptology should be readily detectable (Tripp and Wells, 1978). Finally, the morphological characteristics of vibrissa-sensitive neurons in this nucleus appear quite uniform (Harris, 1986; Belford et al., 1987) so lesion-induced changes in their dendritic arbors should be quite easy to discern. Given these characteristics of the VPM, many of which have been known for a number of years, it is surprising that this nucleus has not been exploited for studies of neuronal plasticity.

D   Lesion-Induced Changes in Receptive Field Properties of Neurons in Primary Somatosensory Cortex

As has been the case with most aspects of sensory development, the functional consequences of neonatal somatosensory system damage have been studied most often at the cortical level, and the literature in this area has been reviewed recently and quite thoroughly by Simons et al. (1984) and Wall and Cusick (1986). While there is general agreement that peripheral lesions in perinatal animals produce substantial cortical functional reorganization, there is considerable variability in the extent and nature of the changes that have been observed. In order to minimize confusion, the types of experiments that have been carried out have been divided into two categories: cauterization of vibrissa follicles and transection of peripheral nerves.

1   Cauterization of Some or All Vibrissa Follicles

This manipulation, as already noted, is essentially a partial transection of the infraorbital nerve, and it has been employed by a number of investigators to examine the effects of peripheral damage upon the functional organization of the primary somatosensory cortex (Welt, 1977; Waite and Taylor, 1978; Killackey et al., 1978; Pidoux et al., 1979; 1980; Simons et al., 1984).

The changes reported by these investigators include an increased representation of adjacent nondenervated hair and skin in "barrel" cortex, increases in the cortical representation of spared vibrissae, and/or adjacent scar tissue and areas in which no cutaneous receptive fields can be mapped. The alterations observed in most of these experiments are extremely difficult to interpret because of the facts that relatively low-resistance electrodes were used to record multiple rather than single units, and the laminar and even tangential locations from which recordings were made were not carefully specified. As noted above, it is also difficult to know the nature of the elements actually being recorded in such experiments. The study in which problems of this nature were minimized by recording only from single units judged to be cells and providing good histological verification of recording sites is that of Simons et al. (1984). It is therefore worthwhile to present the changes that they observed in somewhat more detail.

Their recordings from lamina IV demonstrated that units in the enlarged barrels for the rows adjacent to that where the follicles were cauterized responded primarily to the appropriate vibrissae and that units in the cortical region that corresponded to the damaged row were either unresponsive, activated by vibrissae from the adjacent rows, and/or driven by stimulation of the scar tissue on the region of the face where the vibrissae were removed. The data obtained from the supra- and infragranular laminae followed closely those from lamina IV. The latter point is important because it suggests that the physiological reorganization observed in these animals was due to alterations in the information conveyed from the thalamus to the cortex rather than changes in intracortical connectivity. In fact, Simons et al. (1984) suggest that most or all of the changes that they observed can probably be explained by alterations in the peripheral connections of trigeminal primary afferents. Such a conclusion is certainly consistent with the effects of nerve damage upon the responses of these ganglion cells.

2 Transection of Entire Peripheral Nerves

The alterations in cortical organization that have been observed in these experiments have, as might be expected, generally been more substantial than those that followed cauterization of vibrissa follicles. Transection of the infraorbital nerve (Waite and Cragg, 1982) produced a marked reduction in the vibrissa representation and an "invasion" of the region normally devoted to the mystacial vibrissa by the nose, lower jaw, and supraorbital sinus hair (Figures 10A,B). Surprisingly, Waite and Craggs (1982) did not report the existence of any silent or unresponsive regions. This may have been due to the fact that they used relatively low-impedance electrodes to record multiple- rather than single-unit activity. It is also worth noting that none of the changes that followed nerve transection were observed when the nerve was crushed. In these animals the cortical representation of the infraorbital peripheral field was essentially normal.

The changes observed by Waite (1984) after transection of the infraorbital nerve and prevention of regeneration were different from those reported by Waite and Cragg (1982) after a single transection of this trigeminal branch. In the former animals, there was an invasion of whisker territory by the representation of the lower jaw, the cheek, and the auriculotemporal and supraorbital sinus hairs (Figure 10C). There were also small silent regions and *no change* in the area devoted to the representation of the nose. Why the representation of the nose should change after a single infraorbital nerve transection, but not when regeneration is prevented, is not clear.

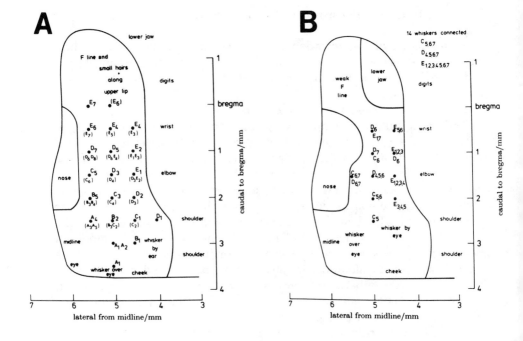

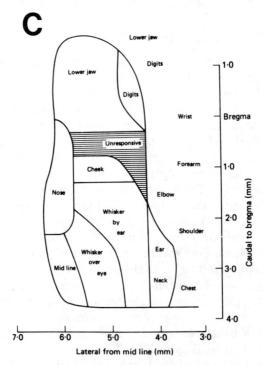

FIGURE 10. (A) Semidiagrammatic map of the facial representation in the primary somatosensory cortex of a normal rat. (B) Data from an animal subjected to a single neonatal transection of the infraorbital nerve. (C) Data from a rat in which the nerve was cut at birth and regeneration prevented. [Adapted from Waite and Cragg (1982) and from Waite (1984).]

The other manipulation that has been used extensively to examine effects of peripheral damage upon cortical functional organization is deafferentation of a paw or a portion thereof. In all of these studies (Kalaska and Pomeranz, 1979; Kelehan et al., 1981; Rasmusson, 1982; Wall and Cusick, 1986) some abnormal cutaneous responsivity was observed in the portion of the cortex that normally represented the deafferented region of the body surface.

One important aspect of the results of these studies in which there has been some variability is whether or not there were cortical regions that remained "disconnected" from the periphery after such lesions. Both Wall and Cusick (1986) and Kalaska and Pomeranz (1979) did report the existence of such areas, but Kelahan et al. (1981) and Rasmusson (1982) did not. This difference in results may be due mainly to the magnitude of the deafferentations that were carried out. Wall and Cusick (1986) transected and ligated the sciatic nerve. Kalaska and Pomeranz (1979) transected and ligated the superficial radial, median, and ulnar nerves to deafferent the entire forepaw. Kelehan et al. (1981) and Rasmusson (1982) amputated only single digits.

One further aspect of the data provided by Wall and Cusick (1986) is worthy of additional mention. They found that the cortical reorganization that followed neonatal transection of the sciatic nerve was *less* extensive than that which occurred after similar deafferentations in adult animals (Wall and Cusick, 1984). Most studies that have compared the effects of neonatal and adult deafferentations upon central somatosensory organization (see the preceding; see also Waite, 1984; Wall and Cusick, 1986) have obtained the opposite result.

E   Conclusions

The data described in this chapter demonstrate clearly that neonatal damage to peripheral nerves produces alterations in somatotopy and changes in the responses of individual neurons at every level of the somatosensory neuraxis. The findings provided to date are at least consistent with the possibility that many or most of the centrally observed changes can be explained by alterations in the connectivity of primary afferent neurons. What should also be clear from this review is that it is exactly these cells that have received the least experimental attention to date. It would therefore seem that an important first step toward identifying the underpinnings of changes that occur centrally following deafferentations of the type described in this chapter would be to determine the effects of such damage upon the peripheral and central connectivity of sensory ganglion cells.

V   SUMMARY

Subject to the technical limitations discussed in the initial portion of this chapter, the available data suggest that the anatomical organization and functional properties of *primary* somatosensory neurons are relatively adult-like by the time of birth. The results obtained from recordings at successively higher levels of the neuraxis are not as clear. The degree to which *brainstem* and *cortical* somatosensory neurons exhibit adult receptive field characteristics depends upon the species examined. Recordings from cat have suggested relatively mature response properties, while those from rat show very definite departures from the organization observed in adult animals. The anomalous responses reported in the rat may reflect the immaturity of central neuronal circuits.

Reorganization of somatotopy and the receptive field properties of individual neurons following neonatal peripheral nerve damage has been well documented at nearly every level of the somatosensory neuraxis. Trigeminal ganglion cells in rats that sustained neonatal transection of the infraorbital nerve show enlarged and sometimes split receptive fields as well as an increase in the likelihood of responding to noxious stimulation. Brainstem neurons occupying central territories normally served by afferents from the mystacial vibrissae display receptive fields on the adjacent cheek and lower jaw. A similar functional reorganization of second-order neurons has been observed in the cuneate nucleus of kittens following denervation of the forepaw. Expansion of the central representation of the periphery adjacent to the site of denervation has also been shown in both thalamus and primary somatosensory cortex. It is not clear whether these central changes represent a reorganization of local circuits in the region of the neurons sampled or simply a faithful reproduction of alterations in the distribution of the peripheral or central axons of primary afferents.

ACKNOWLEDGMENTS

The work from our laboratories and the writing of this chapter were supported in part by DE07734, DE06528, BNS 85 15737 (R. W. R.), DE07662 (M. F. J.), and BNS 84 18715 (H. P. K.) from the National Institutes of Health and the National Science Foundation. Thanks to Patti Vendula for typing the manuscript.

REFERENCES

Andres, K. H. (1966) Uber die feinstruktur der rezeptoren an sinushaaren. Z. Zellforsch. 75:339–365.

Angevine, J. B., and R. L. Sidman (1962) Autoradiographic study of histogenesis in the cerebral cortex of the mouse. Anat. Rec. 142:210.

Armstrong-James, M. (1975) The functional status and columnar organization of single cells responding to cutaneous stimulation in neonatal rat somatosensory cortex SI. J. Physiol. (Lond.) 246:501–538.

Beitel, R. E., J. M. Gibson, and W. I. Welker (1977) Functional development of mechanoreceptive neurons innervating the glabrous skin in postnatal kittens. Brain Res. *129*:213–226.

Belford, G. R., H. P. Killackey, N. L. Chiaia, and R. W. Rhoades (1987) Response characteristics and morphology of vibrissa-sensitive neurons in the ventral posteromedial, thalamic retricular and posterior nuclei of the rat. Soc. Neurosci. Abstr. *271*:4.

Bishop, P. O., W. Burke, and R. Davis (1962) Single unit recording from antidromically activated optic radiation neurones. J. Physiol. (Lond.) *162*:432–450.

Brown, A. G., P. B. Brown, R. E. W. Fyffe, and L. M. Pubols (1983) Effects of dorsal root section on spinocervical tract neurons in the cat. J. Physiol. (Lond.) *337*:589–608.

Clark, H. (1977) A light and electron microscopic analysis of development within the main sensory trigeminal nucleus of the rat. Ph.D. Dissertation, Virginia Commonwealth University. Ann Arbor, Michigan: University Microfilms International.

Dunn, R. C., and L. E. Westrum (1978) Synapse development within the spinal trigeminal nucleus. Brain Res. *143*:421–436.

Ekholm, J. (1967) Postnatal changes in cutaneous reflexes and in the discharge pattern of cutaneous and articular sense organs. Acta Physiol. Scand. *297*:1–130.

Erzurumlu, R. S., and H. P. Killackey (1983) Development of order in the rat trigeminal system. J. Comp. Neurol. *213*:365–380.

Ferrington, D. G., and Rowe, M. J. (1980) Functional capacities of tactile afferent fibres in neonatal kittens. J. Physiol. (Lond.) *307*:335–353.

Ferrington, D. G., and M. J. Rowe (1981) Specificity of tacticle connections in neonatal cuneate nucleus. Dev. Brain Res. *1*:429–433.

Ferrington, D. G., and M. J. Rowe (1982) Specificity of connections and tactile coding capacities in cuneate nucleus of the neonatal kitten. J. Neurophysiol. *47*:622–640.

Fitzgerald, M. (1985) The post-natal development of cutaneous afferent fibre input and receptive field organization in the rat dorsal horn. J. Physiol. (Lond.) *364:*1–18.

Fitzgerald, M. (1987) Spontaneous and evoked activity of fetal primary afferents *in vivo*. Nature *326*:603–605.

Fitzgerald, M., and J. Swett (1983) The termination pattern of sciatic nerve afferents in the substantia gelatinosa of neonatal rats. Neurosci. Lett. *43*:149–154.

Friede, R. L., and T. Samorajski (1968) Myelin formation in the sciatic nerve of the rat. J. Neuropath. Exp. Neurol *27*:546–570.

Fulton, B. P., R. Miledi, and T. Takahashi (1980) Electrical synapses between motoneurones in the spinal cord of the newborn rat. Proc. Royal Soc. (Lond.) B *208*:115–120.

Gibson, J. M., R. E. Beitel, and W. I. Welker (1975) Diversity of coding profiles of mechanoreceptors in glabrous skin of kittens. Brain Res. *86*:181–203.

Harris, R. M. (1986) Morphology of physiologically identified thalamocortical relay neurons in the rat ventrobasal thalamus. J. Comp. Neurol. *251*:491–505.

Harris, R. M., and T. A. Woolsey (1981) Dendritic plasticity in mouse barrel cortex following postnatal vibrissa follicle damage. J. Comp. Neurol. *196*:357–376.

Honig, M. G. (1982) The development of sensory projection patterns in the embryonic chick hind limb. J. Physiol. (Lond.) *330*:175–202.

Hoy, R. R., T. G. Nolen, and G. C. Casaday (1985) Dendritic sprouting and compensatory synaptogenesis in an identified interneuron following auditory deprivation in a cricket. Proc. Natl. Acad. Sci. USA *82*:7772–7776.

Hubel, D. H. (1960) Single unit activity in lateral geniculate body and optic tract of unrestrained cats. J. Physiol. (Lond.) *150*:120–131.

Hubel, D. H., and T. N. Wiesel (1963) Receptive fields of cells in striate cortex of very young, visually inexperienced kittens. J. Neurophysiol. *26*:994–1002.

Ito, M., M. Kawabata, and R. Shoji (1981) Effect of prenatal X-irradiation on sensitivity of cortical neurons responding to vibrissa stimulation. J. Neurophysiol. *46*:716–724.

Jacquin, M. F. (1989) Structure-function relationships in rat brainstem subnucleus interpoloris: V. Functional consequences of neonatal infraorbital nerve section. J. Comp. Neurol. *282*:63–79.

Jacquin, M. F., and R. W. Rhoades (1985) Effects of neonatal infraorbital lesions upon central trigeminal primary afferent projections in rat and hamster. J. Comp. Neurol. *235*:129–143.

Jacquin, M. F., K. Semba, M. D. Egger, and R. W. Rhoades (1983) Organization of HRP-labelled trigeminal mandibular primary afferent neurons in the rat. J. Comp. Neurol. *215*:397–420.

Jacquin, M. F., R. D. Mooney, and R. W. Rhoades (1986a) Morphology, response properties, and collateral projections of trigeminothalamic neurons in brainstem subnucleus interpolaris of rat. Exp. Brain Res. *61*:457–468.

Jacquin, M. F., W. E. Renehan, B. G. Klein, R. D. Mooney, and R. W. Rhoades (1986b) Functional consequences of neonatal infraorbital nerve section in rat trigeminal ganglion. J. Neurosci. *6*:3706–3720.

Jancso, G., E. Kiraly, and A. Jancso-Gabor (1977) Pharmacologically induced selective degeneration of chemosensitive primary sensory neurones. Nature *270*: 22–29.

Kaas, J. H., M. M. Merzenich, and H. P. Killackey (1983) The reorganization of somatosensory cortex following peripheral nerve damage in adult and developing mammals. Ann. Rev. Neurosci. *6*:325–356.

Kalaska, J., and B. Pomeranz (1979) Chronic paw denervation causes an age-dependent appearance of novel responses from forearm in "paw cortex" of kittens and adult cats. J. Neurophysiol. *42*:618–633.

Kalaska, J., and B. Pomeranz (1982) Chronic peripheral nerve injuries alter the somatotopic organization of the cuneate nucleus in kittens. Brain Res. *236*:35–47.

Kelahan, A. M., R. H. Ray, L. V. Carson, C. E. Massey, and G. S. Doetsch (1981) Functional reorganization of adult raccoon somatosensory cerebral cortex following neonatal digit amputation. Brain Res. *223*:151–159.

Kellerth, J. O., A. Mellstrom, and S. Skoglund (1971) Postnatal excitability changes of kitten motoneurones. Acta Physiol. Scand. *83*:31–41.

Killackey, H. P., G. O. Ivy, and T. J. Cunningham (1978) Anomalous organization of SMI somatotopic map consequent to vibrissae removal in the newborn rat. Brain Res. *155*:136–140.

Klein, B. G., W. E. Renehan, M. F. Jacquin, and R. W. Rhoades (1985) Effects of neonatal infraorbital nerve lesion upon the innervation of the vibrissae follicle in the rat. Anat. Rec. 211:99A.

Klein, B. G., G. J. MacDonald, A. M. Szczepanik, and R. W. Rhoades (1986) Topographic organization of peripheral trigeminal ganglionic projections in newborn rats. Dev. Brain Res. 27:257–262.

Kocsis, J. D., J. A. Ruiz, and S. G. Waxman (1983) Maturation of mammalian myelinated fibers: Changes in action-potential characteristics following 4-Aminopyridine application. J. Neurophysiol. 50:449–463.

Levick, W. R., and B. G. Cleland (1974) Selectivity of microelectrodes in recordings from cat retinal ganglion cells. J. Neurophysiol. 37:1387–1393.

McAllister, J. P., and J. Wells (1981) The structural organization of the ventroposterolateral nucleus in the rat. J. Comp. Neurol. 197:271–301.

Malinovsky, L., and J. Sommerova (1972) Die postnatale entwicklung der Vater-Pacinischen korperchen in den fussballen der hauskatze (Felis silvestris f. catus L.). Acta Anat. 76:220–235.

Merrill, E. G., and P. D. Wall (1978) Plasticity of connection in the adult nervous system. In C. W. Cotman (ed.): Neuronal Plasticity. New York: Academic Press.

Naka, K. I. (1964) Electrophysiology of the fetal spinal cord. J. Gen. Physiol. 47:1003–1038.

Otsuka, M., and S. Konishi (1980) Electrophysiology of mammalian spinal cord in vitro. Nature 252:733–734.

Patrizi, G., and B. L. Munger (1966) The ultrastructure and innervation of rat vibrissae. J. Comp. Neurol. 126:423–436.

Pidoux, B., R. Verley, E. Farkas, and J. Scherrer (1979) Projections of the common fur of the muzzle upon the cortical area for mystacial vibrissae in rats dewhiskered since birth. Neurosci. Lett. 11:301–306.

Pidoux, B., M. F. Diebler, C. Savy, E. Farkas, and R. Verley (1980) Cortical organization of the postero-medial barrel-subfield in mice and its reorganization after destruction of vibrissal follicles after birth. Neuropathol. Appl. Neurobiol. 6:93–107.

Pubols, L. M. (1984) The boundary of proximal hindlimb representation in the dorsal horn following peripheral nerve lesions in cats: A reevaluation of plasticity in the somatotopic map. Somatosens. Res. 2:19–32.

Purpura, D. P., R. Shofer, and T. Scarff (1965) Properties of synaptic activities and potentials of neurons in immature neocortex. J. Neurophysiol. 28:925–942.

Rasmusson, D. D. (1982) Reorganization of raccoon somatosensory cortex following removal of the fifth digit. J. Comp. Neurol. 205:313–326.

Renehan, W. E., and B. L. Munger (1986a) Degeneration and regeneration of peripheral nerve in the rat trigeminal system. I. Identification and characterization of the multiple afferent innervation of the mystacial vibrissae. J. Comp. Neurol. 246:129–145.

Renehan, W. E., and B. L. Munger (1986b) Degeneration and regeneration of peripheral nerve in the rat trigeminal system. II. Response to nerve lesion. J. Comp. Neurol. 249:429–459.

Renehan, W. E., and R. W. Rhoades (1984) A quantitative electron microscopic analysis of the infraorbital nerve in the newborn rat. Brain Res. 322:369–373.

Rhoades, R. W., J. M. Fiore, M. F. Math, and M. F. Jacquin (1983) Reorganization of trigeminal primary afferents following neonatal infraorbital nerve section in hamster. Dev. Brain Res. 7:337–342.

Rhoades, R. W., G. R. Belford, and H. P. Killackey (1987a) Receptive field properties of rat VPM neurons before and after selective kainic acid lesions of the trigeminal brainstem complex. J. Neurophysiol. 57:1577–1600.

Rhoades, R. W., N. L. Chiaia, R. D. Mooney, B. G. Klein, W. E. Renehan, and M. F. Jacquin (1987b) Reorganization of the peripheral projections of the trigeminal ganglion following neonatal transection of the infraorbital nerve. Somatosens. Res. 5:35–62.

Rubel, E. W. (1971) A comparison of somatotopic organization in sensory neocortex of newborn kittens and adult cats. J. Comp. Neurol. 143:447–480.

Saito, K. (1979) Development of spinal reflexes in the rat fetus studied in vitro. J. Physiol. (Lond.) 299:581–597.

Saporta, S., and L. Kruger (1977) The organization of thalamocortical relay neurons in the rat ventrobasal complex studied by the retrograde transport of horseradish peroxidase. J. Comp. Neurol. 174:187–208.

Scott, S. A. (1982) The development of the segmental pattern of skin sensory innervation in embryonic chick hind limb. J. Physiol. (Lond.) 330:203–220.

Sedivec, M. J., J. J. Capowski, and L. M. Mendell (1986) Morphology of HRP-injected spinocervical tract neurons: Effect of dorsal rhizotomy. J. Neurosci. 6:661–672.

Shankland, M., D. Bentley, and C. S. Goodman (1982) Afferent innervation shapes the dendritic branching pattern of the medial giant interneuron in grasshopper embryos raised in culture. Dev. Biol. 92:507–520.

Shapley, R., and Y. T. So (1980) Is there an effect of monocular deprivation on the proportions of X and Y cells in the cat lateral geniculate nucleus? Exp. Brain Res. 39:41–48.

Shosaku, A. (1985) A comparison of receptive field properties of vibrissa neurons betwen the rat thalamic retricular and ventro-basal nuclei. Brain Res. 347:36–40.

Simons, D. J. (1978) Response properties of vibrissa units in rat SI somatosensory neocortex. J. Neurophysiol. 41:798–820.

Simons, D. J., D. Durham, and T. A. Woolsey (1984) Functional organization of mouse and rat SmI barrel cortex following vibrissal damage on different postnatal days. Somatosen. Res. 1:207–245.

Smith, C. L. (1983) The development and postnatal organization of primary afferent projections to the rat thoracic spinal cord. J. Comp. Neurol. 220:29–43.

Smith, D. E. (1974) The effect of deafferentation on the postnatal development of Clarke's nucleus in the kitten—a Golgi study. Brain Res. 74:119–130.

Stein, B. E., E. Labos, and L. Kruger (1973) Sequence of changes in properties of neurons of superior colliculus of the kitten during maturation. J. Neurophysiol. 36:667–679.

Stone, J. (1973) Sampling properties of microelectrodes assessed in the cat's retina. J. Neurophysiol. 36:1071–1080.

Tripp, L. N., and J. Wells (1978) Formation of new synaptic terminals in the somatosensory thalamus of the rat after lesions of the dorsal column nuclei. Brain Res. 155:362–367.

Van Exan, R. J., and M. H. Hardy (1980) A spatial relationship between innervation and the early differentiation of vibrissa follicles in the embryonic mouse. J. Anat. 131:643–656.

Verley, R., and I. Onnen (1981) Somatotopic organization of the tactile thalamus in normal adult and developing mice and in adult mice dewhiskered since birth. Exp. Neurol. 72:462–474.

Waite, P. M. E. (1973) The responses of cells in the rat thalamus to mechanical movements of the whiskers. J. Physiol. (Lond.) 228:541–561.

Waite, P. M. E. (1984) Rearrangement of neuronal responsese in the trigeminal system of the rat following peripheral nerve section. J. Physiol. (Lond.) 352:425–445.

Waite, P. M. E., and B. G. Cragg (1982) The peripheral and central changes resulting from cutting or crushing the afferent nerve supply to the whiskers. Proc. Roy. Soc. (Lond.) B 214:191–211.

Waite, P. M. E., and P. K. Taylor (1978) Removal of whiskers in young rats causes functional changes in cerebral cortex. Nature 274:600–602.

Wall, J. T., and C. G. Cusick (1984) Cutaneous responsiveness in primary somatosensory (S-I) hindpaw cortex before and after partial hindpaw deafferentation in adult rats. J. Neurosci. 4:1499–1515.

Wall, J. T., and C. G. Cusick (1986) The representation of peripheral nerve inputs in the S-I hindpaw cortex of rats raised with incompletely innervated hindpaws. J. Neurosci. 6:1129–1147.

Wall, P. D. (1977) The presence of ineffective synapses and the circumstances which unmask them. Phil. Trans. Roy. Soc. (Lond.) B 278:361–372.

Wall, P. D., M. Fitzgerald, J. C. Nussbaumer, H. Van der Loos, and M. Devor (1982) Somatotopic maps are disorganized in adult rodents treated with capsaicin as neonates. Nature 295:691–693.

Wells, J., and L. N. Tripp (1987) Time course of reactive synaptogenesis in the subcortical somatosensory system. J. Comp. Neurol. 255:466–475.

Welt, C. (1977) Physiological organization of the rat cortical barrel field following neonatal vibrissal damage. Soc. Neurosci. Abstr. 3:494.

Woolston, D. C., J. R. La Londe, and J. M. Gibson (1982) Comparison of response properties of cerebellar- and thalamic-projecting interpolaris neurons. J. Neurophysiol. 48:160–173.

Chapter Twelve

PERIPHERAL ALTERATION AND SOMATOSENSORY DEVELOPMENT

THOMAS A. WOOLSEY

Washington University School of Medicine
St. Louis, Missouri

I INTRODUCTION

It has long been known that deafferentation of the somatic periphery can alter brain structure. For instance, Campbell described cell loss in the postcentral gyrus of an individual with a longstanding limb amputation that he called "reaction á distance" (Campbell, 1905). Loss of appropriate nuclear mass in the dorsal column nuclei after experimental limb amputation of opossum pouch young was described in 1972 (Johnson et al., 1972). There is now a sizable literature on the effects of experimental and pathological alterations of the sensory periphery on the central somatosensory system. The purpose of this chapter is to summarize this information for rodents.

The study of "plastic" phenomena in the somatosensory system has lagged significantly behind that on other sensory modalities for a number of important reasons. The somatosensory periphery is anatomically and topologically complex and is highly integrated with the somatic motor system. While not a roadblock to studies of brain function (Mountcastle, 1964), the configuration of the somatosensory system is generally such that experimental manipulations are relatively difficult. For many years the central pathways subserving somatic sensation seemed less favorable in their anatomical arrangement than those for the other sensory modalities. The discovery of certain anatomical features of the rodent cerebral cortex and the functional association of the facial whiskers with them made it possible to undertake more detailed studies of the somatosensory system (Woolsey, 1967). In many respects the system is similar to that demonstrated earlier for the representation of the digits in the raccoon (Welker and Seidenstein, 1959), a demonstration that was critical to the mind set for interpreting the whisker brain–structure relationship (Woolsey and Van der Loos, 1970). When it was shown that manipulation of the peripheral sense organs could alter the brain, the "whisker–barrel" system became especially attractive for studies of neuromorphological and functional plasticity (Van der Loos and Woolsey, 1973).

The rodent trigeminal pathway is described in Chapter 10 (see Figure 1). The main features of this pathway are given here as a frame of reference for this chapter. Most mammals, including man, have specialized tactile organs on the face called sinus hairs because they are surrounded by erectile tissue that may be used to alter their sensitivity. In many species, especially rodents and carnivores, the larger sinus hairs are arranged in species-specific patterns of rows and columns (arcs). These are the whiskers. The behavioral importance of the whiskers as a sensory channel for some animals may be as great as vision is for primates and audition is for bats. Some animals actively move their whiskers in exploratory behaviors (whisking) (Welker, 1964); others do not (Woolsey et al., 1975b). Each whisker is supplied by a stout nerve that is in turn a peripheral branch of the infraorbital nerve (ION) of the maxillary division of the trigeminal nerve. The facial musculature is supplied by the facial nerve. The central processes of the trigeminal ganglion cells enter the pons through the trigeminal root and continue to the caudal brainstem as a relatively pure afferent axon bundle—the trigeminal tract. As the axons descend in the neuraxis, they give off collaterals to four nuclei in the brainstem trigeminal complex (BTC) (Hayashi, 1980), all of which receive anatomically segregated inputs from the whiskers (Bates and Killackey, 1985). The pattern of cell bodies in each nucleus except one is a faithful replica of the pattern of whiskers on the ipsilateral face (Ma and Woolsey, 1983, 1984). Terminals and cell bodies in the contralateral thalamus also replicate the peripheral whisker pattern (Van der Loos, 1976). Thalamic neurons project to the somatosensory cortex of the same side (Bernardo and Woolsey, 1987). In SmI, but not SmII, cortex the pattern of terminals and cell bodies is homeomorphic to the contralateral pattern of whiskers (Woolsey and Van der Loos, 1970; Killackey, 1973). Thus, in this system there is a discrete and regular pattern of behaviorally important peripheral receptors organs—the whiskers. These project to all of the relevant structures along the central somatosensory pathway in which the whisker pattern is faithfully replicated. At each level there is a module consisting of cell bodies, directed dendrites, and segregated afferent inputs called barrels, barreloids, and barrelettes in the cortex, the thalamus, and the brainstem, respectively (Woolsey, 1987). Each barrelette, barreloid, and barrel is mainly associated with a single whisker. At each level in the somatic pathway the modules are arranged in a pattern resembling the order of tactile organs on the face. It is possible to demonstrate the structure and, in some cases, the function of the entire somatosensory pathway by routine neuroanatomical methods within an individual animal (Figures 1 and 2).

The structural features of the whisker–barrel system make it possible to determine in some detail the normal properties of the relevant neurons and to accurately place them in an appropriate context (Lorente de Nó, 1922; Woolsey et al., 1975b; Steffen, 1976; White, 1976). The system is ideal for studies of normal development as patterns of neuronal organization emerge. In many species, the pathway is still undergoing active differentiation in the postnatal period, and the pathway is convenient for studying development of detailed somatotopy in the mammalian brain (Woolsey et al., 1981). The discovery that the development of the pathway can be altered by a number of manipulations in early life attracted considerable interest (Van der Loos and Woolsey, 1973; Weller and Johnson, 1975; Woolsey and Wann, 1976). The status of these studies is the focus of this chapter. In addition, the changes that can be produced in the pathway of adults will be touched on since they are of interest in themselves and have some bearing on the alterations produced in developing animals (e.g., Wong-Riley and Welt, 1980).

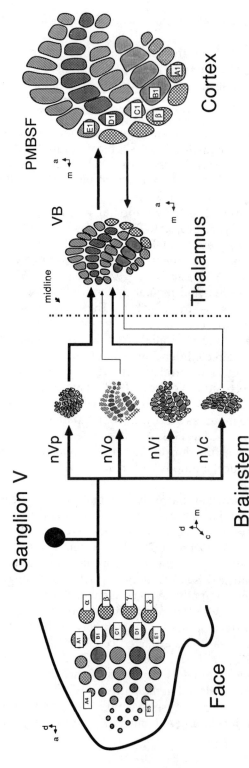

FIGURE 1. Diagram showing the principal components of the rodent trigeminal or whisker–barrel pathway. All parts are shown according to their relative size and orientation. Shading of the whiskers on the face (left) is carried through representations on the pathway to the somatosensory cortex on the right. The whiskers are arranged in five principal *rows* on the face that are labeled A–E in the dorsal to ventral and *arcs* labeled 1 to *n* in the posterior to anterior directions. (See compass at upper left where a = anterior and d = dorsal.) Four caudal whiskers "straddle" the rows and are labeled with the Greek letters alpha, beta, gamma, and delta. A cell in the trigeminal ganglion usually innervates only one whisker but projects to all four subdivisions of the brainstem trigeminal complex (BTC) where the whisker-related patches are called barrelettes. The full pattern illustrated is seen on transverse sections from rostral to caudal. (Compass indicates principal axes: d = dorsal, m = medial; c = caudal.) The whisker pattern is present in trigeminal afferents to all divisions but is not routinely stainable, as indicated by the absence of barrelette outlines in subnucleus oralis (nVo). Other components are the principal nucleus (nVp) and the two other subnuclei of the spinal nucleus of V, the subnucleus interpolaris (nVi) and the subnucleus caudalis (nVc). After injections of HRP in the contralateral thalamus, cells in all parts of the BTC are filled, most are in nVp, many are in nVi, and few are in the other nuclei. This is shown by the thickness of the arrows crossing the midline (in the medial lemniscus) to the ventrobasal complex (VB) of the thalamus. Because of their orientation, the barreloids for the whisker pattern can be seen in transverse and horizontal (see compass) sections through the thalamus. In cortex the barrels are seen in layer IV. The posteromedial barrel subfield (PMBSF) contains the representation of the principal whiskers. The corticothalamic projection is indicated, but many other interconnections of the system components illustrated are not shown.

464

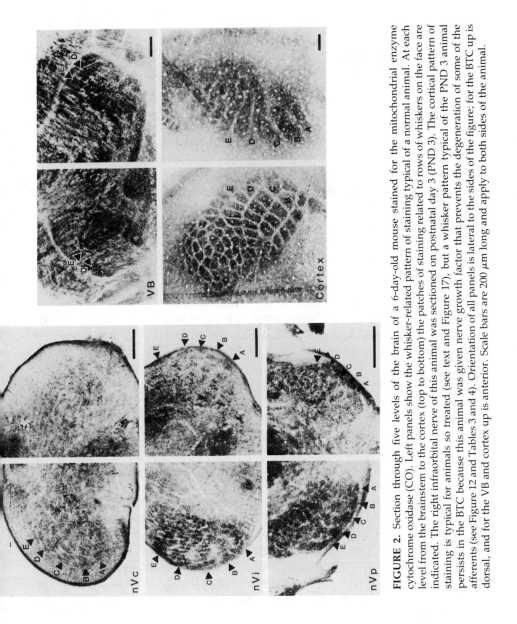

FIGURE 2. Section through five levels of the brain of a 6-day-old mouse stained for the mitochondrial enzyme cytochrome oxidase (CO). Left panels show the whisker-related pattern of staining typical of a normal animal. At each level from the brainstem to the cortex (top to bottom) the patches of staining related to rows of whiskers on the face are indicated. The right infraorbital nerve of this animal was sectioned on postnatal day 3 (PND 3). The cortical pattern of staining is typical for animals so treated (see text and Figure 17), but a whisker pattern typical of the PND 3 animal persists in the BTC because this animal was given nerve growth factor that prevents the degeneration of some of the afferents (see Figure 12 and Tables 3 and 4). Orientation of all panels is lateral to the sides of the figure; for the BTC up is dorsal, and for the VB and cortex up is anterior. Scale bars are 200 μm long and apply to both sides of the animal.

465

II METHODOLOGICAL ISSUES

There are many approaches to the study of the somatic pathways. The purpose here is to highlight some of these and to indicate the advantages each has to offer.

A Animals

The majority of the experimental work has been conducted on the myomorph rodents, principally the laboratory rat (*Rattus norvegicus*) (Belford and Killackey, 1980), the mouse (*Mus musculus*) (Durham and Woolsey, 1984), and to a lesser extent the hamster (*Cricetus cricetus*) (Rhoades et al., 1983). Some work has been done on pouch young of the brush-tailed possum (*Trichosurus vulpecula*) (Weller, 1972). The myomorphs are easily bred in the laboratory and typically have short gestations. Laboratory rodents come from highly inbred stock, reducing interindividual variability for comparisons with different experimental protocols. The supply of animals of known ages is practically limitless.

For mice there are numerous well-characterized genetic stocks that express abnormalities in whisker growth (Yamakado and Yohro, 1979), whisker number (Dun, 1959; Van der Loos et al., 1984), and arrangement of the central nervous system (Sidman et al., 1965; Steindler and Colwell, 1976). Methods to produce tetraperental mice resulting in chimeras offer a number of possibilities that are just beginning to be explored (Goldowitz, 1987). A substantial background on the development of the common laboratory rodents exists (Long and Burlingame, 1938; Woolsey, 1987).

B Lesions

The majority of studies have been based on the consequences of surgical manipulation of the rodent somatosensory system. Because the whiskers are discrete before birth (e.g., Dun and Fraser, 1958; Yamakado and Yohro, 1979; Andres and Van der Loos, 1983) and are arranged in a gridlike pattern, individual receptor organs can be selectively damaged. Originally, individual whisker follicles were destroyed by electrocautery (Van der Loos and Woolsey, 1973). Variations on this theme include excision of selected follicles (Jeanmonod et al., 1977) or the section of the individual follicle nerves (Weller and Johnson, 1975). For follicular damage a wide range of lesion patterns has been employed. These range from damage to one whisker (Van der Loos and Woolsey, 1973) to damage all whiskers except one (Kossut and Hand, 1984) to numerous combinations of lesions to different groups of vibrissae, usually in rows or arcs (see Figure 3; Valentino et al., 1978). A less selective approach is the destruction of the whisker pad without reference to particular individual whiskers (Waite and Cragg, 1979). The extent of the damage produced can be verified with gross anatomical dissection and histology of the whisker pad (Waite and Cragg, 1982; Durham and Woolsey,

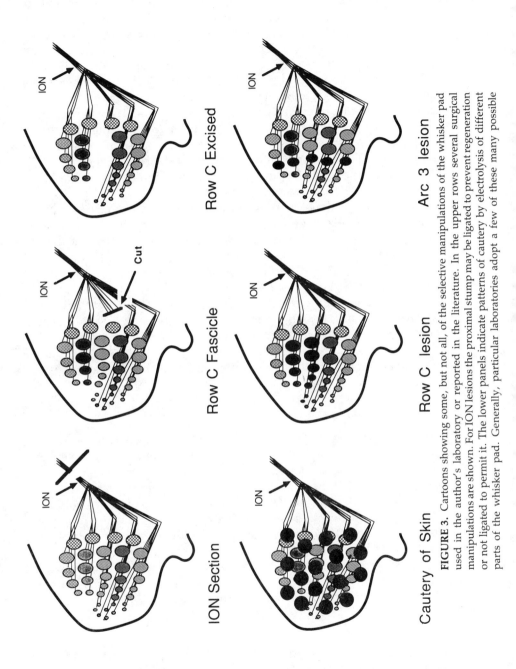

FIGURE 3. Cartoons showing some, but not all, of the selective manipulations of the whisker pad used in the author's laboratory or reported in the literature. In the upper rows several surgical manipulations are shown. For ION lesions the proximal stump may be ligated to prevent regeneration or not ligated to permit it. The lower panels indicate patterns of cautery by electrolysis of different parts of the whisker pad. Generally, particular laboratories adopt a few of these many possible

1984, 1985; Simons et al., 1984; Yip et al., 1987; see Figure 6). One advantage of the rat over the mouse is that the whisker pad is about four times larger (Simons et al., 1984). The ION can be approached directly either at the infraorbital foramen (Yip et al., 1987) or in the floor of the orbit (Jacquin and Ziegler, 1983). If it is transected, the central stump can be ligated (Yip et al., 1987) or left free (Jacquin and Ziegler, 1983) depending on whether or not regeneration of the peripheral fibers is intended.

Destruction of the trigeminal ganglion or the trigeminal root has not been employed in this context. Various parts of the central trigeminal pathway can be surgically or chemically interrupted. The consequences of such lesions to the BTC (Erzurumlu and Killackey, 1980; Erzurumlu et al., 1980), ventrobasal complex (VB) (Wise and Jones, 1978), and cortex (Ito and Seo, 1983; Seo and Ito, 1987) have been reported.

A number studies have employed exogenous agents to disrupt the developing somatosensory system. These include X-irradiation to destroy whiskers or neurons *in utero* (Ito et al., 1981), toxins to eliminate certain neural systems selectively [e.g., capsaisin (Wall et al., 1982) and 6-OH dopamine (Loeb et al., 1987)] or to generally disrupt brain development (Fischer et al., 1972; Wise and Jones, 1978), and local anesthetics and the sodium channel blocker tetrodotoxin (TTX) to alter activity in the pathway (e.g., Jacquin et al., 1984c). Concentrations of naturally occurring substances such as nerve growth factor (NGF) have been changed to alter the system (Hulsebosch and Coggeshall, 1983; Yip et al., 1984; Sikich et al., 1986). Dietary deprivation of the young and their mothers changes the development of the somatic system (Vongdokmai, 1980).

C   Sensory Manipulation

By analogy to studies of the visual system, a "sensory deprivation" can be produced by chronic removal of all or selected whiskers. The whiskers will grow back over a short period of time and the "deprivation" reversed (Dietrich et al., 1982). Section of the facial nerve eliminates the rhythmic motor pattern of the whiskers (called whisking) typical of some species but does not prevent the other aspects of exploratory behavior from being expressed (Welker, 1964). Means have been devised that have the potential for selective and controlled stimulation of the whiskers for extended periods of time (Melzer et al., 1985). Environmental "enrichment" is another potential means by which the somatosensory system could be altered (Diamond et al., 1972; Gustafson and Felbain-Keramidas, 1977).

D   Age Variables

Each species has a consistent developmental time table commencing with conception and punctuated by birth, early postnatal events, sexual maturity, senescence, and death. In the laboratory, the time of impregnation can be determined within minutes and is probably a better index of the developmental progress in an individual than the time of birth (Rice, 1975), but external morphological markers can be used for staging (Long and Burlingame, 1938).

As there are larger numbers of experimental schedules that can be followed, many laboratories have chosen a particular schedule that is standard for that laboratory. For instance, lesions are made at birth; the animals are studied at 60 days of age (Rhoades et al., 1987b). This schedule differs from that employed in other laboratories (Woolsey and Wann, 1976). A particular schedule applied to two species may not be equivalent in terms of the relative development at the time of manipulation or at the time of examination (Renehan and Rhoades, 1984).

E   Morphological Methods

Most of the available morphological methods have been used to characterize the system, and many have been used to examine the consequences of experimentally produced alterations of the system (Cooper and Steindler, 1986) (see Figure 4). For mice cell bodies are well segregated at every station in the pathway and Nissl dyes are used routinely (Woolsey and Van der Loos, 1970; Van der Loos, 1976). The cell groupings are key landmarks for the electron microscope. Stains for the mitochondrial enzymes succinic dehydrogenase (SDH) and cytochrome oxidase (CO) give excellent definition of whisker-related organization at all levels of the central somatic pathway (Friede, 1959; Woolsey, 1967; Wong-Riley and Welt, 1980; Ma and Woolsey, 1984; Yip et al., 1987). Particular advantages of the CO method are that it is compatible with a number of stains (McCasland and Woolsey, 1988a) and it is convenient for electron microscopy (Carroll and Wong-Riley, 1984; Woolsey, 1987). There are several caveats in the use of the mitochondrial stains as markers. First, the intensity of the mitochondrial stains depends on the activity of the system being studied, and for some of the manipulations described in the preceding the stain may not provide the necessary signal (Wong-Riley and Welt, 1980). Second, although the pattern of the stain resembles and apparently reflects the organization of afferent terminals in a region of the brain (Killackey and Belford, 1979), the majority of heavily stained mitochondria are located in postsynaptic elements (Wong-Riley and Welt, 1980; Ma and Woolsey, unpublished data). For instance, in nVp over 50% of highly reactive mitochondria are postsynaptic profiles; only 15% of all mitochondria are in presynaptic profiles.

Anterograde (Killackey, 1973) and retrograde (Grünthal, 1945; Woolsey, 1978a) degeneration methods for tracing axonal connections have been largely supplanted by techniques based on axonal transport, especially autoradiography (ARG) (Cowan et al., 1972), horseradish peroxidase (HRP) (Land and Simons, 1985a), and fluorescent tracers. Fibers have been filled by bulk injections of HRP or intra-axonal injections at various levels in the system (Bates and Killackey, 1985; Ma, 1985; Bernardo and Woolsey, 1987;

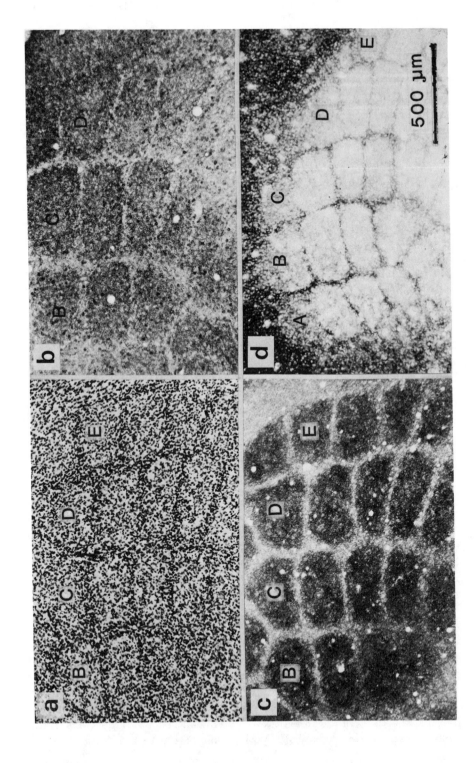

Jensen and Killackey, 1987a,b). Individual neurons at all levels in the pathway have been filled with dyes (Hayashi, 1980; Woolsey and Dierker, 1981; Jacquin et al., 1984b; Harris, 1986), but most of the work on neuronal form has been with the classical methods of Golgi (see Figure 9) (Lorente de Nó, 1922; Åstrom, 1953; Woolsey et al., 1975a; Steffen and Van der Loos, 1980; Ma, 1986). Both can be counterstained so that the architectural context can be determined.

Stains for antigens (see Figure 4) (Kristt and Silverman, 1980; Lin et al., 1985), enzymes (Kristt, 1979; Wallace, 1983; Robertson, 1987), and cell surface markers (Cooper and Steindler, 1986) show a remarkable regional definition for the whisker pathway in normal and developing animals. Some have already proven useful in evaluating sensory alterations. Regional changes in receptor densities (D'Amato et al., 1987), uptake for known or putative transmitters (Søreide and Fonnum, 1980), and concentrations in various nucleotide species (Sutcliffe et al., 1984) are all technically feasible.

F Electrophysiology

Most parts of the somatosensory pathway have been studied with extracellular electrodes. Information can be correlated directly to underlying anatomy with appropriate marking methods (e.g., Welker, 1976; Simons, 1978). Three major kinds of information are obtained. First, the map of the sensory periphery can be determined (Woolsey, 1967; Simons and Woolsey, 1979). Second the receptive field characteristics of individual neurons can be studied (Simons, 1978; Ito, 1981, 1985; Armstrong-James and Fox, 1987). Third, the integrative properties of neurons can be examined (Simons, 1985). Intracellular recording with subsequent intracellular staining with dye (Woolsey and Dierker, 1981; Jacquin et al., 1984a; Harris, 1986) gives precise localization of the recording site and direct information about the morphological characteristics of the functionally characterized neuron.

FIGURE 4. Tangential sections through the somatosensory cortex of the mouse to show four different ways of staining the cortex that demonstrate the whisker–barrels clearly. All sections were cut parallel to the pial surface at 50 μm. All panels are at about the same magnification and in the same orientation with medial up and anterior to the right. (a) Pattern of cell somata as seen with a Nissl dye. The cell rings outline barrels each associated with a contralateral whisker. (b) Pattern of the barrels evident in a subset of presumably inhibitory cortical neurons that stain for the enzyme glutamic acid decarboxylase (GAD). (c) Stain for the mitochondrial enzyme succinic dehydrogenase (SDH). This pattern resembles that of the specific thalamocortical afferents that terminate in the barrel centers. The stain also identifies mitochondria in postsynaptic elements. (d) HRP-tagged peanut agglutinin stains the boundaries between the barrels transiently and is thought to be related to glia. Many of these and numerous other methods can be combined directly in the same section or adjacent sections from the same specimen. The stereotypical pattern of the barrels makes accurate indirect correlations from different preparations easy.

The whisker system permits precisely delivered somatic stimuli with controlled spatial and temporal characteristics (Zucker and Welker, 1969). It has been shown recently that the system is advantageous for studies conducted with the voltage-sensitive dyes introduced by Cohen and colleagues (Orbach et al., 1985). The spatial resolution of this method resembles surface macroelectrode recordings (Woolsey, 1967).

G   Metabolic Markers

The histochemical methods for mitochondrial enzymes mentioned preceding section are also good indicators of long-term changes in regional activity (Wong-Riley and Welt, 1980; Wong-Riley and Riley, 1983; Yip et al., 1987). The same applies to other enzymes that can be demonstrated histochemically or immunocytochemically (e.g., Wallace, 1983). Another approach is to study selected brain regions using microchemical techniques for analysis of small pieces of brain tissue. In sectioned fresh and fixed tissues the relevant structures can be identified without staining under the appropriate illumination (Dietrich et al., 1981; Yip et al., 1987).

Shorter term metabolic events that bridge the gap between days and milliseconds can be followed with the 2-deoxyglucose (2-DG) method as originally described by Sokoloff and colleagues (Sokoloff et al., 1977) and subsequently modified by a number of workers (Durham et al., 1981; McCasland and Woolsey, 1988a). The 2-DG method has been shown to label appropriate parts of the somatosensory system in response to natural (Durham and Woolsey, 1977, 1978) and evoked (Hand, 1981; Melzer et al., 1985) whisker stimulation (see Figure 14). Histology of reasonable quality indicates that the active regions of brain are appropriate to the whiskers stimulated. The resolution of the method and the quality of the underlying histology are improved with systemic fixation (Durham et al., 1981; McCasland and Woolsey, 1988a). Better resolution provides localization of the active elements down to the subcellular level. Since it has been shown that local glucose uptake and utilization is dependent on neuronal activity and may be directly correlated with neuronal firing rates (Kadekaro et al., 1985), the method provides a way to assess active populations of neurons more completely and with greater spatial resolution than is possible with microelectrodes (Durham and Woolsey, 1985).

III   EFFECTS OF VIBRISSA DAMAGE

A   Ganglion Cells

Primary afferent neurons connecting the vibrissae to the brain are trigeminal (Gasserian) ganglion cells. The cell bodies are located in the maxillary—more medial—portion of the ganglion (Zucker and Welker, 1969). Although there is a general topography of these cells, those innervating the ventral vibrissae are lateral to those innervating dorsal vibrissae; there is no strict vibrissa-related order in the ganglion cell bodies (Klein et al., 1986). Recordings from the vibrissa-related ganglion cells in adult rats consistently show that each is activated by one and only one vibrissa (Zucker and Welker, 1969; Rhoades et al., 1983; Simons, 1983). The distal processes of a single afferent have not been individually reconstructed, but the functional data suggest that if they do branch, they do so in relation to a single vibrissa. Central axons of individually labeled vibrissa ganglion cells have been filled and are distributed to all divisions of the BTC (Hayashi, 1980; Jacquin et al., 1984b). The peripheral receptor specializations associated with each vibrissa and the pattern of innervation are known (Andres, 1966; Munger and Rice, 1986; Rice and Munger, 1986). The major innervation is by a single fascicle of fibers from the infraorbital nerve (Dörfl, 1985). This fascicle supplies only one vibrissa; the number of nerve fibers to a particular vibrissa varies little (Lee and Woolsey, 1975; Welker, 1985; Welker and Van der Loos, 1986). Other nerve fibers supplying the skin around a whisker and between whiskers have a more complicated geometry; some are likely related to more than one whisker (Rice et al., 1986).

The ganglion cells are generated early in development, slightly before the whisker primordia can be recognized (Forbes and Welt, 1981). The peripheral and central processes of these cells are in the periphery and in the central nervous system shortly thereafter (Erzurumlu and Killackey, 1982). About 55% of the ganglion cells undergo physiological cell death in the last third of gestation (Davies and Lumsden, 1984). A putative growth factor other than NGF is required for the initial outgrowth of the trigeminal ganglion cells to the whiskers (Lumsden and Davies, 1983); the ganglion cells require NGF to survive during the balance of gestation (Pearson et al., 1983; Davies and Lumsden, 1984). Counts of axons near the ganglion show a one-to-one relationship between them and the number of ganglion cells (Davies and Lumsden, 1984). Counts of axons at the infraorbital foramen show more axons in neonates than in adults and suggest that in development individual fibers branch between the ganglion and the infraorbital foramen (Jacquin et al., 1984a; Renehan and Rhoades, 1984). The branches are apparently not widespread. Double-labeling experiments where one dye is injected into the row E vibrissae and another is injected into the row B vibrissae fail to produce double-labeled cells (Klein et al., 1986). As the animal matures, 20% of these branches are lost. Direct observations on developing infraorbital nerve indicate that individual axons follow independent courses to the periphery (Davies and Lumsden, 1986) and that the consistent fasciculation of the peripheral nerve fibers is not a requirement for appropriate axon targeting (Erzurumlu and Killackey, 1982).

In rats, axons continue to grow into the whiskers and the skin during the first 3 weeks after birth (Munger and Rice, 1986). In the postnatal period both the peripheral and central processes of the ganglion cells increase in diameter and myelinate. In rats, myelination nears completion at the end of the third week after birth (Waite and Cragg, 1979). The ION is silent before spontaneous activity is been recorded in the ION on the second postnatal day (PND 2) (Verley and Axelrad, 1977). Activity correlated with whisker stimulation appears shortly thereafter. Conduction velocity increases have a similar time course to that of nerve myelination. Axons and terminals from primary afferents are in the brainstem at birth (Ma, 1985). These fibers continue to develop over the first 2 weeks of life principally by elaborating their terminals (see Figure 8) (Woolsey, 1987). Based on their spatial location and morphology the terminals associated with each whisker become increasingly elaborate as do the synapses associated with them (unpublished data). Thus, although some of the ganglion cells are connected to the periphery and the central nervous system in early life, increases in peripheral and central myelination, conduction velocity, peripheral axon number, and elaboration of distal and central processes of trigeminal axons continue well after birth.

Section of the infraorbital nerve in adult rats leads to a loss of about 14% of the trigeminal ganglion cells. It is estimated that 30% of ganglion cells with axons in the ION die (Grant and Arvidsson, 1975; Aldskogius et al., 1978). The axons to the vibrissae and the surrounding tissue degenerate within a week after ION section or crush (Renehan and Munger, 1986). Three months after the lesions the whiskers are reinnervated. The pattern of the innervation to individual whiskers after nerve crush appears qualitatively normal while that after nerve section is aberrant. Central degeneration after such a lesion is sparse and is greatest in the laminar portion of the nVc (Gobel and Dubner, 1969). There is no significant central degeneration in the whisker-related parts of the BTC; the available evidence favors the loss of smaller axons as reported for similar experiments on the spinal roots (Tessler et al., 1985).

In contrast to the ganglion cell loss observed with infraorbital nerve lesions in the adult, section of this nerve or damage to all of the individual whiskers and their nerves on the first day of life leads to gross changes in the ganglion (see Figure 5) (Ma, 1985; Jacquin et al., 1986a). The ganglion loses about 35% of its volume (Savy et al., 1981). Counts of ganglion cells show a loss of up to 50% (see Table 1; Savy et al., 1981; Ma, 1985). Based on estimates of the number of ganglion cells with axons in the infraorbital nerve, the neuronal death that follows axotomy probably exceeds 90%. Detailed data are not available on the age dependency of axotomy-produced ganglion cell death between birth and adulthood. From data derived in other parts of the system it may be surmised that many neurons become resistant to lesion-provoked death at about the time the fibers are completely myelinated (Waite and Cragg, 1982). After neonatal infraorbital nerve section about 85% of the myelinated axons are lost when examined in adults (Waite and Cragg, 1982). With nerve crush about twice as many fibers survive, but 70% of the myelinated fibers are gone. Nerve section leads to fiber degeneration in the trigeminal root and the tract of the fifth

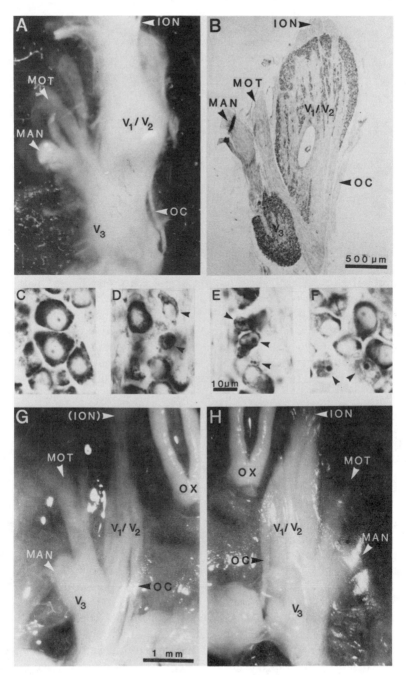

FIGURE 5. The trigeminal ganglion *in situ* and in sections. (*A*) Left ganglion and its branches at birth (in all panels anterior is up). ION, infraorbital nerve; MOT, motor root of V; MAN, mandibular branch of V; OC, IIIrd nerve; OX, optic chiasm; V_1/V_2 = first two divisions of V; V_3 = third division of V. (*B*) Nissl-stained left ganglion showing the ganglion cells intermingled with afferent fibers at birth. (*C*) Normal ganglion cells in a PND 2 animal. (*D–F*) Ganglion cells undergoing degeneration (arrowheads) on PND 2 after an ION lesion on PND 1. (*G*) Left ganglion is shrunken and ION atrophied 30 days after the ION was sectioned on PND 1 as compared to the normal side shown in (*H*).

TABLE 1. Trigeminal Ganglion Cells after PND 1
ION Lesions with and without Exogenous NGF

Age at Sacrifice	Untreated[a]	With NGF (%)
PND 2	73*	85*
PND 5	54**	78
PND 25	54***	63***

[a] Expressed as percentage of unoperated PND 25 ganglion cell counts.

Significance levels: (*) $p \leq 0.05$; (**) $p \leq 0.01$; (***) $p \leq 0.005$.

nerve. Estimates of the magnitude of this loss are similar to that found in the infraorbital nerve. Direct examination of the whisker follicles themselves shows twice as many fibers supplying them as would be expected from the counts in the infraorbital nerves (Waite and Cragg, 1982). Either the distal branches of the ganglion cells that are normally eliminated survive or the surviving axons have sprouted to innervate the deafferented whiskers as they do in adult animals after similar manipulations. Data suggest that surviving cells have peripheral processes in other divisions of the trigeminal nerve (Rhoades et al., 1987b). For instance, one dye injected into the stump of a neonatally transected ION and another in peripheral fields of the other trigeminal branches yielded substantial numbers of doubly labeled neurons in comparison to very few when the same experiment is conducted on an adult. This finding is consistent with receptive fields of central trigeminal axons found in similarly treated animals (Jacquin et al., 1986b).

After ION lesions in neonatal rats and mice the patterns associated with the central terminals of the ganglion cells in three of the trigeminal nuclei disappear (Durham and Woolsey, 1984; Ma, 1985). If the remaining branches of the trigeminal nerve are labeled, their terminal fields are not spread to the denervated territory of the BTC (Jacquin and Rhoades, 1987). Since the target nuclei shrink by about a third in volume, the labeled terminals could appear to encroach on the whisker region of the target nuclei in the BTC. After neonatal ION section, the effected nuclei can be activated by whiskers after all the whiskers become partially reinnervated, although the cross-sectional area of the BTC is very much diminished. The somatotopic pattern is abnormal in that single-unit activity is related to more whiskers than normal and the area for this activity is constricted (Waite and Cragg, 1982). (See what follows also.) In hamsters, which are less fully developed at birth than the mouse or rat, the central processes of the remaining divisions of the trigeminal nerve occupy ION territory after ION section (Jacquin and Rhoades, 1985). A similar experiment on this species at an age that is roughly equivalent to the newborn rat or mouse produces an effect that is similar to the patterns seen in those animals after they are lesioned at birth (Jacquin and Rhoades, 1987). Clearly, from these experiments the alterations that result in the distribution of the central axons of the trigeminal ganglion cells are time dependent.

Considerably less detail is available on the effects of selection disruption of territory *within* the innervation field of the ION. Lesions to individual vibrissae or groups of vibrissae should lead to the death of 10% or less of the ganglion cells, and in the absence of appropriate markers, anatomical changes of this magnitude are hard to detect. Lesions of individual whiskers lead to complete loss of the appropriate whiskers and the innervation to the skin in the lesioned area (see Figure 6: Durham and Woolsey, 1984, 1985).

After lesions of selected whiskers focal gliosis is present in the tract of the Vth nerve generally adjacent to the appropriate target regions of the BTC (see Figure 10; Ma and Woolsey, 1984). If axons of the ION are filled with HRP after whisker row lesions, then the terminals of these axons are missing in the appropriate areas of the brainstem (Bates and Killackey, 1985). After coagulation or cautery of all of the vibrissae at birth, only a modest reduction in the numbers of round vesicle-containing terminals (which include the terminals of primary afferents) has been reported in nVi (Hámori et al., 1986) (see what follows).

For the trigeminal gangion cells and their peripheral and central processes the consequences of surgical lesions to the branches of the trigeminal nerve and to the whiskers have been the most intensively studied. However, other surgical manipulations have been employed, particularly with reference to more central parts of the pathway. Nonetheless, some data are available on the effects of these manipulations on the primary afferents. For instance, after the whisker pad has been rotated *in utero*, the periphery is innervated (Andres and van der Loos, 1985a). Transplants of skin from other body surfaces to the faces have been successful, although a pattern of innervation to them has not been documented.

Different genetic strains of mice are known in which the number of whiskers is either decreased or increased (Dun and Fraser, 1958; Van der Loos et al., 1984). The extent of the peripheral innervation in the latter has been documented and is consistent with the pattern of innervation in normal animals (Welker, 1985). Whether the increased peripheral load of the additional vibrissae reduces Gasserian ganglion cell death is unknown. Irradiation on the twelfth day of gestation can prevent the development of the whiskers (Jacobson, 1966), and this technique could be employed to study the central development of the pathway if damage to the nervous system could be avoided (Ito et al., 1981).

Administration of the active agent in red peppers, capsaisin, either topically or systemically leads to degeneration of the central terminals of substance P containing trigeminal ganglion cells (Wall et al., 1982). The loss of fluoride-resistant acid phosphatase stain in the laminar part of nVc has also been documented after ION section, but the effects on the ganglion cells

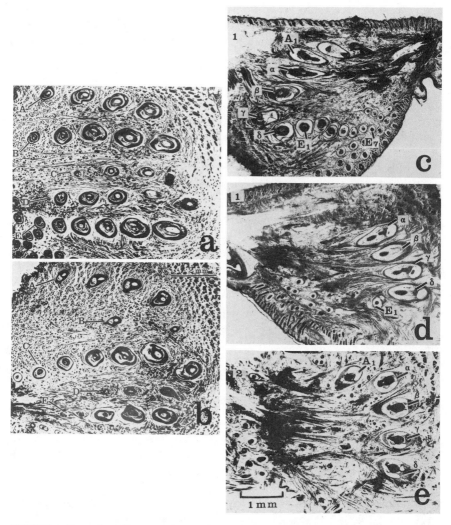

FIGURE 6. Examples of hematoxylin- and eosin-stained sections of the face to demonstrate the pattern of the sensory periphery in adults after lesions in the neonatal period. (*a,b*) Photomicrograph from rats (anterior, left; dorsal, up). (*a*) Row C whiskers were cauterized and are attentuated; (*b*) rows B and D were cauterized. These lesions were made on PND 1. (*c–e*) Sections from the faces of mice where most of the whiskers were cauterized on different postnatal days. Orientation of panels *d* and *e* are as in *a* and *b*; for panel *c* the nose is to the right. The spatial and some quantitative effects of the lesions can be directly assessed from these sections.

and their peripheral processes are not known. One interpretation of the results from central recordings is that ganglion cells innervate more than one whisker. For spinal ganglia, exogenous NGF prevents the capsaisin-produced degeneration of the primary afferents (Csillik et al., 1985).

Nerve growth factor is necessary to maintain trigeminal ganglion cells in later gestation (Davies and Lumsden, 1984). Therefore, it is of interest to examine the effects of altering concentrations of this molecule on the development of the first-order trigeminal neurons. Some guinea pigs develop high antibody titers to murine NGF, which cross-react with guinea pig NGF. These antibodies cross the placenta, depriving the fetus of this growth factor (Johnson et al., 1982). Offspring have severe clinical defects, similar to patients with familial dysautonomia (Riley and Moore, 1966). Nerve growth factor deprivation profoundly effects the cranial ganglia, especially the trigeminal ganglion (Pearson et al., 1983). Such animals, which have fewer than 20% of the normal compliment of ganglion cells, have diminished tactile abilities in neurological examination (Sikich et al., 1986). The number of nerve fibers in the infraorbital nerve and to selected vibrissae is reduced by 50%, which is consistent with a persistance of fetal peripheral branches of the ganglion cells. In spite of this defect, the central axonal patterns in the brainstem as determined by indirect methods seem appropriate in their spatial organization and areal extent.

In contrast, exogenous NGF can retard the profound degeneration of spinal ganglia in newborn rats observed after peripheral nerve section (Yip et al., 1984). If exogenous NGF is given in conjunction with section of the infraorbital nerve in the early postnatal period in mice, it prevents the degeneration of about 50% of the ganglion cells (see Table 1; Ma, 1985). The central processes of these cells are preserved and the thickness of the trigeminal tract is greater with NGF than in lesioned controls (unpublished results). Fewer axons in the tract degenerate with NGF treatment, and their central endings in the brainstem persist (Tables 2 and 3; Figures 2 and 12) for the duration of exogenous NGF treatment. The central axons of the axotomized ganglion cells are myelinated as normally occurs in the time frame between when the nerve is cut and when the animals are sacrificed (unpublished results). There is evidence from studies of spinal ganglia that if the NGF is administered through sexual maturity, then a substantial proportion of the sectioned ganglion cells and presumably their processes—peripheral and central—survive (Yip et al., 1984). This experiment has not been done on the trigeminal system.

TABLE 2. Relative Density of Myelinated Axons in Trigeminal Tract After ION Lesions

Day of Lesion	Lesioned/Control (%)	Degenerating Axons on Lesioned Side (%)
PND 1	64	17
PND 1 + NGF	85	24
PND 3	90	49
PND 3 + NGF	100	10

TABLE 3. Relative Density[a] of Primary
Afferent-Type Terminals in nVp after Lesions of
ION with and without Exogenous NGF

Day of Lesion	Without NGF (%)	With NGF (%)
PND 1	50	70
PND 3	15	32

[a] Animals from timed births; NGF was given subcutaneously at 10 μg/g daily. All animals were sacrificed on PND 6 and were perfused with buffered aldehydes. Vibratome sections through nVp were osmicated, embedded, and thin sectioned. Overlapping photographs covering each nucleus were taken of single sections from formar-coated slotted grids. The number of synapses counted per unit area (measured with a data tablet) is expressed as lesioned/control $\times$ 100.

B Brainstem Neurons

The rodent BTC extends from the rostral pons to the upper cervical segments of the spinal cord. Its position is just under the trigeminal tract, being ventrolateral in the pons and dorsolateral at the closed medulla. In horizontal sections the BTC is easily divided into four nuclei on cytoarchitectonic, histochemoarchitectonic, and myeloarchitectonic bases (Bates and Killackey, 1985; Ma, 1985; see Figures 1 and 2). The principal nucleus (nVp) is rostral, and the spinal nucleus just behind it is divisible into three subnuclei: oralis (nVo), interpolaris (nVi), and caudalis (nVc) from front to back. Neurons in nVp and nVc are smaller than those in nVi, which are smaller than those in nVo. Because of the anatomical layout of the BTC, various authors have chosen to study a particular (sub) nucleus, fully aware that there are differences in structure, connections, and function (e.g., Hámori et al., 1986; Jacquin et al., 1986a). Within each of these subnuclei the trigeminal afferents are somatotopically organized (Hayashi, 1980; Jacquin et al., 1984b; Bates and Killackey, 1985). In particular, there are clusters of fiber terminals associated with each of the vibrissae, which for a given nucleus run as tubes in the rostral caudal direction. The full arrangement can be visualized in transverse sections taken at the appropriate rostral caudal level for any nucleus.

Patterns of afferent terminals and cell bodies related to the whiskers can be demonstrated in all nuclei, except nVo, using Nissl stains and/or histochemical methods for mitochondria. In each nucleus, cell and terminal groupings correspond in a one-to-one fashion with each vibrissa; the organization of the brainstem is homeomorphic to the organization of the receptor periphery. Tracing techniques (Arvidsson, 1982; Jacquin et al., 1983), recording (Waite, 1984), and 2-DG metabolic mapping (Durham et al., 1981;

Melzer et al., 1985) confirm the correspondence between each unit called variously sausage (Belford and Killackey, 1979b), brick (Basbaum and Hand, 1973), or barrelette (Ma, 1985) and the appropriate whisker. In each nucleus the dorsal row of whiskers is represented more ventrally while the ventral row of whiskers is more dorsal. That is, the central representation of the face in the brainstem is inverted. For all nuclei except nVc the caudal whiskers are represented nearer the surface of the brain than the rostral ones. Curiously, in nVc the arrangement is reversed (Arvidsson, 1982; Jacquin et al., 1983). In Golgi preparations the dendrites of many but not all of the neurons in nVp, nVi, and nVc are spatially oriented toward the afferent clusters from the vibrissae (Table 4) (Ma, 1985). Those cells in nVp but not those in nVi (Rhoades et al., 1987a) project to the somatosensory thalamus. The cells of the barrelettes in nVp can be used as whisker-specific markers in thin sections (Figure 7).

In development, the cells of the BTC are the first of the whole whisker system to leave the mitotic cycle; they are born on E-9 to E-11 in mice (Taber Pierce, 1973; Nornes and Morita, 1979). Gradients of neuronogenesis generally resemble those found in the spinal cord (Woolsey et al., 1981). In rats, the histochemical stains show whisker-related groupings at birth (Belford and Killackey, 1979a); they appear in mice on PND 2 (Ma, 1985). In mice the whisker-related cell groupings appear on PND 3 (Ma, 1985) (see Figure 8). In the course of the next 2 weeks the patterns seen with the mitochondrial and cell body stains become more sharply defined. The volume and cross-sectional area of all nuclei at birth is about 30% of that in the adult (Ma, 1985). Throughout the first 3 weeks of life, afferent fibers become increas-

TABLE 4. Golgi-Stained Neurons in Mouse BTC[a]

	Small Neurons (Dendrites Confined to a Barrelette) (%)	Intermediate Neurons (Dendrites Cross Barrelette Boundaries) (%)	Large Neurons (Dendrites Cross Main Boundaries of Nucleus) (%)
Principal sensory Nucleus of V (N = 796)	83	7	10
Subnucleus interpolaris (N = 394)	89	9	2
Subnucleus caudalis (N = 307)	78	10	12

[a] Relative frequency of main neuron types in three divisions of the mouse BTC. Golgi-stained neurons were located in relation to Nissl-stained barrelettes in transverse sections.

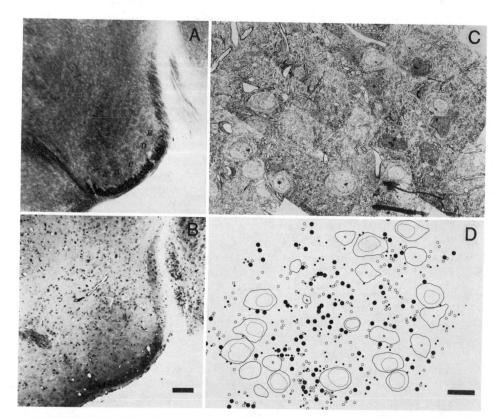

FIGURE 7. Series of panels to show the approach for detailed fine structural analysis in the whisker pathway. (*A*) Vibratome, cut osmicated section through nVp of a PND 6 mouse. Barrelettes are obvious, as is the trigeminal tract on the brain surface to the lower right of the panel. (*B*) Semithin section of the section in (*A*) stained with toluidine blue. Vessels and other markers can be used to find barrelettes in the EM (electron microscope). Scale bar is 100 μm long; panel (*A*) at same magnification. (*C*) Montage from a thin section through an adult nVp showing a barrelette at low tap. (*D*) From the montage various elements were identified and drawn. Neurons have drawn nuclei; glia are marked with upsidedown G's. The large filled dots indicate asymmetrial contacts from primary afferents; smaller circles indicate asymmetrical contacts from other sources; open circles are symmetrical contacts. All are localizable in a precise anatomical context. Scale bar of 100 μm applies to panels (*C*) and (*D*).

ingly complex as do their synapses. The dendrites of the target cells grow longer and are more branched (see Figure 9; Ma, 1986).

In mice and rats, lesions to the infraorbital nerve or selected groups of vibrissae on PND 1 lead to prompt and spatially appropriate degeneration of the primary afferents in all three somatotopically arranged nuclei. The mitochondrial stains pale and the cell bodies fail to organize as barrelettes (see Figures 10 and 11; Ma, 1986). This sequence occurs up to PND 10–15 (Ma and Woolsey, 1984). Thereafter, the same lesions produce paling of the

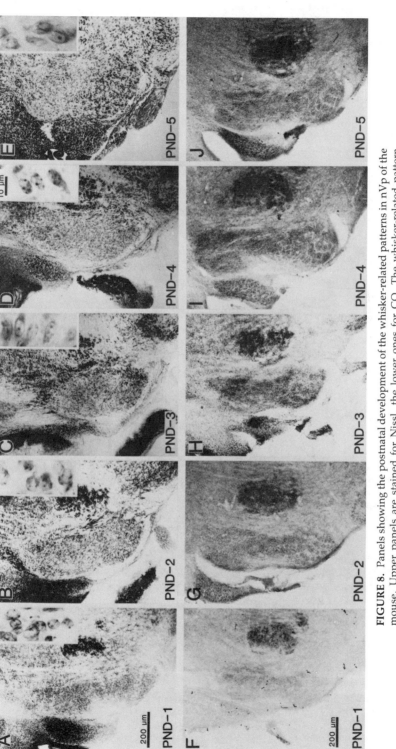

FIGURE 8. Panels showing the postnatal development of the whisker-related patterns in nVp of the mouse. Upper panels are stained for Nissl, the lower ones for CO. The whisker-related pattern appears in the first week of life. At this and all other loci in the system the CO pattern appears before the Nissl staining shows it. The panels for later days show better definition of the whisker pattern associated with the increased size of the representations, their staining density, and the differentiation of the neurons (see insets in upper panels).

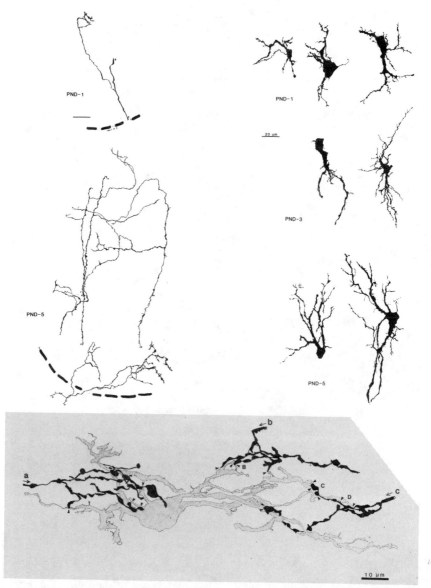

FIGURE 9. Examples of development of neural elements associated with the pattern differentiation seen in the brainstem with the Golgi–Cox method. At the upper left, the afferents from the trigeminal ganglion to the BTC become longer and more elaborate from PND 1 to PND 5. The fibers enter the BTC from the tract of V below the dashed lines. These afferents continue to elaborate for at least another week in postnatal life; bar 20 μm. At the same time target neurons in the brainstem are elaborating their dendritic processes as shown for the large cells at the upper right. Growth and differentiation of the afferents and their targets both contribute to the refinement of the whisker-related patterns in the brainstem. At the bottom, a neuron in nVp presumed to project to VB from a young adult receives numerous contacts from three afferent terminal branches (a–c) at points along its dendrites (arrows and B–D). This cell drawn from a longitudinal section to capture most of its dendrites. These contacts make complex synapses that in the EM resemble mossy fiber contacts in the cerebellum.

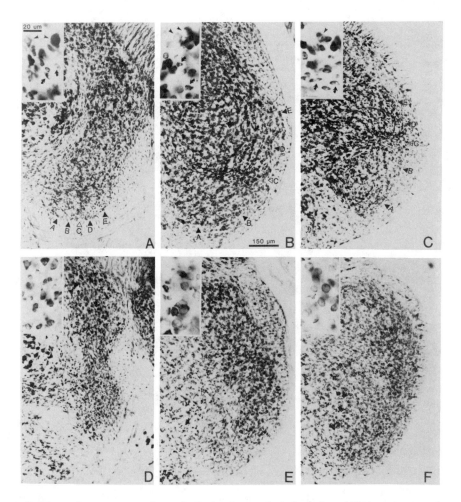

FIGURE 10. Consequences of row C whisker lesions [panels *A–C*) and ION section (panels *D–F*) on the architecture of the BTC. Lesions were made on PND 1 (but similar results are seen for lesions made throughout the first days of life) and the animals sacrificed as young adults. All transverse sections stained from Nissl; insets show shrunken cells related to the deafferented parts of the nuclei (A, D through right nVp; B, D through nVi; C, F through nVc). In all locales the part of the nucleus associated with the missing afferents collapses and the cells are shrunken but many do not degenerate. Other preparations show that these cells where appropriate still project to the thalamus. Compare with Figure 11.

mitochondrial stains, which can recover in several months, and the whisker-related cytoarchitecture persists in all parts of the BTC although the target neurons appear shrunken (Yip et al., 1987). After the later lesions there is a transient rise in the number of glial cells. In young animals the glial response is very rapid and can be missed, as can degenerating neuronal elements. The cell bodies in the BTC associated with the damaged whiskers

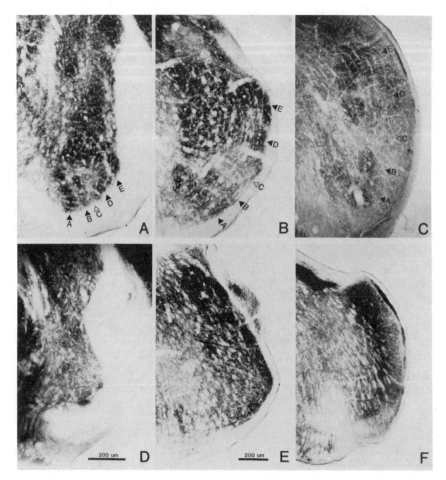

FIGURE 11. Cytochrome-oxidase-stained mouse brainstem after row C (panels *A–C*) and ION (panels *D–F*) lesions. Relevant parts of the BTC are pale with this stain. Other details as in Figure 10.

either shrink and/or fail to grow. The shrinkage of nVi is about 30% after lesions to all of the whiskers, but many of the BTC neurons do not degenerate (see Hámori et al., 1986). In the light microscope the neurons are dark and small (Ramón y Cajal, 1954; see Figure 10); in the electron microscope the cytoplasm is relatively electron dense. The time course over which these changes can be evoked may be correlated with the myelination of the afferents and the development of afferent terminals, synapses, and target cell dendrites (Clark, 1977).

Selected lesions to certain groups of whiskers may provoke an expansion of the territories taken by the afferents associated with intact whiskers based upon the experiments described above in hamsters and in rats operated on *in utero* (Rhoades, personal communication). In our laboratory, it has not been possible to stain the deafferented BTC neurons with Golgi techniques, but Golgi-stained neurons associated with the *intact* afferents appear qualitatively normal and do not have dendrites directed to the deafferented zones. After ION lesions or whisker row lesions, cells in the normal and deafferented parts of nVp and nVi continue to send axons to VB and are retrogradely labeled following injections of tracers in the thalamus (Bates et al., 1982).

The volume of all nuclei associated with the whisker afferents is reduced after ION section (Hámori et al., 1986) and crush as estimated from extracellular tungsten microelectrodes (Waite, 1984). The somatotopy is altered in that activity at a particular recording site is evoked from more whiskers than normal and the representations of many whiskers are missing. The effects of nerve section are more profound than those of nerve crush. Intracellular single-unit recording and labeling with HRP from animals with ION section demonstrates that cells within the vibrissal representation have receptive fields responding to inappropriate parts of the periphery and are activated by abnormally large numbers of whiskers. Dendritic architecture is apparently normal (Stennett et al., 1986).

With *in utero* NGF deprivation the architecture and the whisker-related pattern in nVi is normal as is the volume of the nucleus. This suggests that even though the periphery is substantially underloaded (see the preceding), the remaining afferents are able to direct appropriate development of the nucleus. Other nuclei in the BTC appear normal (Sikich et al., 1986). In contrast to untreated animals, if exogenous NGF is given to mice with ION section on PND 1 and PND 3 patterns demonstrable with CO persist (see Figure 12). In animals with PND 1 lesions, there is no whisker-related pattern, although the CO density is higher with the NGF than without it (Ma, 1985). In animals with PND 3 lesions, a whisker-related pattern remains when exogenous NGF is given (see Figures 2 and 12). The pattern is lighter than on the control side and is less sharply defined. In both cases the pattern that persists qualitatively resembles that seen in normal animals at the time of the ION lesion rather than at the time of sacrifice (Ma, 1985). The NGF apparently prevents the degeneration of some of these fibers and their terminals, but in the absence of a direct connection to the periphery, the differentiation of central patterns halts.

C Thalamic Neurons

The VB, largely equivalent to ventroposterior nuclei (VPL and VPM), is the main thalamic somatosensory relay (Emmers, 1965; Saporta and Kruger, 1977). The external division (VPL) conveys information from spinal segments while the arcuate division (VPM) receives inputs from the head including the trigeminal nerve (Lund and Webster, 1967). Direct somato-

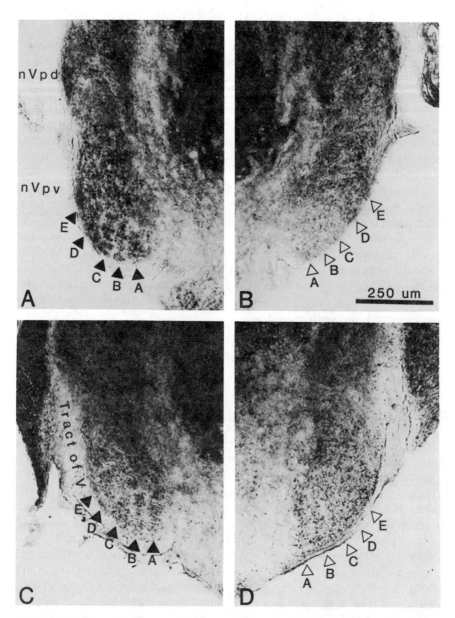

FIGURE 12. Effects of exogenous NGF treatment on altered central patterns of whiskers in animals lesioned on PND 3 and examined on PND 4. (See also Figure 2.) (*A*) The nVp from the intact side of an animal not given NGF; nVpd is the dorsal division of nVp that receives inputs from the mandibular division of the trigeminal nerve; nVpv receives inputs from the other divisions. (*B*) Result of a partial section of the ION (confirmed by dissection) on PND 3 that led to the loss of any whisker-related patterns for rows A–C; fibers to rows D–E were damaged but not completely transected so that the staining is paler than on the control side in panel *A*. (*C*) Intact side of an animal that received daily injections of exogenous NGF; the whisker pattern is essentially normal. (*D*) Whisker pattern after ION lesion on PND 3. Giving NGF causes the pattern to persist, but this does not prevent the lesion-related alterations in the cortex (see Figure 2).

sensory inputs to the arcuate division of VB come principally from the contralateral brainstem nVp, nVo, nVi and marginal cells in the laminar portion of nVc (Erzurumlu et al., 1980). Architectonic whisker representations are recognizable in the arcuate division of VB. Individual whisker-related cell groups, called barreloids, can be demonstrated in adult mice and rats (Van der Loos, 1976; Land and Simons, 1985a). These groups receive clustered afferents from the brainstem (Scheibel et al., 1972); the clusters are presumed to be related to individual whiskers. It is not clear whether the dendrites of thalamic relay cells are confined to individual barreloids (Harris, 1986; Bernardo and Woolsey, 1987). Functional maps of the rat and mouse thalamus are appropriate to the barreloid patterns (Waite, 1973). Under deep anesthesia, one thalamic neuron is activated by only one whisker (Harris, 1986). On the basis of recording, metabolic mapping, and anatomy, the arrangement of the whisker representations is such that caudal whiskers are represented laterally, rostral whiskers medially, dorsal whiskers posteriorly, and ventral whiskers anteriorly (Simons and Woolsey, 1979). The appropriateness of these assignments has recently been confirmed after small injections of HRP into single-whisker territories in the cerebral cortex (Land and Simons, 1985a). The VB also receives inputs from the cortex, to which it projects (Cowan et al., 1972; Woolsey, 1972; Steindler and Colwell, 1976; Hooglund et al., 1987), and from GABAergic (gamma amino butyric acid) neurons in the adjacent reticular nucleus (Harris, 1987; Bernardo and Woolsey, 1987). While some VB cells in the mouse may be interneurons (Woolsey et al., 1979), interneurons are very rare in rat VB (Harris and Hendrikson, 1987). Terminals of the thalamocortical relay cells are located in laminae IV and VI of the somatosensory cortex (see what follows) (Lorente de Nó, 1922; Killackey, 1973; Woolsey, 1978b; Jensen and Killackey, 1987a). Axons arising from functionally similar and anatomically adjacent thalamic neurons, such as a single barreloid, follow widely divergent routes as they course from the thalamus to the cortex (Bernardo and Woolsey, 1987).

Thalamic neurons in the mouse are generated in lateromedial and caudorostral gradients from E-14 to E-16 (Angevine, 1970). This is after the brainstem neurons that project to the thalamus are born. Vibrissa-related patterns emerge in the VB on PND 2 in the rat and appear about a day later in the mouse (Belford and Killackey, 1979a). The patterns have been detected by a number of stains (Woolsey et al., 1979; Steindler and Cooper, 1987). Cells in the VB can be driven by whisker stimuli as early as PND 5 (Verley and Onnen, 1981). In the next week the latencies shorten and the neurons that were initially activated by many whiskers are driven by but one whisker (Verley and Onnen, 1981).

The ION section in mice on PND 1 results in the absence of a whisker pattern in the VB. On PND 2 the pattern is partial, consisting of patches related to whisker rows not segregated into individual barreloids. The ION transection on PND 3 or thereafter does not appear to alter the segregation of the barreloids (see Figure 13; see also Yamakado, personal commu-

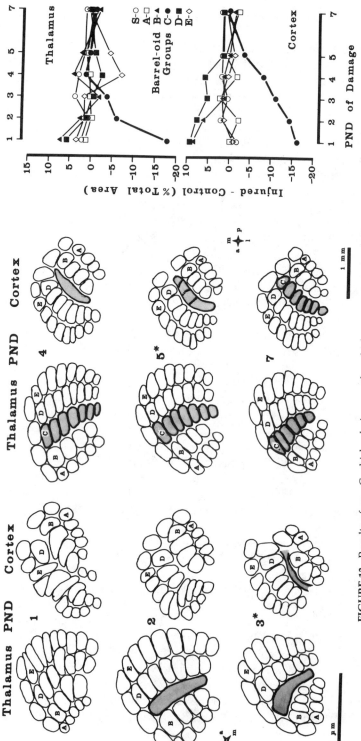

FIGURE 13. Results of row C whisker lesions on the whisker patterns in the thalamus and cerebral cortex. Lesions were made on different postnatal days; the affected portion of the pattern is indicated by the shading. In general, the later the lesion, the less dramatic the effects on the organization of the structure. The period over which these changes can be produced in the cortex is longer than that for the thalamus. Measurements of the barrel and barreloid groups that were normalized are summarized in the graphs on the right. The timing differences between the two structures is obvious. Changes in groups of whisker representations also becomes clear with quantitative assessment. (Adapted from Woolsey et al., 1979.)

nication). With lesions of individual rows of whiskers the time course of the alterations that can be produced in the whisker representations in the thalamus is the same as for the ION lesions. What differs is the pattern related to the whiskers that were not damaged in relation to those that were. The area (volume) for the damaged whiskers is attenuated with respect to normal (Woolsey et al., 1981; Durham and Woolsey, 1984). The patterns associated with the adjacent intact whiskers expand asymmetrically so that the entire volume of the nucleus is unchanged. There is no evidence that the thalamic cells die (Woolsey et al. 1979; but see Hámori, et al., 1986; Yamakado, personal communication). When mitochondrial stains are used, the histochemical reaction is pale after the initial lesions, but staining intensity may return with very long survival times (Durham and Woolsey, 1984; Yip et al., 1987). In the rat and the mouse thalamus the pattern response to whisker lesions differs in several important respects from that seen in the BTC. The pattern can be changed only for a limited period in the animal's postnatal development, is graded as a function of the age of the animal at the time of the peripheral manipulation, and has a component related to the intact whiskers (Belford and Killackey, 1980; Durham and Woolsey, 1984). We have called the latter a "compensation" (Woolsey and Wann, 1976). The period during which the architecture of the thalamus can be modified is called the *critical* or *sensitive* period (see Harwerth et al., 1986; Knudsen and Knudsen, 1986).

Recent findings indicate that after "coagulation" of all of the whiskers there are profound changes in several aspects of the architecture of the VB (Hámori et al., 1986). There is an increase in GAD (glutamic acid decarboxylase) staining puncta. The authors did not speculate on the origin of those punctata, but the thalamic reticular nucleus is an obvious candidate source. In normal animals, the lemniscal terminals from the brainstem to the VB have a characteristic architecture; corticothalamic endings have a different appearance, ending on different portions of the thalamic relay cells (Bernardo and Woolsey, 1987; Hooglund et al., 1987). In the lesioned animals profiles with "lemniscal" structure were demonstrated to be transformed corticothalamic terminals (Hámori et al., 1986). After destruction of all of the whiskers the neurons in the VB are driven by a common hair on the contralateral face (Verley and Onnen, 1981).

D Cortical Neurons

The somatosensory cortex of the rodent is sharply delimited from other cortical areas by its architecture (Woolsey, 1967; Woolsey and Van der Loos, 1970). When this cortex is cut perpendicular to the pia, the granule cells of layer IV related to the face are inhomogeneous and clustered. The region is called area 3 by Caviness (1975). Sections taken parallel to the pia that pass through layer IV demonstrate groupings of granule cells that in aggregate resemble the distorted body form of the animal (Welker, 1976; Dawson and

Killackey, 1985). The regions around the cortical granule cells are dys-granular (Sanderson et al., 1984; Welker et al., 1984; Chapin and Woodward, 1986). These regions receive projections from the corpus callosum (Wise and Jones, 1976; Olavarria et al., 1984). As in the brainstem and the thalamus, cortical layer IV neurons are grouped in a pattern that is homeomorphic to the arrangement of the whiskers on the contralateral face. The whisker groupings are called barrels. Each large barrel is related to a single whisker (but see Dawson and Killackey, 1985). The pattern is such that the dorsal row of whiskers is represented in caudal barrels; the ventral row of whiskers is in rostral barrels; the caudal hairs project medially and the rostral hairs laterally in the cortex (Welker, 1976; Simons and Woolsey, 1979; Nussbaumer and Van der Loos, 1985; McCasland and Woolsey, 1988b). The CO demonstrates similar patterns in upper layer VI (Land and Simons, 1985b) (see Figures 1, 2, and 4). The number of layer IV granule cells is directly proportional to the number of myelinated axons innervating the corresponding whisker but is greater by a factor of 17 (Lee and Woolsey, 1975). The barrel cortex has the usual complement of cortical neuron types, many of which are related by their dendritic and axonal organization to individual barrels (Lorente de Nó, 1922; Simons and Woolsey, 1984). The layer IV stellate cells are of two main types—spiny and smooth (Woolsey et al., 1975a; Steffen, 1976). Some of the smooth stellate cells are GABAergic (Kristt and Waldman, 1981; Lin et al., 1985; Chmielowska et al., 1986b). Twenty to 25% of all synapses in layer IV come from the VB and make asymmetrical contacts on the stellate cells and on all other neurons with processes in layers IV and VI (White, 1979). Single-unit recording (Simons, 1978; Ito, 1985; Simons, 1985; Armstrong-James and Fox, 1987) and 2-DG metabolic mapping (Durham and Woolsey, 1978; Chmielowska et al., 1986a; McCasland and Woolsey, 1988b) demonstrate that most of the cells in a particular barrel are activated by the appropriate contralateral whisker. Neurons in all layers are arranged as functional columns related to individual barrels (see Figure 14; Caviness et al., 1976; Durham and Woolsey, 1978; Simons and Woolsey, 1979). The neurons in nongranular layers are driven by more specific stimuli and have been shown to integrate stimuli moving over the whisker array (Simons, 1985).

The neurons of the mouse somatosensory cortex are generated from E-15 to E-17. Although their postmitotic migration is complete, they are still differentiating at birth (Rice, 1975). In the week after birth the cortex differentiates into six layers (Rice and Van der Loos, 1977; Senft and Woolsey, 1987). Gradients of development in the cortex are from the deep to the superficial layers (Angevine and Sidman, 1961) and from rostrolateral to caudomedial with respect to the cortical mantle (Smart, 1983). The patterns of whisker-related structures appear on the fifth day of life in the mouse and the rat (Rice and Van der Loos, 1977; Killackey and Belford, 1979; Blue and Parnavelas, 1983b). Whisker patches shown by the mitochondrial stains

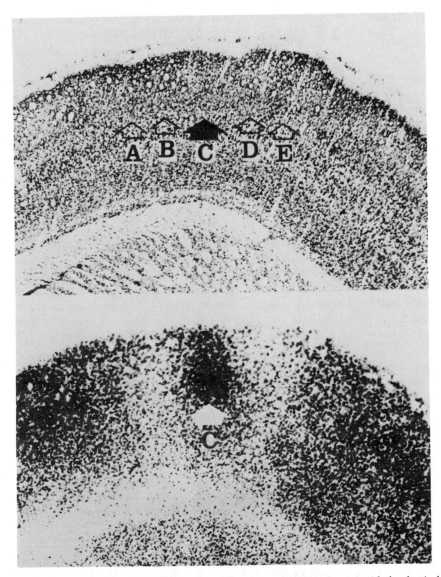

FIGURE 14. Demonstration of the columnar organization of the barrel cortex with the classical Sokoloff [14]C 2-DG film autoradiographic method. A rat had whiskers from all rows except row C clipped prior to receiving an intravenous injection of 2-DG. One hour later the animal was sacrificed, the brain cut in a cryostat, and sections mounted and dried on coverslips and apposed to X-ray film. The developed film is shown below the stained section. Although the histology is poor, the crisp column of activity was directly related to the appropriate barrel row.

appear slightly before the cell bodies are recognizably segregated (as previously described for the BTC). Binding of certain lectins to "glia" has recently been shown to demonstrate a barrel pattern before the layer IV neurons segregate into barrels. The development of these patterns correlates directly with the segregation of the afferents from the thalamus (Senft and Woolsey, 1987; Senft, 1989). The development of synapses and of cortical cell processes has not been studied in detail but, can, by analogy to study of other cortical areas (Blue and Parnavelas, 1983a) and from preliminary studies, continue at least until the fifth postnatal week (i.e., up to sexual maturity).

Lesions of the periphery alter the organization of the whisker-related pattern in this cortex in a time-dependent and lesion-dependent way. The ION section on PND 1 obliterates the barrel pattern in mice (Blue and Parnavelas, 1983b). The outline of the whisker area appears as an interface between the granule cells and the agranular zones surrounding the cortex. After ION lesions on PND 2 the pattern is one of five rows not very sharply divided; lesions on PND 3 lead to a row pattern that has sharper distinctions between the adjacent rows. After a PND 4 lesion the rows are broken into poorly defined barrels that become more sharply defined after lesions on PND 5. Lesions on PND 6 or later do not alter the cortical architecture, except that the intensity of the mitochondrial stains is less (Woolsey, 1987). A similar sequence has been partially described for the rat except that the time table is pushed forward by about a day (see Figure 15) (Killackey and Belford, 1980; Woolsey et al., 1981; Waite and Cragg, 1982). As in the thalamus, there is a period after which the peripheral lesion does not produce an alteration in the pattern of cortical neurons.

The pattern and size of the barrels in animals deprived of NGF *in utero* is normal. For the cortex, as in the brainstem, the peripheral underloading does not reduce the size of the central representation (Sikich et al., 1986). Conversely, peripheral "overloading" does not enlarge the barrel. After ION lesions, in animals given exogenous NGF, which preserves the whisker pattern in the brainstem, the barrel pattern is identical to that of lesioned animals not given NGF (see Figure 2; Ma, 1985).

When selected groups of vibrissae within a row are damaged on different postnatal days, the sequence of architectural segregation in the cortex is similar to that for lesions of the ION (Jeanmonod et al., 1981). However, in

FIGURE 15. Cytochrome-oxidase-stained sections from a 6-day-old rat sustaining left ION section at birth. (*a*) Absence of staining in nVp consistent with a complete section of the ION. (*b*) Normal pattern in nVp. (*c*) Left VB, which receives its input from the right BTC. At this power the barreloids are semidistinct. (*d*) Thalamic barreloids related to the ION section. They are paler than those on the normal side, but some are related to individual whiskers. (*e*) Whisker pattern in the left cortex is normal. (*f*) Rowlike patterns in the right cortex resemble those seen in a mouse with an ION lesion on PND 3. They are different than the pattern shown in the thalamus from this animal in panel D. Scale: (*a, b*) 200 μm; (*c, d*) 500 μm; (*e, f*) 500 μm.

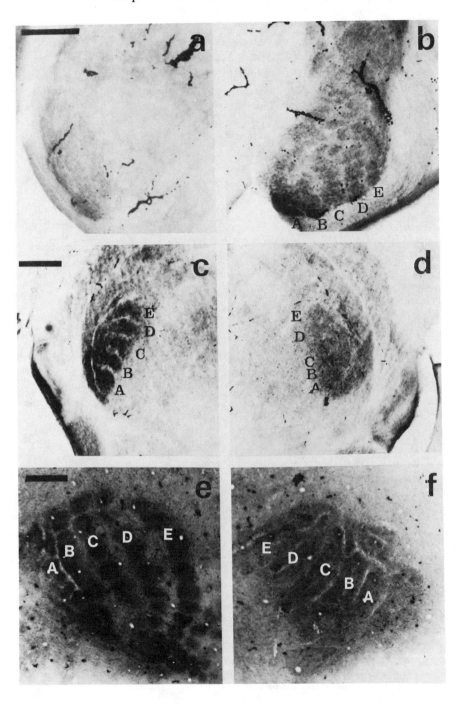

contrast to the ION lesions, the zones associated with the damaged whiskers are narrowed. The narrowing is not due to a loss of cortical space but rather an asymmetrical "compensation" by enlargement of the adjacent barrels with intact vibrissae (Woolsey and Wann, 1976). The asymmetry is such that the more rostral barrels can "compensate" later in development than the more caudal barrels (see Figures 13, 16, and 17). This compensation

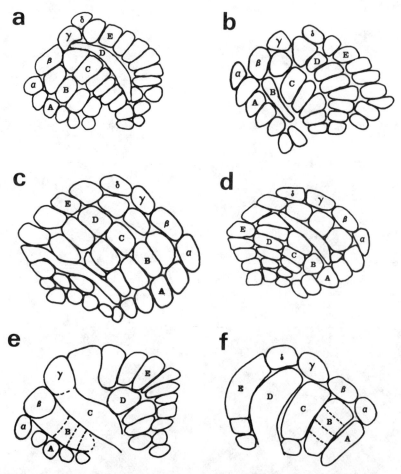

FIGURE 16. Examples of altered patterns of cortical barrels with different types of peripheral lesions in mice on different postnatal days. (*a, b*) Lesions of whisker rows D and B, respectively, on PND 2. The appropriate barrels are attenuated, and there is evidence for a compensation particularly by anterior cortex. (*c, d*) Lesions of whisker arcs 5 and 2, respectively, on PND 1. The appropriate cortex is attenuated, and there is evidence for compensation particularly by medial cortex. (*e*) Most of the whiskers in rows B, C, and D were lesioned on PND 2. The appropriate barrels are missing, and the architecture shows the rows (see Figure 15). (*f*) Most whiskers except the straddlers were lesioned on PND 3. The rowlike organization of the architecture is obvious.

is more obvious in the mouse than in the rat (Woolsey et al., 1981). As in normal animals, the architectural patterns correlate with the pattern of specific projections to this cortex from the VB (Killackey and Leshin, 1975; Woolsey, 1978b). When the thalamus is destroyed after birth, the granule cells do not form whisker-related patterns (Wise and Jones, 1978).

Lesions made across rows produce different results than those along a whisker row. Each whisker within a row is numbered caudal to rostral, and whiskers in different rows having the same number belong to an arc (see Figure 3). If whiskers in an arc are lesioned on different postnatal days, the appropriate barrels are attenuated but do not form groupings independent

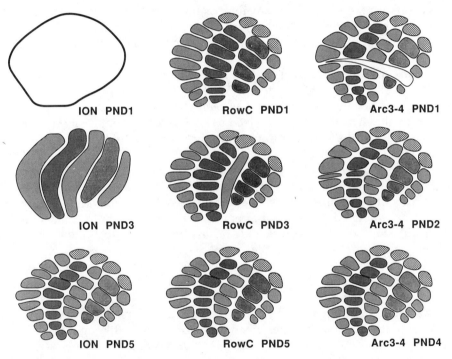

FIGURE 17. Stylized drawings to indicate the patterns of barrel organization that result after lesions of the ION, a whisker row and a whisker arc. In the left-hand column the barrels in mice (in contrast to rats) (see Figure 15) are absent after a PND 1 lesion. The appropriate area can be recognized from the granule cell densities. The same lesion on PND 3 results in patterns to which the straddlers are fused (alpha with row A, beta with row B, etc.). A lesion on PND 5 changes little. For individual whisker row lesions, the barrels may be absent when the lesions are made on PND 1, there is a rowlike tube for lesions on PND 3, which is smaller than that seen with the PND 3 ION lesion and no change for lesions made on PND 5. Arc lesions on PND 1 lead to a tube crossing the rows and medial cortex compensation. Later lesions do not disrupt the "rowness" of the barrels in an arc but lead to the medial compensation. Arc lesions on PND 4 do not appear to change the cortex. Such results are interpreted to indicate a hierarchy of postnatal cortical organization and a competition for cortical space related to developmental gradients in the thalamus and the cortex.

of the rows except when lesions are made on PND 1. The barrels are smaller than normal, with those in more rostral (higher lettered) rows more attenuated than those in more caudal rows (see Figures 16 and 17). The wedge shape of these arc barrels defines the gradient of row compensation described in the preceding. Within a particular row, the more medial barrels, not the lateral ones, are enlarged and compensate for the reduction in size of the barrels associated with the lesioned whiskers (Valentino et al., 1978; Jeanmonod et al., 1981).

Lesions to the ION or all the whiskers produce results that could be interpreted as uncovering a sequence of development of cortical organization in which the fibers from the thalamus first segregate as rows and then divide into individual barrels within those rows (see Figures 2 and 15–17). When many of the whiskers are intact, gradients of compensation are uncovered such that medial and anterior fibers can compensate for the loss of groups of barrels longer than more caudal and lateral barrels (Woolsey et al., 1981).

Lesions affecting one whisker do not perceptibly alter the whisker-related barrel pattern in the cortex (Van der Loos and Woolsey, 1973). Although no histological evidence has been published, it is suggested that lesions to all whiskers except one lead to a single barrel that is larger than normal and that the surrounding architecture is devoid of barrels (Kossut and Hand, 1984; Senft, 1986).

By analogy to studies on development of the limbs (Harrison, 1921) and to the connections from the eye (e.g., Jacobson, 1978), it seems obvious that the effects of surgical rotations or substitutions of the somatic periphery should be examined. Successful attempts have been made to transplant extra whiskers, rotate the whiskers (Andres, 1985), and substitute various cutaneous structures such as back skin, which lacks whiskers, cornea, which lacks hair, and forepaw, which has digits, to the faces of mice *in utero* (Andres, 1985). The whisker pad transplants and rotations have demonstrable innervation. There is not a rotated cortical barrel field after the whisker pad is rotated. In all of these manipulations the barrel fields look like variants of the denervations described in the preceding, although they are not nearly so ordered. It is recognized that the manipulations were carried out too late in fetal development to avoid interrupting the innervation of the periphery; so the experiments are roughly the same as ION section. The animals did not survive similar manipulations tried in younger fetuses.

The anatomy of cortical neurons after lesions of the periphery has been characterized. As in the thalamus there is no evidence for cell loss (Woolsey and Wann, 1976). Whisker lesions reduce the number of spines on apical dendrites of superficial layer V pyramidal cells (Ryugo et al., 1975). Whisker row lesions alter the orientation of layer IV stellate cell dendrites on both types of stellate cells in a temporally graded manner (Harris and Woolsey, 1979; Steffen and Van der Loos, 1980; Harris and Woolsey, 1981, 1983). With lesions on PND 1 the processes of cells that should have been oriented rostrally can be directed caudally. Many of the cells in the zone associated with the missing whiskers send dendrites to adjacent "intact" barrels as if they had been "captured" by the thalamocortical afferents (see Figure 18). These dendrites are straighter than normal and have been interpreted to be longer than normal (Kaas et al., 1983). When dendritic length is sampled at intervals appropriate to their spatial frequency, there is no evidence that dendrites are longer. With lesions on PND 2 or PND 3, the dendrites in the normal barrels are as restricted as normal, and dendrites of cells in the zones for the missing whiskers are confined to those zones. Thus, not only does the expected position of the cells in layer IV change with whisker lesions but so does the direction of growth of the processes of these cells.

Some corticocortical connections are reported to change with whisker damage. Early thalamic lesions do not result in the extensive invasion of would-be barrel territory by callosal axons (Wise and Jones, 1978). However, whisker damage is reported to lead to an increase of the callosal connections terminating in the septa between the barrels (Olavarria et al., 1984).

The functional correlates of the altered barrel patterns are of interest. When all whiskers are removed on PND 1, the barrel cortex in the adult is activated by receptive fields in skin innervated by the intact branches of the trigeminal nerve (Waite and Taylor, 1978). When single rows of whiskers are lesioned on PND 1, PND 3, or PND 5, the whiskers activating cells in the barrels associated with the intact whiskers are appropriate to those barrels (Simons et al., 1984). The zones associated with the lesioned whiskers are relatively silent, and many fewer cells than expected are driven by peripheral stimuli. Those cells that can be driven from the periphery are driven by adjacent whiskers or have receptive fields in adjacent skin. The findings are consistent with receptive fields described for trigeminal ganglion cells after similar but not identical peripheral manipulations (Rhoades et al., 1987b). The properties of neurons in nongranular layers are appropriate to the barrels over or under them and do not seem to be substantially altered by the peripheral manipulation (but see what follows). Cortical cells labeled with 2-DG in similarly prepared animals follow the appropriate barrel boundaries with great precision (Durham and Woolsey, 1985). With the Sokoloff 2-DG technique, it has been reported that the shape and size of the cortical column activated by the remaining whisker when all others have been lesioned at birth exceeds cytoarchitectonic boundaries (Kossut and Hand, 1984).

Small lesions have been made in the barrel cortex or the cortex rotated on PND 1. If the area of the barrel cortex is reduced surgically, the barrels are perfectly formed but smaller (Ito and Seo, 1983; Seo and Ito, 1987). If the barrel cortex is removed and placed back, then barrel patterns form correctly (Andres and Van der Loos, 1985b). Attempts to rotate the cortical piece do not give clear results, which have been attributed to experimental difficulties.

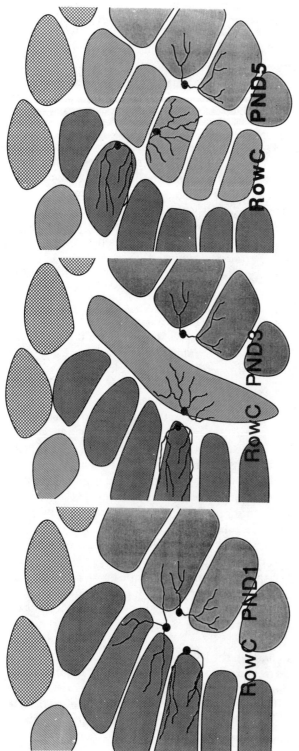

FIGURE 18. Schematic drawings to show the changes in dendritic patterns observed in the cortex after whisker lesions at different postnatal ages. The drawings indicate that the physical location of a cell in the plane of the cortex matters little, but its relationship to the specific thalamocortical afferents to the barrels is critical for dendritic organization. These cells are probably instructed to direct their dendritic growth by the thalamocortical afferents. Single-unit recordings and 2-DG studies from similarly prepared animals indicate that the cortical architectural boundaries, even if changed by the whisker lesions, mark functional boundaries that are appropriate for the intact whiskers projecting to the remaining enlarged barrels.

Several manipulations to the periphery other than damage to the primary afferents are possible. Since the animals actively explore the environment by moving the whiskers back and forth by skeletal muscles supplied by the seventh nerve, section of this nerve eliminates motor behavior and alters the sensory input (Welker, 1964; Zucker and Welker, 1969). No changes in the cortical barrel pattern were observed after seventh nerve section (Rice, 1984). Removing the whisker hairs alone likewise does not alter the architecture of the barrels (Woolsey et al., 1981). However, chronic removal of the whisker hairs alters the response properties of cortical neurons. The cells show higher levels of spontaneous activity, and their spatial tuning is much poorer than in normal animals (Simons and Land, 1987). There is a cortical dependence on whisker hair input for sculpting neuronal response characteristics during development, which may related to changes in the development of intracortical inhibitory pathways.

In adult animals whisker hair removal has been shown to decrease the intensity of mitochondrial stains in appropriate barrels (Wong-Riley and Welt, 1980). When whiskers are chronically clipped in adults, the activities of a number of enzymes associated with aerobic glycolytic metabolism increase on the opposite side of the brain. These results are interpreted as being consistent with the increased use that the animal makes of the intact whiskers (Dietrich et al., 1982).

IV SUMMARY

This account of the effects of peripheral lesions on the whisker–barrel system emphasizes the clear correlation of lesion-related effects with developmental processes. One conclusion is that *peripheral* lesion experiments can be used as a means to study *development* of sensory pathways in the mammalian central nervous system. Assumptions underlying this conclusion are that the changes observed in adult animals reflect processes active at the time the intervention is made. A commitment is made at the earlier time, and subsequent development is carried out according to that commitment. Results from the fully mature brain can be interpreted from a developmental standpoint, and the larger mature brain is much easier to study.

Although the emphasis of this chapter is principally on changes in the brain produced by peripheral manipulations in the young, it is worth noting that lasting changes in the adult brain are produced in response to peripheral lesions and other environmental manipulations (Melville Jones, 1977). Recent extensions of the work on primates (Clark et al., 1988) to the rodent whisker system (Yun et al., 1987) suggests that a form of long-term modifiability of function in adult rodents exists. At the very least this line of investigation may shed light on the mechanisms of use/disuse functional plasticity because of the better definition of cortical anatomy in rodents. The precedent for long-term changes in the adult rodent nervous system after peripheral manipulations is clear. Changes in levels of various metabolic markers including the activity of relevant enzymes follow whisker nerve lesions and simple sensory deprivation produced by whisker clipping (Wong-Riley and Welt, 1980; Dietrich et al., 1982; Ginsberg et al., 1987; Yip et al., 1987). These changes are coupled to activity levels in the system. There is not yet any evidence one way or the other as to whether there are changes in neuronal structure associated with these phenomena. It well may be that the same or similar mechanisms responsible for the lesion-associated changes seen in young animals carry over to adults, a possibility of more than theoretrical interest (Pearson, 1987; Neve et al., 1988).

It is clear that for any part of the rodent whisker pathway a similar sequence of morphological and functional ontogeny occurs differing principally in time. The consequences of the lesions to the periphery in young animals when examined in later life show findings that are remarkably similar to the pattern of structure present at the time of manipulation. It is as if the manipulation led to an *arrest* in the development of the system. Two examples suffice: (1) the pattern of thalamocortical afferents in adult rats with neonatal ION lesions (Jensen and Killackey, 1987b) is very similar to that seen in thalamocortical afferents stained in neonatal animals (Senft and Woolsey, 1987) and (2) the pattern of CO staining preserved by exogenous NGF in the brainstem of ION-sectioned animals is similar to that seen at the time the lesions were made but not to that seen at the time the animals were sacrificed. In both cases it is as if development had reached a certain point but lacked the necessary information and/or drive to complete the task. Where the results are not complicated by afferent degeneration, the relevant elements are suspended; they neither advance nor regress in a developmental sense.

At the time the rodent whisker–barrel system is usually lesioned (i.e., the perinatal period), most of the relevant axons have found their way to target regions and most of the target neurons have finished their major migrations. The interactions between these afferents and the target cells are what develop in the perinatal period, and it is these interactions that the peripheral lesions change. Thus, as important as axonal navigation to the target is, the bulk of the observations summarized here deal with aspects of afferent target interactions. One aspect of this interaction that has become clear from the experiments with altered sensory peripheries is that the process is a competitive one (Woolsey and Wann, 1976; Sikich et al., 1986; Welker and Van der Loos, 1986). The enormous power of this to account for major and minor alterations in this system and others has been indicated elsewhere (Woolsey, 1978b). It is now feasible to examine several possible activity-based mechanisms for this competition, many of which have been proposed or documented in other neural systems (Fawcett and O'Leary, 1985; Cline et al., 1987). One very exciting aspect of future work will be to see whether similar mechanisms can be proven to control development, including its response to peripheral lesions, in the rodent whisker–barrel system, where because of the extent of background of information and because of the clarity of the organization of the system, the relevant data can be collected in mammals at a level of great precision.

Interest in lesion-induced alterations in the developing brain comes particularly from the possibility that these phenomena can be a model of modifiability of the brain by experience. The mechanism, if identified, ought to be of value for explaining phenomena such as learning and for developing strategies for correcting the devastating effects of acquired *lesions*. In one view it is reasonable to sharply divide apparently different phenomena not only for clearly conceptualizing the results but for generating testable hypotheses. It is also possible that different phenomena may result from fundamentally different mechanisms. One such formulation is to consider the brain alterations produced by peripheral lesions as wholly different from those produced by the environment (Belford and Killackey, 1980). In this formulation parts of the brain have periods when they are *sensitive* to lesions that produce a permanent change in brain structure, if not function. This is distinguished from changes produced by interactions with the environment. These may be reversible over different time periods that are *critical* in development. The usefulness of this conceptualization in narrowing the focus of experimental investigations cannot be denied. However, these didactic distinctions, which may be artificial in terms of relevant biological mechanisms, should not obscure the very real and exciting possibility that the development, plasticity, and impressive adaptability of the mammalian brain in fact depend on a small number of robust, simple, and flexible biological mechanisms (Edelman, 1987).

ACKNOWLEDGEMENTS

This work was supported by National Institutes of Health Grant NS 17763, the McDonnell Center for Studies of Higher Brain Function, and a gift from the Spastic Paralysis Foundation of the Illinois–Eastern Iowa District of the Kiwanis International. The author is especially grateful to Ms. Margo Gross for assistance in many phases of preparation of this manuscript and to Mr. Jon Christensen, who assisted in collection and codification of unpublished data, figure preparation, and photography.

REFERENCES

Aldskogius, B. C., J. I. Johnson, and E. M. Ostapoff (1978) Nerve cell degeneration and death in the trigeminal ganglion of the adult rat following peripheral nerve transection. J. Neurocytol. 7:229–250.

Andres, F. L. (1985) Early substitution of whiskerpad by dorsal skin, cornea and palm of forepaw thoroughly modifies structures of barrelfield in mice. Anat. Embryol. 173:157–161.

Andres, F. L. and H. Van der Loos (1983) Cultured embyonic non-innervated mouse muzzle is capable of generating a whisker pattern. Int. J. Dev. Neurosci. *1*:319–338.

Andres, F. L., and H. Van der Loos (1985a) From sensory periphery to cortex: The architecture of the barrelfield as modified by various early manipulations of the mouse whiskerpad. Anat. Embryol. *172*:11–20.

Andres, F. L., and H. Van der Loos (1985b) Removal and reimplantation of the parietal cortex of the neonatal mouse: Consequences for the barrelfield. Dev. Brain Res. *20*:115–121.

Andres, K. H. (1966) Über die Feinstruktur der rezeptoren an sinusharren. Z. Zellforsch. *75*:339–365.

Angevine, J. B. (1970) Time of neuron origin in the diencephalon of the mouse. An autoradiographic study. J. Comp. Neurol. *139*:129–188.

Angevine, J. B., and R. L. Sidman (1961) Autoradiographic study of cell migration during histogenesis of cerebral cortex in the mouse. Nature *192*:766–768.

Armstrong-James, M., and K. Fox (1987) Spatiotemporal convergence and divergence in the rat SI "barrel" cortex. J. Comp. Neurol. *263*:264–281.

Arvidsson, J. (1982) Somatotopic organization of vibrissae afferents in the trigeminal sensory nuclei of the rat studied by transganglionic transport of HRP. J. Comp. Neurol. *211*:84–92.

Åstrom, K. E. (1953) On the central course of afferent fibers in the trigeminal, facial, glossopharyngeal, and vagal nerves and their nuclei in the mouse. Acta Physiol. Scand. (*Suppl.*) *29*:209–320.

Basbaum, A. I., and P. J. Hand (1973) Projections of cervicothoracic dorsal roots to the cuneate nucleus of the rat, with observations on cellular "bricks." J. Comp. Neurol. *148*:347–360.

Bates, C. A., and H. P. Killackey (1985) The organization of the neonatal rat's brainstem trigeminal complex and its role in the formation of central trigeminal patterns. J. Comp. Neurol. *240*:265–287.

Bates, C. A., R. S. Erzurumlu, and H. P. Killackey (1982) Central correlates of peripheral pattern alterations in the trigeminal system of the rat. III. Neurons of the principal sensory nucleus. Dev. Brain Res. *5*:108–113.

Belford, G. R., and H. P. Killackey (1979a) The development of vibrissae representation in subcortical trigeminal centers of the neonatal rat. J. Comp. Neurol. *188*:63–74.

Belford, G. R., and H. P. Killackey (1979b) Vibrissae representation in subcortical trigeminal centers of the neonatal rat. J. Comp. Neurol. *183*:305–322.

Belford, G. R., and H. P. Killackey (1980) The sensitive period in the development of the trigeminal system of the neonatal rat. J. Comp. Neurol. *193*:335–350.

Bernardo, K. L., and T. A. Woolsey (1987) Axonal trajectories between mouse somatosensory thalamus and cortex. J. Comp. Neurol. *258*:542–564.

Blue, M. E., and J. G. Parnavelas (1983a) The formation and maturation of synapses in the visual cortex of the rat. I. Qualitative analysis. J. Neurocytol. *12*:599–616.

Blue, M. E., and J. G. Parnavelas (1983b) The formation and maturation of synapses in the visual cortex of the rat. II. Quantitative analysis. J. Neurocytol. *12*:697–712.

Campbell A. W. (1905) Histological Studies on the Localization of Cerebral Function. Cambridge: Cambridge University Press.

Carroll, E. W., and M. T. T. Wong-Riley (1984) Quantitative light and electron microscopic analysis of cytochrome oxidase-rich zones in the striate cortex of the squirrel monkey. J. Comp. Neurol. 222:1–17.

Caviness, V. S., Jr. (1975) Architectonic map of neocortex of normal mouse. J. Comp. Neurol. 164:247–264.

Caviness, V. S., D. O. Frost, and N. L. Hayes (1976) Barrels in somatosensory cortex of normal and reeler mutant mice. Neurosci. Lett. 3:7–14.

Chapin, J. K., and D. J. Woodward (1986) Distribution of somatic sensory and active-movement neuronal discharge properties in the MI-SI cortical border area in the rat. Exp. Neurol. 91:502–523.

Chmielowska, J., M. Kossut, and M. Chmielowska (1986a) Single vibrissal cortical column in the mouse labeled with 2-deoxyglucose. Exp. Brain Res. 63:607–619.

Chmielowska, J., M. G. Stewart, R. C. Bourne, and J. Hámori (1986b) γ-aminobutgric acid immunoreactivity in mouse barrel field: A light microscopical study. Brain Res. 368:371–374.

Clark, H. C. (1977) A light and electron microscopic analysis of development within the main sensory trigeminal nucleus of the rat. Dissertation, Virginia Commonwealth University, Medical College of Virginia, Richmond, VA.

Clark, S. A., T. Allard, W. M. Jenkins, and M. Merzenich (1988) Receptive field in the body-surface map in adult cortex defined by temporally correlated inputs. Nature 332:444–445.

Cline, H. T., E. A. Debski, and M. Constantine-Paton (1987) N-Methyl-D-aspartate receptor antagonist desegregates eye-specific stripes. Proc. Natl. Acad. Sci. USA 84:4342–4345.

Cooper, N. F., and D. A. Steindler (1986) Lectins demarcate the barrel subfield in the somatosensory cortex of the early postnatal mouse. J. Comp. Neurol. 249:157–169.

Cowan, W. M., D. I. Gottlieb, A. E. Hendrickson, J. L. Price, and T. A. Woolsey (1972) The autoradiographic demonstration of axonal connections in the central nervous system. Brain. Res. 37:21–51.

Csillik, B., M. E. Schwab, and H. Thoenen (1985) Transganglionic regulation of central terminals of dorsal root ganglion cells by nerve growth factor (NGF) Brain Res. 331:11–15.

D'Amato, R. J., M. E. Blue, B. L. Largent, D. R. Lynch, D. J. Ledbetter, M. E. Molliver, and S. H. Snyder (1987) Ontogeny of the serotonergic projection to rat neocortex: Transient expression of a dense innervation to primary sensory areas. Proc. Natl. Acad. Sci. USA 84:4322–4326.

Davies, A. M., and A. G. S. Lumsden (1984) Relation of target encounter and neuronal death to nerve growth factor responsiveness in the developing mouse trigeminal ganglion. J. Comp. Neurol. 223:124–137.

Davies, A. M. and A. G. S. Lumsden (1986) Fasciculation in the early mouse trigeminal nerve is not ordered in relation to the emerging pattern of whisker follicles. J. Comp. Neurol. 252:13–24.

Dawson, D. R., and H. P. Killackey (1985) Distinguishing topography and soma-totopy in the thalamocortical projections of the developing rat. Dev. Brain Res. 17:309–313.

Diamond, M. C., M. R. Rosenweig, E. L. Bennett, B. Lindner, and L. Lyon (1972) Effects of environmental enrichment and impoverishment on rat cerebral cortex. J. Neurobiol. 3:47–64.

Dietrich, W. D., D. Durham, O. H. Lowry, and T. A. Woolsey (1981) Quantitative histochemical effects of whisker damage on single identified cortical barrels in the adult mouse. J. Neurosci. 1:929–935.

Dietrich, W. D., D. Durham, O. H. Lowry, and T. A. Woolsey (1982) "Increased" sensory stimulation leads to changes in energy-related enzymes in the brain. J. Neurosci. 2:1608–1613.

Dörfl, J. (1985) The innervation of the mystacial region of the white mouse. A topograpahical study. J. Anat. 142:173–184.

Dun, R. B. (1959) The development and growth of vibrissae in the house mouse with particular reference to the time of action on the tabby (Ta) and ragged (Ra) genes. Aust. J. Biol. Sci. 12:312–330.

Dun, R. B., and A. S. Fraser (1958) Selection for an invariant character—"vibrissa number"—in the house mouse. Nature 181:1018–1019.

Durham, D., and T. A. Woolsey (1977) Barrels and columnar cortical organization: Evidence from 2-deoxyglucose (2-DG) experiments. Brain Res. 137:169–74.

Durham, D., and T. A. Woolsey (1978) Acute whisker removal reduces neuronal activity in barrels of mouse Sml cortex. J. Comp. Neurol. 178:629–644.

Durham, D., T. A. Woolsey, and L. Kruger (1981) Cellular localization of 2-[^{3}H] deoxy-D-glucose from paraffin embedded brains. J. Neurosci. 1:519–526.

Durham, D., and T. A. Woolsey (1984) Effects of neonatal whisker lesions on mouse central trigeminal pathways. J. Comp. Neurol. 223:424–447.

Durham, D., and T. A. Woolsey (1985) Functional organization in cortical barrels of normal and vibrissae-damaged mice: A (3H)2-deoxyglucose study. J. Comp. Neurol. 235:97–110.

Edelman, G. M. (1987) Neural Darwinism: The theory of neuonal group selection. New York: Basic Books.

Emmers, R. (1965) Organization of the first and second somesthetic regions (SI and SII) in the rat thalamus. J. Comp. Neurol. 124:215–228.

Erzurumlu, R. S., and H. P. Killackey (1980) Diencephalic projections of the sub-nucleus interpolaris of the brainstem trigeminal complex in the rat. Neuroscience 5:1891–1901.

Erzurumlu, R. S., and H. P. Killackey (1982) Order in the developing rat trigeminal nerve. Dev. Brain Res. 3:305–310.

Erzurumlu, R. S., C. A. Bates, and H. P. Killackey (1980) Differential organization of thalamic projection cells in the brainstem trigeminal complex of the rat. Brain Res. 198:427–433.

Fawcett, J. W., and D. D. M. O'Leary (1985) The role of electrical activity in the formation of topographic maps in the nervous system. Trends Neurosci. 8:201–206.

Fischer, M. H., C. Welker, and H. A. Waisman (1972) Generalized growth retardation in rats induced by prenatal exposure to methylazoxymethyl acetate. Teratology 5:223–232.

Forbes, D. J., and C. Welt (1981) Neurogenesis in the trigeminal ganglion of the albino rat. A quantitative autoradiographic study. J. Comp. Neurol. 199:133–147.

Friede, R. L. (1959) Histochemical investigations on succinic dehydrogenase in the central nervous system. III. Atlas of the midbrain of the guinea pig, including pons and cerebellum. J. Neurochem. 4:290–303.

Ginsburg, M. D., W. D. Dietrich, and R. Buston (1987) Coupled forebrain increases of local cerebral glucose utilization and blood flow during physiologic stimulation of a somatosensory pathway in the rat: Demonstration by double-label autoradiography. Neurology 37:11–19.

Gobel, S., and R. Dubner (1969) Fine structural studies of the main sensory trigeminal nucleus in the cat and rat. J. Comp. Neurol. 137:459–494.

Goldowitz, D. (1987) Cell partioning and mixing in the formation of the CNS: Analysis of the cortical somatosensory barrels in chimeric mice. Dev. Brain Res. 35:1–9.

Grant, G., and J. Arvidsson (1975) Transganglionic degeneration in trigeminal primary sensory neurons. Brain Res. 95:265–280.

Grünthal, E. (1945) Die Rindenprojektion der Thalamus Kerne bei der Maus. Eine experimentell-anatomische Untersuchung. Mschr. Psych. Neurol. 110:245–268.

Gustafson, J. W., and S. L. Felbain-Keramidas (1977) Behavioral and neural approaches to the function of the mystacial vibrissae. Psychol. Bull. 84:477–488.

Hámori, J., C. Savy, M. Madarasz, J. Somogyi, J. Takacs, R. Verley, and E. Farkas-Bargeton (1986) Morphological alterations in subcortical vibrissal relays following vibrissal follicle destruction at birth in the mouse. J. Comp. Neurol. 254:166–183.

Hand, P. J. (1981) The 2-deoxyglucose method. In L. Heimer and M. J. Robards (eds.): Neuroanatomical Tract-Tracing Methods. New York: Plenum Press, pp. 511–538.

Harris, R. M. (1986) Morphology of physiologically identified thalamocortical relay neurons in the rat ventrobasal thalamus. J. Comp. Neurol. 251:491–505.

Harris, R. M. (1987) Axon collaterals in the thalamic reticular nucleus from thalamocortical neurons of the rat ventrobasal thalamus. J. Comp. Neurol. 258:397–406.

Harris, R. M., and A. E. Hendrickson (1987) Local circuit neurons in the rat ventrobasal thalamus. A GABA immunocytochemical study. Neuroscience 21:229–236.

Harris, R. M., and T. A. Woolsey (1979) Morphology of Golgi-impregnated neurons in mouse cortical barrels following vibrissae damage at different post-natal ages. Brain Res. 161:143–149.

Harris, R. M., and T. A. Woolsey (1981) Dendritic plasticity in mouse barrel cortex following postnatal vibrissa follicle damage. J. Comp. Neurol. 196:357–376.

Harris, R. M., and T. A. Woolsey (1983) Computer-assisted analyses of barrel neuron axons and their putative synaptic contacts. J. Comp. Neurol. 220:63–79.

Harrison, R. G. (1921) On relations of symmetry in transplanted limbs. J. Exp. Zool. 32:1–136.

Harwerth, R. S., E. L. Smith, III, G. C. Duncan, M. L. J. Crawford, and G. K. Von Noorden (1986) Multiple sensitive periods in the development of the primate visual system. Science 232:235–238.

Hayashi, H. (1980) Distributions of vibrissae afferent fiber collaterals in the trigeminal nuclei as revealed by intra-axonal injection of horseradish peroxidase. Brain Res. 183:442–446.

Hooglund, P. V., E. Welker, and H. Van der Loos (1987) Organization of the projections from barrel cortex to thalamus in mice studied with phaseolus vulgaris-leucoaggutinin and HRP. Exp. Brain Res. 68:73–87.

Hulsebosch, C. E., and R. E. Coggeshall (1983) Age related sprouting of dorsal root axons after sensory denervation. Brain Res. 288:77–83.

Ito, M. (1981) Some quantitative aspects of vibrissa-driven neuronal responses in rat neocortex. J. Neurophysiol. 46:705–715.

Ito, M. (1985) Processing of vibrissa sensory information within the rat neocortex. J. Neurophysiol. 54:479–490.

Ito, M., and M. L. Seo (1983) Avoidance of neonatal cortical lesions by developing somatosensory barrels. Nature 301:600–602.

Ito, M., M. Kawabata, and R. Shoji (1981) Effect of prenatal X-irradiation on sensitivity of cortical neurons responding to vibrissa stimulation. J. Neurophysiol. 46:716–724.

Jacobson, C. M. (1966) A comparative study of the mechanisms by which X-irradiation and genetic mutation cause loss of vibrissae in embryo mice. J. Embryol. Exp. Morphol. 16:369–379.

Jacobson, M. (1978) Developmental Neurobiology (2nd ed.). New York: Plenum Press.

Jacquin, M. F., and R. W. Rhoades (1985) Effects of neonatal infraorbital lesions upon central trigeminal primary afferent projections in rat and hamster. J. Comp. Neurol. 235:129–143.

Jacquin, M. F., and R. W. Rhoades (1987) Development and plasticity in hamster trigeminal primary afferent projections. Dev. Brain Res. 31:161–176.

Jacquin, M. F., and H. P. Ziegler (1983) Trigeminal orosensation and ingestive behavior in the rat. Behav. Neurosci. 97:62–97.

Jacquin, M. F., K. Semba, M. D. Egger, and R. W. Rhoades (1983) Organization of HRP-labelled trigeminal mandibular primary afferent neurons in the rat. J. Comp. Neurol. 215:397–420.

Jacquin, M. F., A. Hess, P. Adamo, G. Yang, M. Math, A. Brown, and R. W. Rhoades (1984a) Oganization of the infraorbital nerve in rat: A quantitative electron microscopic study. Brain Res. 290:131–135.

Jacquin, M. F., R. D. Mooney, and R. W. Rhoades (1984b) Axon arbors of functionally distinct whisker afferents are similar in medullary dorsal horn. Brain Res. 298:175–180.

Jacquin, M. F., R. D. Mooney, and R. W. Rhoades (1984c) Altered somatosensory receptive fields in hamster colliculus after infraorbital nerve section and xylocaine injection. J. Physiol. 348:471–492.

Jacquin, M. F., R. D. Mooney, and R. W. Rhoades (1986a) Morphology, response properties, and collateral projections of trigeminothalamic neurons in brainstem subnucleus interpolaris of rat. Exp. Brain Res. 61:457–468.

Jacquin, M. F., W. E. Renehan, B. G. Klein, R. D. Mooney, and R. W. Rhoades (1986b) Functional consequences of neonatal infraorbital nerve section in rat trigeminal ganglion. J. Neurosci. 6:3706–3720.

Jeanmonod, D., F. L. Rice, and H. Van der Loos (1977) Mouse somatosensory cortex: Development of the alterations in the barrel field which are caused by injury to the vibrissal follicles. Neurosci. Lett. 6:151–156.

Jeanmonod, D., F. L. Rice, and H. Van der Loos (1981) Mouse somatosensory cortex: Alterations in the barrelfield following receptor injury at different early postnatal ages. Neuroscience 6:1503–1535.

Jensen, K. F., and H. P. Killackey (1987a) Terminal arbors of axons projecting to the somatosensory cortex of the adult rat. I. The normal morphology of thalamocortical afferents following neonatal infraorbital nerve cut. J. Neurosci. 7:3529–3543.

Jensen, K. F., and H. P. Killackey (1987b) Terminal arbors of axons projecting to the somatosensory cortex of the adult rat. II. The altered morphology of thalamocortical afferents following neonatal infraorbital nerve cut. J. Neurosci. 7:3544–3553.

Johnson, E. M., P. D. Gorin, P. A. Osborne, R. E. Rydel, and J. Pearson (1982) Effects of autoimmune NGF deprivation in the adult rabbit and offspring. Brain Res. 240:131–140.

Johnson, J. I., T. C. Hamilton, J.-C. Hsung, and P. S. Ulinski (1972) Gracile nucleus absent in adult opossums after leg removal in infancy. Brain Res. 38:421–424.

Kaas, J. H., M. M. Merzenich, and H. P. Killackey (1983) The reorganization of somatosensory cortex following peripheral nerve damage in adult and developing mammals. Ann. Rev. Neurosci. 6:325–356.

Kadekaro, M., A. M. Crane, and L. Sokoloff (1985) Differential effects of electrical stimulation of sciatic nerve on metabolic activity in spinal cord and dorsal root ganglion in the rat. Proc. Natl. Acad. Sci. USA 82:6010–6013.

Killackey, H. P. (1973) Anatomical evidence for cortical subdivisions based on vertically discrete thalamic projections from the ventral posterior nucleus to cortical barrels in the rat. Brain Res. 51:326–331.

Killackey, H. P., and G. R. Belford (1979) The formation of afferent patterns in the somatosensory complex of the neonatal rat. J. Comp. Neurol. 183:285–304.

Killackey, H. P., and G. R. Belford (1980) Central correlates of peripheral pattern alterations in the trigeminal system of the rat. Brain Res. 183:205–210.

Killackey, H. P. and S. Leshin (1975) The organization of specific thalamocortical projections to the posteromedial barrel subfield of the rat somatic sensory cortex. Brain Res. 86:469–472.

Klein, B. G., G. I. MacDonald, A. M. Szczepanik, and R. W. Rhoades (1986) Topographic organization of peripheral trigeminal ganglionic projections in newborn rats. Dev. Brain Res. 27:257–262.

Knudsen, E. I., and P. F. Knudsen (1986) The sensitive period for auditory localization in barn owls is limited by age, not by experience. J. Neurosci. 6:1918–1924.

Kossut, M., and P. Hand (1984) The development of the vibrissal cortical column in the rat: A deoxyglucose study. Neurosci. Lett. 46:7–12.

Kristt, D. A. (1979) Somatosensory cortex: Acetylcholinesterase staining of barrel neuropil in the rat. Neurosci. Lett. 12:177–182.

Kristt, D. A., and J. D. Silverman (1980) Catecholamine cell groups innervating infant rat somatosensory cortex. Neurosci. Lett. 16:181–186.

Kristt, D. A., and J. V. Waldman (1981) Development of neocortical circuitry: GABA-transaminase replaces AChE in the barrel centers. Soc. Neurosci. Abstr. 7:758.

Land, P. W., and D. J. Simons (1985a) Metabolic and structural correlates of the vibrissae representation in the thalamus of the adult rat. Neurosci. Lett. 60: 319–324.

Land, P. W., and D. J. Simons (1985b) Cytochrome-oxidase staining in the rat SmI barrel cortex. J. Comp. Neurol. 258:225–235.

Lee, K. J., and T. A. Woolsey (1975) A proportional relationship between peripheral innervation density and cortical neuron number in the somatosensory system of the mouse. Brain Res. 99:349–353.

Lin, C.-S., S. M. Lu, and D. E. Schmechel (1985) Glutamic acid decarboxylase immunoreactivity in layer IV of barrel cortex of rat and mouse. J. Neurosci. 7:1934–1939.

Loeb, E. P., F.-L. F. Chang, and W. T. Greenough (1987) Effects of neonatal 6-hydroxydopamine treatment upon morphological organization of the posteromedial barrel subfield in mouse somatosensory cortex. Brain Res. 403: 113–120.

Long, J. A., and P. L. Burlingame (1938) The development of the external form of the rat with some observations on the origin of the extraembryonic coelom and foetal membranes. Univ. Calf. Publ. Zool. 43:143–183.

Lorente de Nó., R. (1922) La corteza cerebral del ratón. Trab. Lab. Invest. Biol. Univ. Madrid 20:1–38.

Lumsden, A. G. S., and A. M. Davies (1983) Earliest sensory fibres are guided to peripheral targets by attractants other than nerve growth factor. Nature 306: 786–788.

Lund, R. D., and K. E. Webster (1967) Thalamic afferents from the dorsal column nuclei. An experimental anatomical study in the rat. J. Comp. Neurol. 130:313–328.

Ma, P. K. M. (1985) The barrelettes-architectonic vibrissal representations in the brainstem trigeminal complex of the mouse. Dissertation, Washington University, St. Louis, MO.

Ma, P. K. M., and T. A. Woolsey (1983) Cytoarchitectonic organization of the brainstem trigeminal nuclei in the mouse: Correlation with vibrissal inputs and postnatal development. Soc. Neurosci. Abstr., 9:922.

Ma, P. K. M., and T. A. Woolsey (1984) Cytoarchitectonic correlates of the vibrissae in the medullary trigeminal complex of the mouse. Brain Res. 306:374–379.

McCasland, J. S., and T. A. Woolsey (1988a) New high resolution 2-deoxyglucose method featuring double labeling and automated data collection. J. Comp. Neurol. 278:543–554.

McCasland, J. S., and T. A. Woolsey (1988b) High resolution 2-deoxyglucose mapping of functional cortical columns in mouse barrel cortex. J. Comp. Neurol. 278:555–569.

Melzer, P., H. Van der Loos, J. Dörfl, E. Welker, P. Roberts, D. Emery, and J.-C. Berrini (1985) A magnetic device to stimulate selected whiskers of freely moving or restrained small rodents: Its application in a deoxyglucose study. Brain Res. 348:229–240.

Melville Jones, G. (1977) Plasticity in the adult vestibulo-ocular reflex arc. Phil. Trans. R. Soc. Lond. B., *278:*319–334.

Mountcastle, V. B. (1964) The neural replication of sensory events in the somatic afferent system. In J. C. Eccles (ed.): Brain and Conscious Experience. New York: Springer-Verlag, pp. 85–115.

Munger, B. L., and F. L. Rice (1986) Successive waves of differentiation of cutaneous afferents in rat mystacial skin. J. Comp. Neurol. 252:404–414.

Neve, R. L., E. A. Finch, E. D. Bird, and L. I. Benowitz (1988) Growth-associated protein GAP-43 is expressed selectively in associative regions of the adult human brain. Proc. Natl. Acad. Sci USA 85:3638–3642.

Nornes, H. O., and M. Morita (1979) Time of origin of the neurons in the caudal brain stem of rat: An autoradiographic study. Dev. Neurosci. 2:201–214.

Nussbaumer, J. C., and H. Van der Loos (1985) An electrophysiological and anatomical study of projections to the mouse cortical barrelfield and its surroundings. J. Neurophysiol. 53:686–698.

Olavarria, J., R. C. Van Sluyters, and H. P. Killackey (1984) Evidence for complementary organization of callosal and thalamic connections within rat somatosensory cortex. Brain Res. *291:*364–368.

Orbach, H. S., L. B. Cohen, and A. Grinvald (1985) Optical mapping of electrical activity in rat somatosensory and visual cortex. J. Neurosci. 5:1886–1895.

Pearson, J. C., L. H. Finkel, and G. M. Edelman (1987) Plasticity in the organization of adult cerebral cortical maps: A computer simulation based on neuonal group selection. J. Neurosci. 7:4209–4223.

Pearson, J., E. M. Johnson, and L. Brandeis (1983) Effects of antibodies to nerve growth factor on intrauterine development of derivatives of cranial neural crest and placode in the guinea pig. Dev. Biol. *96:*32–36.

Ramon y Cajal, S. (1954) Neuron Theory or Reticular Theory? (M. U. Purkiss and C. A. Fox, trans.) Madrid: Consejo Superior de Investigationes Cientificas.

Renehan, W. E., and B. L. Munger (1986) Degeneration and regeneration of peripheral nerve in the rat trigeminal system. II. Response to nerve lesion. J. Comp. Neurol. 249:429–459.

Renehan, W. E., and R. W. Rhoades (1984) A quantitative electron microscopic analysis of the infraorbital nerve in the newborn rat. Brain Res. 322:368–373.

Rhoades, R. W., J. M. Fiore, M. F. Math, and M. F. Jacquin (1983) Reorganization of trigeminal primary afferents following neonatal infraorbital nerve section in hamsters. Dev. Brain Res. 7:337–342.

Rhoades, R. W., G. R. Belford, and H. P. Killackey (1987a) Receptive field properties of ventral posterior medial neurons before and after selective kainic acid lesions of the trigeminal brainstem complex. J. Neurophysiol. *57:*1577–1600.

Rhoades, R. W., N. L. Chiaia, R. D. Mooney, B. G. Klein, W. E. Renehan, and M. F. Jacquin (1987b) Reorganization of the peripheral projections of the trigeminal ganglion following neonatal transection of the infraorbital nerve. Somatosen. Res. 5:35–62.

Rice, F. L. (1975) The development of the primary somatosensory cortex in the mouse. 1. A Nissl study of the ontogenesis of the barrels and the barrelfield. 2. A quantitative autoradiographic study of the time of origin and pattern. Dissertation, Johns Hopkins University, Baltimore, MD.

Rice, F. L. (1984) Neonatal facial nerve extirpations fail to produce alterations in the barrel field in the primary somatosensory cortex of mice. Brain Res. *322*:393–395.

Rice, F. L., and B. L. Munger (1986) A comparative light microscopic analysis of the sensory innervation of the mystacial pad. II. The common fur between the vibrissae. J. Comp. Neurol. *252*:186–205.

Rice, F. L., and H. Van der Loos (1977) Development of the barrels and barrel field in the somatosensory cortex of the mouse. J. Comp. Neurol. *171*:545–560.

Rice, F. L., A. Mance, and B. L. Munger (1986) A comparative light microscopic analysis of the sensory innervation of the mystacial pad. I. Innervation of vibrissal follicle-sinus complexes. J. Comp. Neurol. *252*:154–174.

Riley, C. M., and R. H. Moore (1966) Familial dysautonomia differentiated from related disorders. Case reports and discussions of current concepts. Pediatrics *37*:435–446.

Robertson, R. T. (1987) A morphogenic role for transiently expressed acetylcholinesterase in developing thalamocortical systems. Neurosci. Lett. *75*:259–264.

Ryugo, D. K., R. Ryugo, and H. P. Killackey (1975) Changes in pyramidal cell spine density consequent to vibrissae removal in newborn rat. Brain Res. *96*:82–87.

Sanderson, K. J., W. Welker, and G. M. Shambes (1984) Reevaluation of motor cortex and of sensorimotor overlap in cerebral cortex of albino rats. Brain Res. *292*:251–260.

Saporta, S., and L. Kruger (1977) The organization of thalamocortical relay neurons in the rat ventrobasal complex studied by the retrograde transport of horseradish peroxidase. J. Comp. Neurol. *174*:187–208.

Savy, C., S. Margules, C. Farkas-Bargeton, and R. Verley (1981) A morphometric study of mouse trigeminal ganglion after unilateral destruction of vibrissae follicles at birth. Brain Res. *217*:265–277.

Scheibel, M. E., A. B. Scheibel, and T. H. Davies (1972) Some substrates for centrifugal control over thalamic cell ensembles. In T. Frigyesi, E. Rinvik, and M. D. Yahr (eds.): Corticothalamic Projections and Sensorimotor Activities. New York: Raven Press, pp. 131–160.

Senft, S. L. (1986) The barrels of somatosensory cortex are dirichlet domains. Soc. Neurosci. Abstr. *12*:1433.

Senft, S. L. (1989) Development of mouse somatosensory cortex: Anatomical and mathematical descriptions and analyses. Dissertation, Washington University, St. Louis, MO.

Senft, S. L., and T. A. Woolsey (1987) Development of afferents to mouse somatosensory cortex. Soc. Neurosci. Abstr. *13*:308.

Seo, M. L., and M. Ito (1987) Reorganization of rat vibrissa barrelfield as studied by cortical lesioning on different postnatal days. Exp. Brain Res. *65*:251–260.

Sidman, R. L., M. C. Green, and S. H. Appel (1965) Catalog of the Neurological Mutants of the Mouse. Cambridge, MA: Harvard University Press.

Sikich, L., T. A. Woolsey, and E. M. Johnson (1986) Effect of a uniform partial denervation of the periphery on the peripheral and central vibrissal system in guinea pigs. J. Neurosci. *6*:1227–1240.

Simons, D. J. (1978) Response properties of vibrissa units in rat SI somatosensory neocortex. J. Neurophysiol. *41*:798–820.

Simons, D. J. (1983) Multi-whisker stimulation and its effects on vibrissa units on rat SmI barrel cortex. Brain Res. *276*:178–183.

Simons, D. J. (1985) Temporal and spatial integration in the rat SI vibrissa cortex. J. Neurophysiol. *54*:615–635.

Simons, D. J., and P. W. Land (1987) Early experience of tactile stimulation influences organization of somatic sensory cortex. Nature *326*:694–697.

Simons, D. J., and T. A. Woolsey (1979) Functional organization in mouse barrel cortex. Brain Res. *165*:327–332.

Simons, D. J., and T. A. Woolsey (1984) Morphology of Golgi-Cox-impregnated barrel neurons in rat SmI cortex. J. Comp. Neurol. *230*:119–132.

Simons, D. J., D. Durham, and T. A. Woolsey (1984) Functional organization of mouse and rat SmI barrel cortex following vibrissal damage on different postnatal days. Somatosen. Res. *1*:207–245.

Smart, I. H. M. (1983) Three-dimensional growth of the mouse isocortex. J. Anat. *137*:683–694.

Sokoloff, L., M. Reivich, C. Kennedy, M. H. Des Rosiers, C. S. Patlak, K. D. Pettigrew, O. Sakurada, and U. Shinohara (1977) The [^{14}C] deoxyglucose method for the measurement of local cerebral glucose utilization: Theory, procedure, and normal values in the conscious and anesthetized albino rat. J. Neurochem. *28*:897–916.

Søreide, A. J., and F. Fonnum (1980) High-affinity uptake of D-aspartate in the barrel subfield of the mouse somatic sensory cortex. Brain Res. *201*:427–430.

Steffen, H. (1976) Golgi-stained barrel neurons in the somatosensory region of the mouse cerebral cortex. Neurosci Lett. *2*:57–59.

Steffen, H., and H. Van der Loos (1980) Early lesions of mouse vibrissal follicles: Their influence on dendrite orientation in the cortical barrelfield. Exp. Brain Res. *40*:419–431.

Steindler, D. A., and S. A. Colwell, (1976) Reeler mutant mouse: Maintenance of appropriate and reciprocal connections in the cerebral cortex and thalamus. Brain Res. *113*:386–393.

Steindler, D. A., and N. G. F. Cooper (1987) Glial and glycoconjugate boundaries during postnatal development of the central nervous system. Dev. Brain Res. *36*:27–38.

Stennett, R. A., W. E. Renehan, R. W. Rhoades, and M. F. Jacquin (1986) Neonatal deafferentation effects upon structure and function of trigeminal (V) second-order neurons. Soc. Neurosci. Abstr. *12*:543.

Sutcliffe, J. G., R. J. Milner, J. M. Gottesfeld, and W. Reynolds (1984) Control of neuronal gene expression. Science *225*:1308–1315.

Taber Pierce, E. (1973) Time of origin of neurons in the brain stem of the mouse. Prog. Brain Res. *40*:53–65.

Tessler, A., B. T. Himes, N. R. Krieger, M. Murray, and M. E. Goldberger (1985) Sciatic nerve transection produces death of dorsal root ganglion cells and reversible loss of substance P in spinal cord. Brain Res. *332*:209–218.

Valentino, K. L., T. A. Woolsey, and A. J. Wilson (1978) Cytoarchitectonic alterations in mouse cortical barrels following different patterns of early vibrissal damage. Soc. Neurosci. Abstr. *4*:480.

514   Thomas A. Woolsey

Van der Loos, H. (1976) Barreloids in mouse somatosensory thalamus. Neurosci. Lett. 2:1–6.

Van der Loos, H., and T. A. Woolsey (1973) Somatosensory cortex: Structural alterations following early injury to sense organs. Science 179:395–398.

Van der Loos, H., J. Dörfl, and E. Welker (1984) Variation in the pattern of mystacial vibrissae: A quantitative study of mice of ICR stock of several inbred stains. J. Hered. 75:326–336.

Verley, R., and H. Axelrad (1977) Functional maturation of rat trigeminal nerve. Neurosci. Lett. 5:133–139.

Verley, R., and I. Onnen (1981) Somatotopic organization of the tactile thalamus in normal adult and developing mice and in adult mice dewhiskered since birth. Exp. Neurol. 72:462–474.

Vongdokmai, R. (1980) Effect of protein malnutrition on development of mouse cortical barrels. J. Comp. Neurol. 191:283–294.

Waite, P. M. E. (1973) Somatotopic organization of vibrissal responses in the ventrobasal complex of the rat thalamus. J. Physiol. 228:527–540.

Waite, P. M. E. (1984) Rearrangement of neuronal responses in the trigeminal system of the rat following peripheral nerve section. J. Physiol. 352:425–445.

Waite, P. M. E., and B. G. Cragg (1979) The effect of destroying the whisker follicles in mice on the sensory nerve, the thalamocortical radiation and cortical barrel development. Proc. Roy. Soc. (Lond.) B 204:41–55.

Waite, P. M. E., and B. G. Cragg (1982) The peripheral and central changes resulting from cutting or crushing the afferent nerve supply to the whiskers. Proc. Roy. Soc. (Lond.) B 214:191–211.

Waite, P. M. E., and P. K. Taylor (1978) Removal of whiskers in young rats causes functional changes in cerebral cortex. Nature 274:600–602.

Wall, P. D., M. Fitzgerald, J. C. Nussbaumer, H. Van der Loos, and M. Devor (1982) Somatotopic maps are disorganized in adult rodents treated neonatally with capsaicin. Nature 295:691–693.

Wallace, M. N. (1983) Organization of the mouse cerebral cortex: A histochemical study using glycogen phosphorylase. Brain Res. 267:201–216.

Welker, C. (1976) Receptive fields of barrels in the somatosensory neocortex of the rat. J. Comp. Neurol. 166:173–190.

Welker, E. (1985) Brain maps and patterns of sensory organs. A genetical and experimental analysis of the whisker-to-barrel pathway in mice (Mus musculus). Dissertation, University of Amsterdam, Amsterdam, The Netherlands.

Welker, E., and H. Van der Loos (1986) Quantitative correlation between barrel-field size and the sensory innervation of the whiskerpad: A comparative study in six strains of mice bred for different patterns of mystacial vibrissae. J. Neurosci. 6:3355–3373.

Welker, W. I. (1964) Analysis of sniffing in the albino rat. Behaviour 22:223–244.

Welker, W. I., and S. Seidenstein (1959) Somatic sensory representation in the cerebral cortex of the raccoon (Procyon lotor). J. Comp. Neurol. 111:469–502.

Welker, W. I., K. J. Sanderson, and G. M. Shambes (1984) Patterns of afferent projections to transitional zones in the somatic sensorimotor cerebral cortex of albino rats. Brain Res. 292:261–267.

Weller, W. L. (1972) Barrels in somatic sensory neocortex of the marsupial *Tricho-surus vulpecula* (brush-tailed possum). Brain Res. *43*:11–24.

Weller, W. L., and J. I. Johnson (1975) Barrels in cerebral cortex altered by receptor disruption in newborn, but not in five-day-old mice *Cricetidae* and *Muridae*. Brain Res. *83*:504–508.

White, E. L. (1976) Ultrastructure and synaptic contents in barrels of mouse SI cortex. Brain Res. *105*:229–252.

White, E. L. (1979) Thalamocortical synaptic relations: A review with emphasis on the projection of specific thalamic nuclei to the primary sensory areas of the neocortex. Brain Res. Rev. *1*:275–311.

Wise, S. P., and E. G. Jones (1976) Organization and postnatal development of commissural projection of rat somatic sensory cortex. J. Comp. Neurol. *168*:313–344.

Wise, S. P., and E. G. Jones (1978) Developmental studies of thalamocortical and commissural connections in the rat somatic sensory cortex. J. Comp. Neurol. *178*:187–208.

Wong-Riley, M. T. T., and D. A. Riley (1983) The effect of impulse blockage on cytochrome oxidase activity in the cat visual system. Brain Res. *261*:185–193.

Wong-Riley, M. T. T., and C. Welt (1980) Histochemical changes in cytochrome oxidase of cortical barrels after vibrissal removal in neonatal and adult mice. Proc. Natl. Acad. Sci. USA *77*:2333–2337.

Woolsey, T. A. (1967) Somatosensory, auditory and visual cortical areas in the mouse. Johns Hopkins Med. J. *121*:91–112.

Woolsey, T. A. (1972) Organization of corticothalamic projections in the mouse. Anat. Rec. *172*:429.

Woolsey, T. A. (1978a) Lesion experiments: Some anatomical considerations. In S. Finger (ed.): Recovery from Brain Damage: Research and Theory. New York: Plenum Press, pp. 71–89.

Woolsey, T. A. (1978b) Some anatomical bases of cortical somatotopic organization. Brain Behav. Evol. *15*:325–371.

Woolsey, T. A. (1987) Structural, functional and biochemical plasticity in the rodent brain. In C. Chagas, R. Lent, and R. Linden (eds.): Developmental Neurobiology of Mammals. Vatican City: Pontifica Academia Scientiarum, pp. 347–380.

Woolsey, T. A., and M. L. Dierker (1981) Morphometric approaches to neuro-anatomy with emphasis on computer-assisted techniques. In S. L. Palay and V. Chan-Palay (eds.): Cytochemical Methods in Neuroanatomy. New York: Alan R. Liss, pp. 69–91.

Woolsey, T. A., and H. Van der Loos (1970) The structural organization of layer IV in the somatosensory regin (SI) of the mouse cerebral cortex. Brain Res. *17*:205–242.

Woolsey, T. A., and J. R. Wann (1976) Areal changes in mouse cortical barrels following vibrissal damage at different postnatal ages. J. Comp. Neurol. *170*:53–66.

Woolsey, T. A., M. L. Dierker, and D. F. Wann (1975a) Mouse SmI cortex: Qualita-tive and quantitative classification of Golgi-impregnated barrel neurons. Proc. Natl. Acad. Sci. USA *72*:2165–2169.

Woolsey, T. A., C. Welker, and R. Schwartz (1975b) Comparative anatomical studies of the SmI face cortex with special reference to the occurrence of "barrels" in layer IV. J. Comp. Neurol. *164*:79–94.

Woolsey, T. A., J. R. Anderson, J. R. Wann, and B. B. Stanfield (1979) Effects of early vibrissae damage on neurons in the ventrobasal (VB) thalamus of the mouse. J. Comp. Neurol. *184*:363–380.

Woolsey, T. A., D. Durham, R. M. Harris, D. J. Simons, and K. L. Valentino (1981) Somatosensory development. In R. N. Aslin, J. R. Alberts, and M. R. Peterson (eds.): The Development of Perception, Vol. 1. New York: Academic Press, pp. 259–292.

Yamakado, M., and T. Yohro (1979) Subdivision of mouse vibrissae on an embryological basis, with descriptions of variations in the number and arrangement of sinus hairs and cortical barrels in BALB/C (nu/+), nude (nu, nu) and hairless (hr/hr) strains. Amer. J. Anat. *155*:153–174.

Yip, H. K., K. M. Rich, P. A. Lampe, and E. M. Johnson (1984) The effects of nerve growth factor and its antiserum on the postnatal development and survival after injury of sensory neurons in rat dorsal root ganglia. J. Neurosci. *4*:2986–2992.

Yip, V. S., W.-P. Zhang, T. A. Woolsey, and O. H. Lowry (1987) Quantitative histochemical and microchemical changes in the adult mouse central nervous system after section of the infraorbital and optic nerve. Brain Res. *406*:157–170.

Yun, J. T., M. M. Merzenich, and T. Woodruff (1987) Alteration of functional representations of vibrissae in the barrel field of adult rats. Soc. Neurosci. Abstr. *13*:1596.

Zucker, E., and W. I. Welker (1969) Coding of somatic sensory input by vibrissae neurons in the rat's trigeminal ganglion. Brain Res. *12*:138–156.

Part Five

THE CHEMICAL SENSES

Chapter Thirteen

OLFACTORY DEVELOPMENT

PASQUALE P. GRAZIADEI

Florida State University
Tallahassee, Florida

I INTRODUCTION

The behavior of our everyday life is regulated by visual, auditory, and somatosensory cues. We rise at the sound of an alarm clock or to the protestations of our mate, we visually control the time on our watch, and we change from our sleeping position to the activity of the day by means of various somatosensory cues. We would be most surprised, however, to learn that chemical cues are also essential in modulating our behavior and play a major role in our welfare. From a social point of view blindness and

519

deafness are well-recognized medical problems while anosmia and ageusia, if and when these terms are properly interpreted, stimulate curiosity at best; the belief is common that they are not deficits of grave social concern and they are rare! This belief is compounded by the assumption that the olfactory system is a rather primitive one, although it is difficult to meaningfully define "primitive" in a phylogenetic context.

In this chapter we will describe the vertebrate olfactory system, its origin, development, and structure, and the role it plays in early development and maturation of the brain. Because of the current state of knowledge, functional and behavioral aspects will not be dealt with here in much detail; however, early development of olfactory function will be discussed in relation to its role in establishment of precocious behavioral patterns that may have as yet unsuspected but profound effects on the subsequent life-style of the individual. Some emphasis will be placed on the unique characteristics of this system, such as the presence of peripheral, intraepithelial receptor neurons that have a homolateral projection to cerebral cortex without an intervening thalamic way station and on the disposable nature of these sensory neurons. In spite of these uncommon properties, however, several analogies can be established between the olfactory system and other portions of our nervous system, making this part of the central nervous system (CNS) a suitable model for the study of basic neurological problems.

II ANATOMICAL OVERVIEW OF THE OLFACTORY SYSTEM

A Chemoreceptive Apparatus

The peripheral aspect of the olfactory system, the olfactory organ, is deceptively simple in its histological organization, and it is quite unique in the arrangement of its sensory neurons (Allison, 1953; Andres, 1969). The sensory organ is composed of a sensory sheet that lines a portion of the nasal cavities. The configuration of the nasal cavities has different complexity and development in the five vertebrate classes (Parsons, 1971). The neuropithelium, commonly described as pseudostratified, is composed of the sensory neurons, whose axons exit the epithelium to reach the brain, the supporting cells, and the basal cells. Glands specific to the sensory area (the Bowmann's glands) open their duct at the epithelial surface and have their secretory portion (the acini) in the lamina propria. The olfactory epithelium contains well-demonstrated free nerve endings. Discovered by von Brunn in 1882, these free nerve endings are of trigeminal origin (Graziadei and Gagne, 1973) and have been shown to respond not only to mechanical stimuli but also to odors (Tucker, 1971).

The olfactory mucosa lacks a distinct submucosa, and the lamina propria (a layer of loose fibrillar connective tissue, richly vascularized) rests directly on the periostium that covers the bone and cartilage skeleton of the nasal cavities. There are three poorly defined nuclear layers in the sensory epithelium; from the free surface they correspond to the supporting cells, the neurons, and the basal cells (Figure 1).

The supporting cells are typical epithelial secretory elements; their free surface is covered with microvilli but not cilia. The distal portion of the cell is cylindrical and contains the nucleus and cytoplasm; most obviously in lower vertebrates, it shows granules of secretion (Figure 2). The process of exocytosis is dramatized during odor stimulation (Graziadei, 1971a, 1973a). Near the surface each supporting cell shows a junctional complex as observed in other covering epithelia (Graziadei, 1971a). Desmosome attachments are common between neighboring supporting cells, and emidesmosomes are a common feature between the basal portion of these cells and the epithelial basal lamina. The perinuclear portion of the cells is packed with cysternae of the rough and smooth endoplasmic reticulum (Graziadei, 1971a, 1973a). The Golgi complex has a typical perinuclear position. Under the nucleus, namely in the midsection of the epithelium where the perikarya of the neurons are located, the cytoplasm of the supporting cells is laminar or columnar and extends invariably to the basal lamina with one or more processes. The relationship between the olfactory neurons and supporting cells has been extensively studied (Graziadei, 1971b, 1973a; Graziadei and Monti Graziadei, 1979; Rafols and Getchell, 1983) and appears to have functional significance. Under the nucleus the cytoplasm of the supporting cells shows fewer organelles; bundles of filaments extend from the desmosomes, but mitochondria, endoplasmic reticulum, and Golgi profiles are usually sparse. The secretory function of the supporting cells and its putative role in olfactory transduction has been the subject of recent research (Getchell et al., 1984a,b; Getchell, 1977, 1986).

The olfactory neurons are flask-shaped, bipolar elements with a slender, unbranched dendrite reaching the epithelial surface where it protrudes with a ball-like swelling called the olfactory vesicle. The vesicle bears a variable number of cilia some 50–150 μm long. The cilia have an unsynchronous beat that is noticeable only in the proximal portion of the ciliary shaft. The cilia have the classic 9 + 2 set of tubules and a basal body with basal feet or rootlets, at least in mammals. In birds and cold-blooded animals, however, these structures have been reported together with microvilli on the surface of the olfactory vesicle (Graziadei and Bannister, 1967; Graziadei, 1971a, 1973a). Microvilli on the olfactory vesicle are estimated to increase the free surface of the olfactory vesicle in excess of one thousand times when present (Graziadei and Bannister, 1967). The long, often tortuous dendrite of these neurons has prominent tubules and mitochondria; the dendrite often appears in grooves of the supporting cells (Graziadei and Monti Graziadei, 1976, 1979). The diameter of the dendrite is in the range of 2 μm, and the vesicle averages 3 μm. The egg-shaped perikaryon has a diameter of some 8 μm, at least in mammals. The round nucleus occupies most of the perikaryon volume; its chromatin pattern has characteristics

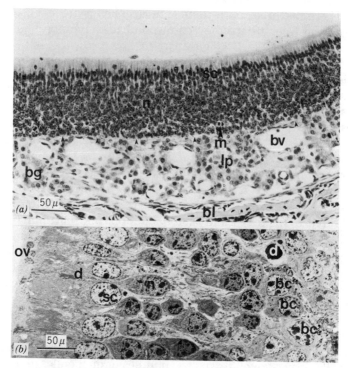

FIGURE 1. (*A*) Normal olfactory epithelium from a 10-day-old mouse stained with Gill's hematoxylin. The base of the epithelium (arrowheads) rests on a loose connective lamina propria (lp) where blood vessels (bv) and the bodies of the Bowmann's glands (bg) are prominent. The lamina propria is in direct contact with the bone lamellae (bl) of the nasal skeleton, without an intervening submucosa. In the epithelium we can distinguish a rather discrete superficial layer of nuclei belonging to the supporting cells (sc). The neuronal layer (n) and the layer of basal cells (bc) do not have a clear boundary. Among the basal cells, however, there are sparse mitotic figures (m) that testify to the ongoing process of neurogenesis occurring in the postnatal period. Mark = 50μm (*B*) Low-power TEM of the mouse olfactory epithelium. At ultrastructural level more details are visible than in (*A*). The supporting cell nuclei (sc) are morphologically different from the nuclei of the neuronal population and more homogeneous in their overall chromatin pattern. On the left of the figure the epithelial surface is covered by the microvilli of the supporting cells and the olfactory vesicles (ov) of the neurons are clearly visible. The mature neurons (n) show an apical dendrite (d) and their flask-shaped perikaryon, even in this low-power picture, shows some rER (rough endoplasmic reticulum) profiles. Toward the base of the epithelium (on the right of the figure) the basal cells have a more varied morphology depending upon the maturation stage. For example, note differences between bc' and bc''. A degenerating element is indicated at (d). Mark = 10μm.

that allow easy differentiation from nuclei of the supporting cells independent of the topographic position in the epithelium. The perinuclear organelles are mitochondria, tubules, free ribosomes, and Golgi profiles (Figure 3).

The rough endoplasmic reticulum is at times conspicuous, but it is never arranged as classic Nissl bodies at the LM level. At the deep pole of the

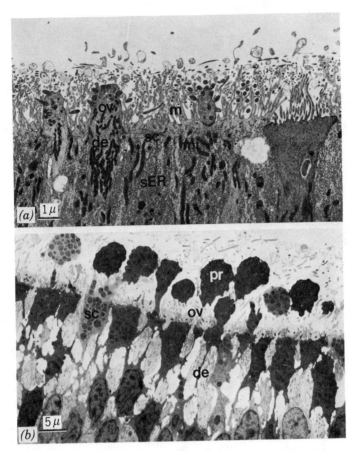

FIGURE 2. (A) Electron micrograph of the surface of the olfactory epithelium from an adult mouse. It shows the microvilli (m) of the supporting cells (sc); mitochondria (mi) and sER (smooth endoplasmic reticulum) fill the distal portion of the cytoplasm of these cells. The apical portions of the neurons' dendrites (de), the so-called olfactory vesicles (ov) protrude from the surface. Mark = 1μm (B) Electron micrograph of the surface of frog olfactory epithelium (*Rana viridis*), fixed while the animal was stimulated with high concentrations of odors. The supporting cells show clublike protrusions (pr) at the free surface that eventually free themselves in the mucous layer covering the epithelium, becoming part of the complex secretion. Olfactory neuron dendrites are also visible with their slightly protruding olfactory vesicles. The phenomenon of secretion with sloughing off of portions of the supporting cell cytoplasm is obvious in many animals and is well documented (see text and Graziadei 1971a). Mark = 5μm.

perikaryon a slender axon exits and soon fasciculates into the epithelium forming small bundles along the basal lamina. Once exiting from the epithelium, these bundles are enclosed in large pockets of the sheat cells (Figure 4); up to several axons can be contained in these pockets (Gasser, 1956, 1958; Graziadei, 1973a).

The basal cells are a morphologically nonhomogeneous population due to the presence of many intermediate stages of differentiation among them

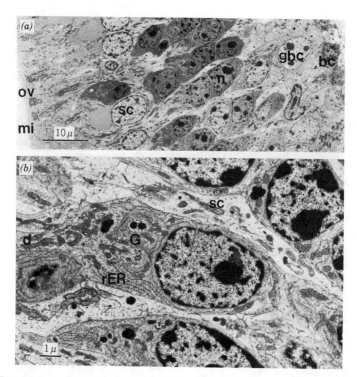

FIGURE 3. (*A*) Low-power electron micrograph of the olfactory epithelium of mouse. The supporting cell nuclei (sc) have a very homogeneous chromatin pattern, well recognizable from the pattern of the mature and immature neuron nuclei (n). The neurons, even in this thin section, show some sign of columnar arrangement that becomes especially evident when serial section studies are performed. In the basal cell compartment there are small, rather electron-dense basal cells (bc) in immediate contact with the basal lamina. Above them the globose basal cells (gbc) show intermediate morphology with mature neurons. The surface is covered by microvilli (m) and the olfactory vesicles (ov). Mark = 10μm (*B*) Detail of two neurons from mouse olfactory epithelium showing a complex Golgi apparatus (G) and rER in the cytoplasm. The emerging dendrite (d) of one neuron will eventually reach the free surface (not shown). The profiles of the supporting cells, which appear among the neurons in the neuronal layer of the epithelium show a laminar outline with characteristic paucity of organelles in contrast to their perinuclear and supranuclear portions (see Figure 2A). Mark = 1μm.

(Graziadei and Monti Graziadei, 1978a,b, 1979). These cells, at least in adult animals, develop into neurons and are not the precursors of the supporting cells; the latter divide *in situ* in the upper third of the epithelium (Graziadei and Monti Graziadei, 1978a, 1979). Among the basal cells the smaller elements are in direct contact with the basal lamina; they have an irregularly shaped nucleus and an electron-dense cytoplasm rich in free ribosomes and epitheliofibrillas. Desmosomes and emidesmosomes are common features among the basal cells and between these basal cells and the epithelial basal lamina (Schwartz et al., 1989). Not necessarily in contact with the basal

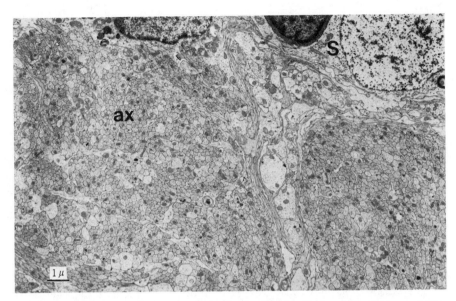

FIGURE 4. Bundles of olfactory axons in the fiber layer of the olfactory bulb of a mouse. In this low-power electron micrograph the small olfactory axons (ax) which average from 0.2 to 0.4μm in diameter, are enclosed in large pockets of the sheath cells (S) with their axolemma in direct contact. Mark = 1μm.

lamina and just above the already described basal cells there are other elements whose cytoplasm is less electron dense, usually lacking bundles of filaments and only sparse desmosomes. The cytoplasm of these cells is characteristically electron clear and filled with free ribosomes. Golgi, mitochondria, and endoplasmic reticulum profiles are not conspicuous and often sparse. These cells increase in number, characteristically, during the phases of regeneration that follow experimental degeneration of the neurons (Graziadei and Monti Graziadei, 1978a,b, 1979; Monti Graziadei and Graziadei, 1979a,b). They have been called *globose basal cells* and are the immediate precursors of the neurons (Graziadei and Monti Graziadei, 1979). Transitional forms exist between the globose basal cells and the basal cells proper and neurons; however, the dynamic relationships between the basal cells proper and the globose basal cells are still not fully understood (Metcalf, 1973; Graziadei and Monti Graziadei, 1978a,b; 1979). Some globose basal cells show a growing dendrite and, from their proximal pole, an emerging axon. It is important to note that the layer of basal and globose basal cells does not have a homogeneous thickness. In some regions it is represented by few elements; in others it is formed by many layers of cells. The regions where the basal and globose cells are sparse and the neuronal layer composed mostly of mature neurons have been termed "quiescent" to indicate a reduced neurogenetic activity. The zones where basal and globose basal cells are numerous have been termed "active" to indicate the intense neurogenetic process leading to the replacement of senescent neurons (Graziadei and Monti Graziadei, 1979).

Present in the olfactory epithelium are also the tubular excretory portions of the glands of Bowmann. These glands, characteristic of the sensory area only, release an abundant, viscous product on the epithelial surface where it mixes with the product of secretion of the supporting cells. These glandular elements and their product have been studied (Bannister, 1974), and the role that these structures and products play in the phenomenon of olfactory perception and transduction seems to be significant (Pelosi and Pisanelli, 1981; Pelosi et al., 1982; Getchell et al., 1984a,b; Bignetti et al., 1985; Pevzner et al., 1985, 1986; Getchell, 1986).

In the olfactory epithelium there are, however sparse in number, other morphological elements that need to be recognized. Some degenerating neurons occur even in the normal epithelium due to their constant turnover. These degenerating cells can be recognized by a picnotic nucleus and vacuolar cytoplasm. Other elements are migrating cells of the connective tissue such as plasma cells, granulocytes, and lymphocytes. True macrophages can be observed during experimental or pathological degeneration of the neurons (Monti Graziadei and Graziadei, 1979a).

In mammals the vomeronasal organ is located in a tubular cavity in the septal area; this organ can also appear as an exposed patch of sensory epithelium in the nasal cavity of some reptiles (Graziadei and Tucker, 1970; Graziadei, 1971a, 1977). The organ is present through vertebrates with the exception of fish and birds. In humans it is rudimentary in the adult but it is present during intrauterine life. The vomeronasal epithelium contains the vomeronasal sensory neurons similar to the olfactory neurons proper; however, they lack cilia. The epithelium as a whole has many analogies with the olfactory epithelium, and it has been described at both light and electron microscope levels by a number of authors (Graziadei and Tucker, 1970; Graziadei, 1971a, 1977; Barber and Raisman, 1978a,b; Wang and Halpern, 1982a,b).

B   Central Pathways

The sensory olfactory sheet sends an exclusively homolateral projection of its sensory axons to an area of the paleocortex called the olfactory bulb. In fact, an italian anatomist, Antonio Scarpa (1785), was the first to clearly prepare and anatomically demonstrate with new, fine dissecting techniques the olfactory nerves (fila olfactoria) in humans which originate intracranially in the olfactory bulb; after passing through the lamina cribrosa, these fibers spread in a fine plexus in the "membrana pituitaria", commonly known as the olfactory neuroepithelium of the nasal cavities (Figure 5). More recently, evidence from anatomical and electrophysiological studies shows a topographical organization for this projection (Clark and Warwick, 1946; Adrian, 1950, 1951; Land et al., 1970; Land, 1973; Land and Shepherd, 1974;

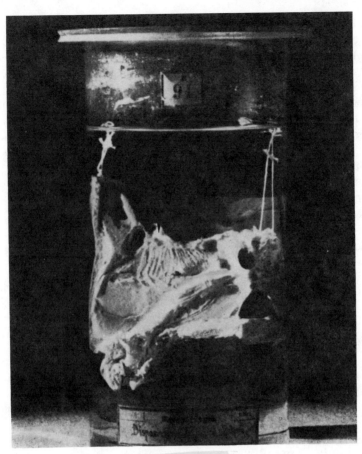

SCARPA

FIGURE 5. Photograph of an original preparation by Antonio Scarpa, now preserved in the Museo per la Storia della Universita di Pavia. It is in the medical school of this university that Scarpa taught as head of the anatomy section and made important contributions to the study of the olfactory and other cranial nerves. This preparation from a human head macroscopically shows the olfactory bulb (arrowhead) and the olfactory nerves that spread in the "membrane pituitaria" the present olfactory mucosa. This specimen was prepared in 1782 as part of a study later presented to the Societé Royal de Medicine in Paris with the approval and under the auspices of Felix Vicq d'Azyr (1748–1794).

Costanzo and Mozell, 1976; Moulton, 1976; Costanzo and O'Connell, 1978, 1980; Jourdan et al., 1980; Kauer, 1981, 1987; Jastreboff et al., 1984; MacKay-Sim and Nathan, 1984; Benson et al., 1985; Clancy et al., 1985; Stewart et al., 1985; Astic and Saucier, 1986; Pedersen et al., 1986; Saucier and Astic, 1986). These studies suggest that a well-established pattern of projections is determinant for odor discrimination. Experimental data support the concept that single glomeruli receive their input from discrete areas of the peripheral epithelium (Graziadei and Monti Graziadei, 1986b). The bulbar area is represented in lower vertebrates and in macroosmatic animals by a large portion of the frontal telencephalon (Papez, 1967). The olfactory bulb, however, can have unconspicuous dimensions, as in humans, where it appears as a small, peduncolate lobe. The peduncle, called the olfactory tract, connects the bulb to the area perforata anterior. The sensory olfactory axons travel unbranched in the fila olfactoria (the olfactory nerve of lower vertebrates) and terminate in the glomerular layer of the olfactory bulb, where they establish synaptic contacts with the apical dendrites of the mitral and tufted cells. These cells are large, typical cortical neurons homologous to the pyramidal cells of other cortical areas.

In the olfactory bulb we can distinguish six discrete morphological layers (Golgi, 1875; Ramon y Cajal, 1955; see Figure 6). From the external surface we have (1) the olfactory nerve layer; (2) the glomerular layer; (3) the external plexiform layer; (4) the mitral cell layer; (5) the internal plexiform layer; and (6) the granule cell layer. The granule cell layer surrounds the ependymal zone and cavity, a remnant of the rostral portion of the frontal projection of the lateral ventricle (Figures 7 and 8A).

The accessory olfactory bulb, the central station where the vomeronasal sensory fibers terminate, is structurally similar to the main olfactory bulb, although its layers are not as recognizable.

The neurons of the olfactory bulb belong to two main categories: (1) output neurons and (b) interneurons. The output neurons connect the olfactory bulb to the more central cortical stations of the telencephalon; the interneurons are all intrinsic to the olfactory bulb and are typical Golgi type II small neurons. Of the output neurons the mitral cells are arranged in a discrete layer that bears their name. They are the larger neurons of the olfactory bulb (Figure 8B). The tufted cells were subdivided by Ramón y Cajal (1955) into at least three categories based on the location of their perikarya in the bulb. The external tufted cells are located close to the glomeruli, mostly in the periglomerular region. The middle tufted cells are found in the outer third of the external plexiform layer, and the internal tufted cells are close to the layer of mitral cell bodies. The topographical location of these cells also correlates with differences in the spatial organization of their dendrites: the internal tufted cells have more numerous sec-

---

FIGURE 6. Reproduction of the original illustration of the work of Camillo Golgi in 1875 on the structure of the olfactory bulb. Golgi himself drafted this figure from material prepared with the newly discovered silver bichromate impregnation method. His characteristically meticulous hand illustrates the cellular and fibrous components of the olfactory bulb of a dog. In (A) the fibrous layer with the sensory axons originates from the sensory neurons of the olfactory mucosa. In (B) there are clearly delineated glomeruli in which sensory axon terminals contribute to the tangle, as do branches of mitral cells, tufted cell dendrites, and the dendrites of periglomerular cells. The mitral cell layer along with granule cells, is clearly represented in (C). This illustration demonstrates the power of the "Golgi" method for study of the nervous system and the painstaking accuracy of the old master. (Reproduced from Golgi, 1875.)

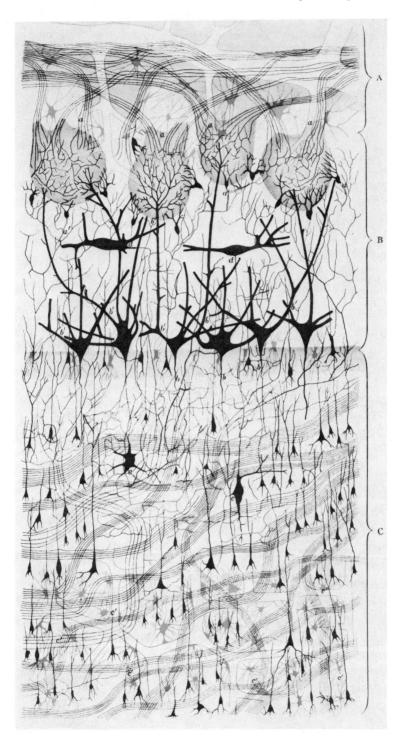

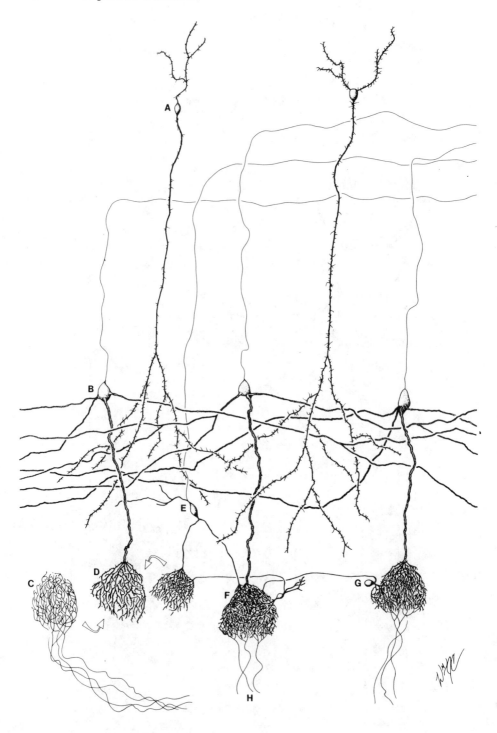

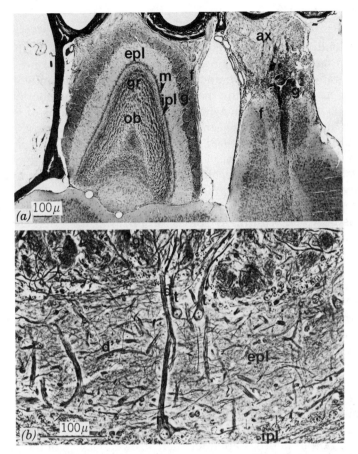

FIGURE 8. (*A*) Horizontal section through the anterior portion of the cranium of an adult mouse. The animal was totally bulbectomized unilaterally (on the right) and sacrificed 30 days after surgery. On the left side of the picture the unoperated olfactory bulb (ob) serves as an internal control and clearly illustrates the layered structure of the olfactory bulb in a rodent: f, nerve fiber layer; g, glomerular layer; epl, external plexiform layer; m, mitral cell layer; ipl, internal plexiform layer; gr, granule cell layer. On the right side, where the olfactory bulb was totally removed, the spared forebrain has extended forward (f) and the olfactory axons (ax) have reached the brain forming ectopic glomeruli (g). See also Figure 15. Mark = 100μm. (*B*) Silver preparation of a segment of the olfactory bulb of a mouse. The olfactory glomeruli (gl) receive the branching dendrites (d) of both the mitral cells (m) and the tufted cells (t). The external plexiform layer (epl) is formed by the lateral dendrites (d') of the mitral cells and by the granule cell processes (see Figure 7); the latter are not specifically impregnated with this method. Below the mitral cell layer there is a portion of the internal plexiform layer (ipl). Mark = 100μm.

FIGURE 7. Simplified diagram of the major components of the olfactory bulb. The glomeruli shown at the bottom of the figure are largely formed by the terminations of the sensory olfactory axons (C, H) and dendrites of the mitral cells (D; soma at B); other contributions from dendrites of tufted (E) and periglomerular (G) cells convey further complexity to the glomerulus as in F. The granule cells (A), which are typical amacrine cells, mediate interdendritic contacts between mitral cell lateral dendrites. Diagram inverted relative to drawing of Golgi shown in Figure 6.

ondary dendrites extending tangentially in the deep portion of the external plexiform layer, while the more external tufted cells have no secondary dendrites and the primary branches are located predominantly in one glomerulus. Centrally, the internal tufted cells have the more extensive projections, which are somewhat similar to the projections of mitral cells (Haberly and Price, 1977; Skeen and Hall, 1977; Macrides and Schneider, 1982; Macrides and Davis, 1983). The interneurons of the olfactory bulb are divided into several categories based on morphological and immunohisto-chemical features. All of the latter neurons are, obviously, intrinsic to the olfactory bulb circuitry. The granule cells are *amacrine* interneurons, which characteristically lack an identifiable axon. The dendrite of this cell class, which is provided with many spines, arborizes in the external plexiform layer where it mediates dendro-dendritic interactions between the large, secondary dendrites of the mitral cells (Rall et al., 1966). The periglomerular cells have their cell bodies located, as the name implies, around the glomerular neuropil. They contact the large output neurons by dendro-dendritic and axo-dendritic synapses in, respectively, the glomerular and external plexiform layers (Macrides and Davis, 1983). Other bulbar neurons are the Blanes and Golgi cells located in the granule cell, internal plexiform, and mitral cell layers. They seem to form axo-somatic and axo-dendritic synapses onto granule cells and short-axon cells in the deep layer of the granule cells. Other short-axon neurons are the Cajal cells located in the internal plexiform and mitral cell layers and the van Gehuchten cells of the internal plexiform, mitral cell, and the external plexiform layers. From the brief description of the neurons intrinsic to the bulb it can be seen that the major output neurons are integrated at several layers of their dendritic tree, and their integration often extends over wide regions of the bulbar cortex.

The main and accessory bulbs send mostly homolateral projections to more central portions of the telencephalon. These two systems have apparent similarity and complementarity of function but do not have overlapping central projections; as a result they provide an anatomical substrate for true dual olfactory processing (Raisman, 1972; Broadwell, 1975; Scalia and Winans, 1975, 1976; Davis et al., 1978). The main olfactory bulb projects through the lateral olfactory tract to all parts of the anterior olfactory nucleus, the olfactory tubercle, the piriform cortex, and the entorhinal area. From these centers other projections reach the amygdala and hypothalamus, various areas of the neocortex, the septum, and the diagonal band (Powell et al., 1965; Scalia, 1968; Davis et al., 1978; Scott et al., 1980; Kosel et al., 1981; Shammah-Lagnado and Negrao, 1981; Macrides et al., 1981, 1985; Scott, 1986). Commissural systems involve connections through the anterior olfactory nucleus from the contralateral bulb as well as those between piriform areas (Singh, 1977; Friedman and Price, 1984). In contrast to the widespread projections of the main olfactory bulb, projections of the accessory olfactory bulb are limited to the amygdaloid region, specifically to a small region of the amygdala termed the "bed nucleus" (Smith, 1935; Broadwell, 1975, 1977; Heimer, 1976; Turner et al., 1977).

Efferent systems to the olfactory bulb are represented by an abundant series of fiber systems that originate in the piriform cortex, hypothalamus–preoptic area, anterior olfactory nucleus, olfactory tubercle, locus coeruleus, and raphe (Price and Powell, 1970; Shipley, 1985; Shiply et al., 1985; Switzer et al., 1985).

The complexity of the olfactory central pathways is not completely understood at present and markedly contrasts with the apparent simplicity of the sensory organ (Figure 9). Indeed, the olfactory message is directly or indirectly transmitted to many CNS sites which clearly underscores the profound but partly ignored complexity of olfactory input on our behavior (Takagi, 1986).

III   DEVELOPMENT OF PERIPHERAL OLFACTORY STRUCTURES

A   Embryology

The anlage of the olfactory organ is determined at very early stages, from early gastrula to neurula; it is consequently determined before many other head structures (Carpenter, 1937). Several embryonic tissue layers have been implicated in the induction of the placode (Yntema, 1955; Haggis, 1956; Reyer, 1962; Jacobson, 1963a,b,c). The mesoderm of the archenteron,

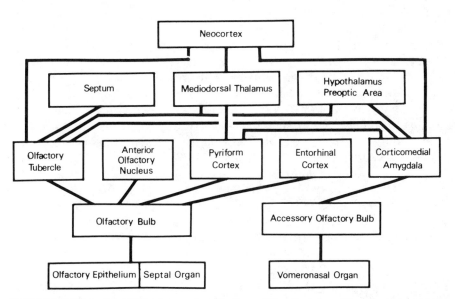

FIGURE 9. Highly simplified scheme of connections of the olfactory and vomeronasal organs and central neural structures.

the pharyngeal entoderm, and the ectoderm of the prospective neural plate seem to play some role either alone or in a complementary way in the development of the olfactory organ. These early studies, mainly based on technically demanding tissue transplantation experiments, have yielded doubtful results. They require cautious interpretation and confirmation with the implementation of more modern approaches such as the use of biological markers (Le Douarin, 1982; Thiebaud, 1983; Kim et al., 1988).

From a morphological point of view the olfactory placode develops from a horseshoe-shaped area of the primitive ectoderm that surrounds the craniolateral aspect of the true neural plate and neural crest (Klein and Graziadei, 1983). On the cranial aspect of the horseshoe-shaped placodal crescent three structures become discrete during development: centrally there is the hypophyseal placode flanked by the paired olfactory placodes. Other placodal structures develop from what is called the placodal thickening at more lateral and caudal positions (Knouff, 1935; McEwen, 1949; Jacobson, 1959; van Oostrom and Verwoerd, 1979; Verwoerd and van Oostrom, 1979; Verwoerd et al., 1981.) It is interesting to note that at very early developmental stages, preceding the closure of the neural tube, the two olfactory placodes laterally border the median hypophyseal anlage from which they become separated later in development. The information briefly summarized in the preceding is mostly derived from studies in amphibia; however, analogous results are demostrated for mammals (van Oostrom and Verwoerd, 1979; Verwoerd and van Oostrom, 1979; Verwoerd et al., 1981).

At the time of neural tube closure the olfactory placode is, in *Xenopus laevis*, composed of two cubic cell layers, and its area shows little difference from the surrounding ectoderm. The morphological differentiation of the two layers begins in the amphibian *Xenopus* following stages 23/24 when the deeper layer shows signs of thickening. This layer is called the nervous, or sensory, layer and derives its name for being anlage to neural plate and neural crest; in the placodal area it will give rise to neural elements of the olfactory organ (Klein and Graziadei, 1983). The superficial layer is also called the epiblast, or nonneural, layer and it will, in the placodal area, give rise to the supporting cells and Bowmann's glands, both specific to the sensory receptive area. Following stages 23/24 the deep sensory layer becomes pluristratified, and the differentiation of neural elements begins. By stage 29/30 the cells of the two layers comingle, and the first olfactory cells begin to differentiate with formation of single dendrites that reach the free surface. It is not until stages 38/39 that the neuroepithelium acquires the typical characteristics of the olfactory neuroepithelium. The first axons to leave the epithelium from the differentiating olfactory cells can be seen between stages 29/30 and 32.

Information in mammals regarding the first stages of olfactory placode differentiation is sparse. In mouse the first sign of neuronal differentiation begins at E10, and the first axons leave the placode at the same time (Figure

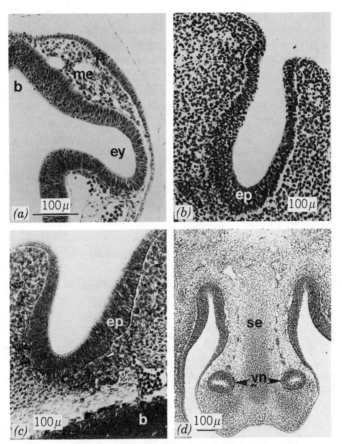

FIGURE 10. Different phases of development of the olfactory organ in mouse from E9 (embryonic day 9) to E12. (A) At 9 days the olfactory placode (p) is evident only as a thickening of the primitive ectoderm. The placode is separated from the primitive brain vesicle (b) by loose mesenchymatic tissue (me). The eye primordium (ey) appears as an extroflexion of the primitive prosencephalic vesicle. At E10 (B) and Ell (C) the placode invaginates forming the primitive nasal cavities and the epithelium becomes thicker and more complex (ep). A few nerve fibers originate from the developing sensory neurons at stages E10 and E11 as indicated by arrowheads. (D) at E12 the primitive nasal septum (se) is formed and the two nasal cavities invaginate further. In the septum notice that two tubular structures are recognized as the primitive vomeronasal organs (vn). The nasal cavities at this early stage (E12) lack the complexity of the turbinates that appear postnatally, as shown in Figures 11A and 12A. Marks = 250μm for (A)–(C) and 100μm for (D.)

10). They seem to reach the presumptive region of the olfactory bulb at E12 (Hinds, 1972a,b; Cuschieri and Bannister, 1975 a,b). In humans the placode begins to differentiate at the end of the first month of gestation, and its sensory fibers begin to contact the brain by the end of the second month (Bossy, 1980).

B Morphogenesis

When the sensory epithelium of the prospective olfactory organ begins to invaginate, what appears to be a dead end cavity results. Depending on the vertebrate considered, this will remain unchanged (e.g., as in fish) or it will communicate posteriorly through the coanal opening with the pharynx. In both groups of animals the cavity will eventually become complicated by a series of foldings, called "rosettes" in fish and "turbinates" in other vertebrates including mammals (Parsons, 1971). The purpose of these folds is complex and not exclusively related to the sensory function of the cavity. The increased area serves to allocate more surface to the sensory organ; however, in various animals, including mammals, it also serves to warm, humidify, and cleanse the atmospheric medium. During development the sensory area undergoes several changes in morphology, physiology, and biochemistry; these changes are directly related to sensory function. For practical purposes the studies here mentioned have been derived from experiments in rodents. However, their significance extends to other mammals and possibly to humans. During the embryonic period and for a variable time postnatally there is considerable expansion of the nasal sensory area and of its neuronal and secretory components (Monti Graziadei et al., 1980b;, Hinds and McNelly, 1977, 1979, 1981; Getchell, 1986). From a functional point of view, in their early maturative stages the olfactory neurons respond nonspecifically to a large variety of odors. Only upon more complete maturation and, presumably, connection with the olfactory bulb do these neurons become selective to specific odors. It is estimated that specificity first appears around the perinatal period, at least in rat (Gesteland et al., 1980, 1982). In fact, peripheral neurons seem to undergo two specific developmental processes; one when they become generally excitable and a second one, possibly related to their synaptic contact, when they can specifically distinguish between odorous compounds with high selectivity (Mair et al., 1982b). From a biochemical point of view the olfactory sensory neurons are reported to contain a specific, low-molecular-weight protein called the olfactory marker protein because of its specificity to these neurons alone (Monti Graziadei et al., 1977: Margolis, 1980). This protein is characteristic of mature neurons (Figure 11); expression of the olfactory marker protein can be demonstrated even in the absence of specific synaptic contacts with the olfactory bulb (Heckroth et al., 1983; Morrison and Graziadei, 1983). The role of this protein is at present unknown. In mice and rats, where most of the studies have so far been conducted, the first positive neurons appear at E14 and E17, respectively (Monti Graziadei et al., 1980b; Farbman and Margolis, 1980). These data correspond approximately to the time when synapses in the olfactory bulb are established between the sensory axon terminals and branches of the main dendrite of mitral cells (Hinds and Hinds, 1976a,b). Temporal coincidence, however, does not mean a relationship of causality. At birth only a small percentage of olfactory neurons are positive to the specific marker,

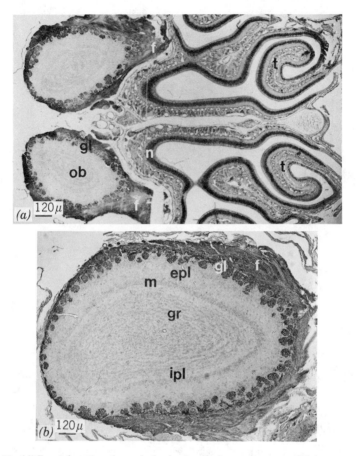

FIGURE 11. (A) Frontal section through the forehead of a young mouse (10 days postnatal) at the level of the olfactory bulbs and the subjacent nasal cavities. The section has been immunostained for the demonstration of the olfactory marker protein (OMP), which is specific to olfactory sensory neurons. Notice the extreme complexity of the nasal turbinates (t). The layer of mature neurons (n) is stained all through the sensory epithelium. The sensory fibers from these sensory neurons reach homolaterally (f) the olfactory bulbs (ob), where they form the typical glomeruli (gl). Mark = 100μm. (B) Detail from the animal is (A). The olfactory bulb is cut frontally, and it has been similarly stained for the demostration of the OMP. The fibrous layer (f) is obviously deeply positive and so are the glomeruli. A slight photographic contrast enhances the other layers of the bulb: epl, external plexiform layer; m, mitral cell layer; ipl, internal plexiform layer; gr, granule cell layer. Mark = 100μm.

and a full complement of positivity is not reached until about postnatal day 30 in mice (Monti Graziadei et al., 1980b; Figures 12 and 13). The presence in culture of an olfactory bulb fragment seems to enhance the quantity of protein in the cotransplanted mucosa (Chuah and Farbman, 1983), although the presence of bulb fragments in culture does not influence the direction of sensory axons toward the bulbar fragments (Gonzales et al., 1985).

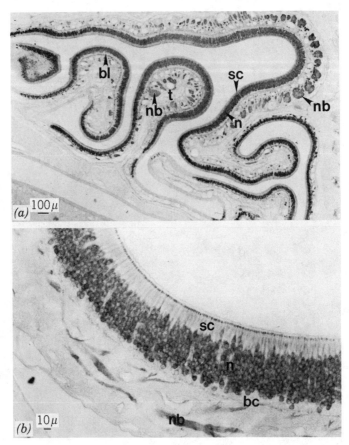

FIGURE 12. (*A*) Detail of the right nasal cavity of mouse stained for OMP. The sensory mucosa shows the intensely positive layer of mature neurons (n); however, the basal layer (bl) where the immature neurons are located is negative. Similarly negative is the distal layer of the epithelium where the bodies of the supporting cells (sc) are located. In the lamina propria there are positive axon bundles of olfactory receptors: t, turbinates; nb, nerve bundles. Mark = 100μm. (*B*) Detail of the olfactory mucosa of mouse-stained for OMP. The mature olfactory neurons and the olfactory nerve bundles in the lamina propria are specifically stained by OMP. The basal cell layer (bc) and the layer of supporting cells are characteristically unstained. Notice the columnar arrangement of the mature olfactory neurons which are perpendicular to the epithelial surface. Mark = 10μm.

In vivo experiments of partial and total bulbectomy suggest that the reduced number of olfactory marker protein positive neurons may be due not so much to the specific effect of the bulb on the neurons but, indirectly, to the effects that a reduced or absent target has on the rate of neuron turnover and, consequently, on the number of mature neurons that exist at any given time (Monti Graziadei, 1983).

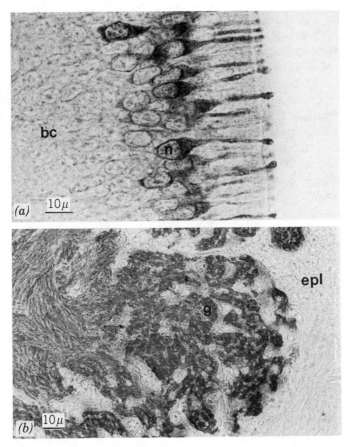

FIGURE 13. (A) This olfactory epithelium from neonatal mouse shows a thick layer of OMP unstained neural cells that have not yet reached maturity (bc). The nucleus of mature neurons (n) stains negative but the perikaryon, the dendrite, and the olfactory vesicle are positive. Mark = 10μm. (B) Detail of a bulbar olfactory glomerulus (g) stained for OMP. The terminals of the olfactory axons are characteristically positive; however, the other components of the glomerulus, namely the dendrites of the mitral, tufted, and periglomerular cells, are negative, giving this complex structure a peculiar marble like appearance. The external plexiform layer (epl) on the right of the figure is completely negative. Mark = 10μm.

C   Ontogenetic Coupling of Epithelium and Olfactory Bulb

During early development of olfactory neurons the olfactory organ is anatomically separated from the brain wall, where olfactory axons will eventually terminate. It is of considerable interest to determine the time sequence of these contacts in order to better understand the phenomena of axon guidance, target recognition, and specificity of interactions that lead the sensory axons from developing epithelium to the brain wall where these fibers may play a role in development of the olfactory bulb (Clairambault,

1971; Stout and Graziadei, 1980; Magrassi and Graziadei, 1985). In amphibians (*Xenopus laevis*) axons begin to exit the epithelium at stage 29/30, and they reach the brain at stages 31/32 (Klein and Graziadei, 1983). In the mouse the first axons exit the epithelium on E11–E12 and reach the forebrain wall at E14 when the first synaptic contacts are observed between the incoming sensory axons and dendritic branches of bulbar neurons (Hinds, 1972a,b; Hinds and Hinds, 1976a,b). In humans the sensory axons seem to contact the brain by the seventh week of gestation (Bossy, 1980). The base of the placode at the time of axon emergence is usually very close to the brain wall, the gap, in most mammals, being in the range of a few micrometers and occupied by loose mesenchyme. It may seem obvious that, due to this close relationship, the axons should reach the brain. However, several processes of guidance and recognition must be involved to assure proper direction and targeting of the sensory input as well as to assure the topological relations that can be demonstrated between the periphery and the glomerular layer. Furthermore, it is clearly demonstrated that when the olfactory axons do not reach the forebrain, severe deficits occur in the development of the olfactory bulb and telencephalon (Prasada Rao and Finger, 1984; Magrassi and Graziadei, 1985).

There are reports indicating that cells derived from the olfactory placode leave their epithelial compartment to accompany axons growing toward the telencephalon. It is not yet established if these cells are neurons or sheath cells, and the possibility exists that some may be neurons of the nervus terminalis (Stanley, 1979). The "terminalis" neurons, indeed, have been observed to follow both olfactory and vomeronasal nerves on their way to CNS adjoining ganglia (van Campenhout, 1936, 1948, 1957; Humphrey, 1940; Pearson, 1941a,b; O'Rahilly, 1967; Stanley, 1979; Farbman and Squinto, 1985). Recently, cells expressing luteinizing hormone-releasing hormone in the brain have been demonstrated to derive, in the mouse, from the olfactory placode (Wray et al., 1989; Schwanzel-Fukuda and Pfaff, 1989). Even in adult rodents, putative neuronal populations have been observed to migrate from the olfactory epithelium along the olfactory nerve and reach the intracranial portion of the first cranial nerve (Monti Graziadei and Graziadei, 1983; Graziadei and Monti Graziadei, 1989). On the other end, peripheral glial progenitor cells, destined to ensheath the olfactory nerve from its origin to its penetration inside the olfactory bulb, are clearly derived from a subpopulation of cells in the olfactory neuroepithelium of mouse embryos. Therefore, the olfactory neuroepithelial matrix has a diverse neurogenetic capacity about which studies have only recently begun (Kim et al., 1988a,b; Kim, 1989).

The mechanisms that govern the orderly pattern of projections from the sensory sheet to the bulbar surface are largely unknown. The growth pattern, however, has been clearly demonstrated by many authors. This pattern may be more complex than at first suspected, and mechanisms specific to the olfactory system may be involved in its formation and maintenance.

So far little is known about underlying substrates that control the orderly establishment of these projections; recently, a major hypothesis for this organizational complexity has been proposed (Graziadei and Monti Graziadei, 1986b).

D   Receptor Turnover

Well before the olfactory neurons were recognized as true neurons, Eckerd in 1855 proposed that basal cells of the olfactory sensory epithelium could serve as replacement elements for the damaged sensory cells. This purely speculative notion persisted in the literature until recently, notwithstanding the lack of any direct evidence. Only within the last 20 years has evidence been presented that in adult vertebrates, including mammals, that olfactory sensory neurons can be replaced when damaged. The phenomenon acquires general biological importance when we consider that the nervous system, an ectodermal derivative, cannot replace its damaged elements (the neurons). In his classification of tissues of the vertebrate body, Bizzozero (1895) reserved the term *"perennial elements"* for neurons to separate them from the *labile* elements of the continuously replacing covering epithelia or from elements of tissues such as muscles and liver that only are replaced under exceptional circumstances; he called the latter the *"stable"* elements. Using ^{3}H-thymidine, Leblond and Walker (1956) and Leblond (1964) decisively confirmed the results outlined by Bizzozero in 1895 (albeit not mentioning them), specifically stating that neurons do not turn over in adult vertebrates nor can they be replaced after injury. These latter observations have been amply supported clinically by neurologists in the past 100 years.

In light of the concept that neurons cannot be replaced when damaged in adult vertebrates, the fact that at least one category of neurons *is* replaceable is of considerable practical and heuristic significance.

Experiments attempting to determine the properties of olfactory neurons after damage date back to the last century. Section of the olfactory nerves was attempted in dogs (Schiff, 1859) and in frogs (Colasanti, 1875). Both authors reported that no change was observed in sensory cells of the olfactory epithelium. However, according to other authors, section of the nerve was followed by terminal degeneration of the receptors in frogs (Hoffmann, 1867; Nakamura, 1916; Takagi and Yajima, 1964, 1965) and mammals (Hofmann, 1867; Baginsky, 1894; Takata, 1929). Removal of the olfactory bulb was reported to produce terminal degeneration of the olfactory sensory neurons in the nasal mucosa (Exner, 1877; Lustig, 1924; Sen Gupta, 1967). Le Gros Clark (1951, 1957) observed that after olfactory bulb removal there was only partial survival of sensory neurons in the epithelium. Degeneration of olfactory receptors in the epithelium of rats produced by local application of zinc sulfate is accompanied by terminal degeneration according to Smith (1938). Later, however, the same author reported that in frogs degeneration of receptors was followed by their reappearance after similar chemical treatment (Smith, 1951). Jackson and Lee (1965), using colchicine, induced degeneration in the olfactory receptors and did not notice regeneration of the elements. Regenerative capacity of the receptors after treatment with zinc sulfate was reported in mammals by Schultz (1941, 1960), Mulvaney and Heist (1971a,b), and Matulionis (1975). The contrasting conclusions of all these experimental studies is largely due to inadequate technical procedures as well as to insufficient understanding of the dynamic complexity of the neuroepithelium under study. The observation that more than others reflects a clear experimental paradigm and a correct interpretation of the experimental data is the one reported in 1940 by Nagahara in an authoritative, yet little recognized contribution. This author reported that section of olfactory axons in adult mouse induces total retrograde degeneration of intraepithelial sensory neurons. From the cells in the basal compartment of the epithelium new neurons were then reformed, thus assuring a reconstitution of the nerve cells. The results of this seminal paper have more recently been amply confirmed by means of more sophisticated and accurate techniques (Graziadei, 1973b).

In the context of all the preceding conflicting results there was a clear need to demonstrate the ablility of olfactory neurons to be replaced using adequate methodology. Once the replacement of neurons could be definitively proven, it was important to determine if this phenomenon was restricted to lower vertebrates or if it could be demonstrated in mammals, including humans. It was important also to know when replacement occurred, if central connections could be reestablished, and what underlying mechansims were involved in this phenomenon. It was also of paramount importance to ascertain if reestablished anatomical connections would be accompanied by return of function and recovery of behavioral ability to respond to odors. During the past 20 years these questions have been addressed, and the answers point to a series of interesting characteristics manifested by the olfactory system.

In 1965 Andres published a photograph of a mitotic figure in the olfactory epithelium of a young cat. The mitotic cell, because of its unspecified morphology, could not be identified as a neuron precursor (in spite of the claim of the author). However, the finding served to repropose the problem of neuronal replaceability in the olfactory epithelium. Many reports followed on the subject. Thornhill (1967) published the first autoradiograph of the olfactory epithelium of salamander where cells were labeled with ^{3}H-thymidine in the basal layer. It was this report that demonstrated replacement of cells, albeit, in a cold-blooded animal. Furthermore, it was not clear if the labeled stem cells were the replacement elements for the neurons or for the supporting cells. Using ^{3}H-thymidine in light microscope preparations, Moulton et al. (1970), Moulton and Fink (1972), and Moulton (1974) determined that cells at the base of the olfactory epithelium of mice became labeled after 24 h survival. The labeled cells eventually migrated upward in the neuronal layer of the epithelium. These observations and their quantitative analysis strongly indicated that olfactory neurons in a normal rodent were being generated and were turning over. According to these authors, the supporting cells were also turning over, albeit at a slower pace. Graziadei and collaborators (Graziadei and Metcalf, 1970, 1971; Graziadei, 1971a; 1973a,b; Graziadei and DeHan, 1973; Metcalf, 1974), using autoradiography at both light and electron microscope levels, were able to identify the basal cells as the only stem cells of the neurons as well as a lineage of morphologically identifiable stages of neuronal maturation. Graziadei and Monti Graziadei (1978a,b, 1979, 1980) extended these observations to mammals and determined that a definite turnover of the olfactory neurons occurs even without obvious intervening pathologic factors. Furthermore, in frogs (Graziadei and DeHan, 1973; Graziadei, 1973b) and in mammals (Monti Graziadei and Graziadei, 1979a,b; Graziadei and Monti Graziadei, 1980) it was possible to demonstrate that severance of olfactory axons in mature animals resulted in retrograde degeneration of the existing mature neurons and reconstitution of a new population of elements (Figure 14) and that these elements reconnected with the olfactory bulb, thus attaining complete morphological recovery of the system. Similar experiments conducted in nonhuman primates gave identical results (Graziadei et al., 1980; Monti Graziadei et al., 1980a). Oley et al. (1975), in birds, also proved that anatomical recovery of the system was accompanied by return of behavioral function. The autoradiographic studies using ^{3}H-thymidine indicated that the neuronal population in the olfactory epithelium of commonly raised animals in standard environment has a limited life span of some 6–8 weeks depending on the age of the animal (Miragall and Monti Graziadei, 1982). The essential facts resulting from the preceding observations then indicate that the olfactory neuron is a disposable element that can be newly generated and rewired to the CNS, even in adult mammals, as a result of several factors (some not completely understood at present) that determine its degeneration. Renewal of olfactory neurons after experimental degeneration has been recently and convincingly demonstrated again by a number of authors in amphibians (Simmons and Getchell, 1981a,b,c), birds (Graziadei and Okano, 1979), and rodents (Harding et al., 1977; Samanen and Forbes, 1984). Similar results were also obtained in complementary experiments using the vomeronasal system (Barber and Raisman, 1978a,b; Barber 1981a,b; Wang and Halpern, 1982a,b).

The possibility that neuronal replacement in the olfactory epithelium could be solely attributed to pathological processes has been mentioned in the literature (Hinds et al., 1984). However, the consistent occurrence of this phenomenon in all vertebrate species so far tested makes it unlikely that the vertebrate phylum as a whole should uniformly suffer from a selective nasal pathology. In fact, recently, contributions from several laboratories have confirmed that in the olfactory epithelium of mammals the neurogenetic matrix persists and is active well into adult life (Miragall et al., 1988; Carr

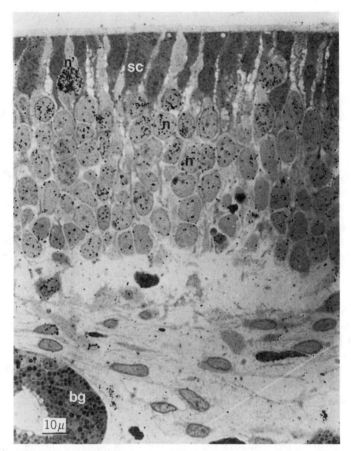

FIGURE 14. Olfactory mucosa from a frog (*Rana viridis*). The animal was subjected to total severance of the olfactory nerve to assure degeneration of mature olfactory neurons. During the period of intense neurogenesis (when the basal cells regrow a new population of neurons), ^{3}H-thymidine was injected and consequently all the neural elements are labeled by radioactive thymidine (n). Some of them closer to the surface and possibly having undergone few divisions after the label have a richer complement of granules (n') than the more basal elements that have undergone repeated divisions. However, all neural elements are labeled, while no supporting cell nucleus (sc) has label, which supports the notion that the two populations have different stem cells. Few Bowman's glands cells have incorporated the label (bg). Mark = 10μm.

et al., 1989; Schoenfeld et al., 1989; Verhaagen et al., 1989; Viereck et al., 1989).

E   Experimental Study of the Olfactory Organ

The presence of a neurogenetic machinery that persists into adult life to continue generating neurons provides an exceptional model for the study of neurogenesis, target recognition, and plasticity that is not possible in other parts of the mature nervous system. A brief account of experimental results will be provided here.

Contrary to what occurs in other sensory pathways, deafferentiation of the olfactory bulb (the first CNS region where the sensory axons terminate) is not a terminal event, but instead recovery usually occurs. Recently, Samanen and Forbes (1984), in confirming our data of 1980 in mice (Graziadei and Monti Graziadei, 1979, 1980) by means of morphometric analysis, demonstrated that following axotomy all mature neurons degenerate and then are reconstituted in a time frame consistent with our previous results. These authors also found that the average life span of olfactory neurons in hamster is in the range of 25–35 days, thus supporting the previous results from the laboratories of Moulton and Graziadei. After clearly establishing the capacity of olfactory neurons to regrow axons back into the primary central target some experiments needed to be conducted to determine if the regenerative process was possible when the olfactory bulb was damaged or partially removed. Removal of even small portions of the olfactory bulb resulted in complex patterns of regrowing olfactory fibers. These new fibers formed glomeruli totally at random in many layers of the olfactory bulb, and while the unlesioned glomeruli persisted, the new glomeruli induced profound changes in the total pattern of the normally orderly layers of the bulb. When large portions of the bulb were removed (in the range of 90% of its total volume), the regenerative ability of the reconstituted neurons was not impaired, and the reformed glomeruli were established in the spared bulbar parenchyma totally at random. In fact, the large bulbar neurons showed a complete rearrangement in orientation of the dendrites toward the newly established ectopic glomeruli (Graziadei and Samanen, 1980; Monti Graziadei and Graziadei, 1984; Graziadei and Monti Graziadei, 1986a,b). These experiments showed that the presumed target of the sensory fibers was playing a minimum role in their orientation and guidance. Behavioral experiments showed that large lesions of the olfactory bulb, resulting in disarrangement of orderly layers and, in fact, removal of up to 90% of the total bulb volume, does not significantly change the ability of the animals to respond to odors or to discriminate among them (Graziadei and Graziadei, unpublished results).

Total removal of the olfactory bulb does not impair the reconstitution of a new population of sensory neurons or their regrowth into the spared CNS (Figure 15). It seems, however, that removal of the target affects their life span (Monti Graziadei, 1983). The olfactory axons, in spite of the absence of their usual target, seem to be able to grow back intracranially and form glomeruli in the forebrain and can also profoundly modify the morphology of the innervated "unconventional" neurons (Graziadei et al., 1978, 1979; Graziadei and Monti Graziadei, 1986a).

Transplantation of occipital and cerebellar cortices in place of removed olfactory bulb results in regrowth of olfactory axons and formation of new glomeruli into these transplanted CNS regions (Graziadei and Kaplan, 1980;

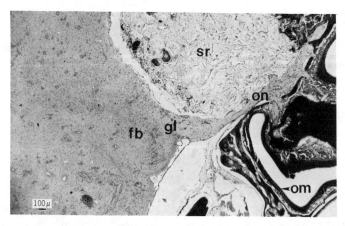

FIGURE 15. Parasagittal section of the forebrain of a mouse that has been totally bulbectomized as an adult and survived the surgery for 30 days. A large scar tissue mass has formed in place of the removed olfactory bulb (sr). In spite of the lack of their normal target (i.e., the olfactory bulb) axons of olfactory neurons of the olfactory mucosa (om) have regrown, forming a single, relatively large olfactory nerve (on) that has penetrated throught the scar tissue to reach the forebrain (fb). There the fibers have formed ectopic glomeruli (gl). For more details see Graziadei and Monti Graziadei, 1986a). Mark = 100µm.

Monti Graziadei and Graziadei, 1984). The preceding results suggest that olfactory neurons can differentiate from their own matrix, independent of a specialized central target, and the glomeruli can also form independent of specific central neurons such as the mitral cells (Graziadei and Monti Graziadei, 1986a). Transplantation of olfactory neuroepithelium in the anterior chamber of the eye or into the large telencephalic ventricles support the preceding conclusions (Graziadei et al., 1980; Morrison and Graziadei, 1983; Heckroth et al., 1983). However, the presence of an adequate and specific target seems to be important to maintain a normal turnover rate of the olfactory neurons (Costanzo and Graziadei, 1983, 1987; Monti Graziadei, 1983).

IV   DEVELOPMENT OF CENTRAL OLFACTORY STRUCTURES

Neurogenetic development that establishes the CNS stations of the olfactory system does not follow a rigid craniocaudal development; rather, the neurons of the interconnecting centers develop in synchrony. In general, the main output neurons of any given neural center are generated before the local interneurons; the former are all generated prenatally while the latter can be generated during postnatal life (Hinds, 1967, 1968; Bayer, 1983). Most of the data on olfactory pathway development have been obtained from studies in rodents (Astic and Saucier, 1982, 1983). According to

Hinds and McNelly (1973, 1977), the olfactory bulb of rats shows a linear increase in volume of approximately 50% from 3 to 24 months. The authors interpret this increase as the continuation of early postnatal growth, in all likelihood due to the acquisition of new granule cells. In mice, axons from the bulbar output neurons which form the lateral olfactory tract establish synapses in the pyriform cortex on E15 (Schwob and Price, 1978, 1984; Luskin and Price, 1983; Schwob et al., 1986). Synaptogenesis in the cortex, however, shows a marked increase during the first and second postnatal weeks. By comparison, fibers do not reach the tubercle and the lateral entorhinal area until the first postnatal week. Ipsilateral intracortical fiber systems begin development prenatally, but a substantial maturative process continues postnatally. Commissural fibers from the anterior portion of pyriform cortex cross the midline at birth in mouse, but their connections with the target neurons in contralateral cortex are established only between the first and second week postnatally (Brunjes and Frazier, 1986; Schwob et al., 1986). These postnatal connections are of special functional importance in the determination of postnatal aspects of behavioral development (Kucharski et al., 1986; Hall and Oppenheim, 1987; Kucharski and Hall, 1986, 1987). Connections between the olfactory cortex and the diencephalon occur at birth; the hypothalamic area innervates the subthalamic nucleus at E18. The fibers of the mediothalamic nucleus enter the stria medullaris by E20 in mouse (Schwob et al., 1986). According to Mair and Gesteland (1982) and Mair et al. (1982a), newborn rats have a complete afferent pathway from receptors to pyriform cortex, although animals at this stage still lack local interneuronal circuitry likely involved in the complex modulation of olfactory behavior as in the adult.

In summary, portions of the central olfactory pathway are relatively well developed at birth, but a considerable degree of maturation occurs well into the postnatal period. For instance, while olfactory bulb projections to olfactory cortex are well developed at birth, connections of the olfactory tubercle and other posterior cortical structures are innervated only postnatally.

V   ONTOGENY OF OLFACTORY BEHAVIOR

Anatomically the olfactory system can be divided into three main sectors: (a) the olfactory mucosa or peripheral sensory organ, where the sensory neuronal perikarya are located; (b) the olfactory bulb, the first paleocortical station where the sensory axons project and where the first large cortical output neurons (mitral and tufted cells) interact with the input neurons; and (c) the areas of olfactory cortex where the large output bulbar neurons project their axons. These areas of projection can be subdivided into several topographically discrete regions. Embryology has demonstrated that these central regions are morphologically advanced, although at different degrees of functional competence, quite early in development. In other words, the machinery for olfactory sensation is in place at and before birth. In mouse the axons of sensory receptors reach the bulb at E14 (Monti Graziadei et al., 1980b), and only subsequent to these contacts do the receptors acquire competence for specific odors (Gesteland et al., 1982; Mair et al., 1982b). It is at postnatal day 1 that mitral cells can be selectively excited by different odors (Mair and Gesteland, 1982). Indeed, the specific time sequence of these anatomical and functional events may vary in different species subject to ethological requirements, while other sensory modalities may also become adept at recording stimuli in different relative time frames during ontogenesis. It is clear that embryos of all vertebrate species respond to a variety of stimuli very early in development (Hamburger, 1963; Gottlieb, 1968; Cheal, 1975; Alberts, 1976, 1981; Blass et al., 1977; 1979; Alberts and May, 1980; Leonard, 1981; Oppenheim, 1982; see Hall and Oppenheim, 1987, for a survey). We know, however, that olfactory behavior is critical in the perinatal period to assure nipple location and attachment and home orientation (Teicher and Blass, 1976, 1977). It is interesting to know that embryos exposed to specific odors during the last days of gestation preferentially attach to nipples with that odor (Pedersen and Blass, 1981, 1982). During the perinatal period when the animal is still blind and deaf, olfactory cues allow the animal to establish feeding and nesting behavior patterns that provide nutrition, temperature-controlled environment, and security essential for survival, especially in altricial animals (Alberts and May, 1980). That the olfactory pathway may be functional *in utero* has been demonstrated using the 2-deoxyglucose technique (Pedersen et al., 1982, 1983, 1985). In fact, experimentally changing the chemical characteristics of the internal milieu determines postnatal behavioral changes (Pedersen and Blass, 1982). Pups avoid odors provided *in utero* in conjunction with intra-peritoneal injection of lithium chloride (Stickrod et al., 1982; Smotherman, 1983a,b; Smotherman et al., 1984; Smotherman and Robinson, 1985). To be sure, the role of perinatal olfaction is at this time not fully explored, nor is the developmental progression of olfactory behavior. However, current experimental evidence points to many avenues of considerable interest for future exploration (Fillion and Blass, 1986).

There is little systematic research on the importance or specific role of olfaction in the perinatal period of humans. While we know that olfactory impairment in adults provides subjective alteration of the "taste" quality of food and exposes the individual to the risk of environmentally dangerous odors, early olfactory experience in humans is still a very open, albeit promising field of investigation.

VI   OLFACTORY SENSORY DEPRIVATION DURING DEVELOPMENT

How experience influences the development, anatomy, and function of the olfactory system has been investigated by a number of authors following two relatively simple experimental procedures. In the first, animals have been raised in a controlled environment where a specific concentration of one odor was maintained. In the second type of experiment, the animals have had one naris obstructed at birth by means of cauterization of the external opening, thus impairing the normal flux of air through the homolateral side. Although some odors may reach the sensory organ through the posterior coana in the latter approach, the stimuli conveyed by the normal respiratory process are reduced to a minimum. In the first procedure (in rat), in which receptors were exposed to a single odor, Doving and Pinching (1973) and Pinching and Doving (1974) reported patterns of degeneration of the mitral cells in the olfactory bulb; the pattern seemed to have a topographic specificity in the mitral cell layer according to the odorant used as a stimulus. Similar results were reported in mice by other authors (Harvey and Cowley, 1984). These experiments left open the possibility that the areas of described mitral cell degeneration could have been overstimulated or, as likely, degeneration could have been determined by lack of stimulation of these same areas (Changeux and Danchin, 1976; Purves and Lichtman, 1980). Laing and Panhuber (1978, 1980) and Laing et al. (1985) raised rats in odorized or deodorized environments and concluded that the animals reared in deodorized experiments were deficient in the detection of specific odors, while rats reared in a specific odorous environment did not lose their acuity for the odor tested. Basically, the interesting finding of these authors was that deprivation could lead to decrease in the sensitivity for the odor tested. The problem is indeed complex, and the techniques used in these studies are varied and not standardized between laboratories, thus casting some doubt on the generality of their conclusions and even on the heuristic value of the data.

The second experimental approach, which involves olfactory deprivation by closure of one external naris, has utilized the contralateral nasal cavity and bulb as an internal control. Since the procedure is implemented unilaterally, it does not impair the total development of the animal or its somatomotor behavior (Meisami, 1976; Brunjes et al., 1985). This deprivation intervention, however, results in size reduction of the homolateral olfactory bulb up to 25% below control values (Fruhwald, 1935; Meisami, 1976; Brunjes and Borror, 1983; Benson et al., 1984; Brunjes, 1985; Meisami and Firoozi, 1985). While the external plexiform layer seems to be most affected by the deprivation procedure, all layers of the bulb suffer a significant reduction in size. Data discrepancies among authors can, however, be detected when specific populations of neurons are considered. Thus, Meisami and Safari (1981) reported reduction of mitral cells in the range of 25–40%, while Benson et al. (1984) did not find significant differences in the number of these cells. Likewise, glomeruli complexity seems to be reduced in mouse (Benson et al., 1984) but not in rats (Meisami and Safari, 1981). It appears that the time of onset of sensory deprivation is important in the development of the olfactory bulb; the effect of deprivation is maximal when implemented during the immediate postnatal period, but it is less severe when initiated later in life, as from postnatal days 10–20 (Brunjes and Borror, 1983; Brunjes, 1985). Biochemical changes in the olfactory bulb have also been reported following sensory deprivation. Meisami and Mousavi (1982) observed that odor deprivation resulted in a decrease in proteins, DNA, and RNA in the affected bulb. Peripheral afferent input has been found to regulate the expression of dopamines in populations of local, intrinsic bulbar neurons, as demonstrated by deafferentiation and reinnervation experiments in rodents (Baker et al., 1983, 1984). Unilateral naris occlusion also reduces by approximately 40% the rate of neurogenesis of the short-lived receptors; this drop in the neurogenetic activity is believed to be due to reduction of toxic agents in the occluded naris (Farbman et al., 1984, 1988). In summary, sensory deprivation seems to affect not only the dynamics of the peripheral population of sensory neurons, but also the biochemical and morphological characteristics of at least the first CNS station, namely, the olfactory bulb.

VII CONCLUSIONS

The olfactory system has a number of unusual characteristics such as the peripheral location of its sensory neurons, the ability of these neurons to be replaced under normal and experimental conditions, and the linkage of sensory neuron axons directly to the brain cortex (the paleocortex of the olfactory bulb) without intervening subcortical stations. The olfactory system also shows an apparent anatomical simplicity, at least at the peripheral and bulbar levels; that contrasts with the highly sophisticated functional performance of this system in detection of an apparently infinite variety of odorous substances. This apparent simplicity also contrasts with its profound behavioral impact on the life of the vertebrate animal. The anatomical organization of at least the two most peripheral portions (the olfactory mucosa and the olfactory bulb), as well as the disposable nature of its sensory neurons, render this system amenable to a number of experimental manipulations even in the adult mammal. As briefly outlined in this chapter, these experiments are not as easily implemented in other portions of the nervous system where regeneration in the adult is either difficult to obtain or thus far believed impossible. Consequently, it is of considerable practical and heuristic value to study this system and to use it as a tool for neurobiological research.

Other aspects of the olfactory pathway merit consideration. The double central projections of the olfactory system proper and the vomeronasal organs are extremely complex and extensive (even more so than the diagram of Figure 13 provides), and this complexity emphasizes the subtle but important role that olfaction plays in our behavior at both conscious and subconscious levels. The relatively new behavioral observations of the intrauterine role of olfaction in postnatal life opens a new field of potentially very interesting avenues that may lead to understanding many complex behaviors. The olfactory system, consequently, not only seems to be ideal as a tool for the study of more general neurobiological problems, but it may also be essential for a more complete understanding of intricate mammalian and human responses to sensory events.

Relatively many references have been provided for the reader interested in different facets of the olfactory system. The references, however, are largely incomplete and serve only as points for further research and understanding. Of course, the view of this system as presented is considerably biased by the limitations of the author, whose knowledge is restricted to the narrow confines of his interests and intellect.

REFERENCES

Adrian, E. D. (1950) Sensory discrimination with some recent evidence from the olfactory organ. Brit. Med. Bull. *6:* 330–333.

Adrian, E. D. (1951) Olfactory discrimination. Annee Psychol. *50:* 107–113.

Alberts, J. R. (1976) Olfactory contribution to behavioral development in rodents. In R. L. Doty (ed.): Mammalian Olfaction, Reproductive Processes and Behavior. New York: Academic Press.

Alberts, J. R. (1981) Ontogeny of olfaction: Reciprocal roles of sensation and behavior in the development of perception. In R. N. Aslin, J. R. Alberts, and M. R. Peterson (eds.): Development of Perception: Psychobiological Perspective, Vol. 1. New York: Academic Press.

Alberts, J. R., and B. May (1980) Ontogeny of olfaction: Development of the rat's sensitivity to urine and amyl acetate. Physiol. Behav. *24:* 965–970.

Allison, A. C. (1953) The morphology of the olfactory system in the vertebrates. Biol Rev. *28:* 193–244.

Andres, K. H. (1965) Differenzierung und regeneration von sinnezellen in der regio olfactoria. Naturwissenschaften *17:* 500.

Andres, K. H. (1969) Der olfactorische saum der katze. Z. Zellforsch. *96:* 250–274.

Astic, L., and D. Saucier (1982) Ontogenesis of the functional activity of rat olfactory bulb: Autoradiographic study with the 2-deoxyglucose method. Dev. Brain Res. *2:* 1243–1256.

Astic, L., and D. Saucier (1983) Ontogenesis of the functional activity of guinea pig olfactory bulb: Autoradiographic study with the 2-deoxyglucose method. Dev. Brain Res. *16:* 257–263.

Astic, L., and D. Saucier (1986) Anatomical mapping of the neuropithelial projection to the olfactory bulb in the rat. Brain Res. Bull. *16:* 445–454.

Baginsky, B. (1894) Uber das verhalten von mervenendorganen nach durchschneidung der zugehorigen merven. Virchows Arch. Path. Anat. *137:* 389–404.

Baker, H., T. Kawano, F. L. Margolis, and T. H. Joh (1983) Transneuronal regulation of tyrosine bydroxylase expression in olfactory bulb of mouse and rat, J. Neurosci. *3:* 69–78.

Baker, H., T. Kawano, V. Albert, T. H. Joh, D. J. Reis, and F. L. Margolis (1984) Olfactory bulb dopamine neurons survive deafferentiation-induced loss of tyrosine hydroxylase. Neuroscience 11: 605–615.

Bannister, L. H. (1974) Possible functions of mucus at gustatory and olfactory surfaces. In T. M. Poynder (ed.): Transduction Mechanisms in Chemoreception. London: Information Retrieval, pp. 39–46.

Barber, P. C. (1981a) Axonal growth by newly-formed vomeronasal neurosensory cells in the normal adult mouse. Brain Res. 216: 229–237.

Barber, P. C. (1981b) Regeneration of vomeronasal nerves into the main olfactory bulb in the mouse. Brain Res. 216: 239–251.

Barber, P. C., and G. Raisman (1978a) Cell division in the vomeronasal organ of the adult mouse. Brain Res. 141: 57–66.

Barber, P. C., and G. Raisman (1978b) Replacement of receptor neurones after section of the vomeronasal nerves in the adult mouse. Brain Res. 147: 297–313.

Bayer, S. A. (1983) ^{3}H-thymidine-radiographic studies of neurogenesis in the rat olfactory bulb. Exp. Brain Res. 50: 329–340.

Benson, T. E., D. K. Ryugo, and J. W. Hinds (1984) Effects of sensory deprivation on the developing mouse olfactory system: A light and electron microscopic, morphometric analysis. J. Neurosci. 4: 638–653.

Benson, T. E., G. D. Burd, C. A. Greer, D. M. D. Landis, and G. M. Shepherd (1985) High-resolution 2-deoxyglucose autoradiography of quick-frozen slaps of neonatal rat olfactory bulb. Brain Res. 339: 67–78.

Bignetti E., A. Cavaggioni, P. Pelosi, K. L. Persaud, R. T. Sorbi, and R. Tirindelli (1985) Purification and characterization of an odorant binding protein from cow nasal tissue. Eur. J. Biochem. 149: 227–231.

Bizzozero, G. (1895) Accrescimento e rigenerazione nell'organismo. Arch. Soc. Med. It. 18: 245–287.

Blass, E. M., M. H. Teicher, C. P. Cramer, J. P. Bruno, and W. G. Hall (1977) Olfactory, thermal and tactile controls of suckling in preauditory and previsual rats. J. Comp. Physiol. Psychol. 91: 1248–1260.

Blass, E. M., E. G. Hall, and M. H. Teicher (1979) The ontogeny of suckling and ingestive behaviors. In J. M. Sprague and A. N. Epstein (eds.): Progress in Psychobiology and Physiological Psychology, Vol. 8. New York: Academic Press.

Bossy, J. (1980) Development of olfactory and related structures in staged human embryos. Anat. Embryol. 161: 225–236.

Broadwell, R. D. (1975) Olfactory relationships of the telencephalon and diencephalon in the rabbit. I. An autoradiographic study of the efferent connections of the main and accessory olfactory bulbs. J. Comp. Neurol. 163: 329–346.

Broadwell, R. D. (1977) Neurotransmitter pathways in the olfactory system. In J. A. Ferrendelli and G. Gurvitch (eds.): Society for Neuroscience Symposia. III. Aspects of Behavioral Neurobiology. Bethesda: Society for Neuroscience, pp. 131–166.

Brunjes, P. C. (1985) Unilateral odor deprivation: Time course of changes in laminar volume. Brain Res. Bull. 14: 233–237.

Brunjes, P. C., and M. J. Borror (1983) Unilateral odor deprivation: Differential effects due to time of treatment. Brain Res. Bull. 11: 501–503.

Olfactory Development   553

Brunjes, P. C., and L. L. Frazier (1986) Maturation and plasticity in the olfactory system of vertebrates. Brain Res. Rev. *11:* 1–45.

Brunjes, P. C., H. D. Schwark, and W. T. Greenough (1982) Olfactory granule cell development in normal and hyperthyroid rats. Dev. Brain Res. *5:* 149–159.

Brunjes, P. C., L. K. Smith-Crafts, and R. McCarty (1985) Unilateral odor deprivations: Effects on the development of olfactory bulb catecholamines and behavior. Dev. Brain Res. *22:* 1–6.

Carpenter, E. (1937) The head pattern in amblystoma studied by vital staining and transplantation methods. J. Exp. Zool. *75:* 103–129.

Carr, V. M., A. I. Farbman, M. S. Lidow, L. M. Colletti, J. L. Hempstead, and J. I. Morgan (1989) Developmental expression of reactivity to monoclonal antibodies generated against olfactory epithelia. J. Neurosci. *9:*1179–1198.

Changeux, J. P., and A. Danchin (1976) Selective stabilisation of developing synapses as a mechanism for the specification of neuronal networks. Nature (Lond.) *264:* 705–712.

Cheal, M. L. (1975) Social olfaction: A review of the ontogeny of olfactory influences on vertebrate behavior. Behav. Biol. *15:* 1–25.

Chuah, M. I., and A. T. Farbman (1983) Olfactory bulb increases marker protein in olfactory receptors cells. J. Neurosci. *3:* 2197–2205.

Clairambault, P. (1971) Les effets de l'ablation bilaterale de la placode nasale sur la morphogenese du telencephale des anoures. Acta Embryol. Exp. *2:* 61–92.

Clancy, A. M., T. A. Schoenfeld, and F. Macrides (1985) Topographic organization of peripheral input to the hamster main olfactory bulb. Chem. Senses *10:* 399.

Clark Le Gros, W. E. (1951) The projection of the olfactory epithelium on the olfactory bulb in the rabbit. J. Neurol. Neurosurg. Psychiat. *14:* 1–10.

Clark Le Gros, W. E. (1957) Inquiries into the anatomical basis of olfactory discrimination. Proc. Roy. Soc. (Lond.) B *146:* 299–319.

Clark Le Gros, W. E., and R. T. T. Warwick (1946) The pattern of olfactory innervation. J. Neurol. Neurosurg. Psychiat. *9:* 101–111.

Colasanti, G. (1875) Untersuchungen uber die durchschneidung des nervus olfactorius bei froschen. Arch. f. Anat. u. Physiol. v. Reichert u. d. Bois Reymond, 469.

Costanzo, R. M., and P. P. C. Graziadei (1983) A quantitative analysis of changes in the olfactory epithelium following bulbectomy in hamster. J. Comp. Neurol. *215:* 370–381.

Costanzo, R. M., and P. P. C. Graziadei (1987) Development and Plasticity. In T. Finger and W. Silver (eds.) Neurobiology of Taste and Smell. New York: John Wiley & Sons, pp. 233–250.

Costanzo, R. M., and M. M. Mozell (1976) Electrophysiological evidence for a topographical projection of the nasal mucosa onto the olfactory bulb of the frog. J. Gen. Physiol. *68:* 297–312.

Costanzo, R. M., and R. J. O'Connell (1978) Spatially organized projections of hamster olfactory nerves. Brain Res. *139:* 327–332.

Costanzo, R. M., and R. J. O'Connell (1980) Receptive fields of second-order neurons in the olfactory bulb of the hamster. J. Gen. Physiol. *76:* 53–68.

Cuschieri, A., and L. H. Bannister (1975a) The development of the olfactory mucosa in the mouse: Electron microscopy. J. Anat. *119:* 471–498.

Cuschieri, A., and L. H. Bannister (1975b) The development of the olfactory mucosa in the mouse: Light microscopy. J. Anat. *119:* 227–286.

Davis, B. J., F. Macrides, W. M. Young, S. P. Schneider, and D. L. Rosene (1978) Efferents and centrifugal afferents of the main and accessory olfactory bulbs in the hamster. Brain Res. Bull. *3:* 59–72.

Doucette, R. (1989) Development of the nerve fibre layer in the olfactory bulb of mouse embryos. J. Comp. Neurol. *285:*514–527.

Doving, K. B., and A. J. Pinching (1973) Selective degeneration of neurones in the olfactory bulb following prolonged odour exposure. Brain Res. *52:* 115–129.

Eckerd, A. (1855) Uber das epithelium, der riechschleimhaut und die wahrschein-liche endging des geruchsnerven. Z. wiss. Zool. *8:* 303–306.

Exner, S. (1877) Forgesetzte Studien uber die Endigungsweise des Geruchsnerven. W.-B. Wien: Akad. 76, Abt. 3.

Farbman, A. I., and F. L. Margolis (1980) Olfactory marker protein during ontogeny: Immunohistochemical localization. Dev. Biol. *74:* 205–215.

Farbman, A. I., and L. M. Squinto (1985) Early development of olfactory receptor cell axons. Dev. Brain Res. *19:* 205–213.

Farbman, A. I., S. M. Ritz, and P. C. Brunjes (1984) The effect of odor deprivation on olfactory epithelium in developing rats. Soc. Neurosci. Abstr. *10:* 530.

Farbman, A. I., P. C. Brunjes, L. Rentfro, J. Michas, and S. Ritz (1988) The effect of unilateral naris occlusion on cell dynamics in the developing rat olfactory epithe-lium. J. Neurosci. *8:*3290–3295.

Fillion, T. J., and E. M. Blass (1986) Infantile experience with suckling odors deter-mines adult sexual behavior in male rats. Science *231:* 729–731.

Friedman, B. and J. L. Price (1984) Fiber systems in the olfactory bulb and cortex: A study in adult and developing rats, using the Timm method with light and electron microscope. J. Comp. Neurol. *223:* 88–109.

Fruhwald, V. (1935) Die folgen des einseitigen masen verschlusses auf die niechsch-leimhaut und auf den bulbus and tractus olfactorius. Arch. Ohren, Nasen and Kehlkopfheilk *139:* 153–173.

Gasser, H. S. (1956) Olfactory nerve fibers. J. Gen. Physiol. *39:* 473–496.

Gasser, H. S. (1958) Comparison of the structure, as revealed by the electron microscope, and the physiology of the unmedullated fibres in the skin nerves and the olfactory nerves. Exp. Cell Res. *5:* 3–17.

Gesteland, R. C., R. A. Yancey, R. G. Mair, G. D. Adamek, and A. I. Farbman (1980) Ontogeny of olfactory receptor specificity. In Olfaction and Taste, Vol. VII. London: IRL Press, pp. 143–146.

Gesteland, R. C., R. A. Yancey, and A. I. Farbman (1982) Development of olfactory receptor neuron selectivity in the rat fetus. Neuroscience *7:* 3127–3136.

Getchell, T. V. (1977) Mechanisms of excitation in vertebrate olfactory receptor sustentacular cells. In Y. Katsuki, M. Sato, S. F. Takagi, and Y. Oomura (eds.): International Symposium on Food Intake and Chemical Senses. Tokyo: Univer-sity of Tokyo Press, pp. 3–13.

Getchell, T. V. (1986) Functional properties of vertebrate olfactory receptor neurons. Physiol. Rev. *66:* 772–818.

Getchell, T. V., F. L. Margolis, and M. L. Getchell (1984a) Perireceptor and receptor events in vertebrate olfaction. Progr. Neurobiol. *23:* 317–3136.

Getchell, M. L., J. A. Rafols, and T. V. Getchell (1984b) Histological and histochemical studies of the secretory components of the salamander olfactory mucosa: effects of isoproterenol and olfactory nerve section. Anat. Rec. *208:* 553–565.

Golgi, C. (1875) Sulla fina struttura dei bulbi olfattorii. Riv. Sperim. Freniat. Medi. Legale *1:*406–425.

Gonzales, F., A. I. Farbman, and R. C. Gesteland (1985) Cell and explant culture of olfactory chemoreceptor cells. J. Neurosci. Meth. *14:* 77–90.

Gottlieb, G. (1968) Prenatal behavior of birds. Quart. Rev. Biol. *43:* 148–174.

Graziadei, P. P. C. (1971a) The olfactory mucosa of vertebrates. In L. M. Beidler (ed.): Handbook of Sensory Physiology, Vol. IV. New York: Springer-Verlag, pp. 27–58.

Graziadei, P. P. C. (1971b) Topological relations between olfactory neurons. Z. Zellforsch. mikrosk. Anat. *118:* 449–466.

Graziadei, P. P. C. (1973a) The ultrastructure of vertebrates olfactory mucosa. In I. Friedmann (ed.): The Ultrastructure of Sensory Organs. Amsterdam-London: North-Holland Publishing, pp. 269–305.

Graziadei, P. P. C. (1973b) Cell dynamics in the olfactory mucosa. Tiss. Cell *5:* 113–131.

Graziadei, P. P. C. (1977) Functional anatomy of the mammalian chemoreceptor system. In D. Muller-Schwarze and M. M. Mozell (eds.): Chemical Signals in Vertebrates. New York: Plenum Press, pp. 435–454.

Graziadei, P., and L. H. Bannister (1967) Some observations on the fine structure of the olfactory epithelium in the domestic duck. Z. Zellforsch. *80:* 220–228.

Graziadei, P. P. C., and R. S. DeHan (1973) Neuronal regeneration in frog olfactory system. J. Cell Biol. *59:* 525–530.

Graziadei, P. P. C., and H. T. Gagne (1973) Extrinsic innervation of olfactory epithelium. Z. Zellforsch. Mikrosk. Anat. *138:* 315–326.

Graziadei, P. P. C., and M. S. Kaplan (1980) Regrowth of olfactory sensory axons into transplanted neural tissue. I. Development of connections with the occipital cortex. Brain Res. *201:* 39–44.

Graziadei, P. P. C., and J. F. Metcalf (1970) Autoradiographic study of frog's olfactory mucosa. Amer. Zool. *10*(4): 716.

Graziadei, P. P. C., and J. F. Metcalf (1971) Autoradiographic and ultrastructural observations on the frog's olfactory mucosa. Z. Zellforsch Mikrosk. Anat. *116:* 305–318.

Graziadei, P. P. C., and G. A. Monti Graziadei (1976) Olfactory epithelium of Necturus maculosus and Ambystoma trigrinum. J. Neurocytol. *5:* 11–32.

Graziadei, P. P. C., and G. A. Monti Graziadei (1978a) Continuous nerve cell renewal in the olfactory system. In M. Jacobson (ed.): Handbook of Sensory Physiology, Vol. IX. Berlin: Springer-Verlag, pp. 55–83.

Graziadei, P. P. C., and G. A. Monti Graziadei (1978b) The olfactory sensory system: A model for the study of neurogenesis and axon regeneration in mammals. In C. W. Cotman (ed.): Neuronal Plasticity. New York: Raven Press, pp. 131–153.

Graziadei, P. P. C., and G. A. Monti Graziadei (1979) Neurogenesis and neuron regeneration in the olfactory system of mammals. I. Morphological aspects of differentiation and structural organization of the olfactory sensory neurons. J. Neurocytol. *8:* 1–18.

Graziadei, P. P. C., and G. A. Monti Graziadei (1979) Plasticity of connections of the olfactory sensory neuron: Regeneration into the forebrain following bulbectomy in the neonatal mouse. Neuroscience 4: 713–727.

Graziadei, P. P. C., and G. A. Monti Graziadei (1980) Neurogenesis and neuron regeneration in the olfactory system of mammals. III. Deafferentiation and reinnervation of the olfactory bulb following section of the fila olfactoria in rat. J. Neurocytol. 9: 145–162.

Graziadei, P. P. C., and G. A. Monti Graziadei (1986a) Neuronal changes in the forebrain of mice following penetration of regenerating olfactory axons. J. Comp. Neurol. 247: 344–356.

Graziadei, P. P. C., and G. A. Monti Graziadei (1986b) Principles of organization of the vertebrate olfactory glomerulus: An hypothesis. Neuroscience 19: 1025–1035.

Graziadei, P. P. C., and G. A. Monti Graziadei (1989) Autoradiographic demonstration of neurons migrating from the olfactory neuroepithelium. Chem. Senses 14:705.

Graziadei, P. P. C., and M. Okano (1979) Neuronal degeneration and regeneration in the olfactory epithelium of pigeon following transection of the first cranial nerve. Acta Anat. 104: 220–236.

Graziadei, P. P. C., and D. W. Samanen (1980) Ectopic glomerular structures in the olfactory bulb of neonatal and adult mice. Brain Res. 187: 467–472.

Graziadei, P. P. C., and D. Tucker (1970) Vomeronasal receptor in turtles. Z. Zellforsch. 105: 498–514.

Graziadei, P. P. C., J. A. Heckroth, and G. A. Monti Graziadei (1986) Ultrastructural observations of olfactory glomeruli without a target. Chem. Senses 11:604.

Graziadei, P. P. C., R. R. Levine, and G. A. Monti Graziadei (1978) Regeneration of olfactory axons and synapse formation in forebrain after bulbectomy in neonatal mice. Proc. Nat. Acad. Sci. USA 75: 5230–5234.

Graziadei, P. P. C., M. D. Karlan, G. A. Monti Graziadei, and J. J. Bernstein (1980) Neurogenesis of sensory neurons in the primate olfactory system after section of the fila olfactoria. Brain Res. 196: 289–300.

Greer, C. A., W. B. Stewart, M. H. Teicher, and G. M. Shepherd (1982) Functional development of the olfactory bulb and a unique glomerular complex in the neonatal rat. J. Neurosci. 12: 1744–1759.

Haberly, L. B., and J. L. Price (1977) The axonal projection patterns of the mitral and tufted cells of the olfactory bulb in the rat. Brain Res. 129: 152–157.

Haggis, A. J. (1956) Analysis of the determination of the olfactory placode in Amblystoma punctatum. J. Embryol. Exp. Morphol. 4: 120–138.

Hall, W. G., and R. W. Oppenheim (1987) Developmental psychobiology: Prenatal, perinatal, and early postnatal aspects of behavioral development. Ann. Rev. Psychol. 38: 91–128.

Hamburger, V. (1963) Some aspects of the embryology of behavior. Quart. Rev. Biol. 38: 342–365.

Harding, J., P. P. C. Graziadei, G. A. Monti Graziadei, and F. L. Margolis (1977) Denervation in the primary olfactory pathway of mice. Brain Res. 132: 11–28.

Harvey, F. E., and J. J. Cowley (1984) Effects of external chemical environment on the developing olfactory bulbs of the mouse (Mus musculus). Brain Res. Bull. 13: 541–547.

Heckroth, J. A., G. A. Monti Graziadei, and P. P. C. Graziadei (1983) Intraocular transplants of olfactory neuroepithelium in rat. Int. J. Dev. Neurosci. *1:* 273–287.

Heimer, L. (1976) The olfactory cortex and the ventral striatum. In O. Livingston and O. Kornykiewicz (eds.). Limbic Mechanisms: The Continuing Evolution of the Limbic System Concept. New York: Plenum Press, pp. 95–189.

Hinds, J. W. (1967) Autoradiographic study of histogenesis in the mouse olfactory bulb. I. Time of origin of neurons and neuroglia. J. Comp. Neurol. *134:* 287–304.

Hinds, J. W. (1968) Autoradiographic study of histogenesis in the mouse olfactory bulb. II. Cell proliferation and migration. J. Comp. Neurol. *134:* 305–322.

Hinds, J. W. (1972a) Early neuron differentiation in the mouse olfactory bulb. I. Light microscopy. J. Comp. Neurol. *146:* 233–252.

Hinds, J. W. (1972b) Early neuron differentiation in the mouse olfactory bulb. II. Electron microscopy. J. Comp. Neurol. *146:* 253–276.

Hinds, J. W., and P. L. Hinds (1976a) Synaptogenesis in the mouse olfactory bulb. I. Quantitative studies. J. Comp. Neurol. *169:* 15–40.

Hinds, J. W., and P. L. Hinds (1976b) Synaptogenesis in the mouse olfactory bulb. II. Morphogenesis. J. Comp. Neurol. *169:* 41–62.

Hinds, J. W., and N. A. McNelly (1973) Aging in the rat olfactory system: Correlation of changes in the olfactory epithelium and maturation of the axon initial segment. J. Comp. Neurol. *151:* 281–306.

Hinds, J. W., and N. A. McNelly (1977) Aging of the rat olfactory bulb: Growth and atrophy of constituent layers and changes in size and number of mitral cells. J. Comp. Neurol. *171:* 345–368.

Hinds, J. W., and N. A. McNelly (1979) Aging in the rat olfactory bulb: Quantitative changes in mitral cell organelles and somato-dendritic synapses. J. Comp. Neurol. *184:* 811–820.

Hinds, J. W., and N. A. McNelly (1981) Aging in the rat olfactory system: Correlation of changes in the olfactory epithelium and olfactory bulb. J. Comp. Neurol. *203:* 441–453.

Hinds, J. W., P. L. Hinds, and N. A. McNelly (1984) An autoradiographic study of the mouse olfactory epithelium: Evidence for long-lived receptors. Anat. Rec. *210:* 375–383.

Hoffmann, C. K. (1867) Uber die Membrana olfactoria. Amsterdam: Inagu.-Diss.

Humphrey, T. (1940) The development of the olfactory and the accessory olfactory formation in human embryos and fetuses. J. Comp. Neurol. *73:* 431–468.

Jackson, R. T., and C. C. Lee (1965) Degeneration of olfactory receptors induced by colchicine. Exp. Neurol. *11:* 483–492.

Jacobson, A. G. (1963a) The determination and positioning of the nose, lens and ear. I. Interactions within the ectoderm and between the ectoderm and underlying tissues. J. Exp. Zool. *154:* 273–284.

Jacobson, A. G. (1983b) The determination and positioning of the nose, lens and ear. II. The role of the endoderm. J. Exp. Zool. *154:* 285–292.

Jacobson, A. G. (1963c) The determination and positioning of the nose, lens and ear. III. Effects of reversing the antero-posterior axis of epidermis, neural plate and neurol fold. J. Exp. Zool. *154:* 293–303.

Jacobson, C. O. (1959) The localization of the presumptive cerebral regions in the neural plate of the Axolotl larva. J. Embryol. Exp. Morphol. *7:* 1–21.

Jastreboff, P. J., P. E. Pederson, C. A. Greer, W. B. Stewart, J. S. Kauer, T. E. Benson, and G. M. Shepherd (1984) Specific olfactory receptor populations projecting to identified glomeruli in the rat olfactory bulb. Proc. Natl. Acad. Sci. U.S.A. *81:* 5250–5254.

Jourdan, F., A. Duveau, L. Astic, and A. Holley (1980) Spatial distribution of [^{14}C] deoxyglucose update in the olfactory bulbs of rats stimulated with two different odours. Brain Res. *188:* 139–154.

Kauer, J.S. (1981) Olfactory receptor cell staining using horseradish peroxidase. Anat. Rec. *200:* 331–336.

Kauer, J.S. (1987) Coding in the olfactory system. In T. E. Finger (ed.): Offprints from Neurobiology of Taste and Smell. New York: Wiley, pp. 205–231.

Kim, H. (1989) The interaction of the sensory organs (olfactory placode and optic vesicles) with brain in *Xenopus* embryos. Ph.D. Dissertation, Florida State University, Tallahassee.

Kim, H., G. A. Monti Graziadei, and P. P. Graziadei (1988a) Eye transplantation experiments in *Xenopus* embryos. Anat. Rec. *220:*53A.

Kim, H., A. G. Monti Graziadei, and P. P. C. Graziadei (1988b) Cell migration after olfactory placode transplantation in *Xenopus*. Soc. Neurosci. Abstr. *14:*1131.

Klein, S. H., and P. P. C. Graziadei (1983) The differentiation of the olfactory placode in *Xenopus laevis:* A light and electron microscope study. J. Comp. Neurol. *217:* 17–30.

Knouff, R. A. (1935) The developmental patterns of ectodermal placodes in Rana pipiens. J. Comp. Neurol. *62:* 17–71.

Kosel, K. C., G. W. Van Hoesen, and J. R. West (1981) Olfactory bulb projections to the parahippocampal area of the rat. J. Comp. Neurol *198:* 467–482.

Kucharski, D., and W. G. Hall (1986) Internasal transfer of unilateral olfactory conditioning in rat pups. Paper presented at the annual meeting of the Eastern Psychological Association, New York.

Kucharski, D., and W. G. Hall (1987) New routes to early memories. Science *238:* 786–788.

Kucharski, D., I. B. Johanson, and W. G. Hall (1986) Unilateral olfactory conditioning in 6-day-old rat pups. Behav. Neur. Biol. *46:* 472–490.

Laing, D. G., and H. Panhuber (1978) Neurol and behavioral changes in rats following continuous exposure to an odor. J. Comp. Physiol. *124:* 259–265.

Laing, D. G., and H. Panhuber (1980) Olfactory sensitivity of rats reared in an odorous or deodorized environment. Physiol. Behav. *25:* 555–558.

Laing, D. G., H. Panhuber, E. A. Pittman, M. E. Willcox, and G. K. Eagleson (1985) Prolonged exposure to an odor or deodorized air alters the site of mitral cells in the olfactory bulb. Brain Res. *336:* 81–87.

Land, L. J. (1973) Localized projections of olfactory nerves to rabbit olfactory bulb. Brain Res. *63:* 153–166.

Land, L. J., and G. M. Shepherd (1974) Autoradiographic analysis of olfactory receptor projections in the rabbit. Brain Res. *70:* 506–510.

Land, L. J., R. P. Eager, and G. M. Shepherd (1970) Olfactory nerve projections to the olfactory bulb in the rabbit: Demonstration by means of a simplified ammonical silver degeneration method. Brain Res. *23:* 250–254.

LeBlond, C. P. (1964) Classification of cell populations on the basis of their proliferative behavior. Nat. Cancer Inst. Monogr. *14:* 119–150.

LeBlond, C. P., and B. E. Walker (1956) Renewal of cell populations. Physiol. Rev. *36:* 255–275.

LeDouarin, N. M. (1982) The Neural Crest. Cambridge: Cambridge University Press.

Leonard, C. M. (1981) Neurological mechanisms for early olfactory recognition. In R. N. Aslin, J. R. Alberts, and M. R. Peterson (eds.): Development of Perception: Psychobiological Perspectives, Vol. 1. New York: Academic Press.

Luskin, M. B., and J. L. Price (1983) The topographic organization of associational fibers of the olfactory system in the rat, including centrifugal fibers to the olfactory bulb. J. Comp. Neurol. *216:* 264–291.

Lustig, A. (1924) Die degeneration des epithels der riechschleimhaut des kaninchens nach zerstorung der riechlappen desselben. W.-B. Wien: Akad. 89, Abt. 2.

MacKay-Sim, A., and M. H. Nathan (1984) The projection from the olfactory epithelium to the olfactory bulb in the salamader Ambystoma trigrinum. Anat. Embryol. *170:* 93–97.

Macrides, F., and B. J. Davis (1983) The olfactory bulb. In P. C. Emson (ed.): Chemical Neuroanatomy. New York: Raven Press, pp. 391–426.

Macrides, F., and S. P. Schneider (1982) Laminar organization of mitral and tufted cells in the main olfactory of the adult hamster. J. Comp. Neurol. *208:* 419–430.

Macrides, F., B. J. Davis, W. M. Young, N. S. Nadi, and F. L. Margolis (1981) Cholinergic and catecholaminergic afferents to the olfactory bulb in the hamster: A neuroanatomical, biochemical and histochemical investigation. J. Comp. Neurol. *203:* 495–514.

Macrides, F., T. A. Schoenfeld, J. E. Marchand, and A. N. Clancy (1985) Evidence for morphologically, neurochemically and functionally heterogeneous classes of mitral and tufted cells in the olfactory bulb. Chem. Senses *10:* 175–202.

Magrassi, L., and P. P. C. Graziadei (1985) Interaction of the transplanted olfactory placode with the optic stalk and diencephalon in Xenopus laevis embryos. Neuroscience *15:* 903–921.

Mair, R. G., and R. C. Gesteland (1982) Response properties of mitral cells in the olfactory bulb of the neonatal rat. Neuroscience *7:* 3117–3125.

Mair, R. G., R. L. Gellman, and R. C. Gesteland (1982a) Postnatal proliferation and maturation of olfactory bulb neurons in the rat. Neuroscience *7:* 3105–3116.

Mair, R. G., R. C. Gesteland, and D. L. Blank (1982b) Changes in morphology and physiology of olfactory receptor cilia during development. Neuroscience *7:* 3091–3103.

Margolis, F. L. (1980) A marker protein for the olfactory chemoreceptor neuron. In R. A. Bradshaw and D. M. Schneider (eds.): Proteins of the Nervous System (2nd ed.). New York: Raven Press, pp. 59–83.

Marin-Padilla, M., and M. R. Amieva B. (1989) Early neurogenesis of the mouse olfactory nerve: Golgi and electron microscopic studies. J. Comp. Neurol. *288:* 339–352.

Math, F., and J. L. Devrainville (1980) Electrophysiological study on the postnatal development of mitral cell activity in the rat olfactory bulb. Brain Res. *190:* 243–247.

Matulionis, D. H. (1975) Ultrastructural study of mouse olfactory epithelium following destruction by $ZnSO_4$ and its subsequent regeneration. Amer. J. Anat. *142:* 67–90.

McEwen, R. S. (1949) A Textbook of Vertebrate Embryology. New York: Hold.

Meisami, E. (1976) Effects of olfactory deprivation on postnatal growth of the rat olfactory bulb utilizing a new method for production of neonatal unilateral anosmia. Brain Res. *107:* 437–444.

Meisami, E., and M. Firoozi (1985) Acetylcholinesterase activity in the developing olfactory bulb: A biochemical study on normal maturation and the influence of peripheral and central connections. Dev. Brain Res. *21:* 115–124.

Meisami, E., and R. Mousavi, R. (1982) Lasting effects of early olfactory deprivation on the growth, DNA, RNA and protein content, and Na-K-ATPase and AChE activity of the rat olfactory bulb. Dev. Brain Res. *2:* 217–229.

Meisami E., and L. Safari (1981) A quantitative study of the effects of early unilateral olfactory deprivation on the number and distribution of mitral and tufted cells and of glomeruli in the rat olfactory bulb. Brain Res. *221:* 81–107.

Messier, B., and C. P. LeBlond (1960) Cell proliferation and migration as revealed by radioautography after injection of thymidine H3 in male rats and mice. Amer. J. Anat. *106:* 247–285.

Metcalf, J. F. (1974) The olfactory epithelium: A model system for the study of neuronal differentiation and development in adult mammals. Ph.D. Dissertation, Florida State University, Tallahassee.

Miragall, F., G. Kadmon, M. Husmann, and M. Schachner (1988) Expression of cell adhesion molecules in the olfactory system of the adult mouse: Presence of the embryonic form of N-CAM. J. Dev. Biol. *129:*516–531.

Miragall, F., and G. A. Monti Graziadei (1982) Experimental studies on the olfactory marker protein. II. Appearance of the olfactory marker protein during differentiation of the olfactory sensory neuron of mouse. An immunohistochemical and autoradiographic study. Brain Res. *239:* 245–250.

Monti Graziadei, G. A. (1983) Experimental studies on the olfactory marker protein. III. The olfactory marker protein in the olfactory neuro-epithelium lacking connections with the forebrain. Brain Res. *262:* 303–308.

Monti Graziadei, G. A., and P. P. C. Graziadei (1979a) Neurogenesis and neuron regeneration in the olfactory system of mammals. II. Degeneration and reconstitution of the olfactory sensory neurons after axotomy. J. Neurocytol. *8:* 197–213.

Monti Graziadei, G. A., and P. P. C. Graziadei (1979b) Studies on neuronal plasticity and regeneration in the olfactory system: Morphologic and functional characteristics of the olfactory sensory neuron. In E. Meisami and M. A. B. Brazier (eds.): Neural Growth and Differentiation. New York: Raven Press, pp. 373–396.

Monti Graziadei, G. A., and P. P. C. Graziadei (1981) Experimental studies on the olfactory marker protein. I. Presence of the olfactory marker protein in tufted and mitral cells. Brain Res. *209:* 405–410.

Monti Graziadei, G. A., and P. P. C. Graziadei (1983) Experimentally induced extraepithelial migration of olfactory neurons in neonatal and adult rodents. Soc. Neurosci. Abstr. *9:*1019.

Monti Graziadei, G. A., and P. P. C. Graziadei (1984) The olfactory organ, neural transplantation. In J. R. Sladek and D. M. Gash (eds.): Neurol Transplants. New York: Plenum Press, pp. 167–186.

Monti Graziadei, G. A., F. L. Margolis, J. W. Harding, and P. P. C. Graziadei (1977) Immunocytochemistry of the olfactory marker protein. J. Histochem. Cytochem. 25: 1311–1316.

Monti Graziadei, G. A., M. S. Karlan, J. J. Bernstein, and P. P. C. Graziadel (1980a) Reinnervation of the olfactory bulb after section of the olfactory nerve in monkey (Saimiri sciureus). Brain Res. 189: 343–354.

Monti Graziadei, G. A., R. S. Stanley, and P. P. C. Graziadei (1980b) The olfactory marker protein in the olfactory system of the mouse during development. Neuroscience 5: 1239–1252.

Morrison, E. E., and P. P. C. Graziadei (1983) Transplant of olfactory mucosa in the rat brain. I. A light microscopic study of transplant organization. Brain Res. 279: 241–245.

Moulton, D. G. (1974) Dynamics of cell populations in the olfactory epithelium. Ann. N.Y. Acad. Sci. 237: 52–61.

Moulton, D. G. (1976) Spatial patterning of responses to odors in the peripheral olfactory system. Physiol. Rev. 56: 578–593.

Moulton, D. G., and R. P. Fink (1972) Cell proliferation and migration in the olfactory epithelium. In D. Schneider (ed.): Olfaction and Taste, Vol. IV. Stuttgart, Germany: Wissenschaftliche Verlagsgesellschaft MHB, pp. 20–36.

Moulton, D. G., G. Celebi, and R. P. Fink (1970) Olfaction in mammals-two aspects: Proliferation of cells in the olfactory epithelium and sensitivity to odors. In G. E. W. Wolstenhome and J. Knight (eds.): Taste and Smell in Vertebrates. London: Churchill.

Mulvaney, B. D., and H. E. Heist (1971a) Centriole migration during regeneration and normal development of olfactory epithelium. J. Ultrastruct. Res. 35: 274–281.

Mulvaney, B. D., and H. E. Heist (1971b) Regeneration of rabbit olfactory epithelium. Amer. J. Anat. 313: 241–252.

Nagahara, Y. (1940) Experimentelle studien ueber die histologischen veranderungen des geruchsorgans nach der olfactoriusdurchschneidung. Beitrage zur kenntnis des feineren baus des geruchsorgans. Jap. J. Med. Sci. Pathol. 5: 165–199.

Nakamura, Y. (1916) Uber die Veranderung des Geruchsorgans nach der Olfactoriusdruchschneidung bei Froschen, Dainihon, Jiji Ih, 22.

Oley, N., R. S. DeHan, D. Tucker, J. C. Smith, and P. P. C. Graziadei (1975) Recovery of structure and function following transection of the primary olfactory nerves in pigeons. J. Comp. Physiol. Psychol. 88: 477–495.

Oppenheim, R. W. (1982) The neuroembryological study of behavior: Progress, problems, perspectives. Curr. Top. Dev. Biol. 17: 257–309.

O'Rahilly, R. (1967) The early development of the nasal pit in staged human embryos. Anat. Rec. 157: 380.

Papez, J. W. (1967) Comparative Neurology. New York: Hafner, pp. 1–509.

Parsons, T. S. (1971) Anatomy of nasal structures from a comparative viewpoint. In L. M. Beidler (ed.): Handbook of Sensory Physiology, Vol. IV. Berlin: Springer-Verlag, pp. 1–23.

Pearson, A. A. (1941a) The development of the olfactory nerve in man. J. Comp. Neurol. *75:* 199–217.

Pearson, A. (1941b) The development of nervus terminalis in man. J. Comp. Neurol. *15:* 39–66.

Pedersen, P. E., and E. M. Blass (1981) Olfactory control over suckling in albino rats. In R. N. Aslin, J. R. Alberts, and M. R. Petersen (eds.): Development of Perception: Psychobiological Perspectives, Vol. 1. New York: Academic Press.

Pedersen, P. E., and E. M. Blass (1982) Prenatal and postnatal determinants of the first suckling episode in the albino rat. Develop. Psychol. *15:* 349–356.

Pedersen, P. E., C. L. Williams, and E. B. Blass (1982) Activation and odor conditioning of suckling behavior in 3-day-old albino rats. J. Exp. Psychol.: Anim. Behav. Proc. *8:* 329–341.

Pedersen, P. E., W. B. Stewart, C. A. Greer, and G. M. Shepherd (1983) Evidence for olfactory function in utero. Science *221:* 478–480.

Pedersen, P. E., C. A. Greer, and G. M. Shepherd (1985) Early development of olfactory function. In E. M. Blass (ed.): Handbook of Behavioral Neurobiology, Vol. 8. New York: Plenum Press, pp. 163–203.

Pedersen, P. E., P. J. Jastreboff, W. B. Stewart, and G. M. Shepherd (1986) Mapping of an olfactory receptor population that projects to a specific region in the rat olfactory bulb. J. Comp. Neurol *250:* 93–108.

Pelosi, P., and A. M. Pisanelli (1981) Binding of [^{3}H]-2-isobutyl-3-methoxypyrazine to cow olfactory mucosa. Chem. Senses *6:* 77–85.

Pelosi, P., N. E. Baldaccini and A. M. Pisanelli (1982) Identification of a specific olfactory receptor of 2-isobutyl-3-methoxypyrazine. Biochem. J. *201:* 245–248.

Pevzner, J., R. R. Trifiletti, S. M. Strittmatter, and S. H. Snyder (1985) Isolation and characterization of an olfactory receptor protein for odorant pyrazines. Proc. Natl. Acad. Sci. USA *82:* 3050–3054.

Pevzner, J., P. B. Sklar, and S. H. Snyder (1986) Odorant-binding protein: Localization to nasal glands and secretions. Proc. Natl. Acad. Sci. USA, *83:* 4942–4946.

Pinching, A. J., and K. B. Doving (1974) Selective degeneration in the rat olfactory bulb following exposure to different odours. Brain Res. *82:* 195–204.

Powell, T. P. S., W. M. Cowan, and G. Raisman (1965) The central olfactory connections. J. Anat. *99:* 791–813.

Prasada Rao, P. D., and T. E. Finger (1984) Asymmetry of the olfactory system in the brain of the whiner flounder, (*Pseudopleuronectes americanus*). J. Comp. Neurol. *225:* 492–510.

Price, J. L., and T. P. S. Powell (1970) An experimental study of the origin and the course of the centrifugal fibers to the olfactory bulb in the rat. J. Anat. *107:* 215–237.

Purves, D., and J. W. Lichtman (1980) Elimination of synapses in the developing nervous system. Science *210:* 153–157.

Rafols, J. A., and T. V. Getchell (1983) Morphological relations between the receptor neurons, sustentacular cells and Schwann cells in the olfactory mucosa of the salamander. Anat. Rec. *206:* 87–101.

Raisman, G. (1972) An experimental study of the projection of the amygdala to the accessory olfactory bulb and its relationship to the concept of a dual olfactory system. Brain Res. *14:* 395–408.

Rall, W., G. M. Shepherd, T. S. Reese, and M. W. Brightman (1966) Dendro-dendritic synaptic pathway for inhibition in the olfactory bulb. Exp. Neurol. *14:* 44–56.

Ramón y Cajal, S. (1955) Histologie du Systeme Nerveux de l'homme et des Verte-bres, Vol. 1, A Maloine, Paris [Reprinted by Consejo Superior de Investigaciones Cientificas, Inst. Ramon y Cajal, Madrid].

Reyer, R. W. (1962) Differentiation and growth of the embryonic nose, lens and corneal anlagen implanted into the larval eye or dorsal fin in Amblystoma punctatum. J. Exp. Zool. *151:* 123–153.

Samanen, D. W., and W. B. Forbes (1984) Replication and differentiation of olfactory receptor neurons following axotomy in the adult hamster: A morphometric anal-ysis of postnatal neurogenesis. J. Comp. Neurol. *225:* 201–211.

Saucier, D., and L. Astic (1986) Analysis of the topographical organization of olfac-tory epithelium projections in the rat. Brain Res. Bull. *16:* 455–462.

Scalia, F. (1968) A review of recent experimental studies on the distribution of the olfactory tracts in mammals. Brain Behav. Evol. *1:* 101–123.

Scalia, F., and S. Winans (1975) The differential projections of the olfactory bulb and accessory olfactory bulb in mammals. J. Comp. Neurol. *161:* 31–56.

Scalia, F., and S. S. Winans (1976) New perspectives on the morphology of the olfactory system: Olfactory and vomeronasal pathways in mammals. In R. L. Doty (ed.): Mammalian Olfaction, Reproductive Processes, and Behavior. New York: Academic Press, pp. 8–28.

Scarpa, A. (1785) Anatomicarum annotationum liber secundus. De organo olfactus praecipuo deque nervis nasalibus interioribus e pari quinto nervorum cerebri. Auctore Antonio Scarpa. Ticini Regii.

Schiff, M. (1859) Der erste hirnnerv ist der geruchsnerv. Moleschotts Untersuch *6:* 254–424.

Schoenfeld, T. A., J. E. Marchand, and F. Macrides (1985) Topographical organiza-tion of tufted cell axonal projections in the hamster main olfactory bulb: An intrabulbar associational system. J. Comp. Neurol. *235:* 503–518.

Schoenfeld, T. A., L. McKerracher, R. Obar, and R. B. Vallee (1989) MAP 1A and MAP 1B are structurally related microtubule associated proteins with distinct developmental patterns in the CNS. J. Neurosci. *9:*1712–1730.

Schultz, E. W. (1941) Regeneration of olfactory cells. Proc. Soc. Exp. Biol. *46:* 41–43.

Schultz, E. W. (1960) Repair of the olfactory mucosa. Amer. J. Path. *37:* 1–19.

Schultze, M. (1856) Uber die Endigungsweise des Geruchsnerven und der Epithe-lialgelbilde der Nasenschleimhaut, Mber. dtsch. Akad. Wiss. Berlin. 21: 504–515.

Schultze, M. (1862) Untersuchungen uber den Bau der Nasenschleimhaut, nament-lich die Strukter and Endigungsweise der Geruchsnerven bei dem Menschen und den Wirbeltieren, Abhandl. Naturforsch, Ges. Halle *7:* 1–100.

Schwanzel-Fukuda, M., and D. W. Pfaff (1989) Origin of luteinizing hormone-releasing hormone neurons. Nature 338:161–164.

Schwob, J. E., and J. L. Price (1978) The cortical projection of the olfactory bulb: Development in fetal and neonatal rats correlated with quantitative variations in adult rats. Brain Res. *151:* 369–374.

Schwob, J. E., and J. L. Price (1984) The development of axonal connections in the central olfactory system of rats. J. Comp. Neurol. *223:* 203–222.

Schwob, J. E., B. Friedman, and J. L. Price (1986) Development of axonal connections in the central olfactory system. In W. Breipohl and R. Apfelbach (eds.): Ontogeny of Olfaction. Berlin: Springer-Verlag, pp. 177–198.

Scott, J. W. (1986) The olfactory bulb and central pathways. Experientia 42: 223–232.

Scott, J. W., R. L. McBride, and S. P. Schneider (1980) The organization of projections from the olfactory bulb to the piriform cortex and olfactory tubercle in the rat. J. Comp. Neurol. 194: 519–534.

Sen Gupta, P. (1967) Olfactory receptor reaction to the lesion of the olfactory bulb. In T. Hayashi (ed.): Olfaction and Taste, Vol. II. New York-London: Pergamon, pp. 193–201.

Shammah-Lagnado, S. J., and N. Negrao (1981) Efferent connections of the olfactory bulb in the opposum (*Didelphis marsupialis autira*): A Fink-Heimer study. J. Comp. Neurol. 201: 51–63.

Sharp, F. R., J. S. Kauer, and G. M. Shepherd (1975) Local sites of activity-related glucose metabolism in rat olfactory bulb during olfactory stimulation. Brain Res. 98: 596–600.

Shipley, M. T. (1985) Transport of molecules from nose to brain: Transneuronal anterograde and retrograde labeling in the rat olfactory system by wheat germ agglutinin-horseradish peroxidase applied to the nasal epithelium. Brain Res. Bull. 15: 129–142.

Shipley, M. T., F. J. Halloran, and J. delaTorre (1985) Surprisingly rich projection from locus coeruleus to the olfactory bulb in the rat. Brain Res. 329: 294–299.

Simmons, P. A., and T. V. Getchell (1981a) Neurogenesis in olfactory epithelium: Loss and recovery of transepithelial voltage transients following olfactory nerve section. J. Neurophysiol. 45: 516–528.

Simmons, P. A. and T. V. Getchell (1981b) Physiological activity of newly differentiated olfactory recpetor neurons correlated with morphological recovery from olfactory nerve section in the salamander. J. Neurophysiol. 45:529–549.

Simmons, P. A., and T. V. Getchell (1981c) Ultrastructional changes in olfactory receptor neurons following olfactory nerve section. J. Comp. Neurol. 197: 237–257.

Singh, S. C. (1977) The development of olfactory and hippocampal pathways in the brain of the rat. Anat. Embryol. 151: 183–199.

Skeen, L. C. and W. C. Hall (1977). Efferent projections of the main and accessory olfactory bulb in the tree shrew (*Tupaia glis*). J. Comp. Neurol. 172: 1–36.

Smith, C. G. (1935) The change in volume of the olfactory and accessory olfactory bulbs of the albino rat during postnatal life. J. Comp. Neurol. 61: 477–508.

Smith, C. G. (1938) Changes in the olfactory mucosa and the olfactory nerves following intranasal treatment with one per cent zinc sulfate. Canad. Med. J. 39: 138–140.

Smith, C. G. (1951) Regeneration of sensory olfactory epithelium and nerves in adult frogs. Anat. Rec. 109: 661–671.

Smotherman, W. P. (1982a) Odor aversion learning by the rat fetus. Physiol. Behav. 29: 769–771.

Smotherman, W. P. (1982b) In utero chemosensory experience alters taste preferences and corticosterone responsiveness. Behav. Neurol. Biol. 36: 61–68.

Smotherman, W. P., and S. R. Robinson (1985) The rat fetus in its environment: Behavioral adjustments to novel, familiar, aversive and conditioned stimuli presented in utero. Behav. Neurosci. *99:* 521–530.

Smotherman, W. P., L. S. Richard, and S. R. Robinson (1984) Techniques for observing fetal behavior in utero: A comparison of chemomyelotomy and spinal transection. Dev. Psychobiol. *17:* 661–674.

Stanley, R. S. (1979) A histological study of the prenatal development of the peripheral olfactory system in the mouse (*Mus musculus*). Thesis, Florida State University, Tallahassee.

Stewart, W. B., P. E. Pedersen, C. A. Greer, and G. M. Shepherd (1985) The topography of olfactory epithelium to olfactory bulb projections in the rat. Chem. Senses *10:* 400.

Stickrod, G. D., Kimble, and W. Smotherman (1982) In uteru taste/odor aversion conditioning in the rat. Physiol. Behav. *28:* 5–7.

Stout, R. P., and P. C. P. Graziadei (1980) Influence of the olfactory placode on the development of the brain in *Xenopus laevis* (Daudin). I. Axonal growth and connections of the transplanted olfactory placode. Neuroscience *5:* 2175–2186.

Switzer, R. C., J. Olmos, and L. Heimer (1985) Olfactory system. In G. Paximos (ed.): The Rat Nervous System, Vol. 1, Forebrain and Midbrain. Australia: Academic Press.

Takagi, S. F. (1971) Degeneration and regeneration in the olfactory epithelium. In L. M. Beidler (ed.): Handbook of Sensory Physiology, Vol. IV. Berlin: Springer-Verlag. pp. 74–79.

Takagi, S. F. (1986) Studies on the olfactory nervous system of the old world monkey. Prog. Neurobiol. *27:* 195–249.

Takagi, S. F., and T. Yajima (1964) Electrical responses to odours of degenerating olfactory epithelium. Nature (Lond.) *202:* 1220.

Takagi, S. F., and T. Yajima (1965) Electrical activity and histological change in the degenerating olfactory epithelium. J. Gen. Physiol. *48:* 559–569.

Takata, N. (1929) Riechnery und geruchsorgan. Arch. Ohren-, Nasen-u, Kehlkopfheilk. *121:* 43–78.

Teicher, M. H., and E. M. Blass (1976) Suckling in newborn rats: Eliminated by nipple lavage, reinstated by pup saliva. Science *193:* 422–525.

Teicher, M. H., and E. M. Blass (1977) The role of olfaction and amniotic fluid in the first suckling response of newborn albino rats. Science *198:* 635–636.

Thiebaud, C. H. (1983) A reliable new cell marker in *Xenopus*. Dev. Biol. *98:* 245–249.

Thornhill, R. A. (1967) The ultrastructure of the olfactory epithelium of the lamprey *Lampetra fluviatilis*. J. Cell Sci. 2: 591–602.

Thornhill, R. A. (1970) Cell division in the olfactory epithelium of the lamprey, *Lampetra fluviatilis*. Z. Zellforsch, Mikrosk. Anat. *109:* 147–157.

Tucker, D. (1971) Nonolfactory responses from the nasal cavity: Jacobson's organ and the trigeminal system. In L. M. Beidler (ed.). Handbook of Sensory Physiology, Vol. IV. New York: Springer-Verlag, pp. 151–177.

Turner, B. H., K. Gupta, M. Mishkin, and M. Kapp (1977) The projections of the olfactory bulb in the monkey (*Macaca mulatta*). Anat. Rec. *187:* 733.

van E. Campenhout, (1936) Origins du nerf olfactif chez le porc. Arch. Anat. Microsc. *32:* 391–407.

van E. Campenhout, (1948) La contribution des placodes epiblastiques au developpement des ganglions des nerfs craniens chez l'embryon humain. Arch. Biol. (Paris) *59:* 253–266.

van E. Campenhout, (1957) Le developement embryonnaire compare des nerfs olfactif et auditif. Acta Otorhinolaryngol. Belg., *11:* 279–287.

Verhaagen, J., A. B. Oestreicher, V. H. Gispen, and F. L. Margolis (1989) The expression of the growth associated protein B50/GAP43 in the olfactory system of neonatal and adult rats. J. Neurosci, *9:*683–691.

Verwoerd, C. D. A., and C. G. van Oostrom (1979) Cephalic neural crest and placodes. In A. Brodal, J. van Limborgh, R. Ortmann, W. Hild, T. H. Schiebler and E. Wolff (eds.): Advances in Anatomy Embryology and Cell Biology *58:* 1–71.

Verwoerd, C. D. A., C. G. van Oostrom and H. L. Veroerd-Verhoef (1981) Otic placode and cephalic neural crest. Acta Otolaryngol. *91:* 431–435.

Viereck, C., R. P. Tucker, and A. Matus (1989) The adult rat olfactory system expresses microtubule-associated proteins found in the developing brain. J. Neurosci. *9:*3547–3557.

Vinnikov, Y. A., and L. K. Titova (1957) The morphology of the olfactory organ. Moscow: Meditsina, p. 295.

von Brunn, A. (1892) Beitrage zur mikroskopischen anatomie der menschlichen nasenhohle. Arch. Mikrosk. Anat. *39:* 632–651.

Van Oostrom, C. G, and C. D. A. Verwoerd (1979) The origin of the olfactory placode. Proc. 92nd Meeting, Amer. Assoc. Anat. Rec. *193:*160.

Wang, R. T., and M. Halpern (1982a) Neurogenesis in the vomeronasal epithelium of adult garter snakes. 1. Degeneration of bipolar neurons and proliferation of undifferentiated cells following experimental vomeronasal axotomy. Brain Res. *237:* 23–39.

Wang, R. T., and M. Halpern (1982b) Neurogenesis in the vomeronasal epithelium of adult garter snakes. 2. Reconstitution of the bipolar neuron layer following experimental vomeronasal axotomy. Brain Res. *237:* 41–59.

Wilson, K. C. P., and G. Raisman (1980) Age-related changes in the neurosensory epithelium of the mouse vomeronsal organ: Extended period of postnatal growth in size and evidence for rapid cell turnover in the adult. Brain Res. *185:* 103–113.

Wray, S., P. Grant, and H. Gainer (1989) Evidence that cells expressing luteinizing hormone-releasing hormone mRNA in the mouse are derived from progenitor cells in the olfactory placode. Proc. Nat. Acad. Sci. USA *86:*8132–8136.

Yntema, C. L. (1955) Ear and Nose. In B. H. Willier, P. A. Weiss, and V. Hamburger (eds.): Sec. VII, Chap. 3. Philadelphia: Saunders pp. 415–428.

Chapter Fourteen

TASTE DEVELOPMENT

CHARLOTTE M. MISTRETTA

University of Michigan
Ann Arbor, Michigan

I INTRODUCTION

The taste system is altered morphologically, neurophysiologically, and behaviorally in profound ways during development. Although there are not the extensive, detailed data that now are available for many parts of the auditory, somesthetic, and visual systems, it is clear that study of the sense of taste will provide insights to complement and supplement emerging principles of sensory system development. Much of the discussion that follows will refer to work on rats and sheep, and therefore a word on use of these two species in taste is warranted. Sheep are an obvious choice for study because they are readily available and have a gestation of reasonable length (about 150 days). Developmental processes do not change radically overnight, and yet gestation is not so lengthy to prohibit approaches that would require longitudinal experiments. The fetuses are a useful size for experiments (about 1000 g at two-thirds of gestation), the pregnant uterus withstands substantial surgical manipulation without subsequent abortion, and amniotic fluid composition is similar to that in humans. Because of these factors, sheep have been used extensively in studies of fetal physiology. Added to this is a developmental time course for taste bud formation that parallels that in the human, with major pre- and postnatal components. For these reasons, sheep were used in the first studies on neurophysiological development of the taste system (Bradley and Mistretta, 1972, 1973a).

On the other hand, rats are suitable for a set of contrary reasons. Development is much shorter so animals do not have to be maintained for months for developmental experiments. Because taste bud development is primarily postnatal, fetal experiments usually are not necessary. There is a wealth of data on the taste system in rats, and developmental studies build on this body of literature. Thus a whole series of experiments on development of taste in rats (Hill and Almli, 1980; Ferrell et al. 1981; Hill et al, 1982, 1983; Hill, 1987a) complement those in sheep.

II OVERVIEW OF TASTE PROCESSING STRUCTURES

The sense of taste is unique among sensory systems because branches of three different cranial nerves (VII, IX, and X) are involved in innervation of receptors and transmission of gustatory sensation. The afferent innervation distributes to taste buds in several lingual and extralingual locations, including nasoincisor ducts, soft palate, and epiglottis (Figure 1). Taste buds in these various oral–pharyngeal locations and their respective innervation are not redundant but have specialized histochemical and functional characteristics (Bradley, 1982, 1988). Although most of this chapter will focus on taste buds in fungiform papillae on the anterior tongue and thus on re-

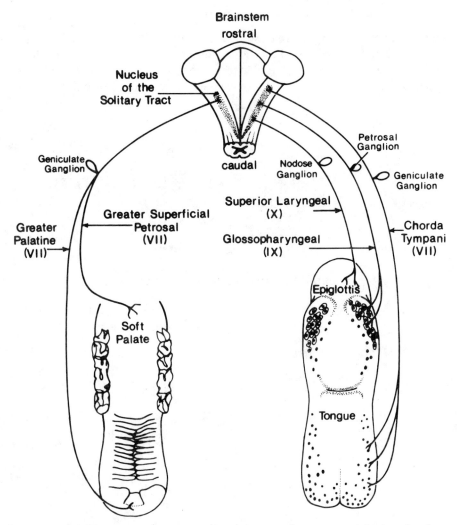

FIGURE 1. Diagram of nerves innervating taste buds on the tongue, epiglottis, soft palate, and nasoincisor duct and relative projections to the nucleus of the solitary tract in the medulla. The drawing is based on the anatomy of the tongue and palate in sheep, but it should be noted that a nasoincisor duct with taste buds, schematically indicated on the anterior hard palate and innervated by the greater palatine nerve, has not yet been reported in this species.

sponses from the chorda tympani nerve and second-order projection neurons of the chorda, this is simply because these are the most frequently studied taste buds. All of the taste receptors presumably have a distinct developmental history, and different processes might play a role in development of the various taste buds.

A   Taste Buds, Papillae, and Innervation

Taste buds on the tongue are contained in epithelial structures called papillae: The *fungiform* are distributed over much of the anterior two-thirds of the tongue; the *foliate* are situated on posterior, lateral borders of the tongue; and the *circumvallate* are located on the posterior tongue (Figures 2 A, B). All

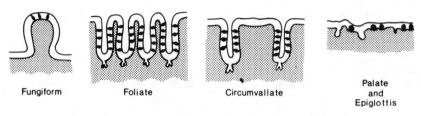

GUSTATORY PAPILLAE AND EPITHELIUM

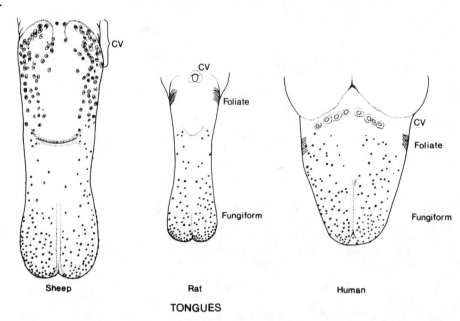

FIGURE 2. (*A*) Diagram of types of lingual gustatory papillae, the fungiform, foliate, and circumvallate, and of gustatory epithelium representative of that on the soft palate and epiglottis. (*B*) Drawings of sheep, rat, and human tongues to illustrate papilla types and distributions. Note that tongue sizes are not drawn to scale. Although foliate papillae are found in posterior, lateral locations of rat and human tongues, there are no foliates in sheep tongue. (From Mistretta, 1989.)

three of these papilla types are present in man and rodents (Figures 2B and 3); some species, such as sheep and cow, have only circumvallate papillae on the posterior tongue and no foliate (Figure 2B). Such species variations are not uncommon and can be reviewed in a chapter by Bradley (1971). Another papilla type on the tongue is the *filiform*. These are heavily keratinized papillae that cover most of the lingual surface area and possibly aid in manipulating food (Figure 3). Filiform papillae do not contain taste buds.

Taste buds in the fungiform papillae are innervated by the *chorda tympani branch of the facial nerve* (cranial nerve VII). In rat there are about 180 fungiform papillae, and they contain one taste bud each; in sheep there are about

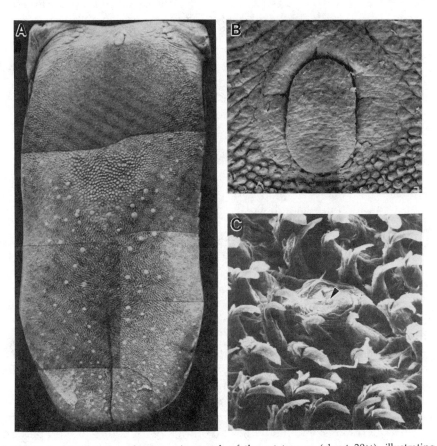

FIGURE 3. (A) Scanning electron micrograph of the rat tongue (about 30×), illustrating nongustatory, filiform papillae on most of the tongue surface. Distributed among the filiform are fungiform papillae that appear as larger, round structures over much of the anterior tongue. On the posterior tongue are located circumvallate and foliate papillae. (B) Micrograph of the circumvallate papilla at higher magnification (140×). (C) Micrograph of a fungiform papilla, with surrounding filiform papillae, at higher magnification (1200×). An arrowhead points to the taste pore in the dorsal surface of the fungiform papilla.

500 fungiform papillae that contain from 1 to 20 taste buds each. In rhesus monkey there are about 320 fungiform papillae on the tongue, and primates and humans generally have several taste buds per fungiform papilla (Bradley et al., 1985). Although taste buds in fungiform papillae have been studied more extensively than those in any other location, they represent only about 15% of total taste buds on the tongue in rats (Miller, 1977), about 20% in rhesus monkeys (Bradley et al., 1985), and about 10% in cows (Davies et al., 1979).

Taste buds in circumvallate papillae are innervated by the *lingual–tonsillar branch of the glossopharyngeal nerve* (cranial nerve IX). In rat there is a single circumvallate papilla with 400–600 buds. In primates and humans there are usually from 4 to 6 circumvallates, and in sheep there are about 20 on each lateral border of the tongue; as in rodent, these papillae can contain a few hundred taste buds each.

Taste buds in the most anterior folds of the foliate papilla are innervated by the *chorda tympani nerve,* and those in the posterior papilla are innervated by the *lingual–tonsillar branch of nerve IX.* In rat each lateral foliate contains about 230 taste buds for a total of 460 (Miller, 1977).

Taste buds in extratongue locations, the nasoincisor duct, soft palate, and epiglottis, are not contained in discrete papillae but are interspersed in the epithelium (Figure 2A). Often these taste buds are situated in close proximity to the opening of a glandular duct. Taste buds in the nasoincisor duct and soft palate are innervated by the *greater palatine* and *greater superficial nerve branches of the facial nerve,* respectively. In rat there are about 40 taste buds in the bilateral, nasoincisor ducts and about 200 on the soft palate.

Taste buds in the epiglottis are innervated by the *superior laryngeal branch of the vagus nerve* (cranial nerve X). There are about 50 of these buds on the epiglottis in rats; in sheep, however, there are 3000 taste buds in the epiglottis. Thus, extratongue taste buds can be numerous and represent a large proportion of an animal's total gustatory receptors. Miller (1977) estimates that in rat 15% of taste buds are in fungiform papillae, 36% in foliate, 28% in the circumvallate, and the remaining 21% in the soft palate and epiglottis.

All taste buds, regardless of location, are contained in stratified epithelium, and the buds themselves are thought to be composed of modified epithelial cells. However, there is no direct evidence to indicate whether gustatory epithelium is of ectodermal or neural crest origin. Taste buds contain about 40–60 cells surrounded by a basement membrane. The cells are arranged like segments within an orange, with an orientation perpendicular to the basement membrane (Figure 4). Most of the cells have apical specializations termed microvilli that extend into a taste pore or pit, which is a channel that penetrates through surface epithelial cells to the oral environment. Although the point of first contact between stimulus and receptor is on the microvilli, there is little known about these membrane specializations or the chemical environment of the taste pore in which the microvilli are

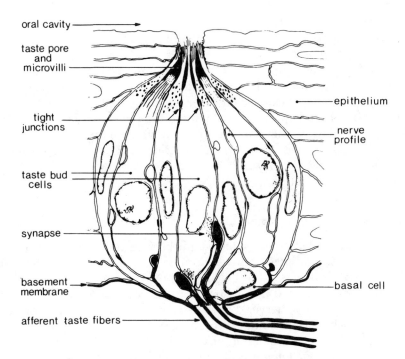

oral cavity

taste pore
and
microvilli

epithelium

tight
junctions

nerve
profile

taste bud
cells

synapse

basement
membrane

basal cell

afferent taste fibers

FIGURE 4. Diagram of the taste bud and associated structures. Although not labeled in the diagram, taste cells are categorized into three types. Type I (dark) cells are diagrammed as those with very long microvilli and large, dense granules near the cell apex. Type II (light) cells have shorter microvilli and membranous vesiculations in the apical region. Type III (intermediate) cells have intermediate structural characteristics. Basal cells, labeled near the basement membrane, are polygonal in shape and are located at the basolateral portions of the taste bud. (From Mistretta, 1989.)

found. Tight junctions are found between taste cells in the apical region of the bud and are thought to prevent direct access of chemicals in the oral environment to the interior of the taste bud.

Investigators still disagree about the number and sources of different cell types within the bud, but all current research indicates that more than two cell types exist, and the old categories of taste cell and supporting cell (still found in some textbooks) are not used. Dark cells (type I) and light cells (type II) generally are described, as are intermediate cells (type III) and basal cells (type IV). Some investigators conclude that all of these types are different ages of a single line of cells (Delay et al., 1986), whereas others conclude that there are discrete types with different lineages. In recent reconstructions of serially sectioned buds, synapses have been found in dark, light, and intermediate cell types (Kinnamon et al., 1985). Therefore, all types are potential taste receptor cells.

As with the olfactory receptor neurons, the taste bud cells turn over and are replaced (Beidler and Smallman, 1965). In rats the life span of a taste bud cell is about 10 days. Thus, peripheral receptor cells must constantly re-establish synaptic connections with afferent fibers and yet maintain order in taste innervation and sensation.

Nerve fibers enter the taste bud by penetrating the basement membrane and establish synapses and other specialized associations with taste cells. The taste fibers branch extensively on entering the taste bud (Beidler, 1969), and taste buds can be innervated by more than one chorda tympani fiber (Miller, 1971). Furthermore, a single chorda tympani fiber innervates from one to several taste buds (Miller, 1971). Therefore, peripheral innervation of taste cells and buds is very complex and provides opportunity for neural interactions in the periphery.

B   Central Taste Pathways

The afferent innervation of the taste buds projects in gustatory branches of the facial, glossopharyngeal and vagus nerves which make their first central synapses in the nucleus of the solitary tract (NST) in the medulla (Figure 1). Projections are arranged in a rostral to caudal direction in the nucleus in order of facial to vagal nerves, but there is overlap among projections from all taste branches. Depending on location of the receptors in various oral–pharyngeal regions, stimulation of taste buds can elicit very different reflexes including swallowing, salivation, the cephalic phase of insulin release, coughing, gagging, and apnea. These reflexes are mediated by short axon connections from the NST to medullary regions that include the salivatory nuclei, nucleus ambiguus, dorsal motor nucleus of the vagus, and the reticular formation.

Taste pathways from the second-order neurons in the NST to other central taste cells take different paths depending on species. In Old World monkeys NST cells project directly to the parvocellular portion of the ventral posteromedial nucleus of the thalamus, and thalamic neurons project to primary gustatory neocortex (Figure 5). (For detailed discussions of the taste pathways in monkeys and interconnections with other central nervous system structures, see Norgren, 1985 and Scott and Yaxley, 1989.) In rats, however, second-order cells project to a taste relay in the parabrachial nucleus in the dorsal pons (Figure 5). From the pons there are bifurcating projections: one to the thalamic–cortical pathway and another to taste areas in the central nucleus of the amygdala, bed nucleus of the stria terminalis, lateral hypothalamus, and caudal substantia innominata. Taste pathways in rat are further complicated because a significant portion of pontine neurons apparently project directly to gustatory neocortex without synapsing in the thalamic taste relay.

At both thalamic and cortical levels the taste nuclei are closely associated with and immediately adjacent to the somatosensory areas for oral sensation. The thalamic taste nucleus is located in the ventromedial tip of the ventral posteromedial thalamus and is distinguished by its small neurons

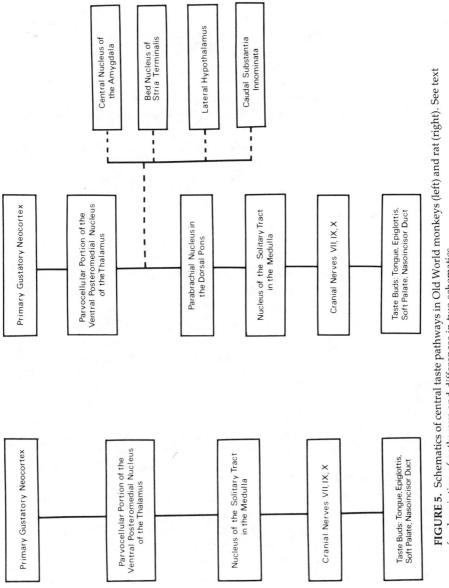

FIGURE 5. Schematics of central taste pathways in Old World monkeys (left) and rat (right). See text for description of pathways and differences in two schematics.

and sparse myelin. Projections from the thalamus to primary gustatory cortex are located immediately ventral to the primary somatosensory cortex. The transition from the somatosensory representation of the tongue to the taste representation of the tongue is at the transition from granular to agranular cortex. The tongue, therefore, is represented in both somatosensory and gustatory cortex; tactile and chemical stimuli activate the two areas, respectively. In rats the gustatory cortex is dorsal to the intersection of the middle cerebral artery and the rhinal sulcus, and in monkeys it is on the dorsal bank of the opercular cortex.

This is only a rudimentary outline of central taste projections. Details and discussion are provided in recent chapters by Finger (1987) and Norgren (1984), from which information in this section is drawn. Finger (1987) emphasizes that information about central taste pathways is based on data from very few species and, therefore, cautions against making firm conclusions about a basic mammalian organization for taste pathways.

C General Taste Physiology

In general, at levels of single taste receptor cells, single afferent fibers, and single neurons in the central nervous system, elements of the taste system respond to more than one class of chemical stimulus (e.g., sweet, salt, sour, or bitter). However, taste buds in different receptor areas complement each other in relative chemical responsiveness (Bradley, 1982). For example, taste buds on the anterior tongue in sheep generally are highly responsive to sodium salts. More posterior lingual taste buds are more responsive to other salts that are bitter or acidic (e.g., KCl and NH_4Cl). Epiglottal taste buds are highly responsive to acids, acidic salts, and water. Interesting recent experiments have demonstrated that taste buds on the soft palate and in the nasoincisor ducts are highly responsive to sugars (Travers et al., 1986; Nejad and Beidler, 1988). Thus, taste receptors throughout the oropharynx are not redundant but respond maximally to different chemicals. This provides a basis for the various taste functions of identification, acceptance or rejection of foods, and initiation of protective reflexes such as gagging, choking, and vomiting.

Because single taste fibers generally respond to more than one chemical stimulus, it was proposed early in the history of the field that quality coding is mediated by an "across-fiber pattern" of neural impulses (Erickson, 1963). Other investigators have espoused a modified "labeled line" idea about coding, emphasizing that single fibers usually respond "best" to chemicals representing one particular taste quality (for a discussion see Bartoshuk, 1978).

In the central nervous system, there can be convergence of input onto one neuron from taste buds that are in apposition to each other in the periphery. So, for example, a single neuron in the NST might receive afferent information from taste buds in both anterior tongue and nasoincisor duct and thus be highly responsive to both sugar and salt in the front of the mouth (Travers et al., 1986). Furthermore, single NST cells can receive afferent input from taste buds on both the anterior tongue and the posterior oral cavity (Sweazey and Smith, 1987). This extensive convergence relates to a major characteristic of NST taste neurons: they generally respond well to chemicals in more than one category of taste quality, and they are even more broadly responsive than peripheral neurons. In rat, taste neurons in the parabrachial nucleus in the pons remain broadly responsive, and there is some evidence that these cells respond with almost equal discharge frequency to a set of chemicals.

Although some investigators note that a substantial portion of taste cells in the thalamus responds to only one chemical quality, others emphasize that neurons usually respond less differentially to chemicals than at lower levels in the taste pathway. Inhibitory taste responses can be recorded from thalamic cells, whereas responses in the NST and pons generally are excitatory only. Cortical taste cells also exhibit more inhibitory responses than those in the brainstem, and as in investigations of thalamic taste responses, there is disagreement about whether data indicate greater or lesser specificity in chemical responses. Recent reviews of central neural taste mechanisms provide details and discussions of taste coding (Norgren, 1984; Travers et al., 1987).

III STRUCTURAL DEVELOPMENT OF TASTE BUDS

A Morphology

Gustatory papillae make an early appearance in the developing lingual epithelium (Figure 6) and subsequently are innervated by taste nerves (for a recent review see Bradley and Mistretta, 1988). After taste nerves reach the appropriate epithelium in apical papilla regions, taste bud cells apparently are induced to differentiate. Although evidence for neural induction of taste buds is based primarily on temporal association of nerve and receptor cell development, other recent data have substantiated this hypothesis. In studies of taste buds in the rat circumvallate papilla after birth, it has been demonstrated with nerve ablation experiments that the full complement of buds is achieved only through the synergistic interaction of the two glossopharyngeal nerves that innervate the papilla and cannot be explained on the basis of temporal associations alone (Hosley et al., 1987). Furthermore, a sensitive period from birth to 10 days postnatal is implied for these taste buds.

Taste buds in fungiform papillae first appear at about 20 days of gestation in the rat (Farbman, 1965; Mistretta, 1972), before 50 days of gestation in sheep (Bradley and Mistretta, 1973a), and at about 55 days of gestation in the human fetus (Bradley and Stern, 1967). There is general agreement that

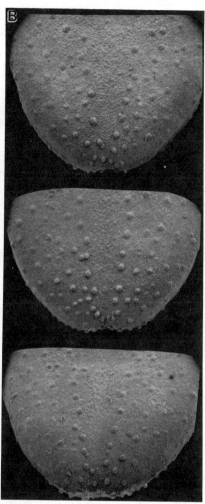

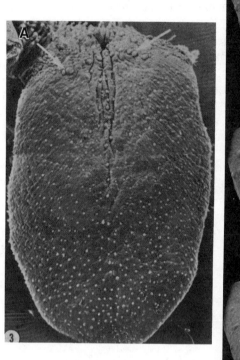

FIGURE 6. Scanning electron micrographs to illustrate initial appearance of fungiform papillae. (*A*) Dorsal tongue surface of a 10-week-old human fetus, ×40. (From Hersch and Ganchrow, 1980.) (*B*) Anterior tongues of three fetal rat littermates, aged 17 days of gestation, ×100. (From Mistretta, 1972.)

the early taste bud is composed of only one cell type. But descriptions of this initial cell type vary, and there is no detailed information on innervation of developing buds. In fact, an in-depth picture of taste bud development at the ultrastructural level in any one species is lacking; at best, only pieces of information are available.

The "presumptive" taste bud in rat, sheep, and human at the stage of first appearance is a localized collection of cells that has no pore and is covered by superficial cells of the tongue epithelium (Figures 7*A* and 8*A*,

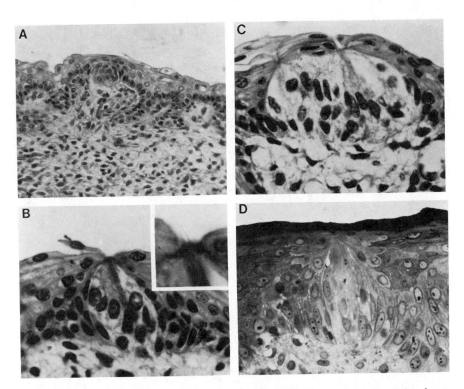

FIGURE 7. Light micrographs of taste buds from human fetuses at various gestational ages and an adult. (*A*) Presumptive taste bud from a fetus at about 12 weeks of gestation. ×400. Taste bud cells are still covered by superficial epithelial cells. (*B*) Taste bud with a taste pore from a fetus at about 16 weeks. ×400. The inset of the taste pore region at higher magnification demonstrates the fine taste microvilli, termed "taste hairs" in the earlier literature. (C) Taste bud from a fetus at about 16 weeks, illustrating presence of more than one pore. ×400. When examined in serial section, this taste bud was noted to have six pores. (*D*) Adult human taste bud. ×400. Although the tongue is covered with cornified cells, this taste bud is similar in general morphology to that in (*B*). [From Bradley and Stern (1977) and Bradley (1972).]

stage A) (Farbman, 1965; Bradley and Stern, 1967; Bradley and Mistretta, 1973a). Gradually the taste bud cells elongate to span the depth of the entire epithelium and a taste pore forms (Figures 7B and 8A, stages B, C, and D), through a process that is not yet understood. In the course of development, some taste buds are noted that have mulitple taste pores, sometimes as many as six (Figures 7C and 8A, stage E) (Bradley and Stern, 1967). Study of taste buds in chickens demonstrates that this general developmental sequence is not peculiar to mammals only (Ganchrow and Ganchrow, 1987).

The development of some of the structural elements in sheep taste buds has been described at the electron microscopic level (Mistretta and Bradley, 1983a). By 80 days of gestation (term = 147 days) apices of taste bud cells are arranged around a taste pit, there are short microvilli and club-shaped

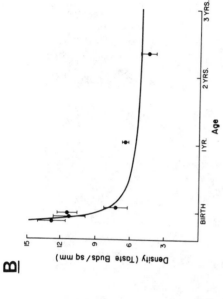

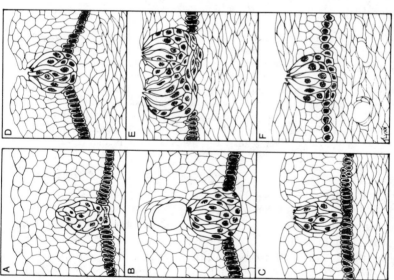

FIGURE 8. (*A*) Diagrammatic representation of key stages in development of taste buds on sheep epiglottis, from 96 days of gestation through birth. Stage A, collection of cells, covered by superficial cells, and no taste pore; B, vacuole above developing taste bud; C, wide taste pore; D, narrow taste pore; E, large taste bud with double pore; F, small taste bud with single, narrow pore. (Drawn from Bradley et al., 1980.) (*B*) The number of taste buds per square millimeter on the laryngeal surface of the epiglottis as a function of age in sheep. Means and standard errors for six age groups are presented. Taste bud density decreases rapidly during early development with growth of the epiglottis. (From Bradley et al., 1980.)

processes present on the cell apices, and tight junctions are observed between cells. Two morphological cell types are present in the taste buds, and numerous nerve profiles are distributed throughout the bud. By 110 days of gestation the microvilli and club-shaped processes on cell apices have increased in length; this could augment the amount of cell membrane accessible for initial interaction with chemical stimuli.

The only study of development of synapses is in fetal macaque taste buds (Zahm and Munger, 1983a,b). Fetuses at about the beginning of the second trimester of gestation have taste bud cells that contain typical afferent synaptic contacts with nerve fibers but no efferent synapses (Zahm and Munger, 1983b). Axoaxonic synapses are especially numerous at this stage of development but are observed less frequently in later fetal stages and not at all in neonatal animals. The investigators also observed degenerating axon profiles in the nerve bundle of some papillae and speculated that axoaxonic synapses could be involved in competitive interactions among axons during development. During the last part of gestation, macaque taste buds have three types of specialized axonal contacts: afferent synapses, efferent synapses, and subsurface cisternae (Zahm and Munger, 1983a). The investigators concluded that the ability of taste bud cells to form afferent synapses precedes ability to elaborate other axon-related membrane specializations.

The scant information on development of taste bud structure is just sufficient to pose intriguing questions for future experiments. Among such questions are: What cell interactions are involved in the process of taste pore formation, during which taste bud cells reportedly elongate and a channel develops in the superficial epithelial cells that cover the bud? Does one initial cell type differentiate into the other taste cell types or do the cell types develop from independent cell lines? Do certain cell types predominate during certain times in development? What is the relation, if any, between taste bud cell type and synapse type? What are the developmental relations between taste cells and synapses?

B Numbers of Taste Buds

In addition to the study of differences in morphology of taste buds, it is also informative to examine developmental differences in numbers of taste buds. In rat there is a single taste bud per fungiform papilla, and therefore once the bud forms, numbers per papilla do not alter. However, in posterior tongue, there are many more taste buds per gustatory papilla (circumvallate or foliate). Collective data from rat and hamster fungiform, circumvallate, and foliate papillae indicate that before 5 days postnatal there are very few mature taste buds on the tongue (Mistretta, 1972; Gottfried et al., 1984; Smith and Miller, 1986; Oakley, 1987). Acquisition of final numbers of mature taste buds is a gradual process over several weeks. In sheep and human, numerous mature taste buds are present prenatally, but the numbers of taste buds continue to increase after birth.

One of the most detailed quantitative studies is of taste buds in the epiglottis of sheep (Bradley et al., 1980). Numbers of taste buds increase developmentally, but because the epiglottis itself grows in size, taste bud density decreases and then plateaus (Figure 8B). From examination of different stages of taste bud development the investigators inferred that the original population of taste buds results from *de novo* formation of buds. The subsequent increase in taste bud number results from division of the original buds. The inference was based on observations that the most immature morphological stages of taste bud development are not observed at later ages when numbers of buds are still increasing. In addition, large taste buds with multiple pores are observed in sheep and human fetuses, and these could divide to form other buds (Figures 7C and 8A, stage E).

On the other hand, others recently have studied development of taste buds in the rat circumvallate and foliate papillae and made quantitative observations on numbers of mature taste buds (possessing a pore) from birth to 90 days (Oakley, 1987). Taste buds with more than one pore were not observed, and investigators concluded that new buds apparently did not form by division of mature buds.

Recently, as part of a study of receptive field development (Mistretta et al., 1988), we have obtained data on the number of taste buds in fungiform papillae of sheep fetuses (130 days of gestation), perinatal animals (about 1 week before or after birth), and postnatal lambs (30–80 days). From about 110 days of gestation through lamb ages, numbers of fungiform papillae on the sheep tongue are constant and total about 500. However, numbers of taste buds per papilla alter. The average number is 3.5 taste buds in fetal, 6.4 in perinatal, and 5.1 in lamb papillae (Figure 9). This is a significant difference across development, and the average number in perinatal animals in fact is larger than that in fetuses or lambs, and the lamb average is larger than that in fetuses. Associated with the perinatal period of increased numbers of taste buds per papilla is the appearance of many large, multipored taste buds. These could be in a process of division or budding (Mistretta et al., 1988).

Overall, then, taste bud number increases developmentally from fetus to lamb, as we have reported previously (Bradley and Mistretta, 1973a). However, because the average number of buds per papilla is greatest at perinatal stages, compared with fetal and lamb, there also must be loss of some taste buds between birth and lamb ages. This loss could be related to developmental differences in number of chorda tympani nerve fibers. Our data (Mistretta et al., 1988) indicate that the number of chorda tympani nerve fibers *increases* between 110 days of gestation and birth but then *decreases* between birth and lamb ages (Figure 9).

In summary, morphological studies demonstrate that the taste bud at time of first appearance is a rather rudimentary structure with one cell type and no direct communication with the oral environment. Maturation involves acquisition of other cell types, formation of a pore at the apex of the

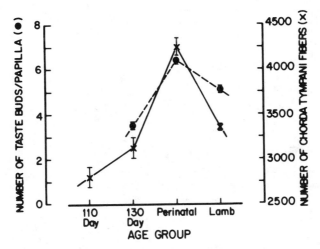

FIGURE 9. Number of taste buds per fungiform papilla in three age groups and total number of chorda tympani nerve fibers in four age groups of sheep. Means and standard errors are shown. Average number of taste buds in fungiform papillae in perinatal sheep is greater than in fetuses or lambs. This peak is associated in time with an apparent increase in number of chorda tympani nerve fibers. (From Mistretta et al., 1988.)

taste bud, progressive elaboration of various types of synapses, and loss of some synapses. Although the organ that contains taste buds, the papilla, develops early and does not change in number developmentally, the numbers of taste buds within papillae are altered. Increasing numbers of taste buds are associated with growth of organs containing the buds, to achieve a final, constant density of receptors. In the context of an overall increase in number of taste buds at least some species also show a loss of buds at one particular stage. This could be related to a loss of chorda tympani nerve fibers. Generally there are complex receptor and neural arrangements in the developing fetal and postnatal taste system. We are just beginning to be aware of the extent of these changes.

IV NEUROPHYSIOLOGICAL DEVELOPMENT OF THE TASTE SYSTEM

In the two species that have been studied extensively, rat and sheep, development of neurophysiological taste responses is characterized by extensive changes at both peripheral and central levels. Although the species are quite disparate, there are some similar developmental changes. However, because in rat there is essentially a postnatal morphological development of taste buds, major neurophysiological changes occur postnatally; in sheep there is pre- and postnatal morphological development of taste buds, and therefore, substantial neurophysiological changes take place before and after birth.

A Peripheral Taste System in Sheep

The first demonstration of neurophysiological taste function in a fetus was published in the early 1970s (Bradley and Mistretta, 1972, 1973a). Summated chorda tympani nerve and single-fiber recordings indicated that the peripheral taste system in sheep is functional for at least the last third of gestation and that fetal taste receptors respond to a variety of stimuli: NH$_4$Cl, KCl, NaCl, LiCl, acetic acid, glycerol, sodium saccharin, glycine, and quinine hydrochloride. In later experiments that focused on salt taste responses, striking developmental differences became apparent (Mistretta and Bradley, 1983a). Recordings were made from the chorda tympani nerve in five age groups of sheep: (1) fetuses at 110 days of gestation (term = 147 days); (2) fetuses at 130 days of gestation; (3) perinatal animals, 1 week before or after birth; (4) lambs, 35–85 days postnatal; and (5) adult sheep. A series of 0.5 M salts, NH$_4$Cl, KCl, NaCl, and LiCl, were used as stimuli.

Significant, substantial changes in taste responses were observed both before and after birth. In the youngest fetuses, NaCl and LiCl elicited much smaller neural response magnitudes than NH$_4$Cl and KCl (Figure 10A). Throughout the rest of gestation and postnatally, the NaCl and LiCl responses gradually increased in magnitude relative to NH$_4$Cl and KCl. In adults, NaCl, LiCl, and NH$_4$Cl all elicited similar, large response magnitudes, and KCl was less effective as a taste stimulus.

A

B

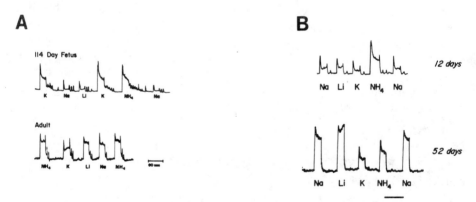

FIGURE 10. (A) Integrated records of multifiber responses from the chorda tympani nerve in a sheep fetus aged 114 days of gestation and an adult ewe. Chemical stimuli applied to the anterior tongue were 0.5 M NH$_4$Cl, KCl, NaCl, and LiCl, in order as indicated under the recordings. (Data from Mistretta and Bradley, 1983a.) (B) Integrated records of multifiber responses from the chorda tympani nerve in rats aged 12 and 52 days postnatal. Chemical stimuli applied to the anterior tongue were 0.1 M NaCl, LiCl, KCl, and, NH$_4$Cl, in order as indicated. (Data from Ferrell et al., 1981.) In both sheep and rat, responses to NaCl and LiCl increase during development relative to NH$_4$Cl and KCl responses.

To further explore factors affecting the emerging taste response to NaCl (and LiCl), receptive fields of single chorda tympani nerve fibers were mapped during development (Mistretta et al., 1986; Nagai et al., 1988). In fetuses (130 days of gestation), perinatal animals (1 week before or after birth) and postnatal lambs (about 1–2 months), punctate electrical stimulation was used to determine the number of fungiform papillae innervated by a single fiber at different ages. Then salt response characteristics of the fiber and its respective receptive field were determined.

Study of receptive fields of chorda tympani nerve fibers demonstrated that receptive field size decreases during development (Nagai et al., 1988). That is, there are fewer fungiform papillae in lamb receptive fields than in fields of younger animals. Median field sizes were 10 papillae per receptive field in fetuses, 14 in perinatal animals, and 9 in lambs, and statistical analyses demonstrated that lamb fields were significantly smaller than those in younger animals (Figure 11A). Second, the NaCl/NH$_4$Cl response ratio increases (Figure 11B), and this is attributed to an increase in the proportion of receptive fields most responsive to NaCl compared to NH$_4$Cl. Fields most responsive to NaCl increased from 12% in fetuses to 41% in lambs (Figure 11B). Third, there is a significant, negative correlation between receptive field size and responsiveness to NaCl. Small receptive fields are more responsive to NaCl, whereas larger receptive fields are more responsive to NH$_4$Cl (Figure 12). Thus, there is a developmental acquisition of small, highly NaCl-responsive, receptive fields in the peripheral taste system that complement existing, larger, highly NH$_4$Cl-responsive receptive fields.

If field size is defined as total number of *taste buds* within the fungiform papillae in a receptive field, it is found that there is an increase in field size in perinatal animals compared to fetuses and a subsequent decrease in numbers of buds per field in lambs (Figure 13A) (Mistretta et al., 1988). As noted in Section III average number of taste buds per fungiform papilla increases to perinatal stages and then decreases in lambs, providing an anatomical basis for the observed increase and decrease in taste buds per field.

Thus, whether defined as number of papillae or number of taste buds within papillae, receptive fields in lambs are smaller than those in younger animals. The decrease in size cannot be attributed to a loss of fungiform papillae on the tongue during development because numbers of papillae are constant over the ages studied (Mistretta et al., 1988). Thus there must be some rearrangement of the peripheral taste innervation that results in acquisition of a greater proportion of small, highly NaCl-responsive, receptive fields.

There is a developmental reorganization of innervation patterns in other parts of the peripheral nervous system, and often this organization involves progression from larger, more diffuse innervation patterns to smaller, more narrow ones. For example, there is a developmental reduction in the number of muscle fibers contacted originally by each motor axon (Brown et al.,

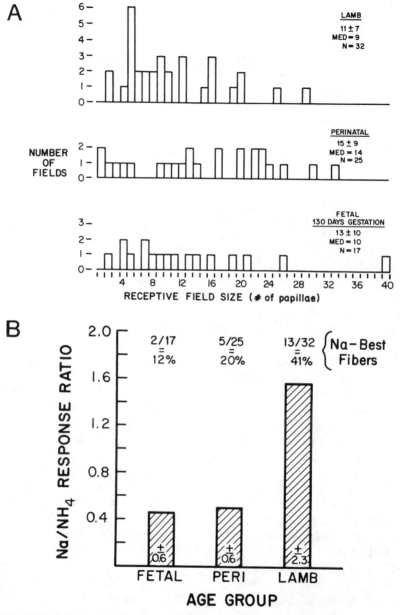

FIGURE 11. (A) Distributions of number of receptive fields of a given size in three age groups of sheep: fetal, perinatal, and postnatal lamb. For each group, data are presented on mean and standard deviation of field size, median field size (MED), and number (N) of receptive fields mapped. Receptive field size (number of fungiform papillae per field) is smaller in lambs than in younger animals. (From Nagai et al., 1988.) (B) The mean NaCl/NH₄Cl response frequency ratio for single chorda tympani nerve fibers innervating receptive fields in three age groups of sheep. Standard deviations are noted within the histogram bars. At the top of the graph are noted numbers and percentages of fibers within each age group that responded with a higher frequency to NaCl than to NH₄Cl (Na best). With age, both the response ratio and the proportion of Na-best fibers increased significantly. (From Nagai et al., 1988.)

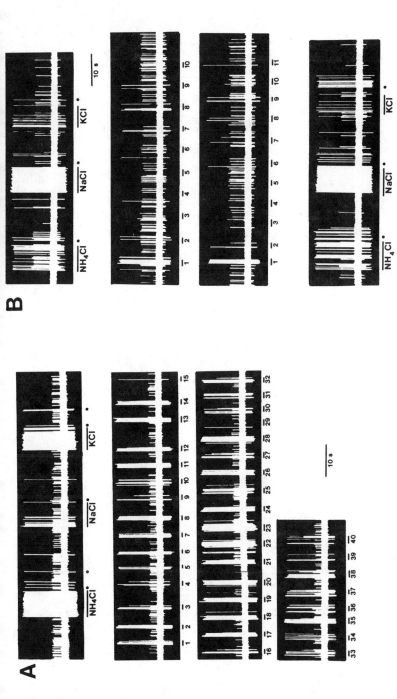

FIGURE 12. Recordings from single chorda tympani nerve fibers in perinatal sheep that respond with highest frequency to NH_4Cl (*A*) and NaCl (*B*). Responses are illustrated to 0.5 *M* NH_4Cl, NaCl, and KCl applied to the anterior tongue and to fungiform papillae in the receptive field area of the fiber. Numbers under the data represent electrical stimulation of individual papillae. Note that the NH_4Cl-responsive fiber in (*A*) has a large receptive field: of 40 papillae that were stimulated with anodal electrical current, 37 responded. In contrast, the NaCl-responsive fiber in (*B*) has a small receptive field: of 10 fungiform papillae that were repeatedly stimulated with anodal current (see two series in this figure), 3 responded. In general, receptive field size correlates negatively with the NaCl/NH_4Cl response ratio. Smaller fields are more responsive to NaCl, larger fields to NH_4Cl.

587

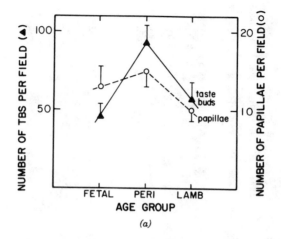

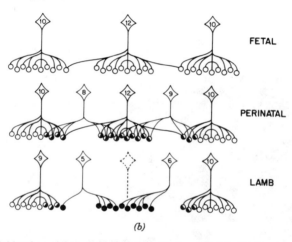

FIGURE 13. (a) Number of taste buds and fungiform papillae in 58 reconstructed receptive fields from sheep. Means and standard errors are presented for three age groups. Average number of taste buds per receptive field is larger in perinatal (PERI) animals than in fetuses or lambs. (From Mistretta el al., 1988.) (b) Model of receptive field development in fetal, perinatal, and postnatal sheep. Chorda tympani neurons are represented as diamonds with the number of papillae in each receptive field noted as a numeral within each diamond. Fungiform papillae are represented as circles; open circles represent papillae with taste buds that have maximum NH_4Cl responsiveness, and filled circles represent maximum NaCl responsiveness. At the top of the model, three fetal chorda tympani neurons are diagrammed with fibers and branches innervating a total of 32 fungiform papillae in three receptive fields that contain 10, 12, and 10 papillae, respectively. Some overlapping innervation among the fields also is illustrated, as has been described in mammalian taste fields. These relatively large receptive fields are to represent the highly NH_4Cl-responsive fields that predominate in early fetal animals. In the second row, the same fungiform papillae are diagrammed at perinatal stages. However, the original chorda neurons are drawn with two new neurons to illustrate new innervation; therefore, a total of five receptive fields now are illustrated that contain 10, 8, 12, 9, and 10 papillae. The model as presented assumes addition of chorda tympani fibers, but additional branching of

1976). Reorganization of peripheral innervation in the taste system provides another example of neural remodeling during development. A model is proposed to account for alterations in taste receptive fields that incorporates neural proliferation, competition, and selective elimination of innervation, and activity-driven specification of chemical response characteristics of fields that occurs as NaCl receptor components are added to taste cell membranes (Figure 13B) (Mistretta, 1988).

In summary, a number of facts now are available about development of the peripheral taste system in sheep. Although the fetus responds to a variety of taste stimuli for at least the last third of gestation (Bradley and Mistretta, 1973a), there are alterations in neural function. Adult taste responses to NaCl and NH_4Cl, two salts with very different tastes, are about equal in magnitude. But in early development, responses to NaCl are of small magnitude. The emerging sensitivity to NaCl is based on an increase in the proportion of chorda tympani nerve fibers that are highly responsive to NaCl and parallels a concomitant decrease in average receptive field size of peripheral afferents. Because small receptive fields are more NaCl responsive than large fields, by inference the system is adding small, Na-sensitive fields. A working model is that these small fields form in association with selective elimination of afferent innervation and in response to developmental alterations in taste membranes.

Although the focus in this chapter has been on anterior tongue taste buds, there also are developmental alterations in responses from taste buds on the back of the tongue (Mistretta and Bradley, 1983b). Recordings have been made from bundles of the glossopharyngeal nerve, which innervates taste buds in circumvallate papillae (Figure 1), in three age groups of sheep fetuses and in lambs and adults. Taste stimuli were NH_4Cl, KCl, NaCl, LiCl, and citric and hydrochloric acids. Responses to NaCl and LiCl increase during development relative to NH_4Cl. But the magnitude of the change is small. On the other hand, KCl responses decrease in magnitude by 50% relative to NH_4Cl. Relative responses to both acids also decrease developmentally.

---

existing fibers could meet the requirements of the overall model. New chorda fibers or branches compete with existing branches to innervate taste buds in the original 32 papillae. It is assumed that additional taste buds that have formed during the perinatal period have acquired receptor membrane that is highly responsive to NaCl compared with NH_4Cl. This NaCl-responsive membrane is noted by changing some of the open papillae to half-filled papillae. In the model, NaCl-responsive membrane could be added under the influence of new innervation or could arise independently and then specify NaCl sensitivity in fibers; or both fibers and membranes could acquire NaCl responsiveness independently and then "match" during the innervation process. Finally, the same fungiform papillae are diagrammed at lamb stages at the bottom of the figure. One neuron has degenerated or been lost during the process of perinatal competition, and fiber branches have new patterns of innervation in receptive fields, acquired through competition for taste buds. A total of four receptive fields remain in the lamb diagram: two of these have 5 and 6 papillae, respectively, and are highly NaCl responsive; two have larger fields of 9 and 10 papillae and are highly NH_4Cl responsive. (From Mistretta, 1988.)

These developmental alterations are different than those for responses from anterior tongue taste buds recorded from the chorda tympani nerve. Anterior tongue responses to NaCl and LiCl change most substantially and those to KCl change much less. The developmental differences for anterior versus posterior tongue responses suggest that the membrane composition of taste buds in the two locations is not the same and that membrane components are present in varying proportions at different developmental stages in anterior and posterior tongue buds.

B Peripheral Taste System in Rat

Between postnatal days 5 and 30 in rat there are profound alterations in responses to chemical stimuli from the chorda tympani nerve (Yamada, 1980; Ferrell et al., 1981; Hill et al., 1982). Changes in salt taste responses are similar to those in sheep. Relative to NH_4Cl and KCl, the NaCl response is very small in early postnatal rats (Figure 10B). Subsequently, there is an increase in the response magnitude to NaCl, and responses to NH_4Cl do not change; those to KCl either remain the same or increase depending on concentration. The changes are effected by developmental alterations in response frequencies of single fibers to the various chemicals and in the proportion of fibers that respond "best" to a particular stimulus (Figures 14A, B). For example, the average, single-fiber response frequency to NaCl increases during development; in addition, the proportion of fibers that respond with highest frequency to NaCl, compared to NH_4Cl, increases developmentally.

As well as developmental differences in salt taste responses, there is a decrease in chorda tympani response magnitudes to citric acid (Figure 14A). Response *latencies* also decrease developmentally (Hill et al., 1982). The decrease in latency parallels the time course of increasing myelination of chorda tympani fibers in postnatal rat (Ferrell et al., 1985).

Thus, in developing rat there are demonstrated differences in neural taste responses to a variety of salt, acid, and sweet stimuli. Although salt responses alter in generally similar directions in rat and sheep, with a notable increase in sensitivity to NaCl, in another rodent there are different changes in salt responses (Hill, 1988a). The adult hamster does not regulate NaCl and internal fluid balance in a manner similar to sheep and rats; it displays neither a taste preference for NaCl nor a salt appetite. Chorda tympani nerve responses to monochloride salts were recorded in postnatal hamsters from 14 to about 90 days. Whereas NaCl responses increase in rat and sheep, relative to NH_4Cl, they decrease developmentally in hamster. Therefore, species adapted to live in different environments, with different internal regulation of salt and fluid, have varying patterns of developmental changes in taste responses.

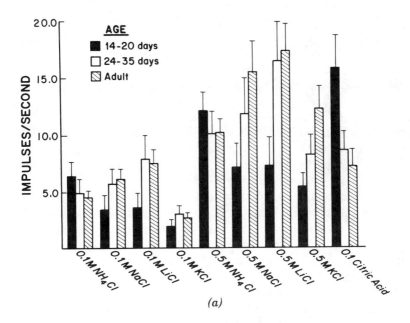

FIGURE 14. (*a*.) Mean response frequencies (and standard errors) for chorda tympani nerve fibers in three age groups of rats to 0.1 and 0.5 *M* salts and 0.1 *M* citric acid. Response frequencies to NH₄Cl remain constant with development, frequencies to NaCl and LiCl increase, and those to citric acid decrease. Although response frequencies to 0.1 *M* KCl do not alter, those to 0.5 *M* KCl increase as a function of age. (*b*) Number of fibers in three age groups categorized according to the stimulus that elicited the maximal response. The proportion of fibers responding maximally to NaCl increases during development. (From Hill et al., 1982.)

C   Receptor Membrane Development and Peripheral Changes in Sheep and Rat

As summarized in preceding paragraphs, substantial changes in salt taste responses take place during development in sheep and rat. The existence of different patterns of developing salt taste responses leads to the inference that there must be different receptor mechanisms for the various salts. That is, if neural responses to NaCl increase while responses to KCl decrease and those to NH$_4$Cl remain the same, different receptor components presumably mediate responses to these stimuli, and these receptor components mature at different rates (Mistretta and Bradley, 1983a).

There are interesting data that provide indirect evidence for developmental alterations in proposed ion channels in taste membranes (Hill and Bour, 1985; Hill, 1987b, 1988b; Formaker and Hill, 1988). Amiloride is a diuretic agent that blocks epithelial transport of sodium. In adult rats, amiloride applied to the tongue depresses the chorda tympani nerve response to NaCl without affecting the response to KCl or NH$_4$Cl. However, in young postnatal rats amiloride does not affect the response to NaCl. Thus, the developmental increase in responsiveness to NaCl is paralleled by an increase in sensitivity to amiloride. This suggests that functional amiloride-sensitive components are added to taste receptor membranes during development and account for the increase in neural taste responses to sodium.

Effects of lingual applications of transport blockers on chorda tympani nerve taste responses cannot demonstrate conclusively that selective ion channels are involved in taste transduction and/or that such channels are added to or deleted from taste membranes developmentally. But the data do suggest a relation between developing taste responses and effectiveness of selective ion channels. Coupled with future acquisition of other, more direct evidence for channels in taste membranes, the demonstration of this relation might eventually be key in clarifying the basis of neural response changes in the taste system.

D   Central Taste System in Sheep

Developmental differences in responses from central taste neurons must occur because peripheral taste responses alter with age. However, central differences might reflect not simply peripheral changes but maturation of central structures as well. In sheep, taste responses have been recorded from the NST in fetuses aged 80 days of gestation through term, postnatal lambs through about 3 months, and adults (Mistretta and Bradley, 1978a; Bradley and Mistretta, 1980). Chemical stimuli included NH$_4$Cl, KCl, NaCl, LiCl, HCl, and citric acid.

In fetuses younger than 114 days of gestation, NH$_4$Cl, KCl, and citric acid elicited a response in all neurons. Responses to HCl were recorded in 33% of cells. Responses to NaCl and LiCl were never elicited. In lambs and adults, NST neurons generally responded to all six chemicals.

Thus, with increasing age, NST cells respond to a broader range of chemicals. But perhaps more important is the demonstration that responses to taste stimuli do not develop randomly but in a specific sequence. Taste neurons respond to NH$_4$Cl and KCl earlier in gestation than to NaCl and

LiCl. Gradually, responses to NaCl and LiCl emerge. At ages when small-magnitude *peripheral* nerve responses to NaCl and LiCl are obtained (i.e., 108–114 days of gestation), no responses to these salts are observed in the NST. The inability of the early fetal central taste system to respond to NaCl and LiCl must relate to factors at the synapse between first- and second-order neurons. Synapses in the central taste pathway might be too inefficient for transmission of low-magnitude responses in young fetuses.

Although there are no data on synapse development in central taste neurons, there now is evidence for a developmental increase in the degree of convergence of afferent input onto NST cells. The increase in convergence implies an increase in number of synapses and/or effectiveness of synapses. Experiments in sheep assessed convergence quantitatively by determining the number of fungiform papillae in receptive fields of NST neurons in fetuses, perinatal animals, and lambs, and by comparing the data to receptive field sizes of peripheral, chorda tympani nerve fibers (Vogt and Mistretta, 1986, 1988). First, responses to $0.5\,M\,NH_4\,Cl$, NaCl, and KCl were recorded from single NST cells. Then a fine platinum probe was used to electrically stimulate individual fungiform papillae with anodal current, and the number and location of papillae in the receptive field were recorded.

In fetuses, perinatal animals, and lambs, average receptive field sizes of central neurons are larger than those of peripheral fibers (Figure 15). This indicates convergence of afferent input onto NST cells. Because the receptive fields of *NST neurons* are larger in lambs than fetuses, whereas receptive fields of *chorda fibers* are smaller in lambs than fetuses, the degree of convergence increases during development from a ratio of about 2 : 1 in fetuses to about 4 : 1 in lambs.

There are other developmental differences in the character of the neural response from NST cells (Bradley and Mistretta, 1980). Latencies of responses to stimulation of the tongue with NH_4Cl, KCl, citric acid, and HCl decrease during gestation, and adult values are reached consistently only after birth (Figure 16). Latency functions for NaCl and LiCl are flat because responses to these chemicals do not occur in fetuses younger than 114 days of gestation. Therefore, when the taste system does acquire the ability to respond to NaCl and LiCl, the developmental latency curve is not reproduced, but response latencies are appropriate for the advanced fetal age.

In parallel with the developmental decrease in response latency is an observed increase in the duration of the neural response discharge (Bradley and Mistretta, 1980). In younger fetuses, responses often adapt to prestimulus, spontaneous activity levels before the stimulus is rinsed from the tongue. Sustained discharges are obtained in older fetuses, lambs, and adults (Figure 16).

In summary, the studies of NST neural function in pre- and postnatal sheep demonstrate developmental differences in number of chemicals that elicit responses, in the size and response characteristics of receptive fields,

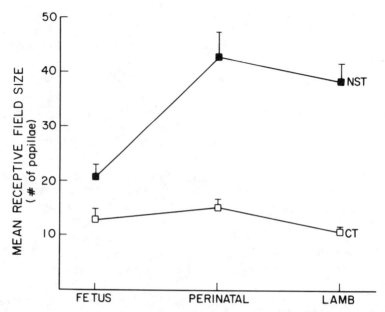

FIGURE 15. Data on receptive field size (number of fungiform papillae) of NST neurons compared with data for chorda tympani nerve fibers (CT). Data are means and standard errors for three age groups of sheep: fetus (130 days of gestation), perinatal, and lamb. The degree of apparent convergence of chorda tympani onto NST is about 2 : 1 in fetuses and about 4 : 1 in lambs. That is, the extent of convergence increases during development.

and in response latency and adaptation characteristics. As in the peripheral taste system, responsiveness to NaCl increases during development.

E   Central Taste System in Rat

Responses from NST neurons have been studied in rats aged 5 days to adult (Hill, et al., 1983). Chemical stimuli were a series of salts, citric and hydrochloric acids, sucrose and sodium saccharin, and quinine hydrochloride. Animals were in five age groups: 5–7 days, 14–20 days, 25–35 days, 50–60 days, and adult.

Several general conclusions can be drawn about central taste development. First, neurons from rats in the youngest age group respond to fewer chemicals than cells in older rats. Second, average response frequencies increase after 35 days of age for NaCl, LiCl, KCl, sucrose, and sodium saccharin. Response frequencies for NH_4Cl, citric and hydrochloric acids, and quinine hydrochloride do not change during development. Third, there are no developmental differences in response latencies in rats aged 14 days and older.

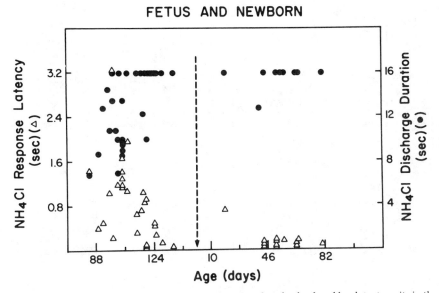

FIGURE 16. Response latency and discharge duration data for fetal and lamb taste units in the NST during stimulation of the tongue with NH₄Cl. Fetal ages are in days of gestation and lamb ages in days after birth. An arrow marks the time of birth. The functions for latency and discharge duration follow a similar time course. Neural response latencies decrease developmentally in temporal association with acquisition of the ability to produce a sustained response discharge. (From Mistretta, 1981.)

The response frequencies of second-order neurons generally reflect developmental changes in first-order afferents; however, increases in frequencies occur comparatively later in development (Figure 17). At all ages, NST responses to monochloride salts include higher response frequencies and a general loss in response specificity compared to chorda tympani fibers. Overall, comparisons of chorda tympani and NST taste data indicate that some of the developmental changes in responses of NST neurons simply reflect peripheral changes, whereas others probably relate to alterations in synapses and morphological characteristics of NST cells.

In rat there also have been developmental studies of taste responses from cells in the parabrachial nucleus (PBN) in the pons (Hill, 1987a). These PBN cells receive projections from second-order NST neurons. Response frequencies to NaCl and LiCl increase progressively in PBN neurons, from 14 days postnatal to adulthood (Figure 18). Response increments to stimulation of the tongue with these chemicals also is observed in chorda tympani and NST neurons, although at each neural level there is a different time course for the developmental increase. It is noteworthy that response fre-

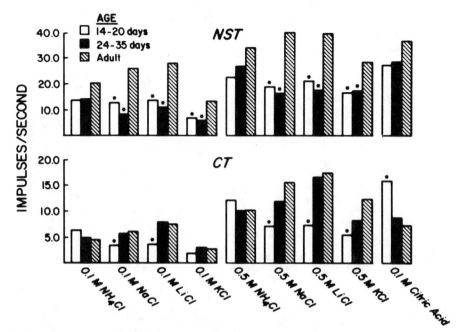

FIGURE 17. Mean response frequencies of neurons in the NST (top) and CT nerve (bottom) from three age groups of rats after stimulation of the tongue with various 0.1 and 0.5 M salts and citric acid. Asterisks denote mean frequencies that are significantly different from the adult mean. Note that ordinates are scaled differently for NST and CT responses. Increases in response frequencies occur later in NST neurons than in CT fibers. (From Hill et al., 1983.)

quencies for NH$_4$Cl also increase in PBN neurons, whereas there is no developmental change in response to this chemical at peripheral or second-order neural levels (Figure 18). Furthermore, response frequencies for citric acid increase during development in PBN, remain constant in NST, and decrease in chorda tympani (Figure 18). The proportion of single PBN cells that respond maximally to specific salts does not change during development, in contrast to chorda tympani and NST neurons.

Developmental studies of PBN taste responses highlight the point that *different* patterns of developmental change can occur at various levels of the nervous system; that is, progressively higher neural centers do not simply mirror, at a later time point, the developmental maturation of lower centers. Recent Golgi studies of PBN neurons suggest that changes in taste responses of these cells are correlated with a period of dendritic outgrowth within the nucleus (Lasiter and Hill, 1988).

F   Summary of Neurophysiological Development

Because there now is rather extensive work on development of neurophysiological taste responses in two species, it is important to highlight key

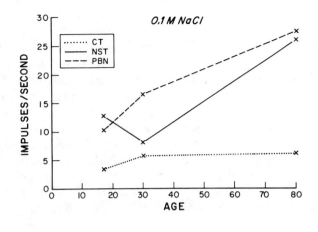

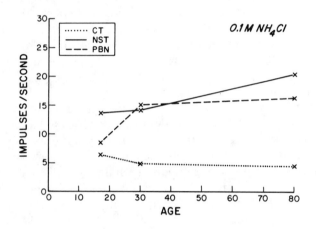

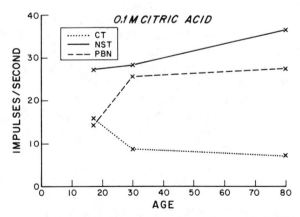

FIGURE 18. Average response frequencies (impulses per second) for CT, NST, and PBN neurons to 0.1 *M* NaCl, NH₄Cl and citric acid in three age groups of rats. Different patterns of developmental change in chemical response frequencies can occur at these three levels of the taste system. (From Hill, 1987a.)

observations. *First,* even in young fetuses or in early postnatal pups, the taste system is functional and responsive to several chemicals. There is taste *function,* although most taste buds are morphologically immature, chorda tympani nerve fibers have not completed development, and pathways in the taste system are not even close to maturity. *Second,* it is notable that neurons at three levels of the gustatory system respond to more chemicals, and to lower concentrations of chemicals, as a function of development. Thus, the breadth of chemical responsiveness that characterizes adult taste cells is acquired gradually. A particular aspect of the limited range of responsiveness in young cells is that at second-order levels of the taste system there are no responses to NaCl or LiCl in early development of sheep and rat.

However, it should be recalled that although gustatory cells of the adult taste system are responsive to a broad range of chemicals at moderate concentrations, there is specificity to the extent that certain chemicals elicit especially high response frequencies from a given neuron. That is, taste neurons often respond best to one chemical or one chemical subset. This leads to the *third* major summary point: that the proportion of neurons especially responsive to NaCl and LiCl, compared to NH_4Cl and KCl, increases during development. This increase usually is accompanied by a developmental increase in neural response frequency to NaCl.

A *fourth* major point is that other characteristics of the taste response alter developmentally, including response latency, which decreases, and length of the neural discharge during chemical stimulation of the tongue, which increases. A *fifth* point is that size of receptive fields alters during development. For peripheral afferents, receptive field sizes *decrease;* for NST cells, fields *increase* in size. Related to field size is the chemosensitivity of afferents or central neurons. Thus, development of chemical responses is accompanied by a reorganization in receptive fields.

Embedded in these general summary points are specific results related to development of salt taste responses. These results lead to the hypothesis that there is a sodium taste system within the sense of taste that develops gradually; it is not present from the moment taste function is first observed. Other evidence for this sodium system is the developmental increase in effectiveness of the sodium transport blocker, amiloride, on the taste response to NaCl and the ability to delay development of NaCl taste responses through diet modifications, without affecting taste responses to other salts (to be discussed in a subsequent section of this chapter).

Although there is great emphasis on salt taste in the current literature, it should not be forgotten that there is evidence for substantial developmental differences in responses to sweet and acidic stimuli as well. There must be extensive further work, however, to begin to describe possible developmental systems for other chemicals.

V DEVELOPMENT OF BEHAVIORAL TASTE RESPONSES AND ROLE OF EARLY EXPERIENCE IN DEVELOPMENT OF NEUROPHYSIOLOGICAL TASTE RESPONSES

Rather than a summary of the complete literature on development of behavioral taste responses, this section will describe some of the more recent studies on salt taste in rats and a selection of the literature on humans that best relates to the neurophysiological data that have been described in the chapter. Also included is a limited discussion of the role of early experience in the development of *neurophysiological* taste responses. More complete reviews of this literature have been published (Mistretta and Bradley, 1978b, 1985; Mistretta, 1981; Hill, 1987c).

A Nonhuman Mammals

Postnatal rats gradually acquire the preference–aversion function for NaCl that is exhibited by adults, in which hypotonic solutions are preferred and hypertonic are rejected (Contreras and Kosten, 1983; Midkiff and Bernstein, 1983; Moe, 1986; Bernstein and Courtney, 1987). Animals have been studied from (a) 3 to 18 days postnatal and intake measured by weighing animals before and after intra-oral infusions (Moe, 1986); (b) 5 to 20 days and intake measured by ingestion of solution from soaked towels (Bernstein and Courtney, 1987); and (c) 25 to 58 days and intake measured by ingestion of NaCl or water from bottles (Midkiff and Bernstein, 1983). The composite data indicate a progressive and gradual shift from preference for, or indifference toward, hypertonic NaCl compared to water, to aversion for hypertonic NaCl compared to water in rats from about 10 through 60 days of postnatal life.

Data from Moe (1986) demonstrate that at 12 days postnatal, rats already exhibit a preference–aversion function for increasing concentrations of NaCl (Figure 19A). By 18 days the preference–aversion function is essentially similar to that in adults. These behavioral measures provide a striking match to neurophysiological data for developing chorda tympani nerve responses to NaCl compared to NH_4Cl (Ferrell et al., 1981). The function for neural development is illustrated in Figure 19B and demonstrates a gradual decrease in NH_4Cl responses relative to NaCl or increase in NaCl responses relative to NH_4Cl. Data from single-fiber studies have shown that, in fact, response frequencies to NaCl *increase* developmentally whereas those to NH_4Cl remain the same (Hill et al., 1982). If two straight lines were drawn through the data points in Figure 19B, the lines would intersect at about 20 days. This estimate of neural "maturation" for chorda tympani responses to NaCl is quite similar to the estimate for behavioral maturation.

On the other hand, Bernstein and Courtney (1987) have concluded that there is a lack of correlation between behavioral and electrophysiological

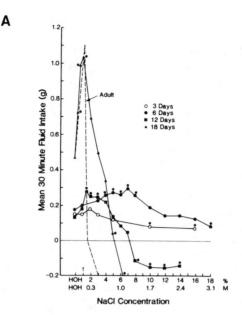

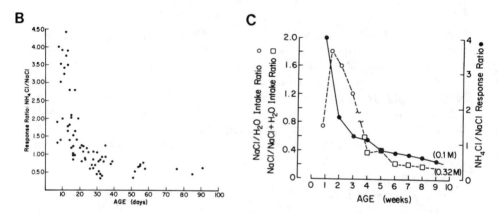

FIGURE 19. (A) Mean intake (grams of fluid ingested) of NaCl solutions by rats aged 3, 6, 12, and 18 days postnatal during 30-min intraoral infusion. Asterisks denote points that are statistically significant compared with water intake. A typical preference-aversion function for NaCl has emerged by 12 days postnatal, and by 18 days the function is very similar to that for adults. (From Moe, 1986.) (B) Ratios of integrated response magnitude from the chorda tympani nerve to 0.1 M NH_4Cl relative to 0.1 M NaCl, plotted as a function of age in rat. A response ratio of 1.00 indicates equal response magnitude for NaCl and NH_4Cl; a ratio greater than 1.00 indicates a larger response magnitude for NH_4Cl than NaCl. Each data point represents responses from one animal. The changes in salt taste responses are gradual and are adequately described by an exponential function. If two straight lines were drawn through the data points, the lines would intersect at about 20 days postnatal age, similar to the age when behavioral "maturation" for NaCl taste responses occurs. (From Ferrell et al., 1981.) (C) NaCl-water intake ratios in rats as a function of age compared with $NH_4Cl/NaCl$ neural response ratios shown in (B). [The intake data for rats up to 3 weeks of age are from Bernstein and Courtney (1987) and data for rats aged 4 weeks and older are from Midkiff and Bernstein (1983).] Functions for neurophysiological and behavioral response maturation are essentially parallel, except for behavioral responses in rats younger than 1 week.

indices of taste sensitivity to salts (NaCl and NH_4Cl). However, when their data are redrawn with data from older rats (Midkiff and Bernstein, 1983) and compared with chorda tympani nerve responses, parallel functions emerge (Figure 19C). The behavioral and neurophysiological data are divergent for very young rats only, less than 1 week old. For example, 5-day pups rejected hypertonic NaCl concentrations relative to water, whereas 10-, 15-, and 20-day rats preferred these solutions, and still older rats began to reject them (Figure 19C; see also Bernstein and Courtney, 1987). In Moe's study (Figure 19A; see also Moe, 1986), 3-day rats rejected very high NaCl concentrations and were indifferent to all other concentrations; 6-day rats preferred or were indifferent to most NaCl concentrations but had begun to express a preference–aversion function that was at least *qualitatively* similar to that of adults.

Investigators apparently have assumed that a perfect fit of neurophysiological and behavioral data requires indifference to, or preference for, hypertonic NaCl solutions in very young rat pups (Bernstein and Courtney, 1987; Moe, 1986). This assumption is based on a further assumption that a low-frequency neural response to NaCl should be associated with indifference or preference for the salt. In this line of reasoning, rejection will occur only with high-frequency neural responses. Although greater neural response frequencies in adults are elicited by higher concentrations of NaCl and higher NaCl concentrations are rejected behaviorally, there are no response-intensity neural data for very young rats and the neural–behavioral association could well be different.

In fact, there are essentially no data on neural taste responses from rats younger than about 10 days postnatal. Hill et al. (1983) have published data on NST responses from 5–7-day pups, but very few responses were recorded, they were multiunit responses, and the data can only demonstrate that the taste system does respond to certain chemicals at this age. The taste buds in rats aged 10 days or younger are so immature morphologically (Farbman, 1965; Mistretta, 1972; Oakley, 1987) that one cannot even assume that neural responses at this age are typical taste responses. Moe (1986) has speculated on a variety of other nongustatory effects of very high NaCl or other salt solutions in the oral cavity of rats younger than 6 days. Trigeminal, osmotic, and postingestional effects all are possible.

In summary, there is converging evidence from various behavioral studies of developing taste function in postnatal rats that demonstrates a close association with emerging neurophysiological responses. That is, a neural basis for changes in salt taste preferences and aversions is clearly demonstrated in the postnatal rat.

1 Role of Early Experience

The developmental phenomenon of increasing neurophysiological responses to NaCl in the postnatal rat can be manipulated by altering dietary experience. Rats were deprived of dietary NaCl in three groups (Hill, et al., 1986): (a) extended depletion—mothers and their pups were fed a NaCl-free diet from the third day of gestation until neurophysiological recordings were made in the pups at 28–48 days postnatal age; (b) shorter depletion—mothers were fed a NaCl-free diet from the third day of gestation until their pups were 12 days of age, at which time mothers and pups were fed a NaCl-replete diet until neurophysiological recordings were made in the pups at 28–45 days postnatal; and (c) no depletion—mothers and their pups were always fed the sodium-replete diet.

There was a specific effect on salt taste responses recorded from the chorda tympani nerve in extended depletion rats compared to other groups. Response magnitudes to high concentrations of NaCl were significantly reduced, but responses to a range of NH_4Cl and KCl concentrations were not affected (Figure 20). Essentially, an extended period of NaCl depletion seems to delay the normal developmental pattern of peripheral taste nerve responses. With a shorter depletion period, from 3 days of gestation to 12 days postnatal, there is no effect on maturation of neurophysiological taste responses.

The specific effect of diet modification on taste responses has been demonstrated recently with pre- and postnatal exposure to a 0.03% NaCl diet also (Hill, 1987b). Chorda tympani nerve responses to NaCl were reduced in rats fed the deficient diet compared with controls fed a sodium-replete diet. Responses to nonsodium salts and nonsalt stimuli were not affected. After early deprived rats were fed a NaCl-replete diet, responses to sodium salts recovered to control response magnitudes within 15 days. There is an apparent sensitive period for the diet modification effect because rats initially fed a sodium-deficient diet as adults have no alteration in chorda tympani nerve taste responses.

The selective effect of dietary sodium deprivation on sodium salt taste responses could be attributable to a reduction in functional, amiloride-sensitive components in taste cell membranes of deprived rats (Hill, 1987b). Application of amiloride on the tongue of deprived rats during electrophysiological experiments was *ineffective* in reducing responses to NaCl, but amiloride reduced sodium responses in control rats to magnitudes observed in deprived animals (Figure 21). Amiloride, therefore, eliminated the difference in response magnitudes to NaCl in deprived and control rats.

These experiments provide an interesting contrast with others in which rat pups aged 4–18 days postnatal were "taste deprived" by an artificial rearing procedure that provided feeding solely through an intragastric route (Bernstein et al., 1986). There was no difference in taste sensitivity or preference for NaCl or sucrose in experimental rats tested at 18 days compared to normally reared animals. As the investigators note, however, saliva and grooming provide other sources of oral taste stimulation. In addition, intragastric animals also would experience intravascular stimula-

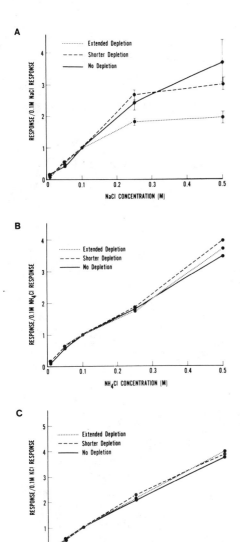
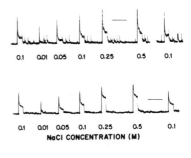

FIGURE 20. *Left.* Magnitude of neurophysiological responses from the chorda tympani nerve to concentration series of NaCl (*A*), NH₄Cl (*B*), and KCl (*C*) from rats in extended NaCl depletion, shorter depletion, and no depletion groups. Responses are expressed relative to the 0.1 *M* response for the respective chemical. Each bar in (*A*) represents standard error of mean. Response magnitudes to high concentrations of NaCl are reduced in extended depletion rats, but responses to a range of NH₄Cl and KCl concentrations are not affected. *Right.* Integrated responses from the chorda tympani nerve in a rat that had extended depletion of dietary NaCl (top) and a rat that had shorter depletion (bottom). Time bars denote 1 min. Note that responses to higher concentrations of NaCl are reduced in the rat that had an extended depletion. (From Hill et al., 1986.)

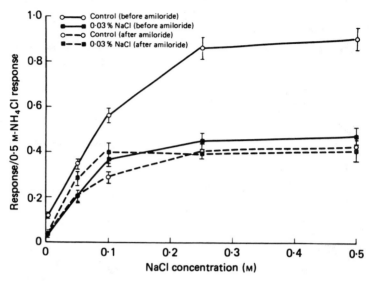

FIGURE 21. Magnitude of chorda tympani nerve responses to NaCl, expressed relative to the response to NH_4Cl, in control and NaCl-deprived rats before and after application of amiloride to the tongue. Standard error bars are shown for each mean. Amiloride reduced sodium responses in control rats to magnitudes observed in deprived animals but was ineffective in reducing NaCl responses in deprived animals. (From Hill, 1987b.)

tion of taste buds via circulating chemicals (Bradley, 1973). Thus, the degree to which experience with tasting NaCl actually was altered is not known.

Although the literature on the role of early experience in taste development generally does not lead to clear conclusions (Mistretta and Bradley, 1978b; Mistretta, 1981), studies of NaCl depletion now demonstrate that functional plasticity can occur in the developing taste system as a result of environmental alterations.

B   Humans

The early intrauterine appearance of taste buds in the human, coupled with demonstration of neurophysiological responses in sheep fetuses, lead to the prediction that the human fetus and newborn have a functional sense of taste. Although there is no direct demonstration of taste responses from the human fetus *in utero*, it has been shown that premature infants can detect some taste stimuli, notably citric acid and glucose (Steiner, 1979; Tatzer et al., 1985). Full-term human infants can respond to and discriminate among a variety of chemical stimuli and apparently exhibit a preference for sugars and an aversion to acid and bitter chemicals (Desor et al., 1973; Weiffenbach and Thach, 1973; Crook and Lipsitt, 1976; Nowlis and Kessen, 1976; Steiner, 1979).

Although premature and term infants clearly have a functional and discriminating sense of taste, there are marked developmental changes in human taste responses after birth. In this section the discussion will center on salt taste, but Cowart (1981) has a recent and comprehensive review of development of human taste perception.

In human newborns it has proved more difficult to demonstrate responses to NaCl than to other chemicals such as sucrose, glucose, citric acid, or quinine. When sucking patterns or tongue movement measures were used, neonatal detection of NaCl was demonstrated (Nowlis, 1973; Crook, 1978); however, there was no indication that newborns discriminated among concentrations of NaCl solutions over a range of 0.10–0.60M. In addition, from intake measures it was concluded that human newborns cannot distinguish between 0.20 M NaCl and water (Maller and Desor, 1973).

Recent work has described acceptability for NaCl solutions in humans over an age range of about 2.5 months through 6 years (Beauchamp et al., 1986; Cowart and Beauchamp, 1986). Infants less than 4 months of age ingest water and 0.20 M NaCl in equal amounts (Figure 22). Between 4 and 7 months of age, 0.20 M NaCl is ingested *preferentially* to plain water. However, children aged about 15 months (range 7–23 months) do not differentiate in consumption of 0.20 M NaCl and water, and children aged 31–60 months *reject* the NaCl relative to water, as do adults. Data comparing intake of water and 0.10 or 0.17 M NaCl in the same children demonstrate similar results. There is, thus, an early acceptance or preference for moderate concentrations of NaCl in water followed by acquistion of an aversion to these solutions compared to water.

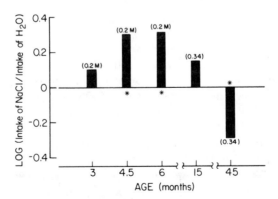

FIGURE 22. Log geometric mean ratios of NaCl intake relative to water intake in five age groups of infants and children: 3 months (2.5–3.9 months); 4.5 months (4.0–5.3 months); 6 months (5.4–6.7 months); 15 months (7–23 months); and 45 months (31–60 months). The molarity of NaCl solution is indicated in parentheses above each bar. An asterisk indicates that the mean for the group differs from zero (zero = no difference between salt and water intake). (Data are redrawn from Beauchamp et al., 1986.)

The investigators (Beauchamp et al., 1986) concluded that the early shift from acceptance of, or preference for, NaCl solutions probably relates to immaturity of neural taste responses to NaCl, as demonstrated in sheep and rat. However, they suggested that the acquisition of the rejection response to NaCl solutions in older children more probably is attributable to experiential effects. Older children may be rejecting the novel solution of salt water because in fact they express a preference for highly salted soup compared to unsalted or moderately salted soup (Cowart and Beachamp, 1986).

Although experience is very likely to influence NaCl taste responses in humans, it also is possible that the total developmental shift from preference to aversion for NaCl relates to neural maturation in the taste system. In sheep, which have a developmental time course for taste bud maturation that is similar to human, relative responses to NaCl from the chorda tympani nerve increase not only prenatally but also postnatally between perinatal and lamb stages and between the lamb and the adult (Mistretta and Bradley, 1983a). Neural maturation is prolonged and spans neonatal to prepubertal periods and prepubertal to adult ages.

Of course, because the time course of neural maturation is so prolonged, there is even more likelihood that experience can have a major role in modifying taste responses. It is therefore very probable that experience interacts with neural development to establish behavioral taste responses to salt. Direct manipulations of early experience with NaCl and subsequent tests of NaCl acceptance have not been performed in humans, but a related study with sucrose has demonstrated that infants fed sweetened water during infancy exhibited greater acceptance of sucrose solutions at 6 months and 2 years of age than other infants not fed sweetened water (Beauchamp and Moran, 1982, 1984).

VI CONCLUSIONS

In mammals with a lengthy gestation, the taste buds are among the first sensory receptors to appear *in utero*. For example, early or presumptive taste buds are first observed in human fetuses at 7–9 weeks of gestation (Bradley and Stern, 1967). This leaves about 7 months of intrauterine maturation for the taste receptors.

During the intrauterine period the taste system has ample opportunity for chemical stimulation (Bradley and Mistretta, 1973b, 1975; Mistretta and Bradley, 1975). The developing fetus lives in an environment of amniotic fluid, composed of water, salts, sugars, acids, amino acids, polypeptides, hormones, and other chemicals that can provide a complex taste environment. Furthermore, amniotic fluid composition is not static but changes throughout gestation and during fetal physiological episodes such as urination *in utero* (Wintour, 1986). Since the fetus swallows large volumes of amniotic fluid during several discrete episodes or bouts throughout the day and night (Figure 23), oral–pharyngeal taste buds frequently are stimulated

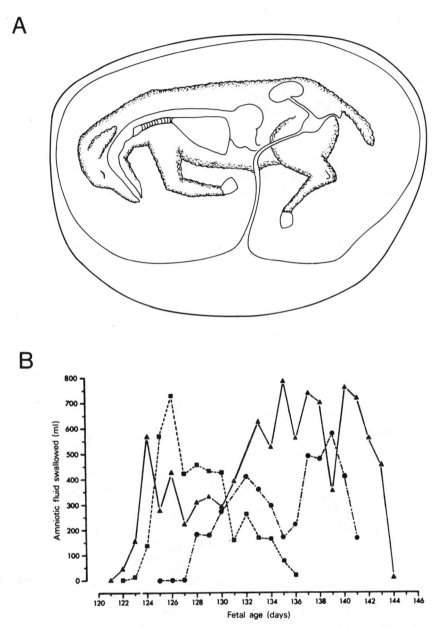

FIGURE 23. (*A*) Diagram of sheep fetus in utero. Avenues for taste bud stimulation during fetal swallowing include gestational changes in amniotic fluid composition and urination. Other sources of chemical stimuli are from oral–pharyngeal glands and the trachea during breathing movements. (*B*) Volume of amniotic fluid swallowed daily by three sheep fetuses during the last third of gestation. Measurements were made after implanting an electromagnetic flow transducer in the esophagus of each fetus. For each animal volumes swallowed were low on the first 2–3 days postoperatively and declined again before the ewes went into labor. All ewes were in labor on the day of the last data point. (From Mistretta and Bradley, 1975.)

with amniotic fluid. In addition, fluids flow into the oral cavity as the fetus produces saliva and other glandular secretions and as it makes breathing movements. Perhaps more than other sensory systems, the sense of taste has extensive natural stimulation *in utero*.

Yet even in mammals with lengthy gestations (e.g., human and sheep), taste buds continue to increase in number and to change in morphology after birth, and as demonstrated in sheep, there are continuing neurophysiological changes during postnatal development. The sense of taste is distinguished, therefore, by a prolonged period of morphological and functional maturation that provides a basis with which dietary experience can interact. Even in adults, the taste bud cells themselves turn over but somehow maintain orderly neural connections. Development never really ends in the sense of taste, and this could explain why patterns of food preferences and aversions, cravings and rejections, are so labile throughout life— in health, disease, and altered physiological states such as pregnancy.

ACKNOWLEDGMENTS

Preparation of this manuscript was supported by National Science Foundation Grant BNS-8311497 and NINCDS, National Institutes of Health Grant NS25825.

REFERENCES

Bartoshuk, L. M. (1978) Gustatory system. In R. B. Masterton (ed.): Handbook of Behavioral Neurobiology, Vol. 1, Sensory Integration. New York: Plenum Press, pp. 503–567.

Beauchamp, G. K., and M. Moran (1982) Dietary experience and sweet taste preference in human infants. Appetite 3: 139–152.

Beauchamp, G. K., and M. Moran (1984) Acceptance of sweet and salty tastes in 2-year old children. Appetite 5: 291–305.

Beauchamp, G. K., B. J. Cowart, and M. Moran (1986) Developmental changes in salt acceptability in human infants. Dev. Psychobiol. 19: 17–25.

Beidler, L. M. (1969) Innervation of rat fungiform papilla. In C. Pfaffmann (ed.): Olfaction and Taste. New York: Rockefeller University Press, pp. 352–368.

Beidler, L. M., and R. L. Smallman (1965) Renewal of cells within taste buds. J. Cell Biol. 27: 263–272.

Bernstein, I. L., and L. Courtney (1987) Salt preference in the preweaning rat. Dev. Psychobiol. 20: 443–453.

Bernstein, I. L., D. P. Fenner, and J. Diaz (1986) Influence of taste stimulation during the sucking period in adult taste preference in rats. Physiol. Behav. 36: 913–919.

Bradley, R. M. (1971) Tongue topography. In L. M. Beidler (ed.): Handbook of Sensory Physiology, Vol. IV, Chemical Senses, Part 2: Taste. Berlin: Springer-Verlag, pp. 1–30.

Bradley, R. M. (1972) Development of the taste bud and gustatory papillae in human fetuses. In J. F. Bosma (ed.): Third Symposium on Oral Sensation and Perception: The Mouth of the Infant. Springfield, Illinois: Thomas, pp. 137–162.

Bradley, R. M. (1973) Electrophysiological investigations of intravascular taste using perfused rat tongue. Amer. J. Physiol. *224:* 300–304.

Bradley, R. M. (1982) The role of epiglottal and lingual chemoreceptors: A comparison. In J. E. Steiner and J. R. Ganchrow (eds.): Determination of Behaviour by Chemical Stimuli. London: IRL Press, pp. 37–45.

Bradley, R. M. (1988) Diversity of taste bud function. In I. J. Miller, Jr. (ed.): Proceedings of the Lloyd M. Beidler Symposium on Taste and Smell. Winston-Salem: Book Service Associates, pp. 33–41.

Bradley, R. M., and C. M. Mistretta (1972) The morphological and functional development of fetal gustatory receptors. In N. Emmelin, and Y. Zotterman (eds.): Oral Physiology. Oxford: Pergamon Press, pp. 239–253.

Bradley, R. M., and C. M. Mistretta (1973a) The gustatory sense in foetal sheep during the last third of gestation. J. Physiol. *231:* 271–282.

Bradley, R. M., and C. M. Mistretta (1973b) Swallowing in fetal sheep. Science *179:* 1016–1017.

Bradley, R. M., and C. M. Mistretta (1975) Fetal sensory receptors. Physiol. Rev. 55: 352–382.

Bradley, R. M., and C. M. Mistretta (1980) Developmental changes in neurophysiological taste responses from the medulla in sheep. Brain Res. *191:* 21–34.

Bradley, R. M., and C. M. Mistretta (1988) Development of taste. In E. Meisami and P. S. Timiras (eds.): CRC Handbook of Human Growth and Developmental Biology, Vol. 1, Part B, Sensory, Motor and Integrative Development. Boca Raton: CRC Press, pp. 63–78.

Bradley, R. M., and I. B. Stern (1967) The development of the human taste bud during the foetal period. J. Anat. *101:* 743–752.

Bradley, R. M., M. L. Cheal, and Y. H. Kim (1980) Quantitative analysis of developing epiglottal taste buds in sheep. J. Anat. *130:* 25–32.

Bradley, R. M., H. M. Stedman, and C. M. Mistretta (1985) A quantitative study of lingual taste buds and papillae in the aging rhesus monkey tongue. In R. T. Davis and C. W. Leathers (eds.): Behavior and Pathology of Aging in Rhesus Monkeys. New York: Alan R. Liss, pp. 187–199.

Brown, M. C., J. K. S. Jansen, and D. Van Essen (1976) Polyneural innervation of skeletal muscle in new-born rats and its elimination during maturation. J. Physiol. *261:* 387–422.

Contreras, R. J., and T. Kosten (1983) Prenatal and early postnatal sodium chloride intake modifies the solution preference of adult rats. J. Nutr. *113:* 1051–1062.

Cowart, B. J. (1981) Development of taste perception in humans: Sensitivity and preference throughout the life span. Psych. Bull. *90:* 43–73.

Cowart, B. J., and G. K. Beauchamp (1986) The importance of sensory context in young children's acceptance of salty tastes. Child Dev. *57:* 1034–1039.

Crook, C. K. (1978) Taste perception in the newborn infant. Infant Behav. Dev. *1:* 52–69.

Crook, C. K., and L. P. Lipsitt (1976) Neonatal nutritive sucking: Effects of taste stimulation upon sucking rhythm and heart rate. Child Dev. *47:* 518–522.

Davies, R. O., M. R. Kare, and R. H. Cagan (1979) Distribution of taste buds on fungiform and circumvallate papillae of bovine tongue. Anat. Rec. *195:* 443–482.

Delay, R. J., J. C. Kinnamon, and S. D. Roper (1986) Ultrastructure of mouse vallate taste buds: II. Cell types and cell lineage. J. Comp. Neurol. *253:* 242–252.

Desor, J. A., O. Maller, and R. E. Turner (1973) Taste in acceptance of sugars by human infants. J. Comp. Physiol. Psychol. *84:* 496–501.

Erickson, R. P. (1963) Sensory neural patterns and gustation. In Y. Zotterman (ed.): Olfaction and Taste. Oxford: Pergamon Press, pp. 205–213.

Farbman, A. I. (1965) Electron microscope study of the developing taste bud in rat fungiform papilla. Dev. Biol. *11:* 110–135.

Ferrell, F., C. M. Mistretta, and R. M. Bradley (1981) Development of chorda tympani taste responses. J. Comp. Neurol. *198:* 37–44.

Ferrell, F., T. Tsuetaki, and R. A. Chole (1985) Myelination in the chorda tympani of the postnatal rat: A quantitative electron microscope study. Acta Anat. *123:* 224–229.

Finger, T. E. (1987) Gustatory nuclei and pathways in the central nervous system. In T. E. Finger and W. L. Silver, (eds.): The Neurobiology of Taste and Smell. New York: Wiley, pp. 331–353.

Formaker, B. K., and D. L. Hill (1988) An analysis of the residual NaCl taste response following amiloride. Amer. J. Physiol. *255:* R1002–1007.

Ganchrow, J. R., and D. Ganchrow (1987) Taste bud development in chickens (*Gallus gallus domesticus*). Anat. Rec. *218:* 88–93.

Gottfried, D. S., C. M. Mistretta, R. M. Bradley and D. L. Hill (1984) Quantitative study of morphological development of rat taste bud. Abstracts of the Association for Chemoreception Sciences, VIth Annaul Meeting.

Hersch, M., and D. Ganchrow (1980) Scanning electron microscopy of developing papillae on the tongue of human embryos and fetuses. Chem. Senses *5:* 331–341.

Hill, D. L. (1987a) Development of taste responses in the rat parabrachial nucleus. J. Neurophysiol. *57:* 481–495.

Hill, D. L. (1987b) Susceptibility of the developing rat gustatory system to the physiological effects of dietary sodium deprivation. J. Physiol. *393:* 413–424.

Hill, D. L. (1987c) Development of the gustatory system and the effects of environmental modifications imposed during development. In T. E. Finger and W. L. Silver (eds.): The Neurobiology of Taste and Smell. New York: Wiley, pp. 379–400.

Hill, D. L. (1988a) Development of chorda tympani nerve taste responses in the hamster. J. Comp. Neurol. *268:* 346–356.

Hill, D. L. (1988b) Development of amiloride sensitivity in the rat peripheral gustatory system: A single fiber analysis. In S. D Roper and J. Atema (eds.): Olfaction and Taste IX. Ann. N.Y. Acad. Sci. *510:* 369–372.

Hill, D. L., and C. R. Almli (1980) Ontogeny of chorda tympani nerve responses to gustatory stimuli in the rat. Brian Res. *197:* 27–38.

Hill, D. L., and T. C. Bour (1985) Addition of functional amiloride-sensitive components to the receptor membrane: A possible mechanism for altered taste responses during development. Dev. Brain Res. *20:* 310–313.

Hill, D. L., R. M. Bradley, and C. M. Mistretta (1983) Development of taste responses in the rat solitary tract. J. Neurophysiol. *50:* 879–985.

Hill, D. L., C. M. Mistretta, and R. M. Bradley (1982) Developmental changes in taste response characteristics of rat single chorda tympani fibers. J. Neurosci. *2:* 782–790.

Hill, D. L., C. M. Mistretta, and R. M. Bradley (1986) Effects of dietary NaCl deprivation during early development on behavioral and neurophysiological taste responses. Behav. Neurosci. *110:* 390–398.

Hosley, M. A., S. E. Hughes, and B. Oakley (1987) Neural induction of taste buds. J. Comp. Neurol. *260:* 224–232.

Kinnamon, J. C., B. J. Taylor, R. J. Delay, and S. D. Roper (1985) Ultrastructure of mouse vallate taste buds. I. Taste cells and their associated synapses. J. Comp. Neurol. *253:* 48–60.

Lasiter, P. S., and D. L. Hill (1988) Histogenesis of pontine taste area neurons in the albino rat. In S. D. Roper, and J. Atema (eds.): Olfaction and Taste IX. Ann. N.Y. Acad. Sci. *510:* 444–446.

Maller, O., and J. A. Desor (1973) Effects of taste on ingestion by human newborns. In J. F. Bosma (ed.): Fourth Symposium on Oral Sensation and Perception: Development of the Fetus and Infant. DHEW Publication No. NIH 73–546. Washington, D.C.: U.S. Government Printing Office.

Midkiff, E. E., and I. L. Bernstein (1983) The influence of age and experience on salt preference of the rat. Dev. Psychobiol. *16:* 385–394.

Miller, I. J., Jr. (1971) Peripheral interactions among single papilla inputs to gustatory nerve fibers. J. Gen. Physiol. *57:*1–25.

Miller, I. J., Jr. (1977) Gustatory receptors of the palate. In Y. Katsuki, M. Sato, S. F. Takagi, and Y. Oomura (eds.): Food Intake and the Chemical Senses. Tokyo: University of Tokyo Press, pp. 173–185.

Mistretta, C. M. (1972) Topographical and histological study of the developing rat tongue palate and taste buds. In J. F. Bosma (ed.): Third Symposium on Oral Sensation and Perception: The Mouth of the Infant. Springfield, Illinois: Thomas, pp. 163–187.

Mistretta, C. M. (1981) Neurophysiological and anatomical aspects of taste development. In R. Aslin, J. R. Alberts, and N. R. Petersen (eds.): The Development of Perception: Psychobiological Perspectives, Vol. I. New York: Academic Press, pp. 433–455.

Mistretta, C. M. (1988) Development of receptive fields of chorda tympani nerve fibers and relation to salt taste sensation. In I. J. Miller, Jr. (ed.): The Lloyd M. Beidler Symposium on Taste and Smell. Winston-Salem: Book Service Associates, pp. 21–31.

Mistretta, C. M. (1989) Anatomy and neurophysiology of the taste system in aged animals. Ann. N. Y. Acad. Sci. *561:* 277–290.

Mistretta, C. M., and R. M. Bradley (1975) Taste and swallowing in utero: A discussion of fetal sensory function. Brit. Med. Bull. *31:* 80–84.

Mistretta, C. M., and R. M. Bradley (1978a) Taste responses in sheep medulla: Changes during development. Science *202:* 535–537.

Mistretta, C. M., and R. M. Bradley (1978b) Effects of early sensory experience on brain and behavioral development. In G. Gottlieb (ed.): Studies on the Development of Behavior and the Nervous System, Vol. 4, Early Influences. New York: Academic Press, pp. 215–247.

Mistretta, C. M., and R. M. Bradley (1983a) Neural basis of developing salt taste sensation: Response changes in fetal, postnatal, and adult sheep. J. Comp. Neurol. 215: 199–210.

Mistretta, C. M. and R. M. Bradley (1983b) Developmental changes in taste responses from glossopharyngeal nerve in sheep and comparisons with chorda tympani responses. Dev. Brain Res. 11: 107–117.

Mistretta, C. M., and R. M. Bradley (1985) Development of taste. In E. M. Blass (ed.): Handbook of Behavioral Neurobiology, Vol. 8. New York: Plenum Press, pp. 205–236.

Mistretta, C. M., T. Nagai, and R. M. Bradley (1986) Relation of receptive field size and salt taste response in chorda tympani fibers during development. Chem. Senses 11: 640.

Mistretta, C. M., S. Gurkan, and R. M. Bradley (1988) Morphology of chorda tympani fiber receptive fields and proposed neural rearrangements during development. J. Neurosci. 8: 73–78.

Moe, K. E. (1986) The ontogeny of salt preference in rats. Dev. Psychobiol. 19: 185–196.

Nagai, T., C. M. Mistretta, and R. M. Bradley (1988) Developmental decrease in size of peripheral receptive fields of single chorda tympani nerve fibers and relation to increasing NaCl taste sensitivity. J. Neurosci. 8: 64–72.

Nejad, M. S., and L. M. Beidler (1988) Taste responses of the cross-regenerated greater superificial petrosal and chorda tympani nerves of the rat. In S. D. Roper, and J. Atema (eds.): Olfaction and Taste IX. Ann. N.Y. Acad. Sci. 510: 523–526.

Norgren, R. (1984) Central neural mechanisms of taste. In I. Darian-Smith (ed.): Handbook of Physiology: The Nervous System, Vol. III, Sensory Processes. Washington D.C.: American Physiological Society, pp. 1087–1128.

Norgren, R. (1985) The sense of taste and the study of ingestion. In D. W. Pfaff (ed.): Taste, Olfaction and the Central Nervous System. New York: The Rockefeller Univ. Press, pp. 233–249.

Nowlis, G. H. (1973) Taste elicited tongue movements in human newborn infants: An approach to palatability. In J. F. Bosma (ed.): Fourth Symposium on Oral Sensation and Perception: Development of the Fetus and Infant. DHEW Publication No. NIH 73–546. Washington, D.C.: U.S. Government Printing Office. pp. 292–310.

Nowlis, G. H., and W. Kessen (1976) Human newborns differentiate differing concentrations of sucrose and glucose. Science 191: 865–866.

Oakley, B. (1987) Taste bud development in rat vallate and foliate papillae. In P. Hnik, T. Soukup, R. Vejsada, and J. Zelena (eds.): Mechanoreceptors: Development, Structure and Function. New York: Plenum Press. pp. 1–6.

Scott, T. R., and S. Yaxley (1989) Interactions of taste and ingestion. In R. H. Cagan (ed.): Neural Mechanisms in Taste. Boca Raton: CRC Press, pp. 147–177.

Smith, D. V., and I. J. Miller, Jr. (1986) Taste bud development in hamster vallate and foliate papillae. Chem. Senses 11: 665.

Steiner, J. E. (1979) Human facial expressions in response to taste and smell stimulation. Adv. Child Dev. Behav. *13:* 257–295.

Sweazey, R. D., and D. V. Smith (1987) Convergence onto hamster medullary taste neurons. Brain Res. *408:* 173–184.

Tatzer, E., M. T. Schubert, W. Timischl, and G. Simbruner (1985) Discrimination of taste and preference for sweet in premature babies. Early Hum. Dev. *12:* 23–30.

Travers, J. B., S. P. Travers, and R. Norgren (1987) Gustatory neural processing in the hindbrain. Ann. Rev. Neurosci. *10:* 595–632.

Travers, S. P., C. Pfaffmann, and R. Norgren (1986) Convergence of lingual and palatal gustatory neural activity in the nucleus of the solitary tract. Brain Res. *365:* 305–320.

Vogt, M. B., and C. M. Mistretta (1986) Converging afferent input on second order taste neurons in sheep during development. Soc. Neurosci. Abstr. *12:* 125.

Vogt, M. B., and C. M. Mistretta (1988) Receptive fields of second order taste neurons in sheep: Convergence of afferent input increases during development. In S. D. Roper and J. Atema (eds.): Olfaction and Taste, Vol. IX. Ann. N.Y. Acad. Sci. *510:* 687–688.

Weiffenbach, J. M., and B. T. Thach (1973) Elicited tongue movements: Touch and taste in the mouth of the neonate. In J. F. Bosma (ed.): Fourth Symposium on Oral Sensation and Perception. Development in the Fetus and Infant. DHEW Publication No. NIH 73–546. Washington, D.C.: U.S. Government Printing Office, pp. 232–244.

Wintour, E. M. (1986) Amniotic fluid—our first environment. News Physiol. Sci. *1:* 95–97.

Yamada, T. (1980) Chorda tympani responses to gustatory stimuli in developing rats. Jap. J. Physiol. *30:* 631–643.

Zahm, D. S., and B. L. Munger (1983a) Fetal development of primate chemosensory corpuscles. I. Synaptic relationships in late gestation. J. Comp. Neurol. *213:* 146–162.

Zahm, D. S., and B. L. Munger (1983b) Fetal development of primate chemosensory corpuscles. II. Synaptic relationships in early gestation. J. Comp. Neurol. *219:* 36–50.

Part Six

DEVELOPMENT OF SENSORY SYSTEMS IN OVERVIEW

Chapter Fifteen

SUMMARY OF EPIGENIC AND EXPERIENTIAL CONTRIBUTIONS UNDERLYING FORMATION OF SENSORY SYSTEMS IN MAMMALS

James R. Coleman

University of South Carolina
Columbia, South Carolina

I GENERAL COMMENTS

Our communication with the outside world is dependent upon the ability of our sensory systems to process the physical energy impinging upon us. Special challenges are evoked in newborn mammals, whose very survival and further development is dependent upon early detection of sensory information. Environmental demands change as mammals mature and the sensory capabilities are altered, presumably to take advantage of essential sensory data available. As described in the preceding chapters, each sensory system has certain unique features in transduction and coding and, to some extent, the development of anatomical and physiological substrates that ultimately provide the processing that leads to perception. Nevertheless, many similar events are occurring as each sensory pathway develops, so as to provide many comparable changes as well as contrasting features. Some of these events are briefly summarized here.

II   EARLY DEVELOPMENTAL GRADIENTS AND CELL INTERACTIONS

The transduction process is vital to sensory coding, so it is of direct concern to identify the properties of receptor and supporting cell development. In the cat retina, receptor and neural cell development is not uniform, as there appears to be a general central-to-peripheral gradient. Likewise, generation and maturation of cochlear hair cells and supporting cells occur as a function of position in the end organ—developmental events are initiated near the base and largely proceed apically. Furthermore, evidence from both the cochlear and vestibular portions of the inner ear indicates that hair cell differentiation is not under primary influence from afferent or efferent neural input. In the gustatory system, however, differentiation of taste buds requires taste nerve innervation (e.g., glossopharyngeal), and there is receptor turnover so that synapses are constantly being established even during adulthood.

One of the major questions relates to the independence of development of particular neural structures along sensory pathways from the influence of innervating fiber systems. First, it is clear that neurogenesis within a sensory structure occurs without influence from other levels of the neuraxis. In the olfactory system neurogenesis largely occurs in synchrony, while in the somatosensory system of rat the trigeminal ganglia and dorsal root ganglia generated on embryonic days 12–14 still overlap production of ventroposterior nucleus neurons on embryonic day 14. In the latter case, dorsal root ganglion axons do not reach the cuneate nucleus until embryonic day 17 so that generation of higher order neurons cannot be influenced by peripheral components. The neurons of auditory nuclei are generated during mainly overlapping periods, although many of the neural elements of some areas such as the cochlear nuclei and medial geniculate body are produced prior to one structure—the auditory cortex where neurons are generated up until around birth in rat. Even in the latter case, thalamic and callosal fibers do not invade auditory cortex until postnatal life and therefore do not impact on initial formation of cortical cells. Consequently, cytogenetic gradients along auditory pathways and most other sensory pathways rely on early genetic expression and local environmental factors rather than on directive influences from other levels of the sensory neuraxis.

Maturation of end organs and peripheral neurons may not fully follow the same time course as central neural components of the sensory system. In fact, the final order of organization in the thalamic and cortical representations (of vibrissae) in the somatosensory system are sequentially dictated by peripheral patterns to provide the initial template that alters preexisting central topography. Organization at each level becomes dependent upon structural patterns of the preceding level. This includes alterations of cortical barrel cells that grow further according to afferent input patterns. At birth, the rat primary peripheral somatosensory neurons show many mature anatomic and functional characteristics, in contrast to neonatal brainstem and forebrain neural pathways. In fact, it is not until after birth that the six-layered neocortex of the different sensory systems develops. Similarly, many aspects of functional maturation in the auditory system follow a centripetal course that is also dependent upon the frequency of stimulation processing.

Another feature of neural development of sensory systems, as well as other regions of the nervous system, is the overproduction of cells and axonal processes. This is especially well documented in the visual system, where many more retinal cells and optic nerve axons are formed early than will survive into adulthood. Following early removal of one eye, exuberant fibers from the remaining eye are sustained and cell death reduced. It is now known that growth factors and other intrinsic substances are essential for neuron survival. Nerve growth factor maintains trigeminal ganglion cells and target brainstem neurons. The presence of nerve growth factor antibody during development promotes ganglion cell loss, while nerve degeneration is retarded by administration of nerve growth factor. The specific factors for neuron survival have not yet been identified in every sensory system.

In the visual system, the source of the cortical projection to the superior colliculus is more widespread during early development. Experimental data also clearly show that developmental organization of lateral geniculate fibers in cortex is dependent upon binocular competition. Loss of retinogeniculate or geniculocortical axons with development is also accompanied by expansion of remaining axon arbors. Also interesting is that unlike retinogeniculate fibers that invade the target relatively quickly, geniculocortical axon invasion of the cortical plate is delayed; the latter may be a general cortical phenomenon, as there is also a protracted cortical invasion of axons from the medial geniculate body and ventrobasal complex.

III MATURATIONAL PROPERTIES

Postnatal development of sensory pathways involves many changes at cellular and subcellular levels. Typical are the retinal ganglion cells in which somal and dendritic growth occurs followed by simplification of dendrites, loss of spines, and reduction in axon collaterals. As in neurons of other pathways, initial dendritic growth of retinal ganglion cells precedes the formation of presynaptic membranes on these cells. At the cortical level, the number of synapses first increases but ultimately declines to a lower density, perhaps related to dendritic spine reduction.

The physiological properties of sensory neurons are typically altered during postnatal life. Universal features include diminished habituation, latency reduction, and more vigorous responses of neurons to sensory stimulation. Factors correlated with latency changes are myelination, redistribution of axonal arbors, and synaptic efficacy. Perhaps most striking are the ontogenic changes in qualitative electrophysiological properties of sensory neurons. The response ratio of NaCl to NH_4Cl responding fibers of the chorda tympani increases with development. Neurons at three levels of the gustatory system respond to a wider range of chemical stimulation at lower concentrations with increased age. These changes reflect developmental alteration of receptor cell membranes in a system in which taste buds turn over throughout life. In the visual system where a high-threshold electroretinogram precedes (by 2 days in cat) the first photic-driven ganglion cell responses, the receptive fields of neurons initially may lack inhibitory mechanisms or possess "silent" surrounds. The acuity of responses of ganglion and geniculate cells show improvement during postnatal development that cannot be solely attributed to changes in vascular membranes of the eye. Furthermore, the X, Y, and W classifications cannot be determined in cat until about the fourth postnatal week due to lack of spatial summation and variability of response latency resulting partly from incomplete myelination. Another feature often observed is a reduction in the size of receptive fields of sensory neurons. For example, gustatory receptive fields of chorda tympani nerve fibers decrease with age, and retinal ganglion cells usually develop smaller response fields attributed to convergence of retinal input rather than dendritic growth. The first receptive fields recorded in rat SI (around postnatal day 7) are very large. It is likely that many of the changes in receptive field properties are due to redistribution of afferent fibers.

IV   EXPERIENTIAL VARIABLES

Some of the effects of stimulus deprivation on development of sensory system properties have been widely recognized. The influence of sensory deprivation during a critical period has been well documented for structural and physiological changes in the visual, auditory, and somatosensory systems. Although considerable research has been conducted on these systems, particularly the ocular dominance pathway, the evidence has now expanded into the chemical senses. For example, neural responses in the chorda tympani to high concentrations of NaCl decrease after rearing on a NaCl-deficient diet. Similar to findings in other sensory pathways, the anatomical consequences of olfactory deprivation are most severe when the deprivation procedure is begun during early postnatal life. Olfactory neurons are, however, unique in that they are regenerated throughout life, and if sensory axons are cut, there is regeneration into the olfactory bulb and other central targets.

In some sensory systems postnatal deprivation, receptor damage, or nerve section all result in greater deficits in lower central structures than those at higher levels of the neuraxis. After vibrissa removal there is cell loss and volume decrease in the nucleus interpositus but not in the ventral posterior nucleus. The pathological effects of such procedures are most pronounced on first-order central neurons. In the visual system, the presence of both eyes are necessary for formation of cortical ocular dominance columns, which nevertheless can form normally without light stimulation. Cortical binocularity is disrupted by any discordant input from the two eyes (e.g., from strabismus) during postnatal life. There is also an age gradient for these effects, the sensitive period, as central pathology is far more severe when these procedures are invoked during early postnatal development compared to the same procedures begun during adulthood.

The timing of acquisition of behavioral sensitivity varies with the system and by species. Evidence in the auditory system suggests that the period of anatomical and physiological maturation may actually exceed that for attaining adult behavioral thresholds to acoustic stimuli. Development of brainstem structures accounts for behavioral threshold sensitivity to sound. However, in the auditory system, as in some other sensory systems, there are anatomical factors that contribute to early elevated sensitivity. Immaturity of external, middle, and inner ear structures or light scatter in the eye all serve to degrade the quality of the stimulus. Although neural mechanisms for binaural localization are present very early, immaturity of the cochlea clearly influences the mechanical coding of sound frequency, particularly limiting the high-frequency response. On the other hand, behavioral thresholds may not be influenced by immaturity of other anatomical features, such as the lack of impact of accommodative inaccuracy on the poor resolution of infant monkeys. It is clear that both the quality and sensitivity of behavioral responses to sensory stimuli change with maturation. In the gustatory system, for example, there is a change in the preference for hypertonic NaCl. In all sensory systems, experiential variables are integrally involved with final pathway organization and sensory capabilities, and they may interact with one another as in the development of the vestibulo-ocular reflex.

V CONCLUDING REMARKS

No matter the level of prococity, the visual system is only exposed to sensory stimuli postnatally—there are no demands for prenatal function. In other systems, however, sensory processing may occur prenatally (e.g., hearing in humans). In fact, the intrauterine environment provides a rich opportunity for chemical stimulation (e.g., water, salts, and sugar) of appropriate receptors. We are just beginning to understand the developmental events that occur prenatally in various mammals with or without sensory function at birth, as this information provides vital insight into mechanisms of development that promote the future organization of the system. There is considerable need for study of prenatal sensory systems as prospective research will establish important anatomical, biochemical, and physiological indices of early formation of sensory tissues. Description of prenatal and postnatal changes of sensory systems provides the framework essential for understanding how mammals acquire the ability to receive and process information from the physical world that permits them to successfully interact with and survive in their environment.

INDEX